# A World without Measles and Rubella: Meeting the Regional Elimination Targets on the Path to Global Eradication

# A World without Measles and Rubella: Meeting the Regional Elimination Targets on the Path to Global Eradication

Guest Editors

**Jon Kim Andrus**
**Mark Papania**
**Sunil Bahl**
**David N. Durrheim**
**Katrina Kretsinger**
**Peter Strebel**
**Paul A. Rota**
**Susan Reef**

MDPI

Basel • Beijing • Wuhan • Barcelona • Belgrade • Novi Sad • Cluj • Manchester

*Guest Editors*
Jon Kim Andrus
George Washington University
Milken Institute of Public Health
Washington, DC
USA

Mark Papania
Centers for Disease Control and Prevention
Atlanta, GA
USA

Sunil Bahl
Formerly with World Health Organization
South-East Asia Regional Office
New Delhi
India

David N. Durrheim
School of Medicine and Public Health
University of Newcastle
Callaghan, NSW
Australia

Katrina Kretsinger
Independent Public Health Consultant Previously with Centers for Disease Control and Prevention
Atlanta, GA
USA

Peter Strebel
Formerly with Centers for Disease Control and Prevention
Atlanta, GA
USA

Paul A. Rota
National Center for Infectious Diseases
Centers for Disease Control and Prevention
Atlanta, GA
USA

Susan Reef
Centers for Disease Control and Prevention
Atlanta, GA
USA

*Editorial Office*
MDPI AG
Grosspeteranlage 5
4052 Basel, Switzerland

This is a reprint of the Special Issue, published open access by the journal *Vaccines* (ISSN 2076-393X), freely accessible at: https://www.mdpi.com/journal/vaccines/special_issues/34BC5B81TS.

For citation purposes, cite each article independently as indicated on the article page online and as indicated below:

Lastname, A.A.; Lastname, B.B. Article Title. *Journal Name* **Year**, *Volume Number*, Page Range.

**ISBN 978-3-7258-4213-1 (Hbk)**
**ISBN 978-3-7258-4214-8 (PDF)**
**https://doi.org/10.3390/books978-3-7258-4214-8**

Cover image courtesy of World Health Organization

# Contents

*vaccines*

MDPI

*Editorial*

# Addressing the Dangerous Consequences of the Resurgence of Measles and Rubella: The Critical Need for a Global Target

**Jon Kim Andrus**

Department of Global Health, Milken Institute of Public Health, George Washington University, Washington, DC 20052, USA; andrus@gwu.edu

I am delighted and honored to be Guest Editor of this *Vaccines* Special Issue on measles and rubella elimination. I was extremely fortunate to have a team of co-editors who assisted with this work. Their experience in the field of immunization, and with the elimination of measles, rubella, congenital rubella syndrome is noteworthy. As evidenced by their biographies, the collective sum of their knowledge and experience is staggering.

On behalf of all the co-editors—Sunil Bahl, David Durrheim, Katrina Kretsinger, Mark Papania, Susan Reef, Paul Rota, and Peter Strebel—I would like to extend my sincerest thanks and appreciation to all the authors of the manuscripts included in this supplement. We are fortunate to have the support of *Vaccines* in publishing this Special Issue, a journal that promotes free and open access to science and boasts a considerable reader rating as a result. In addition to our Editorial Team reviewing the manuscripts, each article underwent another two independent peer review evaluations to be accepted.

I would like to extend special thanks to Xinya Huang and Sydnee Pang from the editorial staff of *Vaccines*, as well as Mark Papania and Amanda McKinnon from CDC, Atlanta, USA, all of whom provided invaluable administrative support. Most importantly, we should to acknowledge all the dedicated government workers, stakeholders, and field workers working for a world free of measles, rubella, and congenital rubella syndrome. I hope you enjoy reading this supplement as much as we enjoyed collating it.

However, this gratitude is dampened by an uneasy feeling of foreboding. This "sense" of gloom is linked to an incredible opportunity missed, stemming from my own personal experience. In the field of public health, a "story" can potentially confer just as much information as a dataset or statistical analysis. With this in mind, please bear with me as I briefly share mine.

My first assignment overseas was in 1985, serving as a Peace Corps volunteer as the District Medical Officer of the Mchinji District Hospital in Malawi, Africa. The 66-bed hospital I supervised as the only doctor in the District had a measles ward that overflowed with children at the start of every annual measles season. With too few beds to meet this overwhelming demand, two or three children were assigned to every bed. Families filled the hallways and were scattered under beds. Mothers mourned the daily death toll, wailing terribly. The noise was overwhelming. Some of the children had peeling skin due to severe protein malnutrition, a foreboding sign. Their fate was an increased risk of death, pneumonia, encephalitis, and blindness. These painful memories of all the deaths and co-morbidities that could have been prevented are forever etched into my soul.

Returning on a World Health Organization (WHO) assignment to Mchinji some 15 years later, after Malawi had conducted a nationwide measles catch-up vaccination campaign, I became convinced that measles could be eliminated, even in some of the most direly affected places in the world. On revisiting during the typical measles season, the ward had been shut down. No more admissions, no more deaths, no more suffering from this dreaded disease. Such was the impact of the catch-up campaign and the consolidation of immunization services implemented here. The catch-up campaign treated every child aged <15 years with a measles containing vaccine (MCV). As described, the results were nothing short of phenomenal.

Unfortunately, there is a caveat to this story. Without follow-up vaccination campaigns being conducted every four years (targeting children aged <5 years with a measles vaccine), measles undoubtedly returns, even despite comparatively high levels of routine coverage. This has indeed played out in Malawi and in other countries in Africa, an oversight requiring swift correction, along with upgrading essential immunization systems, improving the vaccination coverage for other antigens, and optimizing field surveillance.

In absorbing the following research, I hope you share in my sincere belief that the voice of reason resoundingly maintains that global measles rubella elimination (MRE) is feasible, possible, and sustainable [1]. Many, including me, would argue that MRE is a moral imperative [2]. How can we not eliminate a disease so devastating and yet known to be preventable using existing strategies? The measle antigen in current use averts more deaths than any other antigen, and a combined measles–rubella vaccine could also eliminate the leading cause of congenital birth defects due to infectious disease. A global target is required, as pertinently stipulated by all the Chairs of the WHO Regional Verification Commission in their article. No more missed opportunities of this kind can occur. As you read, reflect on the fact that the past two decades of remarkable global progress are at risk of becoming redundant as measles infection reemerges and surges. The question is whether a renewed global commitment to protecting children around the world will be made.

**Funding:** This research received no external funding.

**Conflicts of Interest:** The authors declare no conflict of interest.

## References

1. Cochi, S.L.; Schluter, W.W. What it will take to achieve a world without measles. *J. Infect Dis.* **2020**, *222*, 1073–1075. [CrossRef] [PubMed]
2. Durrheim, D.N.; Andrus, J.K. The ethical case for global measles eradication—Justice and the Rule of Rescue. *Int. Health* **2020**, *12*, 375–377. [CrossRef] [PubMed]

*vaccines*

MDPI

*Commentary*

# Accelerating Global Measles and Rubella Eradication—Saving Millions of Lives, Preventing Disability, and Averting the Next Pandemic

**David N. Durrheim [1,*,†], Jon K. Andrus [2,†], Shahina Tabassum [3,†], David Githanga [4,†], Mira Kojouharova [5,†] and Nadia Talab [6,†]**

1 School of Medicine and Public Health, University of Newcastle, Newcastle 2308, Australia
2 Department of Global Health, Milken Institute of Public Health, George Washington University, Washington, DC 20052, USA; andrusjonkim@yahoo.com
3 Department of Virology, Bangabandhu Sheikh Mujib Medical University, Dhaka 1000, Bangladesh
4 Kenya Paediatrics Association, Nairobi P.O. Box 45820-00100, Kenya
5 National Centre of Infectious and Parasitic Diseases, 1504 Sofia, Bulgaria
6 Regional Office of Eastern Mediterranean, Cairo 11371, Egypt
* Correspondence: david.durrheim@newcastle.edu.au
† The authors are the Chairpersons of the six Regional Measles and Rubella Verification Commissions.

**Abstract:** No vaccine has been more effective in reducing disease burden, especially in preventing child deaths, than measles-containing vaccine. The return on investment makes measles-containing vaccine one of the most cost-effective public health measures available. Exhaustive reviews of biological, technical, economic and programmatic evidence have concluded that measles can and should be eradicated, and by including rubella antigen in measles-containing vaccine, congenital rubella syndrome will also be eradicated. All World Health Organisation Regions have pledged to achieve measles elimination. Unfortunately, not all countries and global partners have demonstrated an appropriate commitment to these laudable public health goals, and the negative impact of the COVID-19 pandemic on coverage rates has been profound. Unsurprisingly, large disruptive outbreaks are already occurring in many countries with a global epidemic curve ominously similar to that of 2018/2019 emerging. The Immunization Agenda 2030 will fail dismally unless measles and rubella eradication efforts are accelerated. Over half of all member states have been verified to have eliminated rubella and endemic rubella transmission has not been re-established in any country to date. In 2023, 84 countries and areas were verified to have sustained elimination of measles. However, without a global target, this success will be difficult to sustain. Now is the time for a global eradication goal and commitment by the World Health Assembly. Having a galvanising goal, with a shared call for action, will demand adequate resourcing from every country government and global partners. Greater coordination across countries and regions will be necessary. Measles, rubella and congenital rubella syndrome eradication should not remain just a technically feasible possibility but rather be completed to ensure that future generations of children do not live under the shadow of preventable childhood death and lifelong disability.

**Keywords:** measles; rubella; congenital rubella syndrome; eradication; elimination

Fifty years after the Expanded Programme on Immunization was launched in 1974, the extraordinary benefits of life-saving vaccines are being enjoyed by millions of children around the world [1]. No vaccine has been more effective in reducing the disease burden (Figure 1), especially in preventing child deaths, than the measles-containing vaccine (MCV). Between 2000 and 2022, the MCV prevented an estimated 57 million deaths globally [2]. Other than perhaps safe water and sanitation and breastfeeding, no other global health initiative can claim such a remarkable impact in averting deaths. Modeling indicates that measles vaccination will prevent 37% of deaths due to vaccination against 14 key pathogens between 2021 and 2030, with a remarkable 18.8 million lives saved in the current decade alone [3]. In addition to the immediate threats posed by measles disease, the subsequent immunosuppression among children who have been infected may last for weeks to months, leading to increased vulnerability to an array of other viral and bacterial infections [4]. Up to half of all infectious disease-related childhood deaths within the first few years of natural measles infection may be explained by this phenomenon. The return on investment makes the MCV one of the most cost-effective public health measures available. The analysis of economic data from 73 low- and middle-income countries on the costs for delivering the measles vaccine suggests that for every USD 1 invested, USD 58 were saved in future costs from 2001 to 2020 [5].

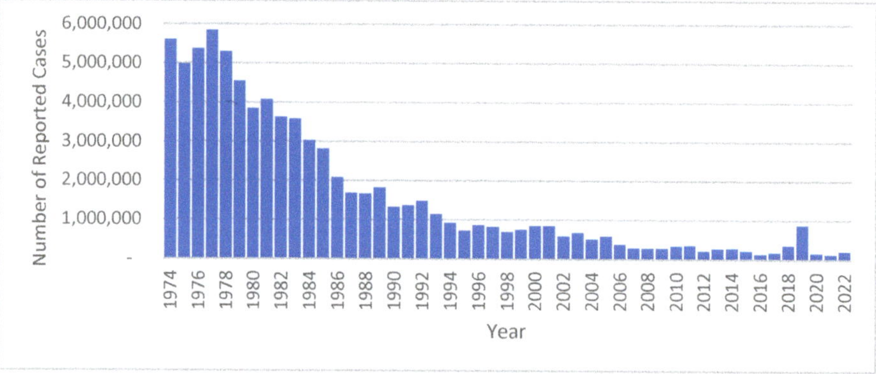


**Figure 1.** Measles reported cases worldwide, 1974–2022. Source: World Health Organization. Global Health Observatory. Measles—number of reported cases (https://www.who.int/), accessed on 29 April 2024.

Congenital rubella syndrome (CRS) is associated with considerable disability, including heart defects, cataracts, hearing loss, and developmental delays, and can occur when a woman is infected with rubella in early pregnancy. The CRS burden is typically low in countries where coverage with rubella-containing vaccines (RCVs) is high and disappears when endemic rubella transmission ceases. Estimates suggest that between 1996 and 2010, the number of children born with CRS decreased from 119,000 to just over 100,000 as the vaccination coverage slowly increased; this is still an intolerable burden of disability given the lower population RCV coverage required to drive this virus to extinction [6]. By including the rubella antigen with the MCV to produce an MR-containing vaccine (MRCV), the elimination of measles will result in the elimination of CRS.

'Measles can and should be eradicated' was the conclusion of the Strategic Advisory Group of Experts (SAGE) Working Group on Immunization to the WHO in 2010 following an exhaustive review of biological, technical, economic, and programmatic evidence [7]. By 2010, all WHO regions had pledged to achieve measles elimination, and this was reflected in the Global Vaccine Action Plan, 2011–2020 (GVAP), implying a global measles eradication agenda by default [8]. The GVAP endorsed by all member states simultaneously committed every region to achieving rubella and CRS elimination. Rubella elimination achievement was verified in the region of the Americas in 2015 and measles elimination in 2016.

Unfortunately, not all countries and global partners have demonstrated an appropriate commitment to these laudable public health goals. The devastating global measles resurgence in 2018/2019 bore testament to a failure to achieve the necessary two-dose MCV coverage required to protect all children. Applying the current criteria, the massive and disruptive measles outbreaks in 2019 in many countries met the criteria for the declaration of a Public Health Emergency of International Concern (PHEIC). The World Health Organization (WHO) did not declare it for measles as another PHEIC, COVID-19's emergence, distracted attention from the measles catastrophe [9]. In contrast with COVID-19, the measles disease burden particularly affects children living in developing countries and so it did not receive the attention and resources devoted to COVID-19, which affected all countries and adult populations. The closure of country borders during the COVID-19 pandemic, coupled with the dramatic decrease in international travel and wide-scale non-pharmaceutical public health measures, significantly obstructed the importation and transmission of measles and rubella viruses and provided an opportunity for accelerated progress towards measles and rubella elimination. However, this would have required concerted and coordinated efforts to close the immunity gaps resulting from the detrimental pandemic impacts on routine immunization program performance and postponed campaigns as a result of COVID-19 [10].

Sadly, only 81% of children born in 2021 received MCV1, the lowest coverage since 2008, leaving 25 million children born that year vulnerable to measles [2]. In 2022, the MCV1 coverage was at 83%, 3% below the pre-pandemic 2019 level of 86%, which had proved inadequate to prevent the epidemic surge at that time. Unsurprisingly, large disruptive outbreaks are already occurring in many countries, with a global epidemic curve ominously similar to that of 2018 and early 2019 (Figure 2), but, additionally, with the knowledge that there is a greater susceptible pool of measles-naïve individuals—both unvaccinated children born since the COVID-19 pandemic and cohorts of older children and young adults who do not enjoy immunity because of historically inadequate routine immunization coverage or sub-optimal campaign performance. It may well be too late to prevent the next measles pandemic.

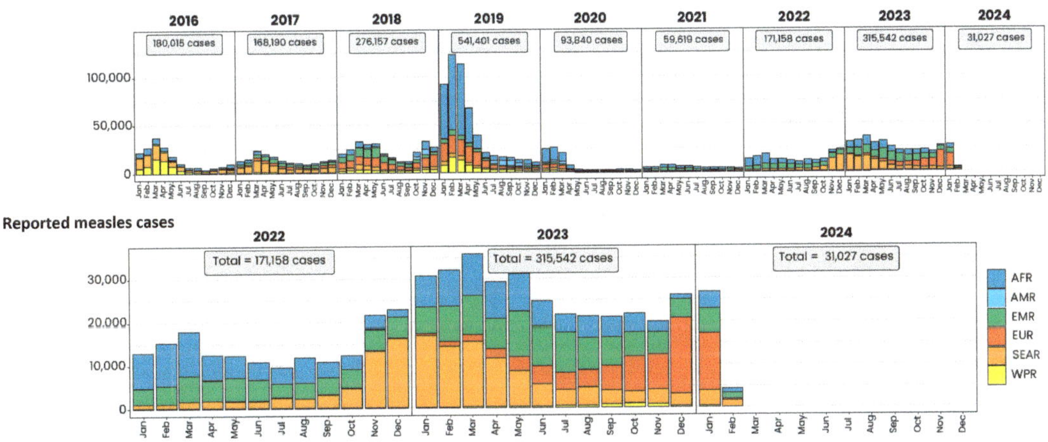


**Figure 2.** Measles reported cases by WHO region, 2016–2024. Source: World Health Organization, used with permission. Based on data received 2024-02—Data Source: IVB Database. These are surveillance data; hence, for the last month(s), the data may be incomplete. Note: The lower panel is an expanded high-resolution representation of years 2022–2024 in the upper panel. AFR = African Region; AMR = Region of the Americas; EMR = Eastern Mediterranean Region; EUR = European Region; SEAR = Southeast Asian Region; WPR = Western Pacific Region.

The Immunisation Agenda 2030 (IA2030) rightly recognizes measles as a tracer of the strength of immunization programs, with strategic priority 3 noting that measles cases and outbreaks should serve to identify weaknesses in immunization programs and guide programmatic planning in identifying and addressing these weaknesses [11]. In reality, IA2030 will inevitably fail unless the measles and rubella eradication efforts are accelerated, including a failure to achieve impact goals 1.1 (deaths averted), 1.2 (endorsed elimination targets), 1.3 (declining trend in number of large or disruptive outbreaks), 2.1 (50% reduction in zero dose children), and 3.1 (90% global coverage with MCV2) [12]. The central tenet of IA2030 is to leave no one behind. As such, the measles virus is the ultimate test of this equity obligation.

Against this bleak backdrop, there are some impressive success stories. Over half of all member states have been verified to have eliminated rubella, and endemic rubella transmission has not been re-established in any country to date (Table 1). This success bodes well for the achievement of global rubella and CRS elimination in the foreseeable future [13], and this progress towards rubella elimination should serve as a catalyst towards measles elimination.

Unfortunately, progress towards global measles elimination has not been homogenous. Only one region has achieved measles elimination, the Americas. This success story has recently been threatened with the loss of 'measles-free' status in Brazil and Venezuela due to a sustained, import-related measles outbreak lasting for longer than 12 months. In the European and Western Pacific Regions, 11 countries were verified to have eliminated measles, but, unfortunately, endemic transmission was then re-established (Table 1).

Without a global target, success is difficult to sustain. The other countries of the Region of the Americas have done so, but authorities recognize the fragility of elimination when the virus circulates elsewhere. To this end, there is great promise appearing on the horizon in each region. For example, in the Americas, Brazil and Venezuela appear to have interrupted measles transmission and are likely to apply for reverification. In the Western Pacific, China continues to make phenomenal steady progress towards measles elimination, and the Pacific Island Countries and Areas [14] and Mongolia are targeting 2025 to apply for verification. In the Eastern Mediterranean region, four countries, including Iran and Egypt, have documented and sustained elimination, and five additional countries are close to being verified.

What are the keys to success in this task? Given that each region has committed to measles and rubella elimination, now is the time for a global eradication goal and commitment by the World Health Assembly.

Having a galvanizing goal, with a shared call for action, will demand adequate resourcing from every country government and global partner. However, in addition to health ministers, we need finance ministers appreciating the return on investment. With many countries delegating health responsibility and funding to provincial or local governments, decentralized governments must embrace the goal as well. Such efforts will attract more local engagement and ownership. By proactively looking for opportunities, measles and rubella elimination will enhance national and local health capacity development and the response to future pandemic threats [15].

Champions are needed as advocates in all communities—this should not be too onerous as every community loves its children. New visionary partners are also needed—the world has become too dependent on single major players. Any country not using a rubella-containing vaccine—currently, there are 19—should immediately do so. No scientific arguments justifying the withholding of the RCV exist that have been proven to outweigh the benefits of CRS elimination.

Greater coordination across countries and regions will be necessary. The approach piloted in the Americas remains valid. Coordinated campaigns and surveillance efforts will foster collaboration between countries and achieve more than individual countries working in isolation could ever achieve alone.

Highly effective measles- and rubella-containing vaccines have shown what is possible. With microarray vaccination patches now in clinical trials, this simplified delivery of effective vaccines may guarantee that outreach to every community and child becomes a practical reality [16].

**Table 1.** Global measles and rubella elimination verification status by country and territory, 2011–2022.

| | | Measles Elimination Verification Status by Year | | | | | | | | | | | |
|---|---|---|---|---|---|---|---|---|---|---|---|---|---|
| **Country** | **WHO Region** | **2011** | **2012** | **2013** | **2014** | **2015** | **2016** | **2017** | **2018** | **2019** | **2020** | **2021** | **2022** |
| Afghanistan | EMR | | | | | | | | | | | | |
| Albania | EUR | | | | | | | | | | | | |
| Algeria | AFR | | | | | | | | | | | | |
| Andorra | EUR | | | | | | | | | | | | |
| Angola | AFR | | | | | | | | | | | | |
| Antigua and Barbuda | AMR | | | | | | | | | | | | |
| Argentina | AMR | | | | | | | | | | | | |
| Armenia | EUR | | | | | | | | | | | | |
| Australia | WPR | | | | | | | | | | | | |
| Austria | EUR | | | | | | | | | | | | |
| Azerbaijan | EUR | | | | | | | | | | | | |
| Bahamas, The | AMR | | | | | | | | | | | | |
| Bahrain | EMR | | | | | | | | | | | | |
| Bangladesh | SEAR | | | | | | | | | | | | |
| Barbados | AMR | | | | | | | | | | | | |
| Belarus | EUR | | | | | | | | | | | | |
| Belgium | EUR | | | | | | | | | | | | |
| Belize | AMR | | | | | | | | | | | | |
| Benin | AFR | | | | | | | | | | | | |
| Bhutan | SEAR | | | | | | | | | | | | |
| Bolivia, Plurinational State of | AMR | | | | | | | | | | | | |
| Bosnia and Herzegovina | EUR | | | | | | | | | | | | |
| Botswana | AFR | | | | | | | | | | | | |
| Brazil | AMR | | | | | | | | | | | | |
| Brunei Darussalam | WPR | | | | | | | | | | | | |
| Bulgaria | EUR | | | | | | | | | | | | |
| Burkina Faso | AFR | | | | | | | | | | | | |
| Burundi | AFR | | | | | | | | | | | | |

**Table 1.** *Cont.*

| | | Measles Elimination Verification Status by Year | | | | | | | | | | | |
|---|---|---|---|---|---|---|---|---|---|---|---|---|---|
| **Country** | **WHO Region** | **2011** | **2012** | **2013** | **2014** | **2015** | **2016** | **2017** | **2018** | **2019** | **2020** | **2021** | **2022** |
| Cabo Verde | AFR | | | | | | | | | | | | |
| Cambodia | WPR | | | | | | | | | | | | |
| Cameroon | AFR | | | | | | | | | | | | |
| Canada | AMR | | | | | | | | | | | | |
| Central African Republic | AFR | | | | | | | | | | | | |
| Chad | AFR | | | | | | | | | | | | |
| Chile | AMR | | | | | | | | | | | | |
| China | WPR | | | | | | | | | | | | |
| Colombia | AMR | | | | | | | | | | | | |
| Comoros | AFR | | | | | | | | | | | | |
| Congo, Republic of | AFR | | | | | | | | | | | | |
| Cook Islands | WPR | | | | | | | | | | | | |
| Country | WHO Region | 2011 | 2012 | 2013 | 2014 | 2015 | 2016 | 2017 | 2018 | 2019 | 2020 | 2021 | 2022 |
| Costa Rica | AMR | | | | | | | | | | | | |
| Côte d'Ivoire | AFR | | | | | | | | | | | | |
| Croatia | EUR | | | | | | | | | | | | |
| Cuba | AMR | | | | | | | | | | | | |
| Cyprus | EUR | | | | | | | | | | | | |
| Czechia | EUR | | | | | | | | | | | | |
| Denmark | EUR | | | | | | | | | | | | |
| Djibouti | EMR | | | | | | | | | | | | |
| Dominica | AMR | | | | | | | | | | | | |
| Dominica Republic | AMR | | | | | | | | | | | | |
| Democratic People's Republic of Korea | SEAR | | | | | | | | | | | | |
| Democratic Republic of the Congo | AFR | | | | | | | | | | | | |
| Ecuador | AMR | | | | | | | | | | | | |
| Egypt, Arab Republic | EMR | | | | | | | | | | | | |

**Table 1.** *Cont.*

| Country | WHO Region | Measles Elimination Verification Status by Year | | | | | | | | | | | |
|---|---|---|---|---|---|---|---|---|---|---|---|---|---|
| | | 2011 | 2012 | 2013 | 2014 | 2015 | 2016 | 2017 | 2018 | 2019 | 2020 | 2021 | 2022 |
| El Salvador | AMR | | | | | | | | | | | | |
| Equatoria Guinea | AFR | | | | | | | | | | | | |
| Eritrea | AFR | | | | | | | | | | | | |
| Estonia | EUR | | | | | | | | | | | | |
| Eswatini (Swaziland) | AFR | | | | | | | | | | | | |
| Ethiopia | AFR | | | | | | | | | | | | |
| Fiji | WPR | | | | | | | | | | | | |
| Finland | EUR | | | | | | | | | | | | |
| France | EUR | | | | | | | | | | | | |
| Gabon | AFR | | | | | | | | | | | | |
| Gambia, The | AFR | | | | | | | | | | | | |
| Georgia | EUR | | | | | | | | | | | | |
| Germany | EUR | | | | | | | | | | | | |
| Ghana | AFR | | | | | | | | | | | | |
| Greece | EUR | | | | | | | | | | | | |
| Grenada | AMR | | | | | | | | | | | | |
| Guatemala | AMR | | | | | | | | | | | | |
| Guinea | AFR | | | | | | | | | | | | |
| Guinea-Bissau | AFR | | | | | | | | | | | | |
| Guyana | AMR | | | | | | | | | | | | |
| Haiti | AMR | | | | | | | | | | | | |
| Honduras | AMR | | | | | | | | | | | | |
| Hungary | EUR | | | | | | | | | | | | |
| Iceland | EUR | | | | | | | | | | | | |
| India | SEAR | | | | | | | | | | | | |
| Indonesia | SEAR | | | | | | | | | | | | |
| Iran, Islamic Republic of | EMR | | | | | | | | | | | | |
| Country | WHO Region | 2011 | 2012 | 2013 | 2014 | 2015 | 2016 | 2017 | 2018 | 2019 | 2020 | 2021 | 2022 |

**Table 1.** *Cont.*

| Country | WHO Region | Measles Elimination Verification Status by Year | | | | | | | | | | | |
|---|---|---|---|---|---|---|---|---|---|---|---|---|---|
| | | 2011 | 2012 | 2013 | 2014 | 2015 | 2016 | 2017 | 2018 | 2019 | 2020 | 2021 | 2022 |
| Iraq | EMR | | | | | | | | | | | | |
| Ireland | EUR | | | | | | | | | | | | |
| Israel | EUR | | | | | | | | | | | | |
| Italy | EUR | | | | | | | | | | | | |
| Jamaica | AMR | | | | | | | | | | | | |
| Japan | WPR | | | | | | | | | | | | |
| Jordan | EMR | | | | | | | | | | | | |
| Kazakhstan | EUR | | | | | | | | | | | | |
| Kenya | AFR | | | | | | | | | | | | |
| Kiribati | WPR | | | | | | | | | | | | |
| Kuwait | EMR | | | | | | | | | | | | |
| Kyrgyz Republic | EUR | | | | | | | | | | | | |
| Lao People's Democratic Republic | WPR | | | | | | | | | | | | |
| Latvia | EUR | | | | | | | | | | | | |
| Lebanon | EMR | | | | | | | | | | | | |
| Lesotho | AFR | | | | | | | | | | | | |
| Liberia | AFR | | | | | | | | | | | | |
| Libya | EMR | | | | | | | | | | | | |
| Lithuania | EUR | | | | | | | | | | | | |
| Luxembourg | EUR | | | | | | | | | | | | |
| Madagascar | AFR | | | | | | | | | | | | |
| Malawi | AFR | | | | | | | | | | | | |
| Malaysia | WPR | | | | | | | | | | | | |
| Maldives | SEAR | | | | | | | | | | | | |
| Mali | AFR | | | | | | | | | | | | |
| Malta | EUR | | | | | | | | | | | | |
| Marshall Islands | WPR | | | | | | | | | | | | |
| Mauritius | AFR | | | | | | | | | | | | |

**Table 1.** *Cont.*

| Country | WHO Region | Measles Elimination Verification Status by Year | | | | | | | | | | | |
|---|---|---|---|---|---|---|---|---|---|---|---|---|---|
| | | 2011 | 2012 | 2013 | 2014 | 2015 | 2016 | 2017 | 2018 | 2019 | 2020 | 2021 | 2022 |
| Mauritania | AFR | | | | | | | | | | | | |
| Mexico | AMR | | | | | | | | | | | | |
| Micronesia, Federated States of | WPR | | | | | | | | | | | | |
| Monaco | EUR | | | | | | | | | | | | |
| Mongolia | WPR | | | | | | | | | | | | |
| Montenegro | EUR | | | | | | | | | | | | |
| Morocco | EMR | | | | | | | | | | | | |
| Mozambique | AFR | | | | | | | | | | | | |
| Myanmar | SEAR | | | | | | | | | | | | |
| Namibia | AFR | | | | | | | | | | | | |
| Nauru | WPR | | | | | | | | | | | | |
| Nepal | SEAR | | | | | | | | | | | | |
| Netherland, The Kingdom of | EUR | | | | | | | | | | | | |
| Country | WHO Region | 2011 | 2012 | 2013 | 2014 | 2015 | 2016 | 2017 | 2018 | 2019 | 2020 | 2021 | 2022 |
| New Zealand | WPR | | | | | | | | | | | | |
| Nicaragua | AMR | | | | | | | | | | | | |
| Niger | AFR | | | | | | | | | | | | |
| Nigeria | AFR | | | | | | | | | | | | |
| Niue | WPR | | | | | | | | | | | | |
| North Macedonia | EUR | | | | | | | | | | | | |
| Norway | EUR | | | | | | | | | | | | |
| Oman | EMR | | | | | | | | | | | | |
| Pakistan | EMR | | | | | | | | | | | | |
| Palau | WPR | | | | | | | | | | | | |
| Panama | AMR | | | | | | | | | | | | |
| Papua New Guinea | WPR | | | | | | | | | | | | |
| Paraguay | AMR | | | | | | | | | | | | |
| Peru | AMR | | | | | | | | | | | | |

**Table 1.** *Cont.*

| | | Measles Elimination Verification Status by Year | | | | | | | | | | | |
|---|---|---|---|---|---|---|---|---|---|---|---|---|---|
| **Country** | **WHO Region** | **2011** | **2012** | **2013** | **2014** | **2015** | **2016** | **2017** | **2018** | **2019** | **2020** | **2021** | **2022** |
| Philippines | WPR | | | | | | | | | | | | |
| Poland | EUR | | | | | | | | | | | | |
| Portugal | EUR | | | | | | | | | | | | |
| Qatar | EMR | | | | | | | | | | | | |
| Republic of Korea | WPR | | | | | | | | | | | | |
| Republic of Moldova | EUR | | | | | | | | | | | | |
| Romania | EUR | | | | | | | | | | | | |
| Russian Federation | EUR | | | | | | | | | | | | |
| Rwanda | AFR | | | | | | | | | | | | |
| Saint Kitts and Nevis | AMR | | | | | | | | | | | | |
| Saint Lucia | AMR | | | | | | | | | | | | |
| Saint Vincent and the Grenadines | AMR | | | | | | | | | | | | |
| Samoa | WPR | | | | | | | | | | | | |
| San Marino | EUR | | | | | | | | | | | | |
| Sao Tome and Principe | AFR | | | | | | | | | | | | |
| Saudi Arabia | EMR | | | | | | | | | | | | |
| Senegal | AFR | | | | | | | | | | | | |
| Serbia | EUR | | | | | | | | | | | | |
| Seychelles | AFR | | | | | | | | | | | | |
| Sierra Leone | AFR | | | | | | | | | | | | |
| Singapore | WPR | | | | | | | | | | | | |
| Slovakia | EUR | | | | | | | | | | | | |
| Slovenia | EUR | | | | | | | | | | | | |
| Solomon Islands | WPR | | | | | | | | | | | | |
| Somalia | EMR | | | | | | | | | | | | |
| South Africa | AFR | | | | | | | | | | | | |
| South Sudan | AFR | | | | | | | | | | | | |
| Country | WHO Region | 2011 | 2012 | 2013 | 2014 | 2015 | 2016 | 2017 | 2018 | 2019 | 2020 | 2021 | 2022 |

**Table 1.** *Cont.*

| Country | WHO Region | Measles Elimination Verification Status by Year | | | | | | | | | | | |
|---|---|---|---|---|---|---|---|---|---|---|---|---|---|
| | | 2011 | 2012 | 2013 | 2014 | 2015 | 2016 | 2017 | 2018 | 2019 | 2020 | 2021 | 2022 |
| Spain | EUR | | | | | | | | | | | | |
| Sri Lanka | SEAR | | | | | | | | | | | | |
| Sudan | EMR | | | | | | | | | | | | |
| Suriname | AMR | | | | | | | | | | | | |
| Sweden | EUR | | | | | | | | | | | | |
| Switzerland | EUR | | | | | | | | | | | | |
| Syrian Arab Republic | EMR | | | | | | | | | | | | |
| Tajikistan | EUR | | | | | | | | | | | | |
| Tanzania, United Republic | AFR | | | | | | | | | | | | |
| Thailand | SEAR | | | | | | | | | | | | |
| Timor-Leste | SEAR | | | | | | | | | | | | |
| Togo | AFR | | | | | | | | | | | | |
| Tokelau | WPR | | | | | | | | | | | | |
| Tonga | WPR | | | | | | | | | | | | |
| Trinidad and Tobago | AMR | | | | | | | | | | | | |
| Tunisia | EMR | | | | | | | | | | | | |
| Türkiye | EUR | | | | | | | | | | | | |
| Turkmenistan | EUR | | | | | | | | | | | | |
| Tuvalu | WPR | | | | | | | | | | | | |
| Uganda | AFR | | | | | | | | | | | | |
| Ukraine | EUR | | | | | | | | | | | | |
| United Arab Emirates | EMR | | | | | | | | | | | | |
| United Kingdom of Great Britain and Northern Ireland | EUR | | | | | | | | | | | | |
| United States of America | AMR | | | | | | | | | | | | |
| Uruguay | AMR | | | | | | | | | | | | |
| Uzbekistan | EUR | | | | | | | | | | | | |
| Vanuatu | WPR | | | | | | | | | | | | |

**Table 1.** *Cont.*

| | | Measles Elimination Verification Status by Year | | | | | | | | | | | |
|---|---|---|---|---|---|---|---|---|---|---|---|---|---|
| **Country** | **WHO Region** | **2011** | **2012** | **2013** | **2014** | **2015** | **2016** | **2017** | **2018** | **2019** | **2020** | **2021** | **2022** |
| Venezuela [1] | AMR | | | | | | | | | | | | |
| Vietnam | WPR | | | | | | | | | | | | |
| Yemen | EMR | | | | | | | | | | | | |
| Zambia | AFR | | | | | | | | | | | | |
| Zimbabwe | AFR | | | | | | | | | | | | |
| Territory/Region | WHO Region | 2011 | 2012 | 2013 | 2014 | 2015 | 2016 | 2017 | 2018 | 2019 | 2020 | 2021 | 2022 |
| American Samoa (US) | WPR | | | | | | | | | | | | |
| French Polynesia (France) | WPR | | | | | | | | | | | | |
| Guam (US) | WPR | | | | | | | | | | | | |
| Hong Kong SAR (China) | WPR | | | | | | | | | | | | |
| Macao SAR (China) | WPR | | | | | | | | | | | | |
| New Caledonia (France) | WPR | | | | | | | | | | | | |
| Northern Mariana Islands (US) | WPR | | | | | | | | | | | | |
| Occupied Palestinian Territories (oPT) | EMR | | | | | | | | | | | | |
| Pitcairn Islands (UK) | WPR | | | | | | | | | | | | |
| Wallis and Futuna (France) | WPR | | | | | | | | | | | | |

| Category | Definition | Code |
|---|---|---|
| Endemic | Continuous transmission of measles and/or rubella that persists for ≥12 months in any defined geographical area and no previous verification of elimination. | |
| Eliminated | Absence of endemic transmission for a continuous period of ≥12 months in the presence of a high-quality surveillance system. | |
| Verified | Verification of elimination for a region requires that all countries in the region document interruption of endemic virus transmission for a period of ≥36 months. | |
| Re-established transmission | Presence of a chain of transmission that continues uninterrupted for ≥12 months in a defined geographical area (region or country) after previous verification of elimination. | |
| No report | National Verification Commission annual report not provided to the Regional Verification Commission for review. | |

[1] (Reverification of Venezuela at the Pan American Health Organization (PAHO)/World Health Organization (WHO) Region of the Americas, Third Annual Meeting of the Measles, Rubella and Congenital Rubella Syndrome Post Elimination Regional Monitoring and Re-Verification Commission held on 14–16 November 2023 and including review of data from first semester of 2023).

**Table 1.** *Cont.*

| Country | WHO Region | Rubella Elimination Verification Status by Year | | | | | | | | | | | |
|---|---|---|---|---|---|---|---|---|---|---|---|---|---|
| | | 2011 | 2012 | 2013 | 2014 | 2015 | 2016 | 2017 | 2018 | 2019 | 2020 | 2021 | 2022 |
| Afghanistan | EMR | | | | | | | | | | | | |
| Albania | EUR | | | | | | | | | | | | |
| Algeria | AFR | | | | | | | | | | | | |
| Andorra | EUR | | | | | | | | | | | | |
| Angola | AFR | | | | | | | | | | | | |
| Antigua and Barbuda | AMR | | | | | | | | | | | | |
| Argentina | AMR | | | | | | | | | | | | |
| Armenia | EUR | | | | | | | | | | | | |
| Australia | WPR | | | | | | | | | | | | |
| Austria | EUR | | | | | | | | | | | | |
| Azerbaijan | EUR | | | | | | | | | | | | |
| Bahamas, The | AMR | | | | | | | | | | | | |
| Bahrain | EMR | | | | | | | | | | | | |
| Bangladesh | SEAR | | | | | | | | | | | | |
| Barbados | AMR | | | | | | | | | | | | |
| Belarus | EUR | | | | | | | | | | | | |
| Belgium | EUR | | | | | | | | | | | | |
| Belize | AMR | | | | | | | | | | | | |
| Benin | AFR | | | | | | | | | | | | |
| Bhutan | SEAR | | | | | | | | | | | | |
| Bolivia, Plurinational State of | AMR | | | | | | | | | | | | |
| Bosnia and Herzegovina | EUR | | | | | | | | | | | | |
| Botswana | AFR | | | | | | | | | | | | |
| Brazil | AMR | | | | | | | | | | | | |
| Brunei Darussalam | WPR | | | | | | | | | | | | |
| Bulgaria | EUR | | | | | | | | | | | | |
| Burkina Faso | AFR | | | | | | | | | | | | |
| Burundi | AFR | | | | | | | | | | | | |

**Table 1.** *Cont.*

| | | Rubella Elimination Verification Status by Year | | | | | | | | | | | |
|---|---|---|---|---|---|---|---|---|---|---|---|---|---|
| Country | WHO Region | 2011 | 2012 | 2013 | 2014 | 2015 | 2016 | 2017 | 2018 | 2019 | 2020 | 2021 | 2022 |
| Cabo Verde | AFR | | | | | | | | | | | | |
| Cambodia | WPR | | | | | | | | | | | | |
| Cameroon | AFR | | | | | | | | | | | | |
| Canada | AMR | | | | | | | | | | | | |
| Central African Republic | AFR | | | | | | | | | | | | |
| Chad | AFR | | | | | | | | | | | | |
| Chile | AMR | | | | | | | | | | | | |
| China | WPR | | | | | | | | | | | | |
| Colombia | AMR | | | | | | | | | | | | |
| Comoros | AFR | | | | | | | | | | | | |
| Congo, Republic of | AFR | | | | | | | | | | | | |
| Country | WHO Region | 2011 | 2012 | 2013 | 2014 | 2015 | 2016 | 2017 | 2018 | 2019 | 2020 | 2021 | 2022 |
| Cook Islands | WPR | | | | | | | | | | | | |
| Costa Rica | AMR | | | | | | | | | | | | |
| Côte d'Ivoire | AFR | | | | | | | | | | | | |
| Croatia | EUR | | | | | | | | | | | | |
| Cuba | AMR | | | | | | | | | | | | |
| Cyprus | EUR | | | | | | | | | | | | |
| Czechia | EUR | | | | | | | | | | | | |
| Denmark | EUR | | | | | | | | | | | | |
| Djibouti | EMR | | | | | | | | | | | | |
| Dominica | AMR | | | | | | | | | | | | |
| Dominica Republic | AMR | | | | | | | | | | | | |
| Democratic People's Republic of Korea | SEAR | | | | | | | | | | | | |
| Democratic Republic of the Congo | AFR | | | | | | | | | | | | |
| Ecuador | AMR | | | | | | | | | | | | |
| Egypt, Arab Republic | EMR | | | | | | | | | | | | |

**Table 1.** *Cont.*

| | | Rubella Elimination Verification Status by Year | | | | | | | | | | | |
|---|---|---|---|---|---|---|---|---|---|---|---|---|---|
| Country | WHO Region | 2011 | 2012 | 2013 | 2014 | 2015 | 2016 | 2017 | 2018 | 2019 | 2020 | 2021 | 2022 |
| El Salvador | AMR | | | | | | | | | | | | |
| Equatoria Guinea | AFR | | | | | | | | | | | | |
| Eritrea | AFR | | | | | | | | | | | | |
| Estonia | EUR | | | | | | | | | | | | |
| Eswatini (Swaziland) | AFR | | | | | | | | | | | | |
| Ethiopia | AFR | | | | | | | | | | | | |
| Fiji | WPR | | | | | | | | | | | | |
| Finland | EUR | | | | | | | | | | | | |
| France | EUR | | | | | | | | | | | | |
| Gabon | AFR | | | | | | | | | | | | |
| Gambia, The | AFR | | | | | | | | | | | | |
| Georgia | EUR | | | | | | | | | | | | |
| Germany | EUR | | | | | | | | | | | | |
| Ghana | AFR | | | | | | | | | | | | |
| Greece | EUR | | | | | | | | | | | | |
| Grenada | AMR | | | | | | | | | | | | |
| Guatemala | AMR | | | | | | | | | | | | |
| Guinea | AFR | | | | | | | | | | | | |
| Guinea-Bissau | AFR | | | | | | | | | | | | |
| Guyana | AMR | | | | | | | | | | | | |
| Haiti | AMR | | | | | | | | | | | | |
| Honduras | AMR | | | | | | | | | | | | |
| Hungary | EUR | | | | | | | | | | | | |
| Iceland | EUR | | | | | | | | | | | | |
| India | SEAR | | | | | | | | | | | | |
| Indonesia | SEAR | | | | | | | | | | | | |
| Country | WHO Region | 2011 | 2012 | 2013 | 2014 | 2015 | 2016 | 2017 | 2018 | 2019 | 2020 | 2021 | 2022 |
| Iran, Islamic Republic of | EMR | | | | | | | | | | | | |

**Table 1.** *Cont.*

| Country | WHO Region | Rubella Elimination Verification Status by Year | | | | | | | | | | | |
|---|---|---|---|---|---|---|---|---|---|---|---|---|---|
| | | 2011 | 2012 | 2013 | 2014 | 2015 | 2016 | 2017 | 2018 | 2019 | 2020 | 2021 | 2022 |
| Iraq | EMR | | | | | | | | | | | | |
| Ireland | EUR | | | | | | | | | | | | |
| Israel | EUR | | | | | | | | | | | | |
| Italy | EUR | | | | | | | | | | | | |
| Jamaica | AMR | | | | | | | | | | | | |
| Japan | WPR | | | | | | | | | | | | |
| Jordan | EMR | | | | | | | | | | | | |
| Kazakhstan | EUR | | | | | | | | | | | | |
| Kenya | AFR | | | | | | | | | | | | |
| Kiribati | WPR | | | | | | | | | | | | |
| Kuwait | EMR | | | | | | | | | | | | |
| Kyrgyz Republic | EUR | | | | | | | | | | | | |
| Lao People's Democratic Republic | WPR | | | | | | | | | | | | |
| Latvia | EUR | | | | | | | | | | | | |
| Lebanon | EMR | | | | | | | | | | | | |
| Lesotho | AFR | | | | | | | | | | | | |
| Liberia | AFR | | | | | | | | | | | | |
| Libya | EMR | | | | | | | | | | | | |
| Lithuania | EUR | | | | | | | | | | | | |
| Luxembourg | EUR | | | | | | | | | | | | |
| Madagascar | AFR | | | | | | | | | | | | |
| Malawi | AFR | | | | | | | | | | | | |
| Malaysia | WPR | | | | | | | | | | | | |
| Maldives | SEAR | | | | | | | | | | | | |
| Mali | AFR | | | | | | | | | | | | |
| Malta | EUR | | | | | | | | | | | | |
| Marshall Islands | WPR | | | | | | | | | | | | |
| Mauritius | AFR | | | | | | | | | | | | |

**Table 1.** *Cont.*

| | | Rubella Elimination Verification Status by Year | | | | | | | | | | | |
|---|---|---|---|---|---|---|---|---|---|---|---|---|---|
| Country | WHO Region | 2011 | 2012 | 2013 | 2014 | 2015 | 2016 | 2017 | 2018 | 2019 | 2020 | 2021 | 2022 |
| Mauritania | AFR | | | | | | | | | | | | |
| Mexico | AMR | | | | | | | | | | | | |
| Micronesia, Federated States of | WPR | | | | | | | | | | | | |
| Monaco | EUR | | | | | | | | | | | | |
| Mongolia | WPR | | | | | | | | | | | | |
| Montenegro | EUR | | | | | | | | | | | | |
| Morocco | EMR | | | | | | | | | | | | |
| Mozambique | AFR | | | | | | | | | | | | |
| Myanmar | SEAR | | | | | | | | | | | | |
| Namibia | AFR | | | | | | | | | | | | |
| Nauru | WPR | | | | | | | | | | | | |
| Nepal | SEAR | | | | | | | | | | | | |
| Country | WHO Region | 2011 | 2012 | 2013 | 2014 | 2015 | 2016 | 2017 | 2018 | 2019 | 2020 | 2021 | 2022 |
| Netherland, The Kingdom of | EUR | | | | | | | | | | | | |
| New Zealand | WPR | | | | | | | | | | | | |
| Nicaragua | AMR | | | | | | | | | | | | |
| Niger | AFR | | | | | | | | | | | | |
| Nigeria | AFR | | | | | | | | | | | | |
| Niue | WPR | | | | | | | | | | | | |
| North Macedonia | EUR | | | | | | | | | | | | |
| Norway | EUR | | | | | | | | | | | | |
| Oman | EMR | | | | | | | | | | | | |
| Pakistan | EMR | | | | | | | | | | | | |
| Palau | WPR | | | | | | | | | | | | |
| Panama | AMR | | | | | | | | | | | | |
| Papua New Guinea | WPR | | | | | | | | | | | | |
| Paraguay | AMR | | | | | | | | | | | | |
| Peru | AMR | | | | | | | | | | | | |

**Table 1.** *Cont.*

| | | Rubella Elimination Verification Status by Year | | | | | | | | | | | |
|---|---|---|---|---|---|---|---|---|---|---|---|---|---|
| Country | WHO Region | 2011 | 2012 | 2013 | 2014 | 2015 | 2016 | 2017 | 2018 | 2019 | 2020 | 2021 | 2022 |
| Philippines | WPR | | | | | | | | | | | | |
| Poland | EUR | | | | | | | | | | | | |
| Portugal | EUR | | | | | | | | | | | | |
| Qatar | EMR | | | | | | | | | | | | |
| Republic of Korea | WPR | | | | | | | | | | | | |
| Republic of Moldova | EUR | | | | | | | | | | | | |
| Romania | EUR | | | | | | | | | | | | |
| Russian Federation | EUR | | | | | | | | | | | | |
| Rwanda | AFR | | | | | | | | | | | | |
| Saint Kitts and Nevis | AMR | | | | | | | | | | | | |
| Saint Lucia | AMR | | | | | | | | | | | | |
| Saint Vincent and the Grenadines | AMR | | | | | | | | | | | | |
| Samoa | WPR | | | | | | | | | | | | |
| San Marino | EUR | | | | | | | | | | | | |
| Sao Tome and Principe | AFR | | | | | | | | | | | | |
| Saudi Arabia | EMR | | | | | | | | | | | | |
| Senegal | AFR | | | | | | | | | | | | |
| Serbia | EUR | | | | | | | | | | | | |
| Seychelles | AFR | | | | | | | | | | | | |
| Sierra Leone | AFR | | | | | | | | | | | | |
| Singapore | WPR | | | | | | | | | | | | |
| Slovakia | EUR | | | | | | | | | | | | |
| Slovenia | EUR | | | | | | | | | | | | |
| Solomon Islands | WPR | | | | | | | | | | | | |
| Somalia | EMR | | | | | | | | | | | | |
| South Africa | AFR | | | | | | | | | | | | |
| Country | WHO Region | 2011 | 2012 | 2013 | 2014 | 2015 | 2016 | 2017 | 2018 | 2019 | 2020 | 2021 | 2022 |
| South Sudan | AFR | | | | | | | | | | | | |

**Table 1.** *Cont.*

| Country | WHO Region | Rubella Elimination Verification Status by Year | | | | | | | | | | | |
|---|---|---|---|---|---|---|---|---|---|---|---|---|---|
| | | 2011 | 2012 | 2013 | 2014 | 2015 | 2016 | 2017 | 2018 | 2019 | 2020 | 2021 | 2022 |
| Spain | EUR | | | | | | | | | | | | |
| Sri Lanka | SEAR | | | | | | | | | | | | |
| Sudan | EMR | | | | | | | | | | | | |
| Suriname | AMR | | | | | | | | | | | | |
| Sweden | EUR | | | | | | | | | | | | |
| Switzerland | EUR | | | | | | | | | | | | |
| Syrian Arab Republic | EMR | | | | | | | | | | | | |
| Tajikistan | EUR | | | | | | | | | | | | |
| Tanzania, United Republic | AFR | | | | | | | | | | | | |
| Thailand | SEAR | | | | | | | | | | | | |
| Timor-Leste | SEAR | | | | | | | | | | | | |
| Togo | AFR | | | | | | | | | | | | |
| Tokelau | WPR | | | | | | | | | | | | |
| Tonga | WPR | | | | | | | | | | | | |
| Trinidad and Tobago | AMR | | | | | | | | | | | | |
| Tunisia | EMR | | | | | | | | | | | | |
| Türkiye | EUR | | | | | | | | | | | | |
| Turkmenistan | EUR | | | | | | | | | | | | |
| Tuvalu | WPR | | | | | | | | | | | | |
| United Arab Emirates | EMR | | | | | | | | | | | | |
| Uganda | AFR | | | | | | | | | | | | |
| Ukraine | EUR | | | | | | | | | | | | |
| United Arab Emirates | EMR | | | | | | | | | | | | |
| United Kingdom of Great Britain and Northern Ireland | EUR | | | | | | | | | | | | |
| United States of America | AMR | | | | | | | | | | | | |
| Uruguay | AMR | | | | | | | | | | | | |
| Uzbekistan | EUR | | | | | | | | | | | | |

**Table 1.** *Cont.*

| | | Rubella Elimination Verification Status by Year | | | | | | | | | | | |
|---|---|---|---|---|---|---|---|---|---|---|---|---|---|
| Country | WHO Region | 2011 | 2012 | 2013 | 2014 | 2015 | 2016 | 2017 | 2018 | 2019 | 2020 | 2021 | 2022 |
| Vanuatu | WPR | | | | | | | | | | | | |
| Venezuela | AMR | | | | | | | | | | | | |
| Vietnam | WPR | | | | | | | | | | | | |
| Yemen | EMR | | | | | | | | | | | | |
| Zambia | AFR | | | | | | | | | | | | |
| Zimbabwe | AFR | | | | | | | | | | | | |
| Territory/Region | WHO Region | 2011 | 2012 | 2013 | 2014 | 2015 | 2016 | 2017 | 2018 | 2019 | 2020 | 2021 | 2022 |
| American Samoa (US) | WPR | | | | | | | | | | | | |
| French Polynesia (France) | WPR | | | | | | | | | | | | |
| Guam (US) | WPR | | | | | | | | | | | | |
| Hong Kong SAR (China) | WPR | | | | | | | | | | | | |
| Macao SAR (China) | WPR | | | | | | | | | | | | |
| New Caledonia (France) | WPR | | | | | | | | | | | | |
| Northern Mariana Islands (US) | WPR | | | | | | | | | | | | |
| Occupied Palestinian Territories (oPT) | EMR | | | | | | | | | | | | |
| Pitcairn Islands (UK) | WPR | | | | | | | | | | | | |
| Wallis and Futuna (France) | WPR | | | | | | | | | | | | |

| Category | Definition | Code |
|---|---|---|
| Endemic | Continuous transmission of measles and/or rubella that persists for $\geq$12 months in any defined geographical area and no previous verification of elimination. | |
| Eliminated | Absence of endemic transmission for a continuous period of $\geq$12 months in the presence of a high-quality surveillance system. | |
| Verified | Verification of elimination for a region requires that all countries in the region document interruption of endemic virus transmission for a period of $\geq$36 months. | |
| Re-established transmission | Presence of a chain of transmission that continues uninterrupted for $\geq$12 months in a defined geographical area (region or country) after previous verification of elimination. | |
| No report | National Verification Commission annual report not provided to the Regional Verification Commission for review. | |

We have no choice—there is a moral imperative to now commit to and achieve measles and rubella eradication [17]. How long will the global community tolerate the ongoing disease burden and preventable deaths due to measles? The rule of rescue demands that if we have effective tools, we should make every effort to save lives. Measles, rubella, and CRS eradication should not remain merely a technically feasible possibility but rather be completed to ensure that future generations of children do not live under the shadow of preventable childhood death and lifelong disability.

**Author Contributions:** Conceptualization, D.N.D., J.K.A., S.T., D.G., M.K. and N.T.; writing—original draft preparation, D.N.D., writing—review and editing, D.N.D., J.K.A., S.T., D.G., M.K. and N.T. All authors have read and agreed to the published version of the manuscript.

**Funding:** This research received no external funding.

**Acknowledgments:** Mahoney F, Deputy Chairperson Regional Measles and Rubella Elimination Verification Commission, European Pacific Region, for his contribution to the conception and review. O'Connor P, Department of Immunization, Vaccines, and Biologicals (IVB). World Health Organization—Geneva, Switzerland, for assisting with the construction and refinement of Table 1.

**Conflicts of Interest:** The authors declare no conflict of interest.

## References

1. World Health Organization. *Essential Programme on Immunisation*; World Health Organization: Geneva, Switzerland, 2024.
2. Minta, A.A.; Ferrari, M.; Antoni, S.; Portnoy, A.; Sbarra, A.; Lambert, B.; Hatcher, C.; Hsu, C.H.; Ho, L.L.; Steulet, C.; et al. Progress toward regional measles elimination—Worldwide, 2000–2022. *MMWR Morb. Mortal. Wkly. Rep.* **2023**, *72*, 1262–1268. [CrossRef] [PubMed]
3. Carter, A.; Msemburi, W.; Sim, S.Y.; Gaythorpe, K.A.; Lambach, P.; Lindstrand, A.; Hutubessy, R. Modeling the impact of vaccination for the immunization Agenda 2030: Deaths averted due to vaccination against 14 pathogens in 194 countries from 2021 to 2030. *Vaccine* 2023, *in press*. [CrossRef] [PubMed]
4. Hübschen, J.M.; Gouandjika-Vasilache, I.; Dina, J. Measles. *Lancet* **2022**, *399*, 678–690. [CrossRef] [PubMed]
5. Ozawa, S.; Clark, S.; Portnoy, A.; Grewal, S.; Stack, M.L.; Sinha, A.; Mirelman, A.; Franklin, H.; Friberg, I.K.; Tam, Y.; et al. Estimated economic impact of vaccinations in 73 low- and middle-income countries, 2001–2020. *Bull. World Health Organ.* **2017**, *95*, 629–638. [CrossRef] [PubMed]
6. Vynnycky, E.; Knapp, J.K.; Papadopoulos, T.; Cutts, F.T.; Hachiya, M.; Miyano, S.; Reef, S.E. Estimates of the global burden of Congenital Rubella Syndrome, 1996–2019. *Int. J. Infect. Dis.* **2023**, *137*, 149–156. [CrossRef] [PubMed]
7. World Health Organization. Meeting of the Strategic Advisory Group of Experts on Immunization, November 2010. Summary, conclusions and recommendations. *Wkly. Epidemiol. Rec.* **2011**, *86*, 1–16.
8. World Health Organization. *Global Vaccine Action Plan, 2011–2020*; World Health Organization: Geneva, Switzerland, 2013.
9. Durrheim, D.N.; Crowcroft, N.S.; Blumberg, L.H. Is the global measles resurgence a "public health emergency of international concern"? *Int. J. Infect. Dis.* **2019**, *83*, 95–97. [CrossRef] [PubMed]
10. Durrheim, D.N.; Andrus, J.K.; Tabassum, S.; Bashour, H.; Githanga, D.; Pfaff, G. A dangerous measles future looms beyond the COVID-19 pandemic. *Nat. Med.* **2021**, *27*, 360–361. [CrossRef] [PubMed]
11. World Health Organization. Immunization Agenda 2030. Available online: https://www.who.int/publications/m/item/immunization-agenda-2030-a-global-strategy-to-leave-no-one-behind (accessed on 27 April 2024).
12. World Health Organization. IA 2030 scorecard–global. In *IA2030 Scorecard for Immunization Agenda 2030*; World Health Organization: Geneva, Switzerland, 2020.
13. Reef, S.E.; Icenogle, J.P.; Plotkin, S.A. The path to eradication of rubella. *Vaccine* **2023**, *41*, 7525–7531. [CrossRef]
14. Durrheim, D.N.; Tuibeqa, I.V.; Aho, G.S.; Grangeon, J.P.; Ogaoga, D.; Wattiaux, A.; Mariano, K.M.; Evans, R.; Hossain, S.; Aslam, S.K. Pacific Island Countries demonstrate the sustained success of a coordinated measles mass vaccination campaign. *Lancet Reg. Health–West. Pac.* **2024**, *42*, 100998. [CrossRef] [PubMed]
15. Andrus, J.K.; Cochi, S.L.; Cooper, L.Z.; Klein, J. Combining global elimination of measles and rubella with strengthening of health systems in developing countries. *Health Aff.* **2016**, *35*, 327–333. [CrossRef] [PubMed]

16. Hasso-Agopsowicz, M.; Crowcroft, N.; Biellik, R.; Gregory, C.J.; Menozzi-Arnaud, M.; Amorij, J.P.; Gilbert, P.A.; Earle, K.; Frivold, C.; Jarrahian, C.; et al. Accelerating the Development of Measles and Rubella Microarray Patches to Eliminate Measles and Rubella: Recent Progress, Remaining Challenges. *Front. Public Health* **2022**, *10*, 809675. [CrossRef]
17. Durrheim, D.N.; Andrus, J.K. The ethical case for global measles eradication-justice and the Rule of Rescue. *Int. Health* **2020**, *12*, 375–377. [CrossRef] [PubMed]

*vaccines*

*Commentary*

# Evolution and Contribution of a Global Partnership against Measles and Rubella, 2001–2023

**Peter Strebel [1,*,†], Mark Grabowsky [2,†], Edward Hoekstra [3,†], Andrea Gay [4,†,‡] and Stephen Cochi [5,†,‡]**

1 Independent Consultant, 1290 Geneva, Switzerland
2 Independent Consultant, Oxford, CT 06478, USA
3 Independent Consultant, New York, NY 11375, USA
4 Washington, DC 20012, USA
5 Atlanta, GA 30345, USA
* Correspondence: peter.strebel@gmail.com
† The authors were in leadership roles for the 5 founding partners of the Measles-Rubella Initiative—American Red Cross (Grabowsky), United States Centers for Disease Control and Prevention (Cochi), United Nations Children's Fund (Hoekstra), United Nations Foundation (Gay), and World Health Organization (Strebel).
‡ Retired.

**Abstract:** This article describes the arc of global measles and rubella elimination since 2000 from the perspective of the founding partners of the Measles Initiative. The Measles Initiative was formed in 2001 as a partnership among the American Red Cross, the Centers for Disease Control and Prevention, UNICEF, the United Nations Foundation, and the World Health Organization with the aim to reduce measles deaths in low-income countries. Recognizing rubella as the leading infectious disease cause of congenital abnormalities globally and achievement of measles and rubella elimination in the region of the Americas, the partnership was renamed the Measles and Rubella Initiative (MRI) in 2012. The goals of the MRI were at least a 95% reduction in global measles mortality and elimination of measles and rubella in at least five of the six WHO regions. In January 2023, the membership of the partnership was expanded to include the Bill and Melinda Gates Foundation (BMGF) and Gavi the Vaccine Alliance, and its name changed to the IA2030 Measles and Rubella Partnership. We describe the role the partnership has had in measles partner effectiveness and its impact on measles and rubella disease burden, including how the partnership has strategically adapted to the evolving immunization landscape. We conclude with lessons learned regarding the role global partnerships can play in furthering the impact of disease control programs within the current global immunization environment.

**Keywords:** Global health partnerships; Epidemiology of measles; Epidemiology of rubella

## 1. The Measles Initiative—The First 10 Years, 2001–2010

Despite substantial progress in the Americas during the 1990s, measles remained the leading cause of vaccine-preventable deaths worldwide, with more than ¾ of a million deaths in 1999 [1]. Ninety-four percent of measles-associated deaths occurred in 47 countries, mainly in Africa [1]. In the late 1990s, seven countries in southern Africa successfully applied PAHO's strategy featuring nationwide mass measles vaccination campaigns, which were country financed and reduced the number of measles-related deaths to near zero in those geographies [2]. Based on those demonstrated successes, other endemic countries were eager to do the same; however, they lacked the resources and technical support to move forward. The Measles Initiative was formed in 2001, with each of the five founding organizations bringing a different perspective and capacity to address these needs.

In its first decade, the Measles Initiative worked with 70 countries, offering financial and technical support to vaccinate more than 900 million children in supplementary immunization activities at a cost of less than USD 1 per child vaccinated [3]. In 2003, with evidence from rapid success in Africa, the World Health Assembly committed to reducing global measles deaths by 50% between 1999 and 2005. Countries outside of Africa expressed interest in mass vaccination strategies, and the Measles Initiative began to support governments worldwide the following year. Not only did the Measles Initiative support vaccination efforts but it also began to support a laboratory network and measles disease surveillance. By the end of 2005, the Measles Initiative, through the committed efforts of national governments, had catalyzed a reduction in global measles deaths by 60% relative to 1999, thereby exceeding the United Nations' target [1]. To continue the momentum, the World Health Assembly endorsed a more ambitious goal—to reduce measles deaths by 90% between 2000 and 2010. By the end of 2008, 2 years ahead of schedule, all countries but one (India) had reached the 2010 goal. Global measles deaths have been reduced by 78% [3]. Between 2000 and 2010, first-dose coverage (Measles vaccination strategies include vaccination coverage of $\geq$95% with the first and second dose of measles vaccine supplemented by wide age range campaigns to vaccinate children who have not had two doses of vaccine) rose from 72% to 84%, and second-dose coverage increased from 17% to 42% [4]. In addition, measles campaigns were successful in delivering more than 41 million insecticide-treated nets, 94 million deworming tablets, 127 million polio vaccines, and 213 million doses of vitamin A [3].

The Measles Initiative initially had an informal but well-coordinated and focused management style. The goal was to provide much-needed technical and financial support to national measles plans, immunization campaigns, and measles surveillance while securing as much national buy in and ownership as possible. Plans were developed at the local and national levels. To supplement national commitment, external funding decisions were made collectively by representatives from each partner in the Measles Initiative. The Measles Initiative functioned without a formal secretariat. As a result, each organization maintained its own internal information systems, and there was no common data repository. The responsibility for managing and coordinating activities was shared equally. Partners jointly mobilized resources and pooled their funds for national program implementation, requiring only a plan of action and report on the activities funded by the Measles Initiative from each country. Each country's single plan and budget prevented parallel funding, ensured joint planning at the country level, and enabled flexibility. This structure streamlined program planning and implementation by lowering transaction costs for governments and partners. New partners at the local level were encouraged. The partnership was inclusive and supported local efforts to improve national immunization programs.

The ensuing rapid expansion, increasing visibility, and growing financial requirements put significant stress on the management of the Measles Initiative. Although the partnership initially experienced a several years-long period of evolutionary continuous growth without a significant setback or internal disruption, after its first decade, the Measles Initiative experienced a period of challenges that required "revolutionary" changes.

## 2. Consolidation of Progress Leads to Increasing Challenges (2011–2020)

The remarkable progress toward measles and rubella elimination during the first decade of the Measles Initiative resulted in heightened political, technical, and programmatic support to pursue measles eradication as the decade of the 2010s began [5]. Recognizing rubella as the leading infectious cause of congenital abnormalities globally, the Measles Initiative was renamed the Measles and Rubella Initiative (MRI) in 2012. In the Americas, the last cases of endemic measles transmission occurred in 2002, and the last cases of rubella and congenital rubella syndrome (CRS) in 2009 [6]. An expert advisory panel convened by the WHO in 2010 concluded that measles can and should be eradicated, and the WHO Strategic Advisory Group of Experts (SAGE) on Immunization endorsed these conclusions. In 2011, the WHO's Executive Board endorsed the SAGE recommendations [5,7]. By 2013, member states of all six WHO regions had voted for regional measles elimination target dates on or before 2020, securing the political commitment of all countries. Countries and regions began pursuing accelerated rubella elimination following the successful verification of rubella elimination in the region of the Americas, which has been sustained until now [5]. Progress in rubella-containing vaccine (RCV) introductions was facilitated by a policy recommendation for the use of a combined measles–rubella (MR) vaccine [8] and the Gavi commitment of USD 500 million for the rubella vaccine introduction that began in 2012. All six WHO regions established regional measles and rubella elimination verification commissions to monitor progress. By mid-decade, the WHO regions and MRI-supported countries were encouraged by the momentum that had been achieved.

Programmatic improvements matched these political and technical commitments. The number of countries providing a second dose of measles vaccine (MCV2) increased markedly from 98 (51%) in 2000 to 182 (94%) in 2020, and the estimated global MCV2 coverage increased from 17% in 2000 to 72% in 2020 [4]. The number of countries providing rubella vaccine increased from 130 (67%) in 2010 to 173 (89%) countries in 2020, and estimated global coverage increased to 70%, resulting in a two-thirds decline in estimated congenital rubella syndrome (CRS) births from 100,000 in 2010 to 32,000 in 2019 and averting an additional 229,000 CRS cases [9]. The introduction and expanded use of RCV in all regions since 1970 averted an estimated 696,859 CRS births globally during 2010–2019 when compared to the situation that might have been expected if RCV had not been introduced anywhere (written communication, Emilia Vynnycky, 30 January 2024). As of March 2024, 19 countries have yet to reduce RCV in their national immunization programs. By 2016, measles incidence and deaths reached record lows compared with rates at the inception of the partnership in 2001. Annual reported measles incidence had decreased by 87%, from 145 to 19 cases per million persons, and annual estimated measles deaths fell by 84% to a record low of 89,780; between 2000 and 2016, measles vaccination prevented an estimated 20.4 million deaths [10].

However, there were clouds on the horizon. Global-level political commitment and momentum for measles and rubella elimination began to dissipate by the middle of the second decade. There was a gradual decline through the end of the decade, despite sustained commitment at the regional level. Impeding factors included (1) a global inability to achieve polio eradication, resulting in disenchantment with eradication initiatives and concerns as to the practical feasibility and true costs of achieving measles eradication; (2) a parallel shift away from vertical health programs; (3) the consolidation of the flow of immunization funding toward Gavi at the expense of disease-specific initiatives; and (4) discontent with the need for, and expense of, frequent mass campaigns (themselves of variable quality) because routine immunization programs were not mature enough to sustain high levels of measles immunity.

Although the strategic approaches to measles and rubella elimination continue to remain valid, they were not fully implemented, mainly due to a lack of global political will, as reflected in inadequate resources and, in some cases, a lack of country ownership [11]. Average annual funding during 2001–2016 was USD 69 million for the MRI, in contrast to USD 818 million for the Global Polio Eradication Initiative [7]. As part of a more comprehensive measles–rubella strategy, Gavi funding increased to USD 820 million (i.e., average annual funding of USD 164 million) for measles–rubella control activities for the strategic period 2016–2020 [12]. However, some key donors expressed reservations about committing additional resources to eliminate measles and rubella. These partners were concerned that committing additional resources to achieve elimination targets in countries that rely on donor support for campaign operational costs would promote mass campaigns over routine service delivery. Subsequently, a worldwide measles resurgence occurred during 2018–2019, the root cause of which was a failure to vaccinate young children, particularly in marginalized communities, as well as school-aged children and young adults facilitated by international spread [13]. The final blow to further progress was the arrival of the COVID-19 pandemic in 2020 with its associated growth in anti-vaccine sentiment and substantial disruption of all immunization services and disease surveillance.

Frustrated by the slow progress toward elimination in other regions and the persistent risk of measles importations, member states of PAHO pushed for establishing a measles eradication goal at the 2017 WHA. A compromise was reached calling for a feasibility assessment of measles and rubella eradication to be presented to the WHA in 2020. Based on a comprehensive review, the feasibility assessment report concluded that while eradicating both measles and rubella was biologically and technically feasible, public, political, and donor support was lacking [14]. Rather than pursue a top-down approach to eradication, the report recommended that the path to measles and rubella eradication should strengthen primary health care and be a pathfinder for the more bottom-up integrated approach laid out in the Immunization Agenda 2030 (IA2030). The conditions for establishing a time-bound measles and rubella eradication goal included setting up a monitoring and accountability framework and achieving predetermined benchmarks, as well as a short and financially feasible end-game strategy.

## 3. Adapting to a Changed Global Immunization Environment (2021 to 2023)

In response to the need for alignment across the global immunization strategy for the coming decade, the MRI partners developed the new Measles and Rubella Strategic Framework 2021–2030 (MRSF2030) with a vision of "A world without measles and rubella" and the goal of achieving and maintaining regional measles and rubella elimination goals [15]. The MRSF2030 called for embedding measles and rubella activities within country immunization and Primary Health Care programs (a key lesson learned from the PAHO approach), a better definition of the roles and responsibilities of stakeholders at each level, strengthening country capacity for outbreak response, and expediting innovative vaccine delivery technologies, such as micro-array patches and rapid diagnostic tests to bolster surveillance. However, the MRSF stopped short of providing an implementation roadmap or a monitoring/accountability framework.

In 2020, the MRI Management Team commissioned a thorough assessment of the global measles and rubella partnership, including recommendations on what would be needed to deliver on the promise of the MRSF2030. The report highlighted the rapid evolution in the global immunization ecosystem characterized by competing country priorities, demand for delivery integration, the growing influence of BMGF and Gavi, and widescale disruption in health care and immunization services due to the COVID-19 pandemic.

To be successful in this new reality, the report recognized that a refreshed partnership would need a sharp strategic focus and more efficient ways of working. Recommendations include (1) integrate the MRI with IA2030 to reap the benefits of linkages with other partners and horizontal approaches; (2) strengthen partnership management by allowing for broader membership in the management team; (3) create a centralized support unit to drive progress and implement new ways of working; (4) commit to monitoring program milestones with regular "stock takes" and take corrective actions; and (5) determine which partnership functions should be incorporated into emerging IA2030 structures.

In the face of a post-pandemic resurgence of measles, implementing key recommendations from the Partnership Assessment has been expedited. As of January 2023, BMGF and Gavi have become full members of the newly renamed IA2030 Measles and Rubella Partnership [16]. The partnership has also created a secretariat to support its strategic activities and goals. However, the IA2030 infrastructure is still under development, and much work remains to effectively integrate the remaining shared functions and adopt more efficient and effective new ways of working.

## 4. Overall Partnership Impact and Lessons Learned

While most partnership support has been directed toward mass vaccination campaigns and improving measles and rubella surveillance, it has also contributed to improvements in routine immunization coverage. Between 2000 and 2022, global MCV1 coverage increased from 72% to 83%, and MCV2 coverage from 17% to 74% [4]. This four-fold increase in MCV2 coverage was driven by the introduction of a routine second dose in ninety-three countries, most of which benefited from Gavi funding that began in 2007. MCV2 still needs to be introduced in six countries. Support from the MR partnership also significantly impacted global RCV coverage, which has increased from 40% in 2012 to 70% in 2020 [9]. This increase was primarily due to the introduction of RCV in countries in the Southeast Asian and Western Pacific Regions. RCV remains to be introduced in 19 countries, mainly in the African Region, and its introduction is being impeded by a lack of agreement on whether RCV can be safely introduced in countries with very weak immunization services [8]. Results from a modeling study by Frey et.al. published in this supplement suggest that this concern may be unfounded.

Over the course of the partnership, reported measles incidence has decreased by 80% from 145 cases per million population in 2000 to 29 in 2022. Similarly, estimated measles deaths have decreased by four-fifths (82%), from 773,000 in 2000 to 136,000 in 2022, with 57 million (recent updates to the mathematical model that include more dynamic approaches to estimating the age distribution of measles cases, as well as age-specific measles case–fatality ratios [17], have shifted cases to younger age groups with higher case-fatality ratios. This resulted in higher overall estimates of the cumulative number of measles deaths averted when compared to estimates that were based on earlier models) cumulative measles deaths averted by vaccination [4]. Global CRS births have declined by more than two-thirds since 2010, from 100,000 in 2010 to 32,000 in 2019 [9], and the use of RCV since 1970 averted an estimated 696,859 CRS births globally during 2010–2019 (written communication, Emilia Vynnycky, 30 January 2024).

Technical and financial support from the partnership has enabled the expansion of the Global Measles and Rubella Laboratory Network (GMRLN) to include 734 national and subnational WHO-certified laboratories, a considerable increase from fewer than 40 laboratories in 1998. The number of measles genotypes detected by GMRLN decreased from thirteen in 2002 to six in 2014, three in 2020, and two (D8 and B3) in 2022, reflecting the increasing pressure of measles vaccination on measles virus transmission and genotype diversity [4].

The first decade of the partnership saw rapid progress due to the rolling out of PAHO measles elimination strategies in Africa and other WHO regions [5,6]. The game-changing approach was conducting catch-up campaigns that targeted multiple cohorts of children and included the vast majority of measles-susceptible individuals (in this context, ages 9 months to 14 years), leading to rapid increases in population immunity. Marked drops in measles incidence and a more than three-quarters reduction in global measles mortality resulted, generating optimism that measles could be eradicated globally. However, failure to achieve polio eradication and competing immunization priorities led to doubts about the political and financial feasibility of eradication. An opportunity to establish a global measles eradication target was missed.

The second decade saw the consolidation of the measles strategy by introducing MCV2, even in settings where MCV1 coverage was low, regular follow-up campaigns, and expansion of the GMRLN. The breakthrough was the 2011 policy decision to link the introduction of RCV to measles elimination efforts and introduce RCV, starting with a broad age range catch-up campaign that would reduce the risk of a paradoxical increase in CRS due to low coverage. Expanding the use of RCV to include low-income countries resulted in a two-thirds reduction in global CRS births by the end of the decade.

As the third decade approached, the sustained success of MRI began to stall. With little further progress toward elimination goals and the absence of new tools or strategies to drive gains, the question was raised by some partners whether the Initiative should be integrated into IA2030, which was championing integrated immunization service delivery. Amid the COVID-19 pandemic, an external assessment of the measles and rubella partnership determined that there were unique functions and essential control strategies that risked being lost if there was no global partnership or common goal.

The first 23 years of the global measles and rubella partnership have generated several lessons learned. The experience has demonstrated the added value of diverse organizations working together toward a shared vision. Dedicated financial and human resources are required for multi-year (2–5 year) program planning. Inter-organizational rivalry and lengthy global policy and strategy discussions can lead to a loss of focus on program performance and country needs, particularly for the most challenging countries. Sustained immunization service delivery requires securing community engagement and demonstrated country ownership, including country ownership of financing, with partners providing supplemental funding rather than sole financing. A common information platform and a sharp focus on regularly tracking performance indicators are needed to identify program weaknesses and allow early course correction. Being responsive to the front-line program needs and "learning from the field" has led to vaccine delivery breakthroughs. While incremental improvements in tactics and best practices will improve program efficiency, new game-changing tools will be needed to change the current trajectory and re-establish momentum [18]. Innovation is urgently needed to address growing anti-vaccine sentiment and the intractable challenge of reaching marginalized communities and vaccinating the more than 20 million infants who miss routine immunization each year. Simpler and safer vaccine delivery technology, such as microarray patches, may help address this inequity and could provide the next leap forward toward regional elimination and eventual eradication of measles and rubella.

**Author Contributions:** Our article is a commentary and each author provided input at the conceptualization, writing and editing phases. All authors have read and agreed to the published version of the manuscript.

**Funding:** This research received no external funding.

**Acknowledgments:** Kendall Krause gave useful feedback on early drafts of the manuscript. Robin Biellik provided information on the importance of countries self-financing their measles catch-up campaigns in the success achieved in the seven southern African countries.

**Conflicts of Interest:** The authors declare no conflict of interest.

## References

1. Wolfson, L.J.; Strebel, P.M.; Gacic-Dobo, M.; Hoekstra, E.J.; McFarland, J.W.; Hersh, B.S. Has the 2005 measles mortality reduction goal been achieved? A natural history modelling study. *Lancet* **2007**, *369*, 191–200. [CrossRef] [PubMed]
2. Christie, A.S.; Gay, A. The Measles Initiative: Moving toward measles eradication. *J. Infect. Dis.* **2011**, *204* (Suppl. 1), S14–S17. [CrossRef]
3. Otten, J.M.W.; Okwo-Bele, J.; Kezaala, R.; Biellik, R.; Eggers, R.; Nshimirimana, D. Impact of Alternative Approaches to Accelerated Measles Control: Experience in the African Region, 1996–2002. *J. Infect. Dis.* **2003**, *187*, S36–S43. [CrossRef] [PubMed]
4. Minta, A.A.; Ferrari, M.; Antoni, S.; Portnoy, A.; Sbarra, A.; Lambert, B.; Hatcher, C.; Hsu, C.H.; Ho, L.L.; Steulet, C.; et al. Progress Toward Measles Elimination—Worldwide, 2000–2022. *MMWR Morb. Mortal Wkly. Rep.* **2023**, *72*, 1262–1268. [CrossRef] [PubMed]
5. Cochi, S.L.; Schluter, W.W. What it will take to achieve a world without measles. *J. Infect. Dis.* **2020**, *222*, 1073–1075. [CrossRef] [PubMed]
6. Andrus, J.K.; de Quadros, C.A.; Solórzano, C.C.; Periago, M.R.; Henderson, D.A. Measles and rubella eradication in the Americas. *Vaccine* **2011**, *29*, D91–D96. [CrossRef] [PubMed]
7. WHO. Report of the 30th meeting of the International Task Force for Disease Eradication, 22 October 2019. *Wkly. Epidemiol. Rec.* **2020**, *95*, 61–68.
8. Rubella Vaccines: WHO Position paper—2011. *Wkly. Epidemiol. Rec.* **2011**, *86*, 301–316.
9. Vynnycky, E.; Knapp, J.K.; Papadopoulos, T.; Cutts, F.T.; Hachiya, M.; Miyano, S.; Reef, S.E. Estimates of the global burden of Congenital Rubella Syndrome, 1996–2019. *Int. J. Infect. Dis.* **2023**, *137*, 149–156. [CrossRef] [PubMed]
10. Dabbagh, A.; Patel, M.K.; Dumolard, L.; Gacic-Dobo, M.; Strebel, P.M.; Mulders, M.N.; Okwo-Bele, J.M.; Kretsinger, K.; Papania, M.J.; Rota, P.A.; et al. Progress toward regional measles elimination—worldwide, 2000–2016. *MMWR Morb. Mortal Wkly. Rep.* **2017**, *66*, 1148–1153. [CrossRef]
11. Orenstein, W.A.; Hinman, A.; Nkowane, B.; Olive, J.M.; Reingold, A. *Measles and Rubella Global Strategic Plan 2012–2020 Midterm Review*; World Health Organization: Geneva, Switzerland, 2016.
12. Available online: https://reliefweb.int/report/world/new-support-measles-vaccine-help-save-more-one-million-lives (accessed on 11 December 2023).
13. Patel, M.K.; Antoni, S.; Nedelec, Y.; Sodha, S.; Menning, L.; Ogbuanu, I.U.; Dobo, M.G. The Changing Global Epidemiology of Measles, 2013–2018. *J. Infect. Dis.* **2020**, *222*, 1117–1128. [CrossRef] [PubMed]
14. Moss, W.J.; Shendale, S.; Lindstrand, A.; O'Brien, K.L.; Turner, N.; Goodman, T.; Kretsinger, K. Feasibility assessment of measles and rubella eradication. *Vaccine* **2021**, *39*, 3544–3559. [CrossRef] [PubMed]

15. Measles and Rubella Strategic Framework: 2021–2030 (who.int). Available online: https://www.who.int/publications/i/item/measles-and-rubella-strategic-framework-2021-2030 (accessed on 11 December 2023).
16. A New Era in the Fight against Measles and Rubella (who.int). Available online: https://www.who.int/news/item/22-02-2023-a-new-era-in-the-fight-against-measles-and-rubella#:~:text=In%202012,%20the%20founding%20partners,and%20Rubella%20Initiative%20(M&RI) (accessed on 11 December 2023).
17. Sbarra, A.N.; Mosser, J.F.; Jit, M.; Ferrari, M.; Ramshaw, R.E.; O'Connor, P.; Krause, L.K.; Rogowski, E.L.; Portnoy, A. Estimating national-level measles case–fatality ratios in low-income and middle-income countries: An updated systematic review and modelling study. *Lancet Glob. Health* **2023**, *11*, e516–e524. [CrossRef] [PubMed]
18. Goodson, J.L.; Rota, P.A. Innovations in vaccine delivery: Increasing access, coverage, and equity and lessons learnt from measles and rubella elimination. *Drug Deliv. Transl. Res.* **2022**, *12*, 959–967. [CrossRef] [PubMed]

*vaccines*

MDPI

*Review*

# Possible Paths to Measles Eradication: Conceptual Frameworks, Strategies, and Tactics

**Amy K. Winter [1] and William J. Moss [2,3,*]**

1 Department of Epidemiology and Biostatistics, College of Public Health, University of Georgia, Athens, GA 30602, USA; awinter@uga.edu
2 International Vaccine Access Center, Department of International Health, Bloomberg School of Public Health, Johns Hopkins University, Baltimore, MD 21205, USA
3 Department of Epidemiology, Bloomberg School of Public Health, Johns Hopkins University, Baltimore, MD 21205, USA
* Correspondence: wmoss1@jhu.edu

**Abstract:** Measles elimination refers to the interruption of measles virus transmission in a defined geographic area (e.g., country or region) for 12 months or more, and measles eradication refers to the global interruption of measles virus transmission. Measles eradication was first discussed and debated in the late 1960's shortly after the licensure of measles vaccines. Most experts agree that measles meets criteria for disease eradication, but progress toward national and regional measles elimination has slowed. Several paths to measles eradication can be described, including an incremental path through country-wide and regional measles elimination and phased paths through endgame scenarios and strategies. Infectious disease dynamic modeling can help inform measles elimination and eradication strategies, and all paths would be greatly facilitated by innovative technologies such as microarray patches to improve vaccine access and demand, point-of-contact diagnostic tests to facilitate outbreak responses, and point-of-contact IgG tests to identify susceptible populations. A pragmatic approach to measles eradication would identify and realize the necessary preconditions and clearly articulate various endgame scenarios and strategies to achieve measles eradication with an intensified and coordinated global effort in a specified timeframe, i.e., to "go big and go fast". To encourage and promote deliberation among a broad array of stakeholders, we provide a brief historical background and key considerations for setting a measles eradication goal.

**Keywords:** measles; eradication; elimination; vaccine

## 1. Introduction

Measles cases are increasing globally, both in countries with endemic measles virus transmission and in those that have eliminated measles. This increase follows historically low reported numbers of measles cases during the early years of the COVID-19 pandemic, as well as disruptions to routine immunization services and delayed measles and rubella vaccination campaigns due to the pandemic. According to the World Health Organization (WHO) and UNICEF, an estimated 23 million children missed routinely administered vaccines in 2020, 3.7 million more than in 2019 [1].

This backsliding is particularly concerning as Member States in all WHO regions adopted measles elimination goals to be reached by or before 2020. Measles elimination refers to the interruption of measles virus transmission in a defined geographic area (e.g., country or region) for 12 months or more, and measles eradication refers to the global interruption of measles virus transmission. To reach elimination, countries seek to achieve ≥95% coverage with two doses of measles-containing vaccine (MCV) [2]; however, as of 2022, only 34% (65 of 194 WHO countries) achieved ≥95% coverage with the first dose of MCV [3]. The Region of the Americas set a measles elimination goal by 2000, was verified to have eliminated measles in 2016, but lost this status in 2018 following the re-establishment of endemic measles in Brazil and Venezuela as measles virus transmission lasted for more than one year [3]. In the Americas, measles elimination was achieved through broad political commitment, coordinated wide-age-range catch-up campaigns, sustained efforts to increase routine vaccination coverage and conduct follow-up campaigns, and the maintenance of sensitive surveillance systems [4]. No other region has achieved measles elimination, although goals to eliminate measles were adopted by the Western Pacific Region by 2012, the European Region by 2015, the African Region by 2020 (revised to 80% of countries by 2030), and the South-East Asian Region by 2020 (revised to 2023). Eighty-three countries were verified to have achieved or maintained measles elimination by the end of 2022 [3]. But measles elimination is a fragile state that is difficult and expensive to sustain in the face of repeated importations, as evidenced by the Americas, where the failure to achieve uniform progress toward a measles eradication goal resulted in repeated measles virus importations through international travel [5,6]. Only measles eradication would obviate the need for continued surveillance, outbreak response, and sustained high measles vaccine coverage.

Measles eradication requires global commitment and coordination. To adopt a measles eradication goal entails an agreed upon resolution by Member States at the World Health Assembly. Deliberation among diverse stakeholders is needed on the setting of a measles eradication goal to garner the necessary political and public support and to foster strategic planning, the consideration of tactical approaches, and creative thinking about how to reach this goal. To encourage and promote deliberation among a broad array of stakeholders, we provide a brief historical background for setting a measles eradication goal, characterize the role of modeling to assess and shape eradication strategies, delineate new tools that could help achieve measles eradication, and discuss a potential framework of endgame scenarios and strategies that could be leveraged to both set an eradication goal and achieve eradication.

## 2. Disease Eradication

Disease eradication is the ultimate public health accomplishment, with a history of remarkable achievements and disappointing failures [7]. The history of disease eradication and its conceptual foundation extend back at least as far as Edward Jenner, who wrote in 1801 with regard to smallpox vaccination that "it now becomes too manifest to admit of controversy, that the annihilation of the Small Pox, the most dreadful scourge of the human species, must be the final result of this practice" [8]. Subsequently, major global efforts to successfully eradicate smallpox virus and rinderpest virus, as well as two of the three wild-type polioviruses as part of the Global Polio Eradication Initiative, and as yet unsuccessful attempts to eradicate malaria, guinea worm, and type 1 poliovirus, were undertaken.

A major advance in the conceptualization of infectious disease eradication was made through the publication in 1993 of the Recommendations of the International Task Force for Disease Eradication (ITFDE) [9]. Eradication was defined as the "reduction of the worldwide incidence of a disease to zero as a result of deliberate efforts, obviating the necessity for further control measures", and criteria for assessing whether a disease could be eradicated were described (Table 1). Eradication was distinguished from elimination, the latter defined as the "cessation of transmission of a disease in a single country, continent or other limited geographic area". Further advances were made at the Dahlem Workshop on The Eradication of Infectious Diseases held in 1997 in Berlin. A similar definition of eradication was adopted, the "permanent reduction to zero of the worldwide incidence of infection caused by a specific agent as a result of deliberate efforts", but a distinction between the elimination of a disease and an infection was added as well as the category of extinction in which a pathogen no longer exists in either nature or the laboratory. Thus, smallpox virus has been eradicated but is not extinct, although the notion of pathogen extinction is muddied by the ability to synthesize pathogens de novo in the laboratory [10,11]. Six preconditions for eradication were identified at the Dahlem Workshop: (1) no animal reservoir is known or suspected; (2) sensitive and specific diagnostic tools are available for surveillance; (3) transmission from one individual to another can be interrupted; (4) non-lethal infection or vaccination confers lifelong immune protection; (5) the disease is a global health priority; and (6) political commitment to eradication exists. These definitions, criteria, and preconditions provide a conceptual framework for thinking about measles eradication. Most experts agree that measles meets the criteria for eradication identified at the Dahlem conference, with the possible exception of broad political commitment.

**Table 1.** Criteria for assessing whether a disease can be eradicated—International Task Force for Disease Eradication, 1993.

| |
|---|
| Scientific feasibility |
| • Epidemiologic characteristics, including the potential existence of non-human reservoirs, ease of spread, induction of natural immunity, and ease of diagnosis;<br>• Availability of an intervention, such as a vaccine, that ideally should be effective, safe, inexpensive, long-lasting, and easily deployed;<br>• Demonstrated feasibility of elimination, such as documented elimination from a defined country or region. |
| Political will and popular support |
| • Perceived burden of disease;<br>• Expected cost of eradication;<br>• Synergy of eradication efforts with other interventions. |

## 3. Measles Eradication

Measles eradication was first discussed and debated in the late 1960's shortly after the licensure of measles vaccines [12,13]. The ITFDE in their 1993 report concluded that measles was "not now eradicable" and cited the lack of an effective vaccine for young infants and public misconceptions of the seriousness of measles as chief obstacles to eradication [9]. The ITFDE subsequently reviewed measles eradication in 2002, 2009, and 2015. In 2002, the ITFDE concluded that "measles eradication is technically feasible, and it is a desirable goal, ultimately". In 2009, the ITFDE reviewed the status of global measles control and regional elimination and focused on the biological feasibility of eradicating measles, particularly in light of the HIV pandemic and the reduced immunogenicity of measles vaccine in children living with HIV and not receiving antiretroviral therapy [14]. The ITDFE concluded that measles eradication is biologically possible using available tools but highlighted the challenges posed by delays in polio eradication and the need to strengthen routine immunization and laboratory-based surveillance. Also highlighted was the need for new tools such as more thermostable, needleless vaccine delivery platforms, vaccines with greater immunogenicity in young infants following a single dose, and field diagnostic tests to confirm measles virus infection and assess population immunity. Despite being written 15 years ago, the need for these tools remains. The ITFDE last reviewed measles eradication in 2015 and concluded that "a paradigm shift will be needed in order to eradicate measles and rubella" and this effort "will require a much more demanding enterprise than the current effort, which has suffered from insufficient resources and wavering political commitment" [15]. The same could be said today.

Measles eradication was also considered by an Ad Hoc Global Measles Advisory Group that was convened by the WHO in 2009, followed by a Global Technical Consultation to Assess the Feasibility of Measles Eradication held in July 2010 [16]. Informed by this consultation, the WHO's Strategic Advisory Group of Experts on immunization concluded that measles can and should be eradicated and that a goal for measles eradication should be established with a proposed target date based on measurable progress made toward existing goals and targets [17]. The Measles and Rubella Global Strategic Plan: 2012–2020 Midterm Review recommended that a "determination should be made, not later than 2020, whether a formal global goal for measles eradication should be set with timeframes for achievement. In the meantime, all regions should work toward achieving the regional elimination goals" [18].

The most recent comprehensive assessment of measles eradication was a report from the World Health Organization titled "Feasibility assessment of measles and rubella eradication" that was drafted prior to the COVID-19 pandemic and published in 2021 [19]. This report was written in part in response to the request of the Director-General at the Seventieth World Health Assembly held on 31 May 2017, during which a resolution on measles eradication was proposed by Colombia on behalf of 18 Pan American Health Organization (PAHO) Member States. This feasibility assessment positioned measles eradication in the broader context of the Sustainable Development Goals, the Global Health Security Agenda, the Global Vaccine Action Plan, Universal Health Coverage, and the Immunization Agenda 2030. The report highlighted the need to link measles and rubella elimination efforts, assessed progress and challenges to achieving measles and rubella elimination goals, and identified important considerations for measles and rubella eradication, including vaccine access and supply, vaccine hesitancy and demand, data needs, the impact of eradication on health systems, the polio transition and lessons from the Global Polio Eradication Initiative, the costs of delaying measles and rubella eradication, and equity and ethical considerations [19]. The report concluded:

> "A time-bound measles and rubella eradication goal should be set only when accelerated progress has been made, benchmarks that establish the conditions for a successful endgame to achieve eradication have been achieved, and there is evidence of a clear trajectory toward the goal. Setting an eradication goal when the endgame is in sight could catalyze a surge in commitment, effort, and resources to complete the task, thus heeding the call to go "big and fast" with measles and rubella eradication, and avoid a premature and drawn-out eradication effort with the potential for unmet goals, delayed milestones, and prolonged input of financial and human resources."

## 4. Infectious Disease Dynamics and Measles Elimination and Eradication

Infectious disease dynamic modeling provides another conceptual framework for thinking about measles elimination and eradication. Standard theory of infectious disease dynamics established the concept of "herd immunity", in which susceptible individuals can be indirectly protected by a reduction in the number of infectious individuals [20]. As a result, it is not necessary to effectively immunize everyone to eliminate or eradicate a pathogen. The critical level of population immunity ($p_c$) is that which is required to reduce the effective reproductive number ($R_{eff}$) to less than one and thus interrupt transmission. The effective reproductive number is estimated as $R_{eff} = R_0(1 - p)$, where $R_0$ is the basic reproductive number and $p$ is the proportion of the population that is immune. The critical level of population immunity can be estimated simply by setting $R_{eff}$ to 1 and solving for $p$, i.e., $p_c = 1 - (1/R_0)$ [20]. For measles virus, $R_0$ is often stated to be between 12 and 18, although this number varies widely in different epidemiological contexts [21]. These estimates result in the frequently cited need to achieve 92% to 95% population immunity to interrupt measles virus transmission and achieve elimination.

While this straightforward estimate of the critical immunity threshold serves as a valuable guide for population immunity goals and vaccination strategies, it is important to recognize several inherent oversimplifications. First, $R_0$ characterizes the number of susceptible individuals a typical infectious individual will infect and is based on an average across potential important differences within population subgroups. Second, this estimate assumes homogenous mixing in which every susceptible individual is equally likely to have contact with every other individual in the population. In fact, age, space, and temporal heterogeneities in populations, transmission, and contacts can significantly impact measles virus transmission dynamics. For example, in the Netherlands in 1999–2000, just five measles cases in a small elementary school triggered an outbreak of 2961 cases, even though reported nationwide vaccination coverage was 96% [22]. Two recent analytic approaches demonstrated the impact of heterogeneities in contacts by age and spatial distribution of susceptible individuals on the critical immunity threshold. Funk et al. combined age-specific mixing patterns and serological data to derive age-contact adjusted immunity levels and found that age-contact adjusted immunity levels better correlated with case numbers [23]. Truelove et al. estimated the critical immunity threshold accounting for the spatial clustering of susceptibility and found that as vaccination coverage and population immunity approach elimination thresholds, the clustering of susceptible individuals results in increases in the critical immunity threshold and the probability of an outbreak after a single introduction of an infectious individual [24]. Some clusters of susceptible individuals, however, may have a low probability of measles virus importation if not well connected through travel to areas of endemic transmission. A study of measles outbreak risk in three under-immunized communities in Virginia, based on population size, location, immunization rates, and network characteristics, showed that one under-immunized community was at lower risk because of low connectivity to other communities [25].

Beyond determining the critical immunity threshold, infectious disease dynamic modeling can be used to assess and shape elimination strategies [26,27]. The transmission (or elimination) of measles virus within a population depends primarily on four factors: the number and distribution of susceptible individuals, the rate at which susceptible individuals are replenished through unvaccinated birth cohorts, the movement patterns of both susceptible and infected individuals, and the rate of effective contact between susceptible and infectious individuals during which virus transmission can occur [21,27–30]. As a result, it is necessary to incorporate sources of epidemiologic variability that impact measles virus persistence, including measles-independent parameters (e.g., demographic characteristics of the population, contact rates, vaccination rates, and correlation of vaccine doses) and measles-dependent parameters (e.g., susceptibility and transmission rates), as well as uncertainty in these estimates [31]. Statistical and geospatial models can be used to estimate model parameters such as vaccination coverage, demographics, and serological profiles necessary to inform models [27]. Models incorporating parameters that impact persistence can: (1) estimate the future spatial, temporal, and age-specific probability of elimination given different vaccination strategies [32,33]; (2) examine how various processes contribute to persistence or elimination (e.g., correlation of measles doses [34], timing of supplemental immunization activities (SIAs), and target age groups [35]); (3) conduct empirical assessments to identify processes that impact persistence or elimination within a particular context (e.g., vaccinating children with personal belief exemptions in the US [36], spatial connectivity in Nigeria [37], changes in birth rates or magnitude of school contact rates in China [38,39]); and (4) assess the impact of plateaued or reversed progress towards measles elimination on programmatically relevant metrics (e.g., increase in the average age of susceptible individuals [40,41]).

Further considerations necessary when using infectious disease dynamic modeling to estimate the spatial, temporal, and age-specific probability of elimination includes how to define "elimination" given that modeled output includes a known *true* number of infections as compared to an observed number of cases. Recent work to estimate the probability of measles elimination in 93 countries defined "elimination" as reaching the conditions for measles elimination, i.e., five infections per million population [32]. This work highlighted the difficulty of achieving measles elimination in many countries even under best-case vaccination scenarios (e.g., by 2050 the probability of elimination would exceed 75% in only 14 to 36 of the 93 modeled countries) and suggested that spatial inequity in routine coverage is a likely driver of continued transmission. The work also made clear the need for future measles transmission models to incorporate feedback responses to outbreaks within the model itself, including outbreak-response vaccination campaigns or behavior change in contact rates. Empirical analyses demonstrated biases in observed case data early in outbreaks [42] and heterogeneity in the impact of outbreak-response vaccination to reach those already vaccinated [43,44], further complicating the inclusion of feedback responses into models.

## 5. New Tools for Measles Eradication

Stalled progress in achieving measles elimination has led to calls to invest in innovative technologies with the potential to facilitate measles elimination and eradication [45,46]. As noted above, the 2009 report of the ITFDE highlighted the need for novel measles vaccine delivery platforms to improve access and demand as well as field diagnostics tests for early outbreak detection and response. Point-of-contact, rapid diagnostics tests to detect measles IgM antibodies have been in development for more than a decade [47], with progress made in evaluating their validity, ease of implementation, and commercialization [48]. Promising results were reported from Brazil evaluating a lateral-flow measles IgM rapid diagnostic test, with a sensitivity and specificity of 95% [49]. However, results from Malaysia showed a much lower-than-desired test sensitivity of only 43% [50]. As measles surveillance and rapid outbreak response will be critical to achieving measles eradication, particularly in areas with limited access to laboratory testing, point-of-contact tests with high sensitivity and specificity for measles IgM and IgG antibodies will be essential tools.

Many experts believe that the intradermal delivery of measles and rubella vaccines through microarray patches will be game changing, improving both vaccine access and demand. Microarray patches were selected for prioritization by the World Health Organization's Vaccine Innovation Prioritisation Strategy (VIPS) group, and extensive efforts have gone into developing target product profiles, use case scenarios, and business case scenarios for measles and rubella microarray patches [51–54]. Microarray patches cause little or no pain, are easily administered and transported, are more thermostable with a less stringent cold-chain requirement, require minimal storage and disposal capacity, do not require reconstitution with diluent, cannot be reused, and do not generate sharps waste. These characteristics make microarray patches a potentially transformative technology to achieve measles and rubella elimination and eradication [55–57]. Human clinical trials using measles microneedle patches are underway, and preliminary results suggest these vaccines are safe and immunogenic [58,59].

## 6. Possible Paths to Measles Eradication

The WHO's Feasibility Assessment identified the need to define clearly articulated paths to measles eradication, with benchmarks, defined endgame scenarios, and strategies to achieve eradication in a defined timeframe. We describe two potential paths and endgame scenarios to achieve measles eradication.

### *6.1. Incremental Path to Measles Eradication through Country-Wide and Regional Elimination*

The standard conceptualization of the path to measles eradication is to achieve 95% coverage with two doses of measles-containing vaccine [60]. This high coverage should be achieved in every birth cohort, every community, and every district to ensure sufficiently high and homogeneous population immunity to interrupt measles virus transmission [2]. Measles eradication would thus be achieved incrementally such that every subnational administrative unit, every country, and every region would achieve elimination and thus collectively achieve measles eradication. High two-dose measles vaccine coverage is, in turn, to be achieved through a strong routine immunization program embedded within a strong primary health-care system with universal access combined with SIAs, periodic intensification of routine immunization (PIRIs; intermittent, enhanced efforts to immunize unvaccinated population with recording of the doses administered), and other focused immunization activities to fill immunity gaps. This strong immunization program needs to be complemented with a sensitive surveillance system with rapid outbreak response to identify and stop chains of measles virus transmission as soon as possible. This combination of strategies has been highly successful in many countries. Using this approach, measles incidence and deaths have significantly declined, and many countries have achieved measles elimination. By the end of 2022, 83 countries, comprising 43% of all countries, were verified by independent regional commissions to have achieved or maintained measles elimination [3]. The Region of the Americas used this combination of strategies, specifically routine vaccination plus catch-up, follow-up, and keep-up campaigns and effective surveillance [61], to interrupt measles virus transmission in November 2002 and was verified to have achieved measles elimination in 2016, making this the only WHO region to have eliminated measles. However, endemic measles virus transmission was reestablished in Venezuela in 2018 and in Brazil in 2019, leading to the loss of measles elimination status in the Americas [62].

In this approach, countries are expected to follow the canonical path to measles elimination. Epidemiological theory and empirical data from countries in Africa and the Americas were used to characterize this path in incidence space made up of two axes: measles incidence and the unpredictability in year-to-year measles cases (captured as a coefficient of variation in measles incidence) [63]. A country's position along this canonical path is associated with birth rates and measles vaccination coverage, which in turn determine the size of the population susceptible to measles (Figure 1). Countries with endemic measles start with high incidence and regular periodic measles epidemics. As vaccination coverage increases, birth rates decline, or both, the susceptible population diminishes, and measles incidence decreases, but measles outbreaks become more irregular and less predictable until incidence reaches very low levels and small outbreaks again become more regular. The canonical path can be used to measure country-specific progress toward measles elimination.

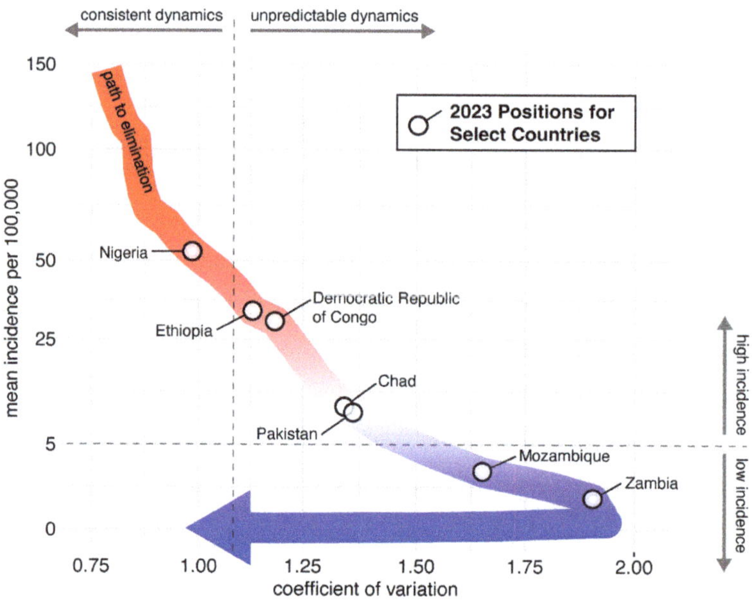


**Figure 1.** The canonical path to measles eradication. Adapted from Graham M, Winter AK, Ferrari M, Grenfell B, Moss WJ, Azman AS, Metcalf CJE, Lessler J. Measles and the canonical path to elimination. *Science* 2019, 364, 584–587 [63]. This two-dimensional plot is known as incidence space. The y-position for each country is determined by averaging the annual WHO reported incidence rates since 1980, weighted by a truncated Gaussian distribution that peaks two years prior. The x-position for each country is calculated as the year-to-year coefficient of variation over the previous 10 years, weighted by the same Gaussian distribution. A country's position in this two-dimensional incidence space is then assigned to the closest point on the canonical path (given a log incidence scale) to determine its country-specific position on the path to elimination. See https://uga-idd.github.io/MeaslesCanonicalPathToElimination_Visual/ (accessed on 3 July 2024) for a visualization of all countries' positions in incidence space in 1990–2023.

Although extremely important as an aspirational strategy and set of tactics, an incremental approach to measles eradication is unlikely to achieve success given the daunting epidemiological, social, political, and economic challenges. In fact, measles virus transmission could be eliminated in all WHO regions without achieving global eradication if transmission persisted for fewer than 12 months in one or more regions but measles virus jumped from one region to another. Importantly, the current geopolitical and financial landscapes are very different from those when smallpox and polio eradication goals were established. Despite extensive efforts to increase global measles vaccine coverage, progress has stalled with backsliding during the COVID-19 pandemic. Global coverage with the first dose of MCV has remained around 85% for the past two decades, reaching 86% in 2019 but declining to 81% in 2021 and 83% in 2022 [3]. Global coverage with the second dose of MCV has steadily increased over the past two decades, largely because more countries introduced the second dose, but reached only 74% in 2022 [3]. Since 2016, endemic measles virus transmission was reestablished in nine countries that had previously been verified to have eliminated measles [3].

At the regional level, progress has been made toward measles elimination in the South-East Asia Region, with five of eleven the countries having verified measles elimination [64]. Importantly, India increased measles and rubella vaccine coverage by strengthening routine immunization services and implementing national and regional strategies, including Mission Indradhanush and phased supplementary immunization activities [65]. Nevertheless, the goal of achieving regional measles elimination in the South-East Asia Region by 2023 was not met, partially thwarted by the negative impact of the COVID-19 pandemic on routine vaccination coverage (i.e., coverage with the first and second doses of measles-containing vaccine decreased from 2019 to 2021 by 8% and 11%, respectively) and the quality of surveillance [66]. An important success story is the progress made by China in the Western Pacific Region in eliminating measles using the WHO strategy of strengthening routine immunization services, periodic supplementary immunization campaigns, and high-quality surveillance [67,68]. However, several other regions are much further from achieving measles elimination. In the Eastern Mediterranean region, all countries pledged in 2015 to achieve measles elimination by 2020, but only four countries achieved this goal [69]. Half of the countries in the region are experiencing conflict or humanitarian crises, significantly hampering measles elimination efforts. During the COVID-19 pandemic from 2019 to 2022, measles incidence increased, and regional coverage with the first dose of MCV was only about 83%, and only 78% for the second dose, far below what is needed to achieve elimination [69]. The African region is even further from achieving measles elimination. After failing to achieve measles elimination by 2020, the Regional Strategic Plan for Immunization 2021–2030 revised the regional goal to elimination in at least 80% of countries by 2030 [70]. Regional coverage with the first dose of MCV was only 68% to 70% between 2017 and 2021, largely driven by low coverage in the populous countries of Nigeria, Ethiopia, and the Democratic Republic of the Congo [70].

Thus, despite some progress toward regional measles elimination, particularly in the Western Pacific Region, the European Region, and the South-East Asia Region, only the Region of the Americas achieved measles elimination but this was not sustained. The Eastern Mediterranean and African Regions face formidable challenges due to conflict, humanitarian crises, and weak immunization systems. These challenges can and should be addressed. Current efforts focus intensely on improving and modifying immunization strategies to identify and reach unvaccinated (zero-dose) children and missed communities, increase coverage with two doses of MCV, and improve measles and rubella surveillance. The Measles and Rubella Strategic Framework 2021–2030, under the umbrella of the Immunization Agenda 2030, envisions a world free from measles and rubella and has as its goal to achieve and sustain regional measles and rubella elimination goals [71]. However, this Strategic Framework recognizes contextual changes, implementation challenges, and the need for strategic pivots. The pivots most germane to a global effort to eradicate measles include: (1) declining interest in vertical disease control programs; (2) the need to shift from a one-size-fits-all approach to approaches tailored to local challenges; (3) embedding measles and rubella immunization activities within primary health care; and (4) accelerating the development and implementation of innovative technologies (such as microarray patches for vaccine delivery and rapid diagnostic tests) and improvements in surveillance [71].

### 6.2. Phased Path to Measles Eradication through Different Endgame Scenarios and Strategies

As stated above, the WHO's Feasibility Assessment concluded that a measles eradication goal should be set when "benchmarks that establish the conditions for a successful endgame to achieve eradication have been achieved, and there is evidence of a clear trajectory toward the goal." The purpose of the benchmarks is to gauge when it is appropriate to set a time-bound measles and rubella eradication target by providing metrics toward achieving the necessary conditions for a successful eradication endgame within a defined period. In contrast to the steady, incremental conceptualization of measles eradication, this path envisions a state of the world at which point an intensive, time-bound, globally coordinated effort to achieve measles eradication is likely to be successful. However, benchmarks should not be barriers to setting a measles eradication goal should the political, epidemiological, or technological landscape change. Rather than being fixed, benchmarks for measles eradication should be adapted and modified to changing circumstances. An example might be the widespread availability of measles and rubella microarray patches that could in turn foster widespread political commitment to measles eradication.

In addition to measuring country-specific progress toward measles elimination, the positions of countries along the measles canonical path to elimination could be used to establish a benchmark for eradication (e.g., some proportion of countries or regions at specified thresholds of mean incidence and variation). For example, given that a country's position on the path is linked to the age distribution of susceptible individuals, with a broader age range of susceptible individuals as incidence decreases, placement along the path could be used to target vaccination efforts. As the authors conclude, "Both path progress and position in incidence space could serve as important features for classifying or taxonomizing countries on the basis of their measles situation and progress toward elimination" [63].

Two technical consultations were convened by teleconference by the WHO on establishing benchmarks for setting a future measles and rubella eradication goal. Participants represented the WHO, Centers for Disease Control and Prevention, Institute for Disease Modeling, and several academic institutions. The first, held on 27 March 2020, asked the question of what the world will need to look like to be ready to attempt measles eradication and began discussions of conceptualizing a benchmarking framework. The second, held on 30 April 2020, began discussions of potential domains for indicators and triggers for an eradication endgame. Although the minutes and subsequent report were not published or disseminated, a few key points are summarized here.

During these consultations, the path to measles eradication was conceptualized as divided into three phases (Figure 2). The first phase consists of employing efforts to incrementally improve measles vaccination coverage, vaccination data quality, surveillance systems, and outbreak responses while recognizing that these alone will not achieve eradication. The second phase involves setting the time-bound eradication goal to "go big and go fast" when the global measles and rubella epidemiological situation has reached an endgame scenario for which endgame strategies can realistically achieve eradication within a defined time frame (e.g., five years), sufficient political and public support have been garnered, financial commitments have been made, and adequate vaccine supply to sustain the endgame strategy through to completion is ensured. The third phase comprises the endgame strategy itself, consisting of a globally coordinated, intensive effort designed to interrupt all chains of measles virus transmission within the specified time frame of setting the goal. Different endgame scenarios, each with a unique endgame strategy, may be developed, but one would be actualized.

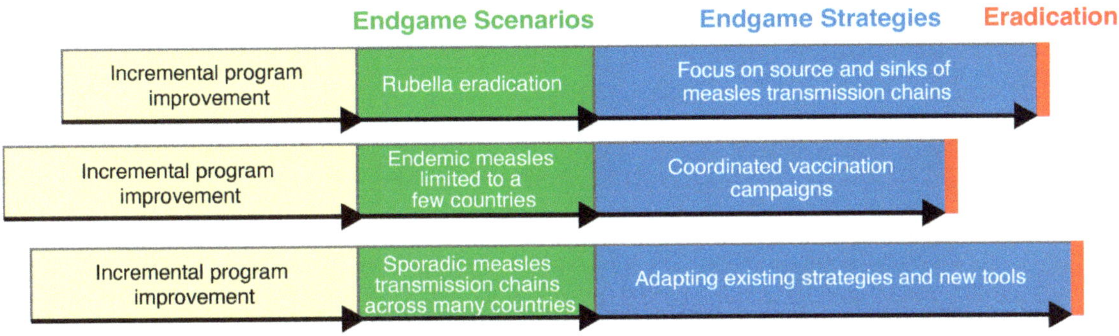


**Figure 2.** Examples of phased paths to measles eradication through different endgame scenarios and endgame strategies.

Further stakeholder discussions at the regional and global levels are needed to advance and achieve this vision of phased paths to measles eradication and to identify key benchmarks, endgame scenarios, and endgame strategies. Here, we briefly propose several endgame scenarios and strategies that could be considered; however, creative thinking by diverse stakeholders will be needed to fully articulate the array of endgame scenarios and strategies.

Endgame scenario #1: Rubella eradication: A first type of endgame scenario for a "go big and go fast" measles eradication effort would be when rubella eradication has been achieved. Countries that have introduced rubella vaccination use a combined measles–rubella-containing vaccine in their childhood immunization programs. Rubella virus is less contagious than measles virus, with an $R_0$ of 6 to 7 and a herd immunity threshold of 80–85% [72]. Thus, lower vaccine coverage is needed to interrupt rubella virus transmission. Furthermore, rubella vaccines are more immunogenic than measles vaccines, resulting in >95% protection after a single dose [72]. Because measles and rubella vaccines can and should be administered in combination through all routine immunization and supplementary immunization activities, rubella eradication could constitute an endgame scenario for measles eradication. Such a scenario would ensure that measles and rubella vaccination programs are effective enough to achieve rubella eradication and that fever–rash surveillance systems are sufficiently sensitive to verify eradication. Additionally, efforts to introduce rubella-containing vaccines and eliminate rubella through wide age range campaigns can also facilitate measles eradication. In the Region of the Americas, vaccination campaigns targeting a wide age range (including children up to 15 years old) were critical in achieving measles elimination. Currently, Gavi, the Vaccine Alliance, funds wide-age-range campaigns to support the integration of rubella vaccines into routine childhood vaccination programs in eligible countries.

Progress has been made in eliminating rubella at the country and regional levels. All regions but one (the Eastern Mediterranean Region) have rubella and congenital rubella elimination goals, and the Region of the Americas was verified as having eliminated rubella in 2015 [73]. Rubella-containing vaccines have been introduced in 90% of the 194 countries by 2022, and rubella elimination was verified in half of all countries, although no country in the African Region has eliminated rubella [73]. Achieving rubella eradication will require that the remaining 19 countries introduce rubella-containing vaccines (16 of which are eligible for Gavi support) and that coverage with measles and rubella vaccines increase [74,75]. The verification of rubella eradication could thus be an endgame scenario when a measles eradication goal is set, although measles could be endemic in many countries and regions despite rubella eradication.

Endgame scenario #2: Endemic measles limited to several countries or WHO regions: A different type of endgame scenario for a "go big and go fast" measles eradication effort would be when endemic measles virus transmission is restricted to several countries in one or two WHO regions, with measles having been eliminated in other countries and regions. The remaining endemic countries will likely be the result of conflict or humanitarian crises preventing effective vaccination programs and/or inaccessible or migrant populations maintaining measles virus transmission, but vaccine refusal could also play a role in some communities. Countries and regions that eliminated measles would need to strengthen surveillance, given the continued risk of viral importations, and implement rapid outbreak responses. Although experience in the Region of the Americas has shown how expensive and challenging it can be to maintain measles elimination, low connectivity of the remaining measles endemic countries could lower the risk of exportations.

Endgame scenario #3: Sporadic measles virus transmission chains across many or all WHO regions: In this endgame scenario, endemic measles virus transmission would be interrupted in all countries, but persistent transmission chains among clusters of susceptible individuals, lasting less than one year, would hinder eradication. These pockets of susceptible individuals would need to be well connected and have sizable populations to sustain limited transmission and export the virus to other susceptible communities [26].

*6.3. Endgame Strategies*

The endgame strategies would consist of intensive, time-bound, globally coordinated efforts to eradicate measles that are matched to specific endgame scenarios and possibly differ from the strategies used to make incremental progress and program improvements. We present some potential endgame strategies but this exercise also will require creative input from diverse stakeholders to fully articulate the array of endgame strategies.

Endgame strategy #1: Adapting existing strategies and new tools: One set of endgame strategies could rethink how we use current vaccination tools to make them more efficient and effective in different endgame scenarios, i.e., routine immunization, SIAs, PIRIs, preventative vaccination campaigns, and outbreak-response vaccination campaigns. For example, ring vaccination outbreak response around hard-to-reach and isolated populations would be appropriate in endgame scenario 3. Endgame strategies would be greatly facilitated by innovative technologies such as house-to-house vaccination using microarray patches [56], point-of-contact diagnostic tests to facilitate outbreak responses [48], or point-of-contact IgG tests to identify susceptible populations. The benefits of these technologies would be to increase access to populations that would otherwise not be reached by routine or supplementary immunization programs or would not be identified through facility-based fever-rash surveillance. These technologies would be particularly useful in endgame scenarios 2 and 3 described above, in which transmission chains prove difficult to interrupt.

Endgame strategy #2: Coordinated vaccination campaigns: A second potential endgame strategy would leverage coordinated vaccination campaigns to synchronize periods of absent or low transmission across countries or regions, reducing rates of reintroduction and allowing a longer time prior to the importation of measles virus. This approach could be deployed in endgame scenarios 1 and 2 to either establish the conditions for eradication or shift populations from endemic to non-endemic transmission. Measles virus transmission dynamics can be conceptualized using a meta-population framework in which the spatial and temporal distribution of susceptible individuals (the patches) either achieves elimination or incurs outbreaks following the reintroduction of measles virus, driven by the size of the susceptible population and contact patterns between patches [76]. While this framework is most helpful in understanding the timing of outbreaks in settings with endemic measles virus transmission, the relative impact of vaccination strategies can also be explored [77]. Unsynchronized vaccination results in a loss of correlation in the timing of measles outbreaks between patches, promoting the persistence of infection because virus transmission is always found in at least one patch. However, synchronized or pulse vaccination can synchronize measles outbreaks [78,79], which in turn can promote measles elimination by synchronizing measles elimination across patches over time and space. An endgame strategy can be envisioned with a similar goal. Coordinated vaccination campaigns can act as pulsed vaccinations to synchronize periods of absent to low transmission, i.e., honeymoon periods. If all populations interrupt measles virus transmission at the same time, elimination is achieved. In a more likely scenario, measles virus transmission chains may persist in a few populations, but most will have achieved elimination with effective, coordinated campaigns. During these synchronized troughs of absent or low transmission, there is lower risk of measles virus importation from infectious individuals. Even though susceptible individuals continue to accumulate (and $R_{eff}$ can be > 1) in eliminated populations, the risk of measles outbreaks is low because of the reduced probability of measles virus importation. This also allows more time for elimination programs to identify and interrupt remaining transmission chains.

Endgame strategy #3: Sources and sinks: A third endgame strategy could be to first focus on sources and sinks of measles virus transmission based on measles risk assessments and connectivity networks. Clusters of susceptible individuals known to be linked to other communities or countries through transportation networks would be prioritized over clusters of susceptible individuals less likely to export measles virus because of limited connectivity (e.g., isolated rural communities). From the perspective of measles eradication, it may be permissible (but not ideal) to allow susceptible individuals to accumulate in communities with low connectivity if the risk of measles virus importation or exportation is low. An example of such a situation is found in the United States, where measles elimination has been maintained since 2000 despite occasional small outbreaks. Clusters of susceptible individuals remain free of measles because the probability of an infectious individual entering that community is low. To demonstrate how a source–sink framework might be applied, a predictive risk model was constructed in 2019 of the expected relative size of a measles outbreak in each county in the United States based on international air travel volume into the county (the sinks), non-medical exemption rates in the county as a measure of unvaccinated persons, the county population, and the incidence of measles at the country of origin for international travel (the sources) [80]. Model predictions were consistent with the actual number and location of measles outbreaks in the United States through 15 April 2019. Also identified were the countries of origin that contributed most to measles risk in the United States. Similar results were obtained when the model was applied to measles outbreaks in the United States from 2011 to 2018 [80]. This analysis was later expanded to include a spatial diffusion model to distribute arriving travelers to counties near international airports (including counties without an airport) and a comprehensive county-level measles vaccination rate for 40 states to replace non-medical exemptions [81]. The counties at highest risk of measles outbreaks (sinks) and the countries most likely to export measles (sources) were identified, with the limitation that the analysis did not fully account for the risk of domestic spread within the United States [81]. This work provides an approach to conceptualizing an endgame strategy for measles eradication using a source–sink framework at the global rather than regional level. Prioritizing vaccination efforts at sources and sinks could interrupt measles virus transmission without the need to achieve 95% coverage with two doses of measles vaccine in every district, country, and region.

## 7. Conclusions

Eradication goals can be aspirational, pragmatic, or a combination of these elements. An aspirational eradication goal seeks to garner political, social, and economic support for an eventual eradication effort in the future without necessarily having achieved the preconditions, or perhaps even having the tools and strategies in place, to achieve eradication. An example might be the setting of a malaria eradication goal by 2050 [82]. A more pragmatic approach seeks to achieve the necessary preconditions and define the endgame scenarios and strategies to "go big and go fast" to achieve eradication within a defined timeframe. There are strong epidemiologic, economic, and ethical arguments to set a measles eradication goal [83,84], and many share the vision for a world free of measles and rubella. There are also costs for delaying measles eradication [85]. In addition to the tragedy of preventable illness, hospitalization, and death due to measles, as well as the financial costs of surveillance and outbreak response, measles eradication could become increasingly difficult to achieve as immunity gaps increase among older age groups [40,86]. It is time to regain the momentum that began prior to the COVID-19 pandemic [19,87] to engage with multiple stakeholders, including civil society organizations, politicians, policy makers, donors, vaccine manufacturers, and public health professionals, to articulate and agree upon the paths to measles eradication and the endgame scenarios and strategies.

**Author Contributions:** Conceptualization, A.K.W. and W.J.M.; Methodology, A.K.W. and W.J.M.; Writing—original draft, A.K.W. and W.J.M.; Writing—review & editing, A.K.W. and W.J.M. All authors have read and agreed to the published version of the manuscript.

**Funding:** This research received no external funding.

**Conflicts of Interest:** The authors declare no conflict of interest.

## References

1. UNICEF. COVID-19 Pandemic Leads to Major Backsliding on Childhood Vaccinations, New WHO, UNICEF Data Shows. 2021. Available online: https://www.unicef.org/press-releases/covid-19-pandemic-leads-major-backsliding-childhood-vaccinations-new-who-unicef-data (accessed on 29 April 2024).
2. World Health Organization. Measles vaccines: WHO position paper—April 2017. *Wkly. Epidemiol. Rec.* **2017**, *92*, 205–227.
3. Minta, A.A.; Ferrari, M.; Antoni, S.; Portnoy, A.; Sbarra, A.; Lambert, B.; Hatcher, C.; Hsu, C.H.; Ho, L.L.; Steulet, C.; et al. Progress toward measles elimination—Worldwide, 2000–2022. *MMWR* **2023**, *72*, 1262–1268. [CrossRef]
4. De Quadros, C.A.; Andrus, J.K.; Danovaro-Holliday, M.C.; Castillo-Solórzano, C. Feasibility of global measles eradication after interruption of transmission in the Americas. *Expert. Rev. Vaccines* **2008**, *7*, 355–362. [CrossRef] [PubMed]
5. Pike, J.; Leidner, A.J.; Gastañaduy, P.A. A review of measles outbreak cost estimates from the United States in the postelimination era (2004–2017): Estimates by perspective and cost type. *Clin. Infect. Dis.* **2020**, *71*, 1568–1576. [CrossRef] [PubMed]
6. Pike, J.; Melnick, A.; Gastañaduy, P.A.; Kay, M.; Harbison, J.; Leidner, A.J.; Rice, S.; Asato, K.; Schwartz, L.; DeBolt, C. Societal costs of a measles outbreak. *Pediatrics* **2021**, *147*, e2020027037. [CrossRef] [PubMed]
7. Stepan, N.L. *Eradication. Riding the World of Diseases Forever*; Cornell University Press: Ithica, NY, USA, 2011.
8. Jenner, E. *The Origin of Vaccine Inoculation*; D.N. Shury: London, UK, 1801.
9. Recommendations of the International Task Force for Disease Eradication. *MMWR* **1993**, *42*, 1–38.
10. Cello, J.; Paul, A.V.; Wimmer, E. Chemical synthesis of poliovirus cDNA: Generation of infectious virus in the absence of natural template. *Science* **2002**, *297*, 1016–1018. [CrossRef] [PubMed]
11. Noyce, R.S.; Lederman, S.; Evans, D.H. Construction of an infectious horsepox virus vaccine from chemically synthesized DNA fragments. *PLoS ONE* **2018**, *13*, e0188453. [CrossRef] [PubMed]
12. Sencer, D.J.; Dull, H.B.; Langmuir, A.D. Epidemiologic basis for eradication of measles in 1967. *Public Health Rep.* **1967**, *82*, 253–256. [CrossRef]
13. Albrecht, R.M. Can measles be eradicated? *Science* **1967**, *156*, 1029. [CrossRef]
14. Moss, W.J.; Scott, S.; Mugala, N.; Ndhlovu, Z.; Beeler, J.A.; Audet, S.A.; Ngala, M.; Mwangala, S.; Nkonga-Mwangilwa, C.; Ryon, J.J.; et al. Immunogenicity of standard-titer measles vaccine in HIV-1-infected and uninfected Zambian children: An observational study. *J. Infect. Dis.* **2007**, *196*, 347–355. [CrossRef] [PubMed]
15. Meeting of the International Task Force for Disease Eradication, November 2015. *Wkly. Epidemiol. Rec.* **2016**, *91*, 61–71.
16. World Health Organization. Proceedings of the Global Technical Consultation to assess the feasibility of measles eradication, 28–30 July 2010. *J. Infect. Dis.* **2011**, *204* (Suppl. S1), S4–S13. [CrossRef] [PubMed]
17. World Health Organization. Meeting of the Strategic Advisory Group of Experts on Immunization, November 2010. Summary, conclusions and recommendations. *Wkly. Ep Rec* **2011**, *86*, 1–16.
18. Orenstein, W.A.; Cairns, L.; Hinman, A.; Nkowane, B.; Olivé, J.M.; Reingold, A.L. *Measles and Rubella Global Strategic Plan* 2012–2020 Mid-Term Review. *Vaccine* **2018**, *36*, A35–A42. [CrossRef] [PubMed]
19. Moss, W.J.; Shendale, S.; Lindstrand, A.; O'Brien, K.L.; Turner, N.; Goodman, T.; Kretsinger, K.; Measles, S.W.G.O.; Rubella, V.; Measles; et al. Feasibility assessment of measles and rubella eradication. *Vaccine* **2021**, *39*, 3544–3559. [CrossRef] [PubMed]
20. Fine, P.; Eames, K.; Heymann, D.L. "Herd immunity": A rough guide. *Clin. Infect. Dis.* **2011**, *52*, 911–916. [CrossRef] [PubMed]
21. Guerra, F.M.; Bolotin, S.; Lim, G.; Heffernan, J.; Deeks, S.L.; Li, Y.; Crowcroft, N.S. The basic reproduction number ($R_0$) of measles: A systematic review. *Lancet. Infect. Dis.* **2017**, *17*, e420–e428. [CrossRef] [PubMed]
22. Centers for Disease Control and Prevention (CDC). Measles outbreak—Netherlands, April 1999–January 2000. *MMWR* **2000**, *49*, 299–303.
23. Funk, S.; Knapp, J.K.; Lebo, E.; Reef, S.E.; Dabbagh, A.J.; Kretsinger, K.; Jit, M.; Edmunds, W.J.; Strebel, P.M. Combining serological and contact data to derive target immunity levels for achieving and maintaining measles elimination. *BMC Med.* **2019**, *17*, 180. [CrossRef]

24. Truelove, S.A.; Graham, M.; Moss, W.J.; Metcalf, C.J.E.; Ferrari, M.J.; Lessler, J. Characterizing the impact of spatial clustering of susceptibility for measles elimination. *Vaccine* **2019**, *37*, 732–741. [CrossRef] [PubMed]
25. Afroj Moon, S.; Marathe, A.; Vullikanti, A. Are all underimmunized measles clusters equally critical? *R. Soc. Open Sci.* **2023**, *10*, 230873. [CrossRef] [PubMed]
26. Gay, N.J. The theory of measles elimination: Implications for the design of elimination strategies. *J. Infect. Dis.* **2004**, *189* (Suppl. S1), S27–S35.
27. Cutts, F.T.; Dansereau, E.; Ferrari, M.J.; Hanson, M.; McCarthy, K.A.; Metcalf, C.J.E.; Takahashi, S.; Tatem, A.J.; Thakkar, N.; Truelove, S.; et al. Using models to shape measles control and elimination strategies in low- and middle-income countries: A review of recent applications. *Vaccine* **2020**, *38*, 979–992. [CrossRef] [PubMed]
28. Ferrari, M.J.; Grenfell, B.T.; Strebel, P.M. Think globally, act locally: The role of local demographics and vaccination coverage in the dynamic response of measles infection to control. *Philos. Trans. R. Soc. London. Ser. B Biol. Sci.* **2013**, *368*, 20120141. [CrossRef] [PubMed]
29. Trentini, F.; Poletti, P.; Merler, S.; Melegaro, A. Measles immunity gaps and the progress towards elimination: A multi-country modelling analysis. *Lancet. Infect. Dis.* **2017**, *17*, 1089–1097. [CrossRef] [PubMed]
30. Yang, W.; Li, J.; Shaman, J. Characteristics of measles epidemics in China (1951–2004) and implications for elimination: A case study of three key locations. *PLoS Comput. Biol.* **2019**, *15*, e1006806. [CrossRef] [PubMed]
31. Bansal, S.; Grenfell, B.T.; Meyers, L.A. When individual behaviour matters: Homogeneous and network models in epidemiology. *J. R. Soc. Interface* **2007**, *4*, 879–891. [CrossRef] [PubMed]
32. Winter, A.K.; Lambert, B.; Klein, D.; Klepac, P.; Papadopoulos, T.; Truelove, S.; Burgess, C.; Santos, H.; Knapp, J.K.; Reef, S.E.; et al. Feasibility of measles and rubella vaccination programmes for disease elimination: A modelling study. *Lancet. Glob. Health* **2022**, *10*, e1412–e1422. [CrossRef]
33. Hao, L.; Glasser, J.W.; Su, Q.; Ma, C.; Feng, Z.; Yin, Z.; Goodson, J.L.; Wen, N.; Fan, C.; Yang, H.; et al. Evaluating vaccination policies to accelerate measles elimination in China: A meta-population modelling study. *Int. J. Epidemiol.* **2019**, *48*, 1240–1251. [CrossRef]
34. McKee, A.; Ferrari, M.J.; Shea, K. Correlation between measles vaccine doses: Implications for the maintenance of elimination. *Epidemiol. Infect.* **2018**, *146*, 468–475. [CrossRef]
35. Prada, J.M.; Metcalf, C.J.E.; Takahashi, S.; Lessler, J.; Tatem, A.J.; Ferrari, M. Demographics, epidemiology and the impact of vaccination campaigns in a measles-free world—Can elimination be maintained? *Vaccine* **2017**, *35*, 1488–1493. [CrossRef] [PubMed]
36. Glasser, J.W.; Feng, Z.; Omer, S.B.; Smith, P.J.; Rodewald, L.E. The effect of heterogeneity in uptake of the measles, mumps, and rubella vaccine on the potential for outbreaks of measles: A modelling study. *Lancet. Infect. Dis.* **2016**, *16*, 599–605. [CrossRef]
37. Bharti, N.; Djibo, A.; Ferrari, M.J.; Grais, R.F.; Tatem, A.J.; McCabe, C.A.; Bjornstad, O.N.; Grenfell, B.T. Measles hotspots and epidemiological connectivity. *Epidemiol. Infect.* **2010**, *138*, 1308–1316. [CrossRef]
38. Li, S.; Ma, C.; Hao, L.; Su, Q.; An, Z.; Ma, F.; Xie, S.; Xu, A.; Zhang, Y.; Ding, Z.; et al. Demographic transition and the dynamics of measles in six provinces in China: A modeling study. *PLoS Med.* **2017**, *14*, e1002255. [CrossRef] [PubMed]
39. Wang, H.; Zhu, Z.; Duan, X.; Song, J.; Mao, N.; Cui, A.; Wang, C.; Du, H.; Wang, Y.; Li, F.; et al. Transmission pattern of measles virus circulating in China during 1993–2021: Genotyping evidence supports that China is approaching measles elimination. *Clin. Infect. Dis.* **2023**, *76*, e1140–e1149. [CrossRef] [PubMed]
40. Patel, M.K.; Antoni, S.; Nedelec, Y.; Sodha, S.; Menning, L.; Ogbuanu, I.U.; Gacic Dobo, M. The changing global epidemiology of measles, 2013–2018. *J. Infect. Dis.* **2020**, *222*, 1117–1128. [CrossRef]
41. Anderson, R.M.; May, R.M. Age-related changes in the rate of disease transmission: Implications for the design of vaccination programmes. *J. Hyg. (Lond)* **1985**, *94*, 365–436. [CrossRef]
42. Graham, M.; Suk, J.E.; Takahashi, S.; Metcalf, C.J.; Jimenez, A.P.; Prikazsky, V.; Ferrari, M.J.; Lessler, J. Challenges and opportunities in disease forecasting in outbreak settings: A case study of measles in Lola Prefecture, Guinea. *Am. J. Trop. Med. Hyg.* **2018**, *98*, 1489–1497. [CrossRef]
43. Minetti, A.; Hurtado, N.; Grais, R.F.; Ferrari, M. Reaching hard-to-reach individuals: Nonselective versus targeted outbreak response vaccination for measles. *Am. J. Epidemiol.* **2014**, *179*, 245–251. [CrossRef]
44. Grout, L.; Conan, N.; Juan Giner, A.; Hurtado, N.; Fermon, F.; N'Goran, A.; Grellety, E.; Minetti, A.; Porten, K.; Grais, R.F. Local discrepancies in measles vaccination opportunities: Results of population-based surveys in Sub-Saharan Africa. *BMC Public. Health* **2014**, *14*, 193. [CrossRef] [PubMed]
45. Grant, G.B.; Masresha, B.G.; Moss, W.J.; Mulders, M.N.; Rota, P.A.; Omer, S.B.; Shefer, A.; Kriss, J.L.; Hanson, M.; Durrheim, D.N.; et al. Accelerating measles and rubella elimination through research and innovation—Findings from the Measles & Rubella Initiative research prioritization process, 2016. *Vaccine* **2019**, *37*, 5754–5761. [PubMed]
46. Goodson, J.L.; Rota, P.A. Innovations in vaccine delivery: Increasing access, coverage, and equity and lessons learnt from measles and rubella elimination. *Drug Deliv. Transl. Res.* **2022**, *12*, 959–967. [CrossRef] [PubMed]
47. Warrener, L.; Slibinskas, R.; Chua, K.B.; Nigatu, W.; Brown, K.E.; Sasnauskas, K.; Samuel, D.; Brown, D. A point-of-care test for measles diagnosis: Detection of measles-specific IgM antibodies and viral nucleic acid. *Bull. World Health Organ.* **2011**, *89*, 675–682. [CrossRef] [PubMed]

48. Brown, D.W.; Warrener, L.; Scobie, H.M.; Donadel, M.; Waku-Kouomou, D.; Mulders, M.N.; Rota, P.A. Rapid diagnostic tests to address challenges for global measles surveillance. *Curr. Opin. Virol.* **2020**, *41*, 77–84. [CrossRef] [PubMed]
49. Warrener, L.; Andrews, N.; Koroma, H.; Alessandrini, I.; Haque, M.; Garcia, C.C.; Matos, A.R.; Caetano, B.; Lemos, X.R.; Siqueira, M.M.; et al. Evaluation of a rapid diagnostic test for measles IgM detection; accuracy and the reliability of visual reading using sera from the measles surveillance programme in Brazil, 2015. *Epidemiol. Infect.* **2023**, *151*, e151. [CrossRef] [PubMed]
50. Senin, A.; Noordin, N.M.; Sani, J.A.M.; Mahat, D.; Donadel, M.; Scobie, H.M.; Omar, A.; Chem, Y.K.; Zahari, M.I.; Ismail, F.; et al. A measles IgM rapid diagnostic test to address challenges with national measles surveillance and response in Malaysia. *PLoS ONE* **2024**, *19*, e0298730. [CrossRef] [PubMed]
51. Hasso-Agopsowicz, M.; Crowcroft, N.; Biellik, R.; Gregory, C.J.; Menozzi-Arnaud, M.; Amorij, J.P.; Gilbert, P.A.; Earle, K.; Frivold, C.; Jarrahian, C.; et al. Accelerating the development of measles and rubella microarray patches to eliminate measles and rubella: Recent progress, remaining challenges. *Front. Public Health* **2022**, *10*, 809675. [CrossRef] [PubMed]
52. Ko, M.; Malvolti, S.; Cherian, T.; Mantel, C.; Biellik, R.; Jarrahian, C.; Menozzi-Arnaud, M.; Amorij, J.P.; Christiansen, H.; Papania, M.J.; et al. Estimating the future global dose demand for measles-rubella microarray patches. *Front. Public Health* **2022**, *10*, 1037157. [CrossRef]
53. Malvolti, S.; Ko, M.; Menozzi-Arnaud, M.; Mantel, C.; Jarrahian, C.; Amorij, J.P.; Giersing, B.; Hasso-Agopsowicz, M. Exploring potential applications of measles and rubella microarray patches (MR-MAPs): Use case identification. *Front. Public Health* **2023**, *11*, 1165110. [CrossRef]
54. Fu, H.; Abbas, K.; Malvolti, S.; Gregory, C.; Ko, M.; Amorij, J.P.; Jit, M. Impact and cost-effectiveness of measles vaccination through microarray patches in 70 low-income and middle-income countries: Mathematical modelling and early-stage economic evaluation. *BMJ Glob. Health* **2023**, *8*, e012204. [CrossRef] [PubMed]
55. Peyraud, N.; Zehrung, D.; Jarrahian, C.; Frivold, C.; Orubu, T.; Giersing, B. Potential use of microarray patches for vaccine delivery in low- and middle- income countries. *Vaccine* **2019**, *37*, 4427–4434. [CrossRef] [PubMed]
56. Richardson, L.C.; Moss, W.J. Measles and rubella microarray array patches to increase vaccination coverage and achieve measles and rubella elimination in Africa. *Pan Afr. Med. J.* **2020**, *35*, 3. [CrossRef]
57. Prausnitz, M.R.; Goodson, J.L.; Rota, P.A.; Orenstein, W.A. A microneedle patch for measles and rubella vaccination: A game changer for achieving elimination. *Curr. Opin. Virol.* **2020**, *41*, 68–76. [CrossRef] [PubMed]
58. Baker, B.; Bermingham, I.M.; Leelasena, I.; Hickling, J.; Young, P.R.; Muller, D.A.; Forster, A.H. Safety, tolerability, and immunogenicity of measles and rubella vaccine delivered with a high-density microarray patch: Results from a randomized, partially double-blinded, placebo-controlled phase I clinical trial. *Vaccines* **2023**, *11*, 1725. [CrossRef] [PubMed]
59. Adigweme, I.; Yisa, M.; Ooko, M.; Akpalu, E.; Bruce, A.; Donkor, S.; Jarju, L.B.; Danso, B.; Mendy, A.; Jeffries, D.; et al. A measles and rubella vaccine microneedle patch in The Gambia: A phase 1/2, double-blind, double-dummy, randomised, active-controlled, age de-escalation trial. *Lancet* **2024**, *403*, 1879–1892. [CrossRef] [PubMed]
60. Gastañaduy, P.A.; Goodson, J.L.; Panagiotakopoulos, L.; Rota, P.A.; Orenstein, W.A.; Patel, M. Measles in the 21st century: Progress toward achieving and sustaining elimination. *J. Infect. Dis.* **2021**, *224*, S420–S428. [CrossRef]
61. De Quadros, C.A.; Hersh, B.S.; Nogueira, A.C.; Carrasco, P.A.; da Silveira, C.M. Measles eradication: Experience in the Americas. *Bull. World Health Organ.* **1998**, *76* (Suppl. S2), 47–52. [PubMed]
62. Patel, M.K.; Goodson, J.L.; Alexander, J.P., Jr.; Kretsinger, K.; Sodha, S.V.; Steulet, C.; Gacic-Dobo, M.; Rota, P.A.; McFarland, J.; Menning, L.; et al. Progress toward regional measles elimination—Worldwide, 2000–2019. *MMWR* **2020**, *69*, 1700–1705. [CrossRef]
63. Graham, M.; Winter, A.K.; Ferrari, M.; Grenfell, B.; Moss, W.J.; Azman, A.S.; Metcalf, C.J.E.; Lessler, J. Measles and the canonical path to elimination. *Science* **2019**, *364*, 584–587. [CrossRef]
64. Khanal, S.; Kassem, A.M.; Bahl, S.; Jayantha, L.; Sangal, L.; Sharfuzzaman, M.; Bose, A.S.; Antoni, S.; Datta, D.; Alexander, J.P., Jr. Progress toward measles elimination—South-East Asia Region, 2003–2020. *MMWR* **2022**, *71*, 1042–1046. [CrossRef] [PubMed]
65. Murugan, R.; VanderEnde, K.; Dhawan, V.; Haldar, P.; Chatterjee, S.; Sharma, D.; Dzeyie, K.A.; Pattabhiramaiah, S.B.; Khanal, S.; Sangal, L.; et al. Progress toward measles and rubella elimination—India, 2005–2021. *MMWR* **2022**, *71*, 1569–1575. [CrossRef] [PubMed]
66. Bahl, S.; Khanal, S.; Sangal, L.; Tabassum, S.; Ungchusak, K.; Andrus, J. Measles and rubella elimination: Protecting children through immunization in South-East Asia Region (SEAR). *Lancet Reg. Health Southeast. Asia* **2023**, *18*, 100303. [CrossRef]
67. Ma, C.; Rodewald, L.; Hao, L.; Su, Q.; Zhang, Y.; Wen, N.; Fan, C.; Yang, H.; Luo, H.; Wang, H.; et al. Progress toward measles elimination—China, January 2013-June 2019. *MMWR* **2019**, *68*, 1112–1116. [PubMed]
68. Durrheim, D.N.; Xu, A.; Baker, M.G.; Hsu, L.Y.; Takashima, Y. China has the momentum to eliminate measles. *Lancet Reg. Health West. Pac.* **2023**, *30*, 100669. [CrossRef]
69. Musa, N.; Ghoniem, A.; Hsu, C.H.; Mubarak, S.; Sume, G.; Sharifuzzaman, M.; Bak, J.; Hutin, Y.; Teleb, N.; Crowcroft, N.; et al. Progress toward measles elimination—World Health Organization Eastern Mediterranean Region, 2019–2022. *MMWR* **2024**, *73*, 139–144. [CrossRef] [PubMed]
70. Masresha, B.G.; Hatcher, C.; Lebo, E.; Tanifum, P.; Bwaka, A.M.; Minta, A.A.; Antoni, S.; Grant, G.B.; Perry, R.T.; O'Connor, P. Progress toward measles elimination—African Region, 2017-2021. *MMWR* **2023**, *72*, 985–991. [CrossRef] [PubMed]
71. World Health Organization. *Measles and Rubella Strategic Framework 2021–2030*; World Health Organization: Geneva, Switzerland, 2020.
72. Winter, A.K.; Moss, W.J. Rubella. *Lancet* **2022**, *399*, 1336–1346. [CrossRef] [PubMed]

73. Ou, A.C.; Zimmerman, L.A.; Alexander, J.P., Jr.; Crowcroft, N.S.; O'Connor, P.M.; Knapp, J.K. Progress toward rubella and congenital rubella syndrome elimination—Worldwide, 2012-2022. *MMWR* **2024**, *73*, 162–167. [CrossRef]
74. Plotkin, S.A. Rubella eradication: Not yet accomplished, but entirely feasible. *J. Infect. Dis.* **2021**, *224*, S360–S366. [CrossRef]
75. Reef, S.E.; Icenogle, J.P.; Plotkin, S.A. The path to eradication of rubella. *Vaccine* **2023**, *41*, 7525–7531. [CrossRef] [PubMed]
76. Grenfell, B.; Harwood, J. (Meta)population dynamics of infectious diseases. *Trends Ecol. Evol.* **1997**, *12*, 395–399. [CrossRef] [PubMed]
77. Keeling, M.J.; Grenfell, B.T. Understanding the persistence of measles: Reconciling theory, simulation and observation. *Proc. Biol. Sci.* **2002**, *269*, 335–343. [CrossRef] [PubMed]
78. Earn, D.J.; Rohani, P.; Grenfell, B.T. Persistence, chaos and synchrony in ecology and epidemiology. *Proc. Biol. Sci.* **1998**, *265*, 7–10. [CrossRef] [PubMed]
79. Nokes, D.J.; Swinton, J. Vaccination in pulses: A strategy for global eradication of measles and polio? *Trends Microbiol.* **1997**, *5*, 14–19. [CrossRef] [PubMed]
80. Sarkar, S.; Zlojutro, A.; Khan, K.; Gardner, L. Measles resurgence in the USA: How international travel compounds vaccine resistance. *Lancet. Infect. Dis.* **2019**, *19*, 684–686. [CrossRef] [PubMed]
81. Gardner, L.; Dong, E.; Khan, K.; Sarkar, S. Persistence of US measles risk due to vaccine hesitancy and outbreaks abroad. *Lancet. Infect. Dis.* **2020**, *20*, 1114–1115. [CrossRef] [PubMed]
82. Feachem, R.G.A.; Chen, I.; Akbari, O.; Bertozzi-Villa, A.; Bhatt, S.; Binka, F.; Boni, M.F.; Buckee, C.; Dieleman, J.; Dondorp, A.; et al. Malaria eradication within a generation: Ambitious, achievable, and necessary. *Lancet* **2019**, *394*, 1056–1112. [CrossRef] [PubMed]
83. Durrheim, D.N.; Andrus, J.K. The ethical case for global measles eradication-justice and the Rule of Rescue. *Int. Health* **2020**, *12*, 375–377. [CrossRef]
84. Durrheim, D.N. Measles eradication-retreating is not an option. *Lancet. Infect. Dis.* **2020**, *20*, e138–e141. [CrossRef]
85. Durrheim, D.N.; Crowcroft, N.S. The price of delaying measles eradication. *Lancet Public. Health* **2017**, *2*, e130–e131. [CrossRef] [PubMed]
86. Bolotin, S.; Osman, S.; Hughes, S.L.; Ariyarajah, A.; Tricco, A.C.; Khan, S.; Li, L.; Johnson, C.; Friedman, L.; Gul, N.; et al. In Elimination Settings, Measles antibodies wane after vaccination but not after infection: A systematic review and meta-analysis. *J. Infect. Dis.* **2022**, *226*, 1127–1139. [CrossRef] [PubMed]
87. Durrheim, D.N.; Andrus, J.K.; Pfaff, G.; Tabassum, S.; Bashour, H.; Githanga, D. Eradicating measles: A call for an exceptional coordinated global effort. *J. Infect. Dis.* **2019**, *220*, 1870–1872. [CrossRef] [PubMed]

*vaccines*

*Article*

# The Health and Economic Benefits of United States Investments in Measles and Rubella Control and Elimination

**Kimberly M. Thompson**

Kid Risk, Inc., Orlando, FL 32819, USA; kimt@kidrisk.org

**Abstract: Background:** Prior to measles vaccine introduction in 1963, measles virus caused hundreds of thousands of annual reported cases, which led to substantial US morbidity, mortality, and costs. Similarly, congenital rubella syndrome (CRS) led to highly visible and tragic lifelong disability for thousands of Americans, before rubella vaccine introduction in 1969. The US certified national virus transmission elimination of indigenous measles in 2000 and rubella in 2004. **Methods:** Applying an existing integrated transmission and economic model, this analysis characterizes the net benefits of US investments in measles (1963–2030) and rubella (1969–2030) immunization assuming continued high routine immunization coverage. Due to importation risks, the US maintains two doses of both vaccines in its routine immunization schedule. **Results:** This analysis estimates total US costs of 8.1 billion (economics reported in 2023 US dollars) for measles immunization for 1963–2023 and 14.1 billion for rubella immunization for 1969–2023. The analysis estimates an additional approximately 1.2 billion for measles immunization and 1.5 billion for rubella immunization expected for 2024–2030. Historical and future US investments prevented an estimated approximately 237 million measles infections, 228,000 measles deaths, 193 million rubella infections, and 166,000 CRS cases. These investments imply net benefits (from avoided treatment costs minus immunization costs) of approximately 310 billion for measles and 430 billion for rubella and CRS, even without incorporating avoided productivity losses and intangible costs. **Conclusions:** US investments in measles and rubella immunization continue to provide enormous savings of human and financial costs and to prevent substantial mortality and morbidity.

**Keywords:** measles; rubella; vaccine; United States; health economic; modeling

## 1. Introduction

Aggressive control and elimination measures successfully ended the transmission of indigenous measles and rubella viruses in the US, but the importation of both viruses remains a concern for public health authorities despite over 55 years of the use of measles and rubella vaccines. Prior to vaccine introduction, the US annually incurred significant morbidity, mortality, and costs associated with the reported hundreds of thousands of measles cases and tens of thousands of rubella cases, and many more cases most likely went unreported. Measles infections cause rash and fever, and can lead to serious complications, including encephalitis, blindness, and death [1]. Infections with rubella virus (also known as German measles) similarly cause rash and fever illnesses that present clinically like measles infections. However, rubella infections generally lead to more mild clinical symptoms than measles infections for most individuals, with some rubella infections occurring asymptomatically. Unfortunately, when women experience a rubella infection during early pregnancy, the rubella virus can infect the fetus and cause a wide range of birth defects collectively referred to as congenital rubella syndrome (CRS) that can lead to lifelong disability [1,2].

Shortly after the introduction of measles vaccines in 1963, a March 1967 presidential statement launched the first US national measles elimination goal [3]. The first national measles elimination strategy notably included (i) the routine immunization of infants,

(ii) the immunization of unvaccinated children entering school, (iii) improved disease surveillance, and (iv) the containment of outbreaks with immune globulin treatment and the immunization of susceptible individuals [4]. A 1963–1965 rubella epidemic led to highly visible and tragic cases of CRS that motivated intensive vaccine development efforts, which led to the introduction of rubella vaccines in 1969 [5]. Over time, two other national measles elimination initiatives followed in 1978 [6] and 1993 [7–9]. The US most likely stopped indigenous measles transmission by 1993 [10] and it convened an expert consultation that certified the accomplishment in 2000 [11]. After eliminating measles, the US turned its sights on rubella, and it successfully stopped indigenous rubella virus transmission by the early 2000s with the certification of the achievement in October 2004 [5].

Building on the success of the US and other countries, the entire western hemisphere (i.e., the Americas), led by the Pan American Health Organization (PAHO), set a goal in 1994 to eliminate regional indigenous measles virus transmission by the year 2000 [12], and established a goal in 2003 to eliminate indigenous rubella virus transmission by the year 2010 [13]. PAHO certified the accomplishment of the regional elimination of indigenous rubella transmission in 2015 [13] and indigenous measles transmission in 2016 [12]. These regional efforts helped to decrease the number of importations of both viruses into the US and reduced the risks of transmission restarting.

Despite these accomplishments, importations of measles and rubella viruses from other parts of the world continue(d) to pose a threat to Americans. The US continues to report measles cases associated with these importations, which lead to costly US measles outbreak response efforts [14–19]. In 2018, PAHO lost its regional measles elimination status due to the reestablished transmission of imported measles viruses in the Bolivarian Republic of Venezuela [20] and Brazil [21], and the US came close to losing its national measles elimination status due to a 2018–2019 outbreak in New York [22]. As of 2024, the national and regional elimination status of indigenous rubella transmission remains, although the US periodically reports clinical rubella and CRS cases associated with individuals infected outside the US.

*1.1. US Measles and Rubella Vaccine and Immunization Policies*

Measles and rubella immunization policies evolved over time. In 1963, the initial indication for the measles vaccine included healthy children 9 months and older and individuals in high-risk groups, who could receive one dose of a live attenuated measles vaccine or three doses of an inactivated measles vaccine given in monthly intervals, with the inactivated vaccine preferred only for individuals contraindicated for the live attenuated measles vaccine [23]. In 1965, the newly established Advisory Committee on Immunization Practice (ACIP) approved a routine immunization schedule that recommended the measles vaccine for children 12 months or older, due to interference between maternal antibodies and the live attenuated vaccine [24]. ACIP issued a 1965 statement in support of achieving high levels of immunization to achieve national measles elimination [25]. In 1966, ACIP changed its schedule to not recommend the inactivated measles vaccine, except for individuals contraindicated for the live attenuated measles vaccine [26]. In 1967, ACIP completely removed the inactivated measles vaccine from its list of recommended vaccines due to the evidence of atypical measles reported in children who received the inactivated measles vaccine and the limited effectiveness of the inactivated vaccine in immunocompromised children [27]. In 1969, ACIP recommended one dose of the rubella vaccine for children 12 months through puberty [28]. Following successful introduction and the prevention of rubella infections in children, ACIP extended its recommendation to include immunizing susceptible non-pregnant adolescent and adult women who agreed to prevent pregnancy for 3 months after receiving the vaccine, ideally with susceptibility to rubella demonstrated by serologic testing prior to immunization [29].

The separate administration of measles and rubella vaccines largely ended within a few years of rubella vaccine introduction. Following the licensure and demonstration of the non-inferiority of protection provided by combination vaccines containing both live attenuated measles and rubella antigens compared to the single antigen counterparts, ACIP recommended the use of the measles–rubella (MR) vaccine in 1971 [30]. This recommendation reduced the number of vaccine administrations and eliminated the previously recommended spacing of one month between doses of the single antigen live virus vaccines [30]. In the context of numerous outbreaks, ACIP made specific recommendations in 1971 for vaccinating or revaccinating children who lacked sufficient evidence of immunity, and encouraged restricting unvaccinated children from school attendance during outbreaks [31]. In 1976, ACIP recommended the measles–mumps–rubella (MMR) vaccine and further reconsidered the strategy of administration of more than one live virus vaccine antigen (e.g., MMR and the oral poliovirus vaccine) during a single clinical visit [32]. ACIP also changed the recommended age for receiving measles-containing vaccines (MCVs), MR and MMR at the time, to 15 months in 1976, with the further increase in age again due to interference with measles maternal antibodies [33]. In 1978, ACIP reconfirmed 15 months as the recommended age of receiving an MCV and its preference for the MMR formulation for childhood vaccination, and further emphasized the importance of vaccinating or revaccinating individuals lacking immunological protection from measles (including those who may have previously received the inactivated measles vaccine) [34].

The expansion of ACIP recommendations continued since the 1980. In 1982, ACIP added an international travel indication for measles vaccination for those born after 1956 without evidence of measles immunity [35]. In 1987, ACIP recommended that colleges require proof of measles vaccination for students prior to matriculation and that medical facilities require proof of measles vaccination for all employees born since 1956 and all employees with potential occupational exposure to measles virus [36]. Responding to the epidemiology of the time, in January 1989 ACIP issued a supplementary statement that recommended areas with recurrent measles outbreaks give infants a dose of a measles single antigen (i.e., monovalent measles) vaccine at 9 months of age in addition to the recommended MMR dose at 15 months [37]. In December 1989, ACIP changed its recommendation to a two-dose MMR schedule for all children: one dose at 15 months (or as early as 12 months in areas with recurrent outbreaks) and one dose at the age of school entry [38]. In 1998, ACIP changed the two-dose schedule to specify the delivery of the first MMR dose between 12 and 15 months and the second dose between 4 and 6 years of age, and it set a goal for all states to achieve the delivery of two MMR doses to all children prior to school entry by 2001 [39]. In 2005, the ACIP schedule recommended that children aged 12 months–12 years receive two doses of the MMR vaccine at least 1 month apart (with the recommended target ages for both doses unchanged from the 1998 recommendations [39]). The licensure of a combination vaccine that included measles–mumps–rubella–varicella (MMRV) in 2005 offered an alternative to separate MMR and varicella vaccines [40]. ACIP subsequently issued several related recommendations that did not impact the measles vaccine schedule or the choice of MMR or MMRV, henceforth MMR(V), and ACIP recommended administering the first doses at 12–47 months and second doses at 5–12 years of age [41–44]. As of 2024, the US routine immunization schedule continues to recommend two doses of MMR(V), with two vaccine formulations available: MMR (M-M-R-II™, North Wales, PA, USA and Priorix™, Philadelphia, PA, USA) and MMRV (ProQuad™, North Wales, PA, USA), with administration at ages of 12–15 months and 4–6 years and clearly indicated age ranges for catch-up [45].

### 1.2. Economic Analyses

Economic analyses of measles and rubella vaccines in the US performed over time emphasized the significant benefits of the vaccines, and many explored different immunization policy changes [46]. For measles, a 1969 economic analysis projected significant savings of lives and costs for the first 6 years of US measles immunization compared to no immunization with estimated net benefits of USD 423 million (USD 1962, which equals approximately USD 4.3 billion in USD 2023) [47]. A 1975 update strengthened the health and economic case for supporting measles immunization in the US during the first 10 years [48]. A 1978 economic analysis estimated a benefit–cost ratio of 10.3 and net benefits exceeding USD 1.1 billion (USD 1972, or USD 8.0 billion USD 2023) for the national measles elimination efforts between 1966 and 1974 [49]. Several economic analyses reported sustained significant net benefits of measles vaccination for the first 20 years of its use in the US [50–52], and characterized the savings associated with the shared administration of combination vaccines that included measles (i.e., MR and MMR) [51]. Consistent with the epidemiological importance of outbreaks around 1990, several economic analyses explored different options for outbreak response and the costs of outbreaks [53–56]. Around 2000, studies demonstrated significant potential savings for the US associated with the cessation of measles vaccination after global measles eradication [57], and emphasized the need to identify cost-effective strategies to increase measles immunization coverage [58].

Similarly, soon after the introduction of the rubella vaccine, economic analyses began exploring its health and financial benefits and the impacts of different US rubella immunization policies [46]. Based on an extrapolation of the costs of the 1963–65 rubella epidemic, an economic analysis of the US national rubella immunization policy of immunizing children 1–12 years old to avert the next expected rubella epidemic in the 1970s suggested that rubella immunization would need to cost more than USD 1 billion (USD 1964, USD 9.8 billion USD 2023) for the costs to exceed the benefits [59]. Two additional economic analyses estimated significant net benefits for the first 20 years of US rubella vaccine use [51,52]. An unpublished economic analysis in 1994 showed positive benefits of a two-dose MMR schedule, with the incremental costs of a second dose of MMR not exceeding the expected incremental benefits due to high first-dose coverage [60]. An analysis suggested that US rubella vaccination would provide benefits at least eight times greater than costs, with higher benefit–cost ratios associated with the use of MMR combination vaccines instead of the monovalent rubella vaccine and with various immunization policies and coverage assumptions [61].

Economic analyses of the current full childhood immunization schedule, including MRCVs, continue to show significant health and economic benefits compared to no vaccination [62–64] and the costs associated with importation-associated outbreaks [14–19]. Despite the numerous static economic analyses of the US investments in measles immunization [47–52,57,58,60,62–64] and rubella immunization [46,51,52,59,62–64] and many measles and rubella transmission models [65], no studies using a dynamic transmission model demonstrate the economic benefits of the more than five decades of the US use of measles and rubella vaccines. Prior studies demonstrated the importance of using dynamic models instead of static models to characterize the economics of interventions of communicable diseases theoretically [66,67] and for real diseases [68]. Guidelines for economic analyses recommend the use of dynamic transmission models for economic analyses for vaccine-preventable diseases [69–71]. This analysis fills the gap of using a dynamic transmission model to characterize the health and economic benefits of the US measles and rubella immunization programs.

## 2. Materials and Methods

To characterize the health and economic outcomes of the actual US program, this analysis considered the reported measles and rubella cases and estimates of cases using an existing dynamic disease transmission model for measles and rubella [72]. Briefly, the model tracked the births, deaths, aging, and immunity of all individuals in the US population as it evolves through the following immunity states: maternally immune (i.e., infection-induced and vaccine-induced tracked separately), susceptible, exposed, infected (and infectious), recovered, or vaccinated. The model also tracked the progression of pregnancies to simulate the impacts of infections on pregnancy outcomes and cases of CRS [72]. This analysis updated the time-related model inputs for epidemiology, demographics, immunization, and costs through the end of 2023. The model time horizon extended from 1963 to 2030, and assumed the prospective use of two doses of MMR(V) for 2024–2030. The analysis used standard methods to characterize the societal health and financial costs, including the use of a discount rate of 3% and the computation of incremental cost-effectiveness ratios (ICERs) as well as incremental net benefits (INBs). The model estimates provided comparisons between the actual historical US immunization program use of MRCVs (i.e., including all of the changes that occurred over time in schedules and formulation changes) and a counterfactual world with no measles or rubella vaccine use.

### 2.1. Transmission Model Input Updates

Measles became a notifiable disease in the United States in 1912, with 19 states reporting initially, all states reporting by 1928, and the US Centers for Disease Control and Prevention (CDC) taking on the responsibility for data collection and synthesis starting in 1961 [73]. Due to their similar clinical presentation, prior to the 1960s, reported measles cases probably included some rubella cases. Rubella became a reportable disease in 1966 with the widespread utilization of laboratory testing facilitating its distinction from other fever and rash diseases [73]. Figure 1 shows the steady and substantial increase in the estimated size of the US population [74–76] for (a) 1912–2023 along with reported measles cases [73,77–81] and deaths [78,79,82], and (b) 1966–2023 along with reported rubella and CRS cases [73,77,80,82]. While the US population increased by a factor of 3, Figure 1a shows the rate of measles incidence and deaths varied significantly prior to the introduction of the measles vaccine in 1963, and then dropped significantly following its introduction. These data imply a substantial reduction in the reported measles case fatality rate over time, which most likely reflects improvements in health care (e.g., detection, treatment, case management, and overall health systems). Similarly, rates of rubella and CRS incidence declined significantly over time following the introduction of the rubella vaccine in 1966 (Figure 1b).

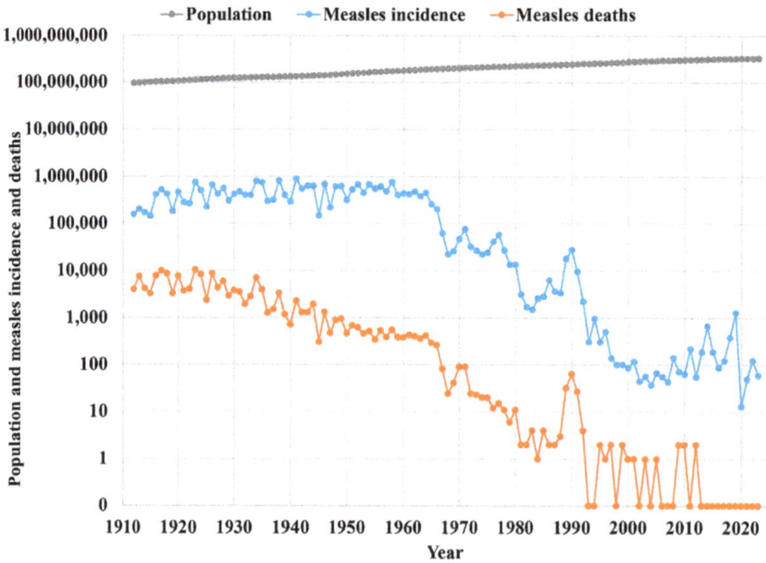


(a)

**Figure 1.** *Cont.*

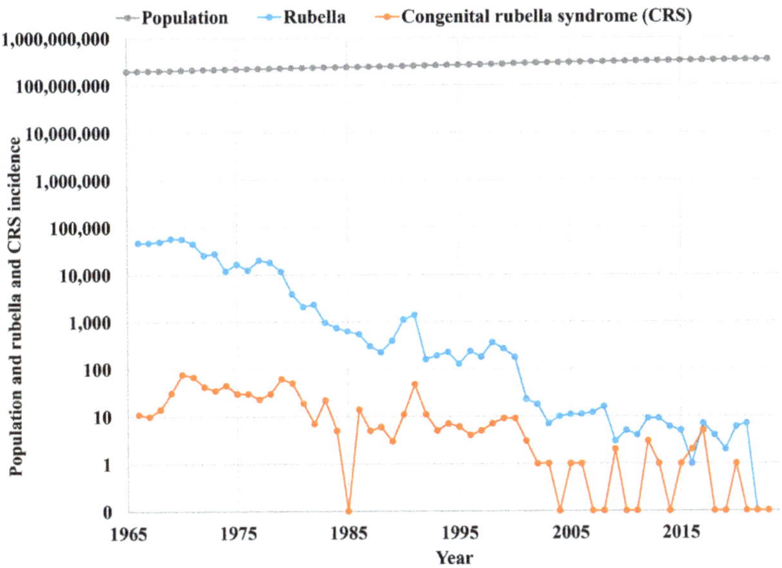


(**b**)

**Figure 1.** Trends for US population growth [74–76] and (**a**) reported measles incidence [73,77–81] and deaths [78,79,82] between 1912 and 2023 and (**b**) reported rubella incidence and congenital rubella syndrome (CRS) cases [73,77,80,82] between 1965 and 2023.

The quality of measles surveillance in the US changed significantly over time. Estimates suggest that in the pre-vaccine era through the early 1970s, reporting most likely captured less than 10% of all cases [83–85]. A review of the completeness of measles reporting during the 1980s and 1990s suggested a wide range of 3–58% [86]. Given the substantial underreporting, the early measles incidence data (Figure 1a) most likely provide some indication of the years of major outbreaks (i.e., the peaks and troughs of cases), but not the absolute numbers of cases. However, some uncertainty related to the peak years comes from the potential impact of major rubella epidemics contributing to measles case counts due to the reliance on syndromic surveillance [72]. In contrast to measles, given the relatively short period of time between rubella becoming notifiable and the introduction of the rubella vaccine, relatively little information exists to assess the extent of the underreporting of rubella infections prior to vaccine introduction. However, given the substantial underreporting for measles, the use of syndromic surveillance for both diseases, and the relatively less severe clinical presentation of rubella, substantial underreporting most likely occurred for rubella and CRS. As the US pursued and achieved the elimination of indigenous measles and rubella transmission, surveillance continued to improve (as required to confirm the achievement of the goals), but some underreporting of cases still occurs. Nonetheless, improvements in laboratory methods allowed the US to document the end of the transmission of indigenous rubella lineages [87] and measles lineages and identify the likely sources of imported measles and rubella viruses after the national elimination of indigenous transmission [10,88]. Given the uncertainty about the timing, location, and transmission of future importations of measles and rubella into the US, for 2024–2030 this analysis prospectively assumed 250 annual measles cases, 4 annual rubella cases, and 1 annual CRS case. These assumptions may over- or under-estimate the cases that will occur, because the actual size of outbreaks depends on the timing of introduction and the level of under-immunization in the outbreak communities. For example, as shown in Figure 1a, relatively larger recent measles outbreaks occurred during the winters of

2014–2015 and 2018–2019, and cases dropped substantially in 2020 due to reductions in social mixing and travel during the COVID-19 pandemic.

This analysis started with estimates of historical routine immunization coverage for MCVs (i.e., monovalent measles, MR, MMR, and MMRV) and rubella-containing vaccines (RCVs, i.e., monovalent rubella, MR, MMR, and MMRV) in the US based on prior work [72,89]. A closer review of the use of measles and rubella vaccines in the US and the evolution of ACIP policies (described above) led to some additional considerations for the model. In 1963, the US introduced two types of licensed injectable measles vaccines: inactivated and live attenuated. The inactivated vaccine represented about one-third of total doses used in 1963 and required 3 doses per child, which implied a higher cost per fully immunized child. The model accounted for this requirement of multiple doses for the inactivated vaccine in the coverage estimates for 1963–1966. Many recipients (approximately 50%) of the initial live attenuated measles vaccine developed symptoms of fever and rash, which motivated the development of a further attenuated live measles vaccine with significantly lower side effects [90]. Similarly, the initial rubella vaccines introduced varied with respect to their immunogenicity and reactivity, but by 1979 the RA27/3 rubella vaccine emerged as the national preference [91].

In the US, individuals receive health care (including immunizations) paid for by public sources (i.e., the government) or private sources (e.g., self-pay or employer-based health insurance). Figure 2a shows the estimated number of MCV doses purchased by year in the US since 1963 by payer type and in total, and Figure 2b shows the estimated number of RCV doses purchased by year in the US since 1969 by payer type and in total. For the rubella dose estimates in 1969 and 1970, this analysis apportioned the estimated total rubella vaccine doses purchased by 1970 as equivalent for 1969 and 1970 and assumed 90% public purchase and 10% private purchase. The CDC began purchasing MCV doses following the approval of federal funds for 1966–1968 [92] to support national measles elimination in 1967 [4]. After the licensure of the rubella vaccine in 1969, Congress allocated federal funds for RCV purchase, instead of for measles immunization, between 1969 and 1971, since it prioritized the introduction of the rubella vaccine [92]. Following a resurgence of measles incidence in 1969–1971, federal funds began to support the public purchase of measles and rubella vaccines individually and then in the combination MR formulations. The purchase of MRCVs increased as school immunization requirements started to come into effect in some states in the early 1970s.

In 1989 and 1990, vaccine demand increased consistent with the shift to a two-dose immunization schedule. The demand increase included just over 1 million monovalent live measles vaccine doses, which aimed to increase measles protection in adolescents and young adults who received the inactivated measles vaccine as children. In addition, the US military delivered one dose of MCV to all military recruits (i.e., approximately 200,000 doses per year) between 1980 [93] and the mid-2000s [94], after which time the military services began screening recruits and selectively vaccinating only those lacking immunity. Based on data prior to 2015, this analysis assumed a public purchase of 45% of total doses for 2016–2024. Although the fraction of all MRCV doses in Figure 2 given to Americans of different ages remains uncertain, consistent with immunization recommendations for travel, military personnel, unvaccinated women of childbearing age, and health care providers, this analysis assumed that 5–10% of the annual MRCV doses have gone to individuals over 17 years old after 1980.

Figure 3 summarizes (a) MCV and (b) RCV routine immunization coverage estimates by year by the age of vaccine delivery [89]. For 2023 on, this analysis assumed the same routine immunization schedule and coverage rates as occurred in 2022 and that the other vaccine doses purchased include supplemental immunization activities, including campaigns performed to introduce both vaccines, outbreak response, and the catch-up of older individuals (e.g., military and women of childbearing age) as well as wastage. For 1977 to 1988, this analysis included a second opportunity for unvaccinated children aged 5 years to receive the vaccine, to account for the increasing adoption of school immunization requirements (see * in Figure 3). The administration costs of MCVs and RCVs depended on the number of antigens in the vaccine formulation, because the multiple antigens share the costs for the single injection.

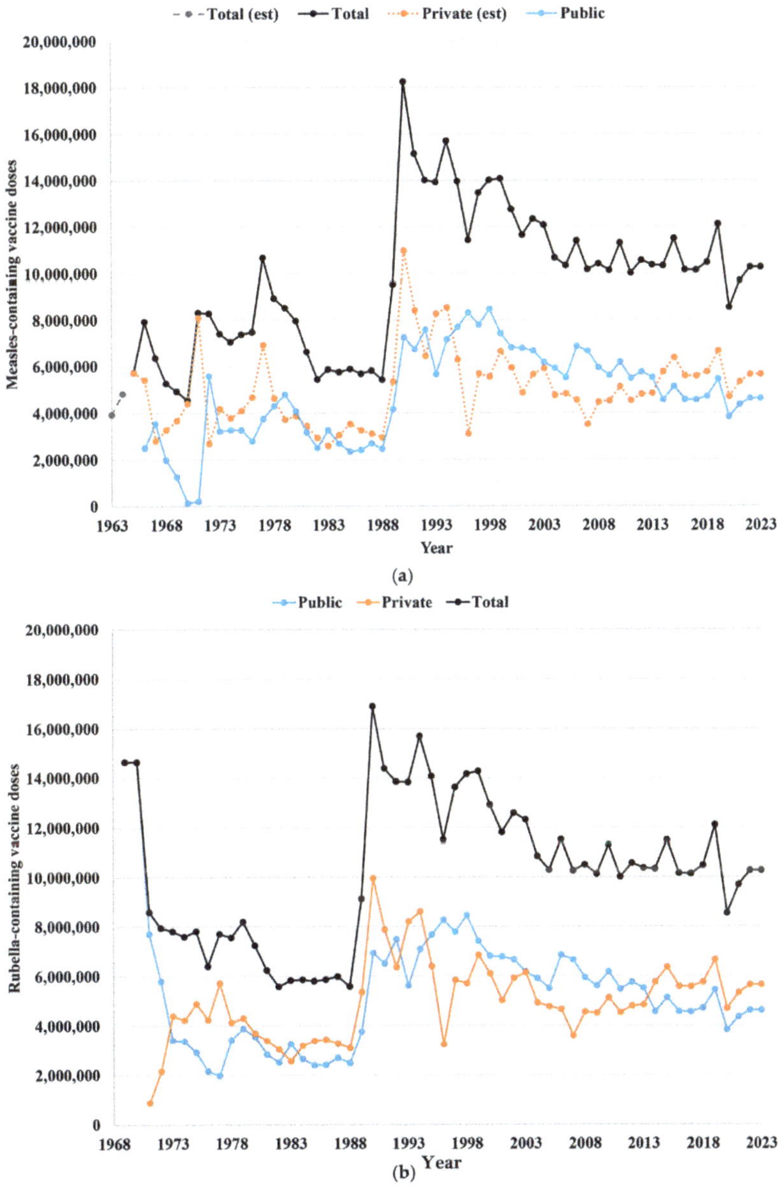


**Figure 2.** Number of vaccine doses by payer type and in total in the United States for (**a**) measles-containing vaccine doses since 1963 and (**b**) rubella-containing vaccine doses since 1969 with dashed lines showing estimates (see acknowledgments at the end). Total measles doses for 1963 and 1964 estimated [48]; reporting of total measles doses started in 1965; reporting of public doses started in 1966; reporting of total rubella doses started in 1969; and public doses estimated as 45% of total for 2016–2022.

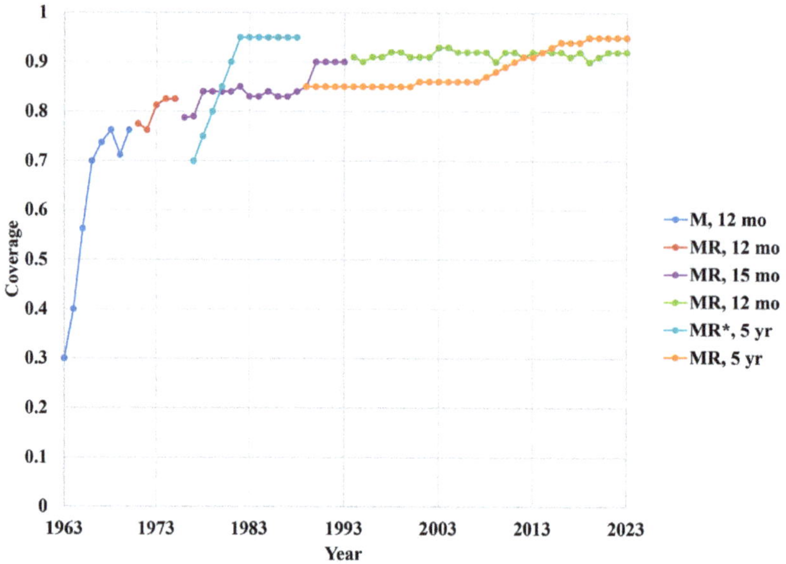


**Figure 3.** Assumptions about routine immunization coverage of measles- and rubella-containing vaccines by year and age of administration. * Second opportunity for unvaccinated children aged 5 years to receive the measles vaccine, to account for the increasing adoption of school immunization requirements (not a second dose).

Figure 4 shows the fractions of the different MRCV formulations used for the public sector doses by year. Slow uptake and supply disruptions of MMRV explain some of the variation in the fractions of MMR and MMRV in Figure 4. For 2016 on, this analysis assumed the public delivery of 65% of all MMR doses and 35% of all MMRV doses.

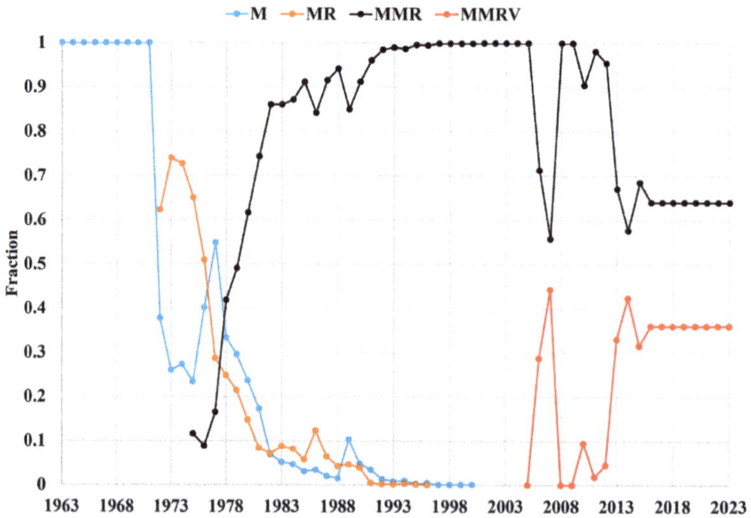


(a)

**Figure 4.** *Cont.*

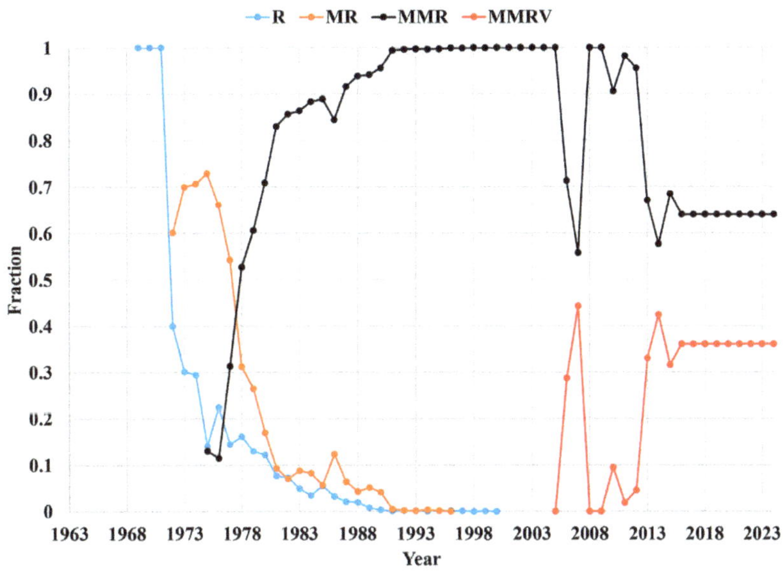


(b)

**Figure 4.** Fractions of the different (**a**) measles- and (**b**) rubella-containing vaccine formulations used in the public sector by year since 1963.

### 2.2. Cost Input Updates

For consistency, the analysis reported all costs in 2023 US dollars (noted USD 2023) adjusted using the consumer price index [95]. Figure 5 summarizes the (a) measles component price for MCVs and (b) rubella component price for RCVs for the public and private sectors (converted to USD 2023) based on data obtained from the published literature [96] and unpublished data provided to the CDC by vaccine manufacturers. The cost estimates accounted for the estimated numbers of doses for each vaccine presentation (Figures 2 and 4), the applicable federal excise taxes, and the estimated cost of the specific antigen component in the combination vaccines. In 1987, vaccine purchases (both public and private) became subject to a federal excise tax [97] used to create a fund to support the Vaccine Injury Compensation Program [98]. A federal excise tax of USD 4.44 per dose (nominal) applied for MMR for 1987–1992 [97]. On August 10, 1993, the federal excise tax became permanent [99] and the amount for MMR of USD 4.44 per dose (nominal) resumed. In August 5, 1997, the Taxpayer Relief Act of 1997 [100] lowered the federal excise tax to USD 0.75 per antigen (nominal, i.e., USD 2.25 per MMR dose), and the tax continues at that amount to date. This analysis assumed that the nominal federal excise tax will continue to be USD 0.75 per antigen in perpetuity, which implies a gradual decline in real cost over time. The drop in the cost in 1993 in Figure 5 reflects the absence of a federal excise tax for part of that year (the analysis assumed the tax applied to 50% of the MRCV vaccine supply in 1993, which includes tax applied to the 40% of annual doses sold after 9 August 1993 and 10% more to account for some of the floor tax imposed for doses held on 10 August 1993). To obtain the cost of the measles component in the mixture of all MCVs each year, the analysis assumed that the measles component accounts for 60% of the antigen cost of MR and 30% of the antigen cost of MMR, and the same cost for the measles component in MMR and MMRV for both the public and private sector costs. The model assumed that the rubella component accounts for 40% of the antigen cost of MR, 30% of the antigen cost of MMR, and the same cost for the rubella component in MMR and MMRV for both the public and private sectors. The Vaccines for Children program [99] mandates that the contract price for public purchases of some vaccines (including MRCVs) cannot increase more than the pre-excise tax public price of the vaccine in 1 May 1993 adjusted using the consumer price index [95], which explains the slightly decreasing public real cost of MRCVs (in USD 2023) in Figure 5 after 1993. The analysis assumed a constant public cost for the measles and rubella components of MRCVs from 2023 through the rest of the analytical time horizon. In contrast, consistent with the trend in Figure 5, the model assumed that the private cost will increase at a rate of USD 0.36 per year from 2023 to 2030 (based on a linear regression of historical private cost increases, $R^2 = 0.96$).

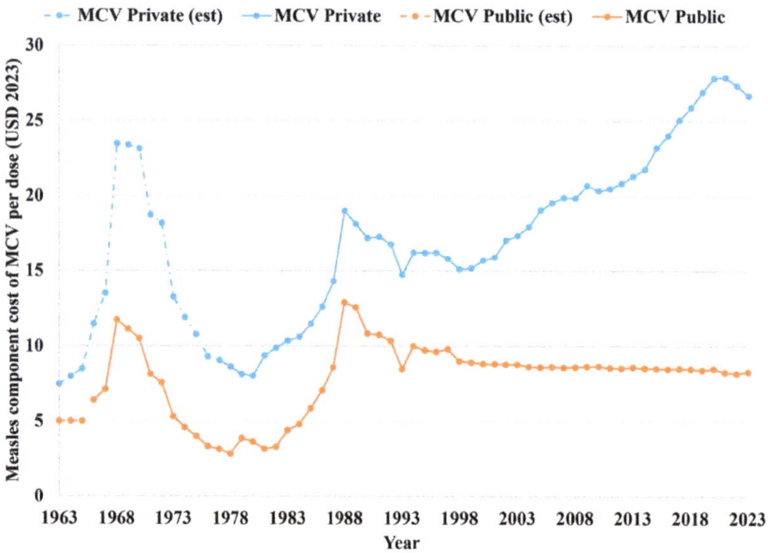


(a)

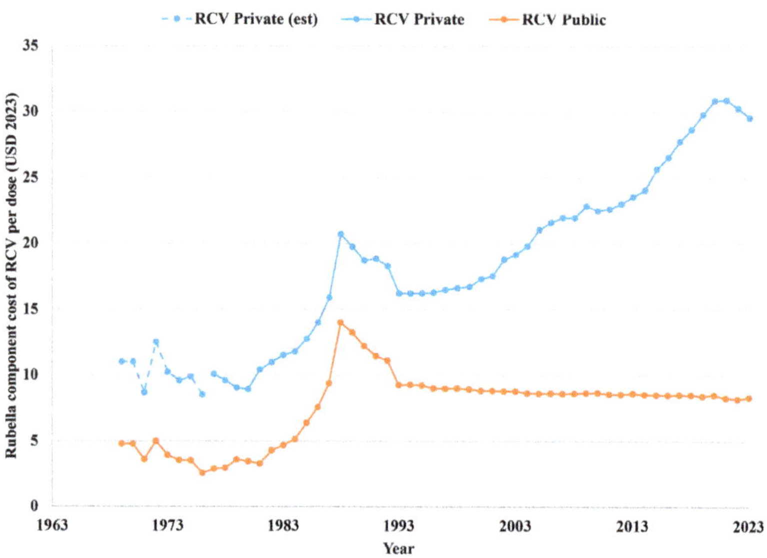


(b)

**Figure 5.** Estimated cost per dose of the (**a**) measles component and (**b**) rubella component by public and private purchase.

This analysis based its non-vaccine cost and valuation estimates on the values for high-income countries reported previously [1]. Table 1 summarizes the updated or new estimates for non-vaccine costs per injection (including administration, needle disposal, etc.) and other costs per measles or rubella infection or per dose for MRCVs, all appropriately updated to USD 2023. The baseline analysis did not include costs related to measles or rubella research, surveillance, or program management related to achieving the national control and elimination goals (i.e., programmatic costs).

**Table 1.** Costs and effectiveness of measles immunization programs in the United States (USD 2023).

| Metric | Measles | | Rubella | |
|---|---|---|---|---|
| Introduction *–2023 | No vaccine | Vaccine | No vaccine | Vaccine |
| Infections (millions) | 228 | 20 | 172 | 5 |
| Measles deaths (thousands) | 222 | 20 | | |
| CRS cases (thousands) | | | 152 | 7 |
| Treatment costs (billions) | 307 | 26 | 400 | 13 |
| DALYs lost (millions) | 17 | 1 | 8 | 0.2 |
| Vaccine doses (millions) | | 583 | | 546 |
| Immunization costs (billions) | | 8 | | 14 |
| Productivity losses (billions) | 985 | 55 | 516 | 10 |
| 2024–2030 | | | | |
| Infections (millions) | 30 | 0.002 | 25 | 0.00003 |
| Measles deaths (thousands) | 26 | 0.003 | | |
| CRS cases (thousands) | | | 21 | 0.007 |
| Treatment costs (billions) | 38 | 0.003 | 59 | 0.009 |
| DALYs lost (millions) | 2 | 0.00009 | 1 | 0.0001 |
| Vaccine doses (millions) | | 72 | | 56 |
| Immunization costs (billions) | | 1 | | 2 |
| Productivity losses (billions) | 167 | 0.007 | 104 | 0.01 |
| **Economic analysis summary** | **Measles** | **Rubella** | **Total** | |
| Introduction *–2030 | | | | |
| Incremental immunization costs (billions) | 9 | 16 | 25 | |
| Incremental treatment cost (billions) | −320 | −446 | −765 | |
| Incremental cost–effectiveness ratio | CLS | CLS | CLS | |
| Incremental net benefits (INBs) (billions) | 310 | 430 | 740 | |
| Productivity costs saved (billions) | 1097 | 610 | 1706 | |
| INB with productivity costs (billions) | 1407 | 1040 | 2447 | |

Abbreviations: CRS, congenital rubella syndrome; DALY, disability adjusted life years; INB, incremental net benefits. * Introduction year 1963 for measles vaccine and 1969 for rubella vaccine.

## 3. Results

Figure 6 shows the model estimates of prevented cases of measles and rubella (left axis) and CRS (right axis) by the US immunization program (compared to no measles or rubella vaccines). The results show the increase in prevented cases following the introduction of the measles vaccine in 1963 and rubella vaccine in 1969, with the measles cases prevented approaching the size of the annual US birth cohort. A comparison of the prevented rubella (left axis) and CRS (right axis) cases shows a slight shift to the right for the CRS cases, which corresponds with the time between early trimester infections and CRS diagnosis after live births. In Figure 6, after the national elimination of the transmission of indigenous viruses, this analysis subtracts the reported cases from the estimated cases from the modeled counterfactual with no immunization up to and through 2023 and assuming average imported cases for 2024–2030 (see Section 2.1).

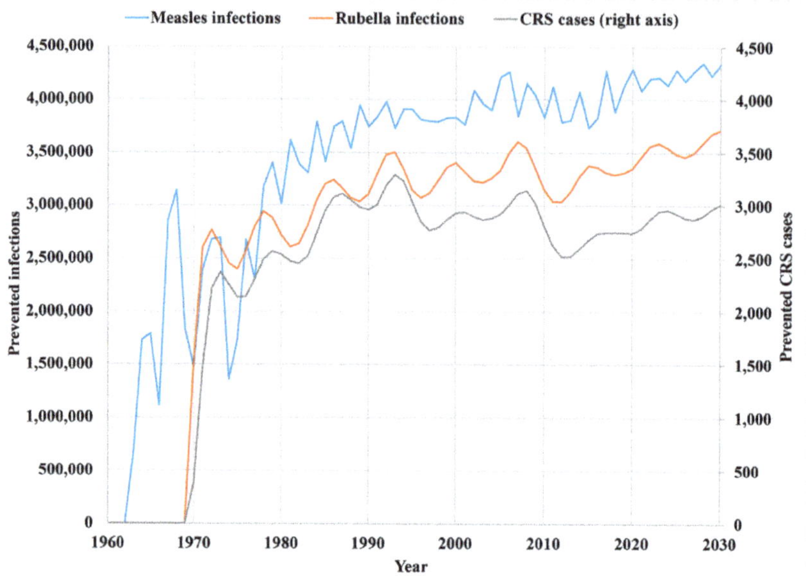


**Figure 6.** Estimates of prevented annual measles and rubella cases (left axis) and CRS cases (right axis) in the United States for 1963–2030 based on differences between the modeled US immunization program and the counterfactual scenario of no immunization.

Table 1 summarizes the results of the economic analyses. For the program of actual US investments, Table 1 shows total costs for US investments in measles immunization for 1963–2023 of USD 8.1 billion and in rubella immunization for 1969–2023 of USD 14.1 billion. The analysis estimates an additional approximately USD 1.2 billion for measles immunization and USD 1.5 billion for rubella immunization expected for 2024–2030. Historical and future US investments prevented an estimated approximately 237 million measles infections, 228,000 measles deaths, 193 million rubella infections, and 166,000 CRS cases. These investments imply net benefits (from avoided treatment costs minus immunization costs) of approximately USD 310 billion for measles and USD 430 billion for rubella and CRS, even without incorporating avoided productivity losses and intangible costs. Including productivity savings estimated by valuing each DALY lost as equivalent to per capita gross national income [1], this analysis estimates incremental net benefits of immunization in the US compared to no immunization of over USD 1.2 trillion for measles for 1963 to 2023 (with USD 200 billion additionally anticipated for 2024–2030) and over USD 880 billion for rubella for 1969 to 2023 (with USD 160 billion additionally anticipated for 2024–2030). Due to importations, the US continues to incur some financial costs associated with investigations by public health authorities, particularly for measles outbreaks. Since 1980, this analysis estimates that cumulative outbreak response costs most likely exceeded USD 30 million. US investments in measles and rubella immunization continue to provide enormous savings of human and financial costs, and global eradication of both diseases would offer some additional savings due to avoided outbreaks, if achievable.

## 4. Discussion

US investments in measles and rubella immunization continue to provide enormous net savings of human and financial costs for Americans. While these results apply to the US, the wealth of economic analyses related to measles immunization imply similar expectations of significant savings for other countries, regions, and globally [46]. A 2016 analysis that characterized the benefits of vaccines for 94 low- and middle-income countries for

2011–2020 reported approximately USD 58 (USD 2010) returned per dollar spent on measles vaccination, and showed the measles vaccine as the most net beneficial vaccine delivered among the 10 commonly delivered childhood vaccines considered in the analysis [101]. A recent analysis identified reductions in measles mortality as responsible for over 80% of the global reduction in mortality by all vaccine-preventable diseases during the first 50 years of the Expanded Program on Immunization (EPI) [102].

Despite regional measles and rubella elimination efforts, importations of measles and rubella viruses into the US remain an ongoing threat due to the possibility of any unvaccinated American coming into contact with an infected individual (e.g., while traveling in measles- and/or rubella-endemic countries or with an infected individual traveling within the US). Recent outbreaks demonstrate the potential for restarting transmission in under-vaccinated communities. By extension, this and other analyses suggest that the global eradication of measles and rubella virus transmission could lead to significant savings for the US and globally, and this continues to motivate national investments in the global immunization and potential eradication of measles and rubella. However, the US appears unlikely to ever stop its immunization with MRCVs, and consequently, recognizing an eradication dividend largely depends on potential savings of avoided treatment costs and national outbreak response.

Although relatively minor with respect to both health and economic impacts, this analysis includes the quantification of very rare, but still non-zero, adverse vaccine-associated events. In theory, with global eradication (i.e., no more measles or rubella transmission or infections), the costs of these rare events could exceed the consequences of infections in the US, which might lead to discussions about ending immunization. However, as of 2024, global concerns about biological agents remain heightened by the recent emergence of the SARS-CoV-2 virus that led to the global COVID-19 pandemic. Ending immunization for measles and/or rubella in the US would not likely find support with US public health authorities.

All models come with limitations. Given the limited information and the need to reconstruct historical information for retrospective model inputs and extrapolate for future model inputs, the model results inherently include uncertainty about how well the model estimates represent the past and/or will predict the future. The model includes numerous assumptions that simulate transmission artificially (e.g., assuming more homogeneity in the population than exists), but produces estimates consistent with the available evidence. In addition, the results of any economic analysis depend on the assumptions made related to valuation over time (e.g., discounting future costs and benefits). The major insight of very significant benefits remains highly robust to changes in the assumptions: measles and rubella immunization lengthens and improves the quality of lives and saves money. Thus, this analysis emphasizes the overwhelming results of substantial health and economic savings from measles and rubella vaccine use in the US, while noting some uncertainty about the absolute numbers and the lack of inclusion of all costs (e.g., unquantified non-vaccine-related programmatic costs).

Combining this analysis with a similar analysis for polio [68] and prospective analyses of the full national childhood immunization program, the US has benefitted and continues to benefit very significantly from its investments in childhood immunization programs. Given the ability of measles and rubella vaccines to prevent bad and costly outcomes, Americans do not experience the events that do not happen. While fortunately enjoying the benefits of prevention, this unfortunately leads to some lack of appreciation of the important health and economic benefits of these vaccines. Studies like this should help provide some insights about what might occur in the absence of vaccines. Those who remember and/or understand the tragic outcomes caused by vaccine-preventable diseases will need to continue to help those with no or little experience with the diseases to fully appreciate the value of vaccines. Measles and rubella importations remain a very real threat, and all individuals remain vulnerable to the potential adverse health outcomes associated with measles and rubella infections so long as they remain unprotected.

## 5. Conclusions

US investments in measles and rubella immunization continue to provide enormous savings of human and financial costs and to prevent substantial mortality and morbidity.

**Funding:** This research received no external funding.

**Institutional Review Board Statement:** Not applicable.

**Informed Consent Statement:** Not applicable.

**Data Availability Statement:** No new data were created or analyzed in this study. Data sharing is not applicable to this article.

**Acknowledgments:** The author acknowledges unrestricted donations to Kid Risk, Inc that supported this manuscript and thanks the US Centers for Disease Control and Prevention for supporting prior related work under Cooperative Agreement Number 6NU2RGH001913-01-02. For information related to Figures 2 and 4, the author thanks Robert Synder for discussions in 2001, John Grabenstein, Bruce Weniger, and Jeanne Santoi for discussions in 2017, and Jeanne Santoli for additional discussions in 2024. The author also thanks Kevin Agnew, James Alexander, Stephen Cochi, Louis Cooper (posthumously), John Grabenstein, Sam Katz (posthumously), Narayan Nair, Mark Papania, Stanley Plotkin, Susan Reef, and Jim Robinson for helpful information and comments over many years.

**Conflicts of Interest:** The author declares no conflicts of interest.

## References

1. Thompson, K.M.; Odahowski, C.L. The costs and valuation of health impacts of measles and rubella risk management policies. *Risk Anal.* **2016**, *36*, 1357–1382. [CrossRef] [PubMed]
2. Simons, E.A.; Reef, S.E.; Cooper, L.Z.; Zimmerman, L.; Thompson, K.M. Systematic review of the manifestations of Congenital Rubella Syndrome in infants and characterization of Disability-Adjusted Life Years (DALYs). *Risk Anal.* **2016**, *36*, 1297–1314. [CrossRef] [PubMed]
3. Sencer, D.J. A program to eradicate measles. *Am. J. Public Health Nations Health* **1967**, *57*, 729–730. [CrossRef] [PubMed]
4. Sencer, D.J.; Dull, H.B.; Langmuir, A.D. Epidemiologic basis for eradication of measles in 1967. *Public Health Rep.* **1967**, *82*, 253–256. [CrossRef]
5. Centers for Disease Control and Prevention. Achievements in public health: Elimination of rubella and congenital rubella syndrome—United States, 1969–2004. *MMWR* **2005**, *54*, 279–282.
6. Hinman, A.R.; Brandling-Bennett, A.D.; Nieburg, P.I. The opportunity and obligation to eliminate measles from the United States. *JAMA* **1979**, *242*, 1157–1162. [CrossRef]
7. Robinson, C.A.; Sepe, S.J.; Lin, K.F. The president's child immunization initiative--a summary of the problem and the response. *Public Health Rep.* **1993**, *108*, 419–425.
8. Orenstein, W.A.; Papania, M.J.; Wharton, M.E. Measles elimination in the United States. *J. Infect. Dis.* **2004**, *189* (Suppl. S1), S1–S3. [CrossRef]
9. Hinman, A.R.; Orenstein, W.A.; Papania, M.J. Evolution of measles elimination strategies in the United States. *J. Infect. Dis.* **2004**, *189* (Suppl. S1), S17–S22. [CrossRef]
10. Bellini, W.J.; Rota, P.A. Genetic diversity of wild-type measles viruses: Implications for global measles elimination programs. *Emerg. Infect. Dis.* **1998**, *4*, 29–35. [CrossRef]
11. Katz, S.L.; Hinman, A.R. Summary and conclusions: Measles elimination meeting, 16–17 March 2000. *J. Infect. Dis.* **2004**, *189* (Suppl. S1), S43–S47. [CrossRef] [PubMed]
12. Pan American Health Organization. Region of the Americas Is Declared Free of Measles. Available online: http://www.paho.org/hq/index.php?option=com_content&view=article&id=12528:region-americas-declared-free-measles (accessed on 24 January 2024).
13. Pan American Health Organization. Americas Region Is Declared the World's First to Eliminate Rubella. Available online: http://www.paho.org/hq/index.php?option=com_content&view=article&id=10798:2015-americas-free-of-rubella&Itemid=1926&lang=en (accessed on 24 January 2024).
14. Dayan, G.H.; Ortega-Sanchez, I.R.; LeBaron, C.W.; Quinlisk, M.P. The cost of containing one case of measles: The economic impact on the public health infrastructure—Iowa, 2004. *Pediatrics* **2005**, *116*, e1–e4. [CrossRef]
15. Sugerman, D.E.; Barskey, A.E.; Delea, M.G.; Ortega-Sanchez, I.R.; Bi, D.; Ralston, K.J.; Rota, P.A.; Waters-Montijo, K.; Lebaron, C.W. Measles outbreak in a highly vaccinated population, San Diego, 2008: Role of the intentionally undervaccinated. *Pediatrics* **2010**, *125*, 747–755. [CrossRef] [PubMed]
16. Chen, S.Y.; Anderson, S.; Kutty, P.K.; Lugo, F.; McDonald, M.; Rota, P.A.; Ortega-Sanchez, I.R.; Komatsu, K.; Armstrong, G.L.; Sunenshine, R.; et al. Health care-associated measles outbreak in the United States after an importation: Challenges and economic impact. *J. Infect. Dis.* **2011**, *203*, 1517–1525. [CrossRef] [PubMed]

17. Ortega-Sanchez, I.R.; Vijayaraghavan, M.; Barskey, A.E.; Wallace, G.S. The economic burden of sixteen measles outbreaks on United States public health departments in 2011. *Vaccine* **2014**, *32*, 1311–1317. [CrossRef] [PubMed]
18. Wendorf, K.A.; Kay, M.; Ortega-Sanchez, I.R.; Ismael, R.; Munn, M.; Duchin, J.L. Cost of measles containment in an ambulatory pediatric clinic. *Pediatr. Infect. Dis. J.* **2015**, *34*, 589–593. [CrossRef]
19. Pike, J.; Leidner, A.J.; Gastañaduy, P.A. A Review of Measles Outbreak Cost Estimates from the United States in the Postelimination Era (2004–2017): Estimates by Perspective and Cost Type. *Clin. Infect. Dis.* **2020**, *71*, 1568–1576. [CrossRef]
20. Pan American Health Organization. PAHO Urges Rapid Increase in Vaccination Coverage to Stop Spread of Measles in the Americas. Available online: https://www.paho.org/en/news/24-8-2018-paho-urges-rapid-increase-vaccination-coverage-stop-spread-measles-americas (accessed on 25 July 2024).
21. Pan American Health Organization. Regional Framework for the Monitoring and Re-Verification of Measles, Rubella, and Congenital Rubella Syndrome Elimination in the Americas. Available online: https://iris.paho.org/handle/10665.2/55074 (accessed on 25 July 2024).
22. Zucker, J.R.; Rosen, J.B.; Iwamoto, M.; Arciuolo, R.J.; Langdon-Embry, M.; Vora, N.M.; Rakeman, J.L.; Isaac, B.M.; Jean, A.; Asfaw, M.; et al. Consequences of undervaccination—Measles outbreak, New York City, 2018–2019. *N. Engl. J. Med.* **2020**, *382*, 1009–1017. [CrossRef]
23. Terry, L.L. Statement on the status of measles vaccines. *J. Am. Med. Assoc.* **1963**, *183*, 1112–1113.
24. Communicable Disease Center. Recommendations of the Public Health Service Advisory Committee on Immunization Practice. II. Measles vaccine—Status and recommendations for use. *MMWR Morb. Mortal. Wkly. Rep.* **1965**, *14*, 64–67.
25. Communicable Disease Center. Statement prepared by the Public Health Service Advisory Committee on Immunization Practice: The importance of measles and methods for achieving high levels of measles immunization in the community. *MMWR Morb. Mortal. Wkly. Rep.* **1965**, *14*, 310–316.
26. Communicable Disease Center. Recommendations of the Public Health Service Advisory Committee on Immunization Practice. I. Measles vaccines—Status and recommendations for use. *MMWR Morb. Mortal. Wkly. Rep.* **1966**, *15*, 135–137.
27. Communicable Disease Center. Recommendations of the Public Health Service Advisory Committee on Immunization Practice. Measles vaccine. *MMWR Morb. Mortal. Wkly. Rep.* **1967**, *16*, 269–271.
28. Centers for Disease Control. Recommendation of the Public Health Service Advisory Committee on Immunization Practices. *Am. J. Biotechnol.* **1969**, *18*, 124–126.
29. Centers for Disease Control and Prevention. Rubella vaccine—Recommendation of the U.S. Public Health Service Advisory Committee on Immunization Practices. *MMWR Morb. Mortal. Wkly. Rep.* **1977**, *26*, 385–391.
30. Centers for Disease Control. Combination live virus vaccines--measles and rubella, measles mumps and rubella. *MMWR Morb. Mortal. Wkly. Rep.* **1971**, *20*, 145.
31. Centers for Disease Control. Recommendation of the Public Health Service Advisory Committee on Immunization Practices. Measles outbreak control. *MMWR Morb. Mortal. Wkly. Rep.* **1977**, *26*, 294–299.
32. Centers for Disease Control. Recommendation of the Public Health Service Advisory Committee on Immunization Practices. General recommendations on immunization. *MMWR Morb. Mortal. Wkly. Rep.* **1976**, *25*, 349–355.
33. Centers for Disease Control. Recommendation of the Public Health Service Advisory Committee on Immunization Practices. Measles vaccine. *MMWR Morb. Mortal. Wkly. Rep.* **1976**, *25*, 359–365.
34. Centers for Disease Control. Recommendation of the Public Health Service Advisory Committee on Immunization Practices. Measles prevention. *MMWR Morb. Mortal. Wkly. Rep.* **1978**, *27*, 427–435.
35. Centers for Disease Control. Recommendation of the Immunization Practices Advisory Committee. Measles prevention. *MMWR Morb. Mortal. Wkly. Rep.* **1982**, *31*, 217–231.
36. Centers for Disease Control. Recommendations of the Immunization Practices Advisory Committee. Measles prevention. *MMWR Morb. Mortal. Wkly. Rep.* **1987**, *36*, 405–423.
37. Centers for Disease Control. Recommendations of the Immunization Practices Advisory Committee. Measles prevention: Supplementary statement. *MMWR Morb. Mortal. Wkly. Rep.* **1989**, *38*, 1, 11–14.
38. Centers for Disease Control. Recommendations of the Immunization Practices Advisory Committee. Measles prevention. *MMWR Morb. Mortal. Wkly. Rep.* **1989**, *38* (Suppl. S9), 1–18.
39. Centers for Disease Control and Prevention. Measles, mumps, and rubella—Vaccine use and strategies for elimination of measles, rubella, and congenital rubella syndrome and control of mumps. *MMWR Morb. Mortal. Wkly. Rep.* **1998**, *47*, 1–57.
40. Centers for Disease Control and Prevention. Notice to readers: Licensure of a combined live attenuated measles, mumps, rubella, and varicella vaccine. *MMWR Morb. Mortal. Wkly. Rep.* **2005**, *54*, 1212–1214.
41. Centers for Disease Control and Prevention. Recommendations from the Advisory Committee on Immunization Practices (ACIP): Prevention of varicella. *MMWR Morb. Mortal. Wkly. Rep.* **2007**, *56*, 1–40.
42. Centers for Disease Control and Prevention. Update: Recommendations from the Advisory Committee on Immunization Practices (ACIP) regarding administration of combination MMRV vaccine. *MMWR Morb. Mortal. Wkly. Rep.* **2008**, *57*, 258–260.
43. Marin, M.; Broder, K.R.; Temte, J.L.; Snider, D.E.; Seward, J.F. Use of combination measles, mumps, rubella, and varicella vaccine: Recommendations of the Advisory Committee on Immunization Practices (ACIP). *MMWR Recomm. Rep.* **2010**, *59*, 1–12.

44. McLean, H.Q.; Fiebelkorn, A.P.; Temte, J.L.; Wallace, G.S. Prevention of measles, rubella, congenital rubella syndrome, and mumps, 2013: Summary recommendations of the Advisory Committee on Immunization Practices (ACIP). *MMWR Recomm. Rep.* **2013**, *62*, 1–34.
45. Centers for Disease Control and Prevention. Recommended Immunization Schedule for Children and Adolescents Aged 18 Years or Younger, United States. 2017. Available online: https://www.cdc.gov/vaccines/schedules/hcp/imz/child-adolescent.html (accessed on 20 May 2024).
46. Thompson, K.M.; Odahowski, C.L. Systematic review of health economic analyses of measles and rubella immunization interventions. *Risk Anal.* **2016**, *36*, 1297–1314. [CrossRef]
47. Axnick, N.W.; Shavell, S.M.; Witte, J.J. Benefits due to immunization against measles. *Public Health Rep.* **1969**, *84*, 673–680. [CrossRef] [PubMed]
48. Witte, J.J.; Axnick, N.W. The benefits from 10 years of measles immunization in the United States. *Public Health Rep.* **1975**, *90*, 205–207. [PubMed]
49. Albritton, R.B. Cost-benefits of measles eradication: Effects of a federal intervention. *Policy Anal.* **1978**, *4*, 1–21. [PubMed]
50. Bloch, A.B.; Orenstein, W.A.; Stetler, H.C.; Wassilak, S.G.; Amler, R.W.; Bart, K.J.; Kirby, C.D.; Hinman, A.R. Health impact of measles vaccination in the United States. *Pediatrics* **1985**, *76*, 524–532. [CrossRef]
51. White, C.C.; Koplan, J.P.; Orenstein, W.A. Benefits, risks and costs of immunization for measles, mumps and rubella. *Am. J. Public Health* **1985**, *75*, 739–744. [CrossRef]
52. Koplan, J.P.; White, C.C. An update on the benefits and costs of measles and rubella immunization. 1986. In *Immunizing Against Mental Disorders: Progress in the Conquest of Measles and Rubella*; Gruenberg, E.M., Lewis, C., Goldston, S., Eds.; Oxford University Press: Oxford, UK, 1986; pp. 117–127.
53. Davis, R.M.; Markowitz, L.E.; Preblud, S.R.; Orenstein, W.A.; Hinman, A.R. A cost-effectiveness analysis of measles outbreak control strategies. *Am. J. Epidemiol.* **1987**, *126*, 450–459. [CrossRef]
54. Mast, E.E.; Berg, J.L.; Hanrahan, L.P.; Wassell, J.T.; Davis, J.P. Risk factors for measles in a previously vaccinated population and cost-effectiveness of revaccination strategies. *JAMA* **1990**, *264*, 2529–2533. [CrossRef]
55. Shlian, D.M.; Matchar, D.; Seymann, G.B. Cost-effectiveness evaluation of measles immunization strategies on a college campus. *Fam. Pract. Res. J.* **1991**, *11*, 193–207.
56. Chavez, G.F.; Ellis, A.A. Pediatric hospital admissions for measles lessons from the 1990 epidemic. *West. J. Med.* **1996**, *165*, 20–25.
57. Miller, M.A.; Redd, S.; Hadler, S.; Hinman, A. A model to estimate the potential economic benefits of measles eradication for the United States. *Vaccine* **1998**, *16*, 1917–1922. [CrossRef] [PubMed]
58. Zwanziger, J.; Szilagyi, P.G.; Kaul, P. Evaluating the benefits of increasing measles immunization rates. *Health Serv. Res.* **2001**, *36*, 885–909. [PubMed]
59. Sencer, D.J.; Axnick, N.W. Utilization of cost/benefit analysis in planning prevention programs. *Acta Medica Scand.* **1975**, *197*, 123–128. [CrossRef]
60. Hatziandreu, E.J.; Brown, R.E.; Halpern, M.T. A cost-benefit analysis of the measles-mumps-rubella (MMR) vaccine. In *Report Prepared for the National Immunization Program, Centers for Disease Control and Prevention*; Batelle: Arlington, VA, USA, 1994.
61. Schoenbaum, S.C.; Hyde, J.N.J.B.L.; Crampton, K. Benefit-cost analysis of rubella vaccination policy. *N. Engl. J. Med.* **1976**, *294*, 306–310. [CrossRef]
62. Zhou, F.; Reef, S.; Massoudi, M.; Papania, M.J.; Yusuf, H.R.; Bardenheier, B.; Zimmerman, L.; McCauley, M.M. An economic analysis of the current universal 2-dose measles-mumps-rubella vaccination program in the United States. *J. Infect. Dis.* **2004**, *189* (Suppl. S1), S131–S145. [CrossRef]
63. Zhou, F.; Shefer, A.; Wenger, J.; Messonnier, M.; Wang, L.Y.; Lopez, A.; Moore, M.; Murphy, T.V.; Cortese, M.; Rodewald, L. Economic evaluation of the routine childhood immunization program in the United States, 2009. *Pediatrics* **2014**, *133*, 577–585. [CrossRef]
64. Zhou, F.; Jatlaoui, T.C.; Leidner, A.J.; Carter, R.J.; Dong, X.; Santoli, J.M.; Stokley, S.; Daskalakis, D.C.; Peacock, G. Health and economic benefits of routine childhood immunizations in the era of the Vaccines for Children Program —United States, 1994–2023. *MMWR Morb. Mortal. Wkly. Rep.* **2024**, *73*, 682–685. [CrossRef]
65. Thompson, K.M. Evolution and use of dynamic transmission models for measles and rubella. *Risk Anal.* **2016**, *36*, 1383–1403. [CrossRef]
66. Edmunds, W.J.; Medley, G.F.; Nokes, D.J. Evaluating the cost-effectiveness of vaccination programmes: A dynamic perspective. *Stat. Med.* **1999**, *18*, 3263–3282. [CrossRef]
67. Brisson, M.; Edmunds, W.J. Economic evaluation of vaccination programs: The impact of herd-immunity. *Med. Decis. Mak.* **2003**, *23*, 76–82. [CrossRef]
68. Thompson, K.M.; Tebbens, R.J. Retrospective cost-effectiveness analyses for polio vaccination in the United States. *Risk Anal.* **2006**, *26*, 1423–1440. [CrossRef] [PubMed]
69. World Health Organization. WHO guide for standardization of economic evaluations of immunization programmes. In *Geneva: Initiative for Vaccine Research, Department of Immunization, Vaccine, and Biologicals*; Report No.: WHO/IVB/0814; World Health Organization: Geneva, Switzerland, 2008.
70. Pitman, R.; Fisman, D.; Zaric, G.S.; Postma, M.; Kretzschmar, M.; Edmunds, J.; Brisson, M. Dynamic transmission modeling. *Med. Decis. Mak.* **2012**, *32*, 712–721. [CrossRef] [PubMed]

71. Initiative for Vaccine Research of the Department of Immunization Vaccines and Biologicals. In *WHO Guide for Standardization of Economic Evaluations of Immunization Programmes*; World Health Organization: Geneva, Switzerland, 2019.
72. Thompson, K.M.; Badizadegan, N.D. Modeling the transmission of measles and rubella to support global management policy analyses and eradication investment cases. *Risk Anal.* **2017**, *37*, 1109–1131. [CrossRef] [PubMed]
73. Koo, D.T.; Dean, A.G.; Slade, R.W.; Knowles, C.M.; Adams, D.A.; Fortune, W.K.; Hall, P.A.; Fagan, R.F.; Panter-Connah, B.; Holden, H.R.; et al. MMWR Summary of Notifiable Diseases, United States, 1993. *MMWR Morb. Mortal. Wkly. Rep.* **1994**, *42*, 1–73.
74. Population Estimates Program, U.S. Census Bureau Population Division. Historical National Population Estimates: July 1, 1900 to July 1, 1999. Available online: https://www2.census.gov/programs-surveys/popest/tables/1900-1980/national/totals/popclockest.txt (accessed on 24 January 2024).
75. Population Estimates Program, U.S. Census Bureau Population Division. Table 1. Intercensal Estimates of the Resident Population by Sex and Age for the United States: April 1, 2000 to July 1, 2010. Available online: https://www2.census.gov/programs-surveys/popest/tables/2000-2010/intercensal/national/us-est00int-01.xls (accessed on 24 January 2024).
76. Population Estimates Program, U.S. Census Bureau Population Division. Table 1. Annual Estimates of the Resident Population for the United States, Regions, States, and Puerto Rico: April 1, 2010 to July 1, 2016. Available online: https://www2.census.gov/programs-surveys/popest/tables/2010-2016/state/totals/nst-est2016-01.xlsx (accessed on 24 January 2024).
77. Hall-Baker, P.A.; Nieves, E.; Jajosky, R.A.; Adams, D.A.; Sharp, P.; Andersen, W.J.; Aponte, J.J.; Jones, G.F.; Aranas, A.E.; Rey, A.; et al. Summary of Notifiable Diseases—United States, 2007. *MMWR Morb. Mortal. Wkly. Rep.* **2009**, *56*, 1–94.
78. Vaccination News. Reported Measles Cases, Deaths, Death-to-Cases Ratio and Estimated Population United States 1912–1948. Available online: www.vaccinationnews.org/sites/default/files/DailyNews/January2002/CDCMeaslesDataPage1.pdf (accessed on 24 January 2024).
79. Vaccination News. Reported Measles Cases, Deaths, Death-to-Cases Ratio and Estimated Population United States 1949–1984. Available online: www.vaccinationnews.org/sites/default/files/DailyNews/January2002/CDCMeaslesDataPage2.pdf (accessed on 24 January 2024).
80. Centers for Disease Control and Prevention. MMWR: Summary of Notifiable Infectious Diseases. Available online: https://www.cdc.gov/mmwr/mmwr_nd/index.html (accessed on 24 January 2024).
81. Centers for Disease Control and Prevention. Yearly Measles Cases (Data 1985–2024 as of August 31, 2024). Available online: https://www.cdc.gov/measles/data-research/index.html#cdc_data_surveillance_section_5-yearly-measles-cases (accessed on 31 August 2024).
82. Centers for Disease Control and Prevention. CDC WONDER Compressed Mortality File Underlying Cause-Of-Death. Available online: https://wonder.cdc.gov/mortSQL.html (accessed on 24 January 2024).
83. Center for Disease Control. *Measles Surveillance*; Report No 9. Issued August, 1973; DHEW Publication Number 74-8253: Washington, WA, USA, 1973.
84. Barkin, R.M.; Conrad, J.L. Current status of measles in the United States. *J. Infect. Dis.* **1973**, *128*, 353–356. [CrossRef]
85. Hinman, A.R.; Brandling-Bennet, A.D.; Bernier, R.H.; Kirby, C.D.; Eddins, D.L. Current features of measles in the United States: Feasibility of measles elimination. *Epidemiol. Rev.* **1980**, *2*, 153–170. [CrossRef]
86. Harpaz, R. Completeness of measles case reporting: Review of estimates for the United States. *J. Infect. Dis.* **2004**, *189* (Suppl. S1), S185–S190. [CrossRef]
87. Icenogle, J.P.; Frey, T.K.; Abernathy, E.; Reef, S.E.; Schnurr, D.; Stewart, J.A. Genetic analysis of rubella viruses found in the United States between 1966 and 2004: Evidence that indigenous rubella viruses have been eliminated. *Clin. Infect. Dis.* **2006**, *43*, S133–S140. [CrossRef]
88. Rota, J.S.; Rota, P.A.; Redd, S.B.; Redd, S.C.; Pattamadilok, S.; Bellini, W.J. Genetic analysis of measles viruses isolated in the United States, 1995–1996. *J. Infect. Dis.* **1998**, *177*, 204–208. [CrossRef]
89. Thompson, K.M.; Odahowski, C.L.; Goodson, J.L.; Reef, S.E.; Perry, R.T. Synthesis of evidence to characterize national historical measles and rubella exposure and immunization histories. *Risk Anal.* **2016**, *36*, 1427–1458. [CrossRef] [PubMed]
90. Krugman, S.; Giles, J.P.; Jacobs, A.M.; Friedman, H. Studies with a further attenuated live measles-virus vaccine. *Pediatrics* **1963**, *31*, 919–928. [CrossRef] [PubMed]
91. Parkman, P.D. Making vaccination policy: The experience with rubella. *Clin. Infect. Dis.* **1999**, *28* (Suppl. S2), S140–S146. [CrossRef]
92. Hinman, A.R.; Kirby, C.D.; Eddins, D.L.; Orenstein, W.A.; Bernier, R.H.; Turner, P.M.; Bart, K.J. Elimination of indigenous measles from the United States. *Rev. Infect. Dis.* **1983**, *5*, 538–545. [CrossRef] [PubMed]
93. Centers for Disease Control. Measles—U.S. military. *MMWR Morb. Mortal. Wkly. Rep.* **1981**, *30*, 314–315.
94. Grabenstein, J.D.; Pittman, P.R.; Greenwood, J.T.; Engler, R.J.M. Immunization to Protect the US Armed Forces: Heritage, Current Practice, and Prospects. *Epidemiol. Rev.* **2006**, *28*, 3–26. [CrossRef]
95. Bureau of Labor Statistics, U.S. Department of Labor. Consumer Price Index. Available online: http://www.usinflationcalculator.com/inflation/consumer-price-index-and-annual-percent-changes-from-1913-to-2008/ (accessed on 2 June 2024).
96. Sing, M.; Kaye, W.M. An overview of the market and regulatory context. In *Supplying Vaccines: An Economic Analysis of Critical Issues*, 1st ed.; Pauly, M.V., Robinson, C.A., Sepe, S.J., Sing, M., Willian, M.K., Eds.; IOS press: Amsterdam, The Netherlands, 1996; pp. 45–99.

97. 100th U.S. Congress (1987–8). H.R.3545–Omnibus Budget Reconciliation Act of 1987. Available online: https://www.gpo.gov/fdsys/pkg/GOVPUB-T22-aea199473486be343141837068bc0f08/pdf/GOVPUB-T22-aea199473486be343141837068bc0f08-3.pdf (accessed on 24 January 2024).
98. U.S. Department of Health and Human Services, H.S.R.A. About the National Vaccine Injury Compensation Program. Available online: https://www.hrsa.gov/vaccinecompensation/about/index.html (accessed on 24 January 2024).
99. 103rd U.S. Congress (1993–4). H.R.2264–Omnibus Budget Reconciliation Act of 1993. Available online: https://www.congress.gov/bill/103rd-congress/house-bill/2264/text (accessed on 24 January 2024).
100. 105th Congress (1997–8). Public Law 34, Taxpayer Relief Act of 1997. Available online: https://www.gpo.gov/fdsys/pkg/PLAW-105publ34/html/PLAW-105publ34.htm (accessed on 24 January 2024).
101. Ozawa, S.; Clark, S.; Portnoy, A.; Grewal, S.; Brenzel, L.; Walker, D.G. Return on investment from childhood immunization in low- and middle-income countries, 2011–2020. *Health Aff.* **2016**, *35*, 199–207. [CrossRef]
102. Shattock, A.J.; Johnson, H.C.; Sim, S.Y.; Carter, A.; Lambach, P.; Hutubessy, R.C.W.; Thompson, K.M.; Badizadegan, K.; Lambert, B.; Ferrari, M.J.; et al. Contribution of vaccination to improved survival and health: Modelling 50 years of the Expanded Programme on Immunization. *Lancet* **2024**, *403*, 2307–2316. [CrossRef]

*vaccines*

MDPI

*Article*

# Global Status Report for the Verification of Measles and Rubella Elimination, 2022

**Patrick O'Connor [1,*], Balcha Masresha [2], Desirée Pastor [3], Nasrin Musa [4], José Hagan [5], Sudhir Khanal [6], Chung-Won Lee [7] and Natasha Crowcroft [1]**

1 World Health Organization, Headquarters, 1211 Geneva, Switzerland; crowcroftn@who.int
2 World Health Organization, Regional Office for Africa, Brazzaville P.O. Box 06, Congo; masreshab@who.int
3 World Health Organization, Regional Office for Americas, Washington, DC 20037, USA; dpastor@paho.org
4 World Health Organization, Regional Office for the Eastern Mediterranean, Cairo 11371, Egypt; musan@who.int
5 World Health Organization, Regional Office for Europe, 2100 Copenhagen, Denmark; haganj@who.int
6 World Health Organization, Regional Office for South-East Asia, New Delhi 110002, India; khanals@who.int
7 World Health Organization, Regional Office for Western Pacific, Manila 1000, Philippines; leech@who.int
* Correspondence: oconnorp@who.int

**Abstract:** Since the World Health Assembly (WHA) in 2012 endorsed the Global Vaccine Action Plan (GVAP), which included regional measles and rubella elimination goals by 2020, global progress towards verification of measles and rubella elimination has been incremental. Even though the 2020 elimination goals were not achieved, commitment towards achieving measles and rubella elimination has been firmly established in the Immunization Agenda 2030 (IA2030) and the Measles and Rubella Strategic Framework (MRSF) 2021–2030. In 2023, the six Regional Verification Commissions for measles and rubella elimination (RVCs) reviewed data as of 31 December 2022 and confirmed that 82 (42%) Member States have been verified for measles elimination, and 98 (51%) Member States have been verified for rubella elimination. The six RVCs are composed of independent public health and immunization experts who are well-placed to support accelerating measles and rubella elimination. RVCs should be leveraged not only to review elimination documents but also to advocate for and champion public health programming that supports measles and rubella activities. The verification of elimination process is one of many tools that should be deployed to reinforce and accelerate efforts towards achieving a world free of measles and rubella.

**Keywords:** measles; rubella; elimination; verification

## 1. Introduction: History, Background, and Context

There has been considerable progress towards achieving measles and rubella elimination and reducing the burden caused by measles and rubella since the World Health Organization (WHO) convened an expert advisory panel in 2010, which concluded measles can and should be eradicated [1]. In November 2010, the WHO Strategic Advisory Group of Experts on Immunization (SAGE) endorsed the conclusion of the expert advisory panel; and in 2012, the World Health Assembly (WHA) endorsed the Global Vaccine Action Plan (GVAP), which included measles and rubella elimination goals by 2020 [2,3]. The ambitious regional elimination goals of GVAP were not attained and the Region of the Americas (AMR) was the only WHO region to achieve and maintain its regional rubella elimination goal [4,5]. However, the global, regional, and national commitment to achieve these goals continues through the implementation of the Immunization Agenda 2030 (IA2030) and the Measles and Rubella Strategic Framework (MRSF) with the ultimate goal of a world free of measles and rubella [6,7]. Immunization activities aimed at achieving and maintaining measles and rubella elimination will advance the following: (1) the IA2030 goal to prevent 50 million deaths by 2030; modeling estimates that measles vaccine will account for 37% of deaths averted between 2021–2030; and, (2) the MRSF goal to complete the introduction of rubella vaccines into routine immunization schedules and prevent the estimated 32,000 cases of congenital rubella syndrome, which is the leading cause of vaccine-preventable birth defects [8,9].

As of April 2024, all six WHO Regions have Regional Committee resolutions with endorsement by Member States and commitment to achieve measles elimination [10–15]. Because of the range in immunization coverage and disease burden across Member States, the target dates for regional measles elimination goals vary. In addition, five of the six WHO Regions have Regional Committee resolutions with endorsement by Member States and commitment to achieve rubella elimination. The sixth region, WHO Eastern Mediterranean Region (EMR), the final region, is in the process of developing a regional rubella elimination goal that will be presented at a future Regional Committee for consideration and endorsement. Despite not having a rubella elimination goal yet, several countries in the EMR have already been verified for the elimination of rubella. This report provides a global update on the current situation on measles and rubella elimination, challenges, and potentials for acceleration.

## 2. Materials and Methods

The verification statuses of measles and rubella elimination for WHO Member States were reviewed from the meeting reports of the six regional verification commissions (RVCs) that were conducted in 2023. The RVCs reviewed immunization and surveillance data submitted by National Verification Committees (NVCs) as of 31 December 2022. Relevant measles and rubella elimination documents and guidance were also reviewed to provide context and historical perspective. Guidance for the verification of measles and rubella elimination including lines of evidence, suggested composition of RVCs and NVCs, and documentation is outlined in the Weekly Epidemiological Record (WER) report of October 2018 [16].

## 3. Results: Measles and Rubella Elimination Progress 2022

The regional verification commissions (RVCs) are responsible for reviewing the national reports prepared and submitted by the National Verification Committees (NVCs) and provide an assessment of the elimination status for each Member State. The Weekly Epidemiological Record (WER) report of October 2018 provides the most recent guidance on the agreed process for evaluating measles and rubella elimination status [16]. Throughout 2023, all six of the RVCs reviewed the elimination status of the 194 WHO Member States and 11 territories for data ending 31 December 2022. During the COVID-19 pandemic, many of the RVCs held virtual meetings; 2023 was the first year that all the RVCs held in-person meetings:

- the African Regional Verification Commission (AF-RVC) met in May 2023 [17];
- the South-East Asian Regional Verification Commission (SEA-RVC) in June 2023 [18];
- the Western Pacific Regional Verification Commission (WP-RVC) in September 2023 [19];
- the European Regional Verification Commission (EU-RVC) in September 2023 [20];
- the Region of the Americas—measles, rubella, and congenital rubella syndrome post-elimination Regional Monitoring and Re-Verification Commission in November 2023 [21];
- and the Eastern Mediterranean Regional Verification Commission (EM-RVC) in December 2023 [22].

While some of the regions have developed elimination classifications and categories to guide national immunization programmes and provide actionable feedback to Member States, the guidance outlined in the 2018 WER report has four elimination categories: (1) endemic—continuous transmission of measles and/or rubella that persists for greater than or equal to 12 months in any defined geographic area and no previous verification of elimination; (2) eliminated—absence of endemic transmission or a continuous period of greater than or equal to 12 months in the presence of high-quality surveillance systems; (3) verified—no endemic virus transmission for a continuous period of greater than or equal to 36 months in the presence of a high-quality surveillance system and confirmed by the RVC;

and (4) re-established endemic transmission post-verification—the presence of a chain of transmission that continues uninterrupted for greater than or equal to 12 months in a defined geographic area (region or country) after previous verification of elimination [15]. Classifications provided in the 2022 regional verification reports have been aligned with the WER 2018 guidance.

Table 1 summarizes the current measles and rubella elimination status and is based on data as of 31 December 2022. For measles elimination, the results are as follows: 82 (42%) Member States were classified as verified, 21 (11%) Member States were classified as eliminated, 85 (43%) Member States were classified as endemic, 5 (3%) Member States were classified as re-established endemic transmission post-verification, and 1 (1%) Member State did not submit a report for review. For rubella elimination, the results were as follows: 98 (50%) Member States were classified as verified, 13 (7%) Member States were classified as eliminated; 82 (42%) Member States were classified as endemic; no (0%) Member States were classified as re-established endemic transmission post-verification; and 1 (1%) Member State did not submit a report for review.

**Table 1.** Summary of WHO Member States' measles and rubella elimination status by elimination categories and total populations, 2022.

| Category * | Measles Elimination Category (%) | Total Population 2021 (Thousands) † (%) | Rubella Elimination Category (%) | Total Population 2021 (Thousands) † (%) |
|---|---|---|---|---|
| Verified | 82 (42%) | 1,561,166 (20%) | 98 (50%) | 2,214,852 (28%) |
| Eliminated | 21 (11%) | 381,881 (5%) | 13 (7%) | 2622 (<1%) |
| Endemic | 85 (43%) | 5,641,186 (71%) | 82 (42%) | 5,644,853 (71%) |
| Re-established endemic transmission post-verification | 5 (3%) | 278,094 (3%) | 0 (0%) | 0 (0%) |
| No report | 1 (1%) | 8900 (<1%) | 1 (1%) | 8900 (<1%) |
| Total | 194 | 7,871,227 | 194 | 7,871,227 |

Abbreviation: WHO = World Health Organization. [* Categories for classifying the elimination status of countries and territories and definitions are derived from the Weekly Epidemiological Record (WER) 12 October 2018 (93): 544–552 [16]. Guidance for evaluating progress towards elimination of measles and rubella. https://iris.who.int/bitstream/handle/10665/275394/WER9341-544-552.pdf?sequence=1&isAllowed=y (accessed on 30 April 2024). † United Nations, Department of Economic and Social Affairs, Population Division (2022). World Population Prospect 2022, Online Edition. World Population Prospects—Population Division—United Nations].

Analyzing the measles and rubella elimination classifications by total population provides an additional lens on global progress and the challenges particularly for large countries to achieve and maintain measles and rubella elimination [Figure 1]. For measles elimination, the numbers were as follows: 1,561,166,000 (20%) persons reside in Member States classified as verified; 381,881,000 (5%) persons reside in Member States classified as eliminated; 5,641,186,000 (72%) persons reside in Member States classified as endemic; 278,094,000 (4%) persons reside in Member States classified as re-established endemic transmission post-verification; and 8,900,000 (<1%) persons reside in a Member State that did not provide a report. For rubella elimination, the numbers were as follows: 2,214,852,000 (28%) persons reside in Member States classified as verified; 2,622,000 (<1%) persons reside in Member States classified as eliminated; 5,644,853,000 individuals reside in Member States classified as endemic (71%); no (0%) persons reside in Member States classified as re-established endemic transmission post-verification; and 8,900,000 (<1%) persons reside in a Member State that did not provide a report. Tables 2 and 3 summarize the 2022 measles and rubella elimination status by WHO Region and elimination status, respectively. Table 4 summarizes the 2022 measles and rubella elimination status by WHO Member State and national population. Currently, the only regional elimination goal that has been achieved and maintained is rubella elimination in the WHO AMR, which has maintained this status since 2015.

**Table 2.** Summary of measles elimination status by WHO Region and elimination categories, 2022.

| Category * | WHO Region | | | | | |
|---|---|---|---|---|---|---|
| | African Region (AFR) | Region of the Americas (AMR) | Eastern Mediterranean Region (EMR) | European Region (EUR) | South-East Asia Region (SEAR) | Western Pacific Region (WPR) |
| Verified | 0 | 34 | 4 | 33 | 5 | 6 |
| Eliminated | 0 | 0 | 0 | 8 | 0 | 13 |
| Endemic | 47 | 0 | 17 | 9 | 6 | 6 |
| Re-established endemic transmission post-verification | 0 | 1 | 0 | 2 | 0 | 2 |
| No report | 0 | 0 | 0 | 1 | 0 | 0 |
| Total | 47 | 35 | 21 | 53 | 11 | 27 |

Abbreviation: WHO = World Health Organization. [* Categories for classifying the elimination status of countries and territories and definitions are derived from the Weekly Epidemiological Record (WER) 12 October 2018 (93): 544–552 [16]. Guidance for evaluating progress towards elimination of measles and rubella. https://iris.who.int/bitstream/handle/10665/275394/WER9341-544-552.pdf?sequence=1&isAllowed=y] (accessed on 30 April 2024).

**Table 3.** Summary of rubella elimination status by WHO Region and elimination categories, 2022.

| Category * | WHO Region | | | | | |
|---|---|---|---|---|---|---|
| | African Region (AFR) | Region of the Americas (AMR) | Eastern Mediterranean Region (EMR) | European Region (EUR) | South-East Asia Region (SEAR) | Western Pacific Region (WPR) |
| Verified | 0 | 35 | 4 | 49 | 5 | 5 |
| Eliminated | 0 | 0 | 0 | 0 | 0 | 13 |
| Endemic | 47 | 0 | 17 | 3 | 6 | 9 |
| Re-established endemic transmission post-verification | 0 | 0 | 0 | 0 | 0 | 0 |
| No report | 0 | 0 | 0 | 1 | 0 | 0 |
| Total | 47 | 35 | 21 | 53 | 11 | 27 |

Abbreviation: WHO = World Health Organization. [* Categories for classifying the elimination status of countries and territories and definitions are derived from the Weekly Epidemiological Record (WER) 12 October 2018 (93): 544–552 [16]. Guidance for evaluating progress towards elimination of measles and rubella. https://iris.who.int/bitstream/handle/10665/275394/WER9341-544-552.pdf?sequence=1&isAllowed=y (accessed on 30 April 2024)].

**Table 4.** Measles and rubella elimination status of WHO Member State by elimination categories and total population, 2022.

| WHO Member States | WHO Region | Measles Elimination Category 2022 * | Rubella Elimination Category 2022 * | Total Population 2021 (Thousands) † |
|---|---|---|---|---|
| Afghanistan | EMR | | | 40,099 |
| Albania | EUR | | | 2855 |
| Algeria | AFR | | | 44,178 |
| Andorra | EUR | | | 79 |
| Angola | AFR | | | 34,504 |
| Antigua and Barbuda | AMR | | | 93 |
| Argentina | AMR | | | 45,277 |
| Armenia | EUR | | | 2791 |

**Table 4.** *Cont.*

| WHO Member States | WHO Region | Measles Elimination Category 2022 * | Rubella Elimination Category 2022 * | Total Population 2021 (Thousands) † |
|---|---|---|---|---|
| Australia | WPR | | | 25,921 |
| Austria | EUR | | | 8922 |
| Azerbaijan | EUR | | | 10,313 |
| Bahamas, The | AMR | | | 408 |
| Bahrain | EMR | | | 1463 |
| Bangladesh | SEAR | | | 169,356 |
| Barbados | AMR | | | 281 |
| Belarus | EUR | | | 9578 |
| Belgium | EUR | | | 11,611 |
| Belize | AMR | | | 400 |
| Benin | AFR | | | 12,997 |
| Bhutan | SEAR | | | 777 |
| Bolivia, Plurinational State of | AMR | | | 12,079 |
| Bosnia and Herzegovina | EUR | | | 3271 |
| Botswana | AFR | | | 2588 |
| Brazil | AMR | | | 214,326 |
| Brunei Darussalam | WPR | | | 445 |
| Bulgaria | EUR | | | 6886 |
| Burkina Faso | AFR | | | 22,101 |
| Burundi | AFR | | | 12,551 |
| Cabo Verde | AFR | | | 588 |
| Cambodia | WPR | | | 16,589 |
| Cameroon | AFR | | | 27,199 |
| Canada | AMR | | | 38,155 |
| Central African Republic | AFR | | | 5457 |
| Chad | AFR | | | 17,180 |
| Chile | AMR | | | 19,493 |
| China | WPR | | | 1,425,893 |
| Colombia | AMR | | | 51,517 |
| Comoros | AFR | | | 822 |
| Congo, Republic of | AFR | | | 5836 |
| Cook Islands | WPR | | | 17 |
| Costa Rica | AMR | | | 5154 |
| Côte d'Ivoire | AFR | | | 27,478 |
| Croatia | EUR | | | 4060 |
| Cuba | AMR | | | 11,256 |
| Cyprus | EUR | | | 1244 |
| Czechia | EUR | | | 10,511 |
| Democratic People's Republic of Korea | SEAR | | | 25,972 |
| Democratic Republic of the Congo | AFR | | | 95,894 |
| Denmark | EUR | | | 5854 |
| Djibouti | EMR | | | 1106 |
| Dominica | AMR | | | 72 |
| Dominica Republic | AMR | | | 11,118 |
| Ecuador | AMR | | | 17,798 |

**Table 4.** *Cont.*

| WHO Member States | WHO Region | Measles Elimination Category 2022 * | Rubella Elimination Category 2022 * | Total Population 2021 (Thousands) † |
|---|---|---|---|---|
| Egypt, Arab Republic | EMR | | | 109,262 |
| El Salvador | AMR | | | 6314 |
| Equatoria Guinea | AFR | | | 1634 |
| Eritrea | AFR | | | 3620 |
| Estonia | EUR | | | 1329 |
| Eswatini (Swaziland) | AFR | | | 1192 |
| Ethiopia | AFR | | | 120,283 |
| Fiji | WPR | | | 925 |
| Finland | EUR | | | 5536 |
| France | EUR | | | 64,531 |
| Gabon | AFR | | | 2341 |
| Gambia, The | AFR | | | 2640 |
| Georgia | EUR | | | 3758 |
| Germany | EUR | | | 83,409 |
| Ghana | AFR | | | 32,833 |
| Greece | EUR | | | 10,445 |
| Grenada | AMR | | | 125 |
| Guatemala | AMR | | | 17,608 |
| Guinea | AFR | | | 13,532 |
| Guinea-Bissau | AFR | | | 2061 |
| Guyana | AMR | | | 805 |
| Haiti | AMR | | | 11,448 |
| Honduras | AMR | | | 10,278 |
| Hungary | EUR | | | 9710 |
| Iceland | EUR | | | 370 |
| India | SEAR | | | 1,407,564 |
| Indonesia | SEAR | | | 273,753 |
| Iran, Islamic Republic of | EMR | | | 87,923 |
| Iraq | EMR | | | 43,534 |
| Ireland | EUR | | | 4987 |
| Israel | EUR | | | 8900 |
| Italy | EUR | | | 59,240 |
| Jamaica | AMR | | | 2828 |
| Japan | WPR | | | 124,613 |
| Jordan | EMR | | | 11,148 |
| Kazakhstan | EUR | | | 19,196 |
| Kenya | AFR | | | 53,006 |
| Kiribati | WPR | | | 129 |
| Kuwait | EMR | | | 4250 |
| Kyrgyz Republic | EUR | | | 6528 |
| Lao People's Democratic Republic | WPR | | | 7425 |
| Latvia | EUR | | | 1874 |
| Lebanon | EMR | | | 5593 |
| Lesotho | AFR | | | 2281 |
| Liberia | AFR | | | 5193 |
| Libya | EMR | | | 6735 |

**Table 4.** *Cont.*

| WHO Member States | WHO Region | Measles Elimination Category 2022 * | Rubella Elimination Category 2022 * | Total Population 2021 (Thousands) † |
|---|---|---|---|---|
| Lithuania | EUR | | | 2787 |
| Luxembourg | EUR | | | 639 |
| Madagascar | AFR | | | 28,916 |
| Malawi | AFR | | | 19,890 |
| Malaysia | WPR | | | 33,574 |
| Maldives | SEAR | | | 521 |
| Mali | AFR | | | 21,905 |
| Malta | EUR | | | 527 |
| Marshall Islands | WPR | | | 42 |
| Mauritania | AFR | | | 4615 |
| Mauritius | AFR | | | 1299 |
| Mexico | AMR | | | 126,705 |
| Micronesia, Federated States of | WPR | | | 113 |
| Monaco | EUR | | | 37 |
| Mongolia | WPR | | | 3348 |
| Montenegro | EUR | | | 628 |
| Morocco | EMR | | | 37,077 |
| Mozambique | AFR | | | 32,077 |
| Myanmar | SEAR | | | 53,798 |
| Namibia | AFR | | | 2530 |
| Nauru | WPR | | | 13 |
| Nepal | SEAR | | | 30,035 |
| Netherlands, The Kingdom of the | EUR | | | 17,502 |
| New Zealand | WPR | | | 5130 |
| Nicaragua | AMR | | | 6851 |
| Niger | AFR | | | 25,253 |
| Nigeria | AFR | | | 213,401 |
| Niue | WPR | | | 2 |
| North Macedonia | EUR | | | 2103 |
| Norway | EUR | | | 5403 |
| Oman | EMR | | | 4520 |
| Pakistan | EMR | | | 231,402 |
| Palau | WPR | | | 18 |
| Panama | AMR | | | 4351 |
| Papua New Guinea | WPR | | | 9949 |
| Paraguay | AMR | | | 6704 |
| Peru | AMR | | | 33,715 |
| Philippines | WPR | | | 113,880 |
| Poland | EUR | | | 38,308 |
| Portugal | EUR | | | 10,290 |
| Qatar | EMR | | | 2688 |
| Republic of Korea | WPR | | | 51,830 |
| Republic of Moldova | EUR | | | 3062 |
| Romania | EUR | | | 19,329 |
| Russian Federation | EUR | | | 154,103 |

**Table 4.** *Cont.*

| WHO Member States | WHO Region | Measles Elimination Category 2022 * | Rubella Elimination Category 2022 * | Total Population 2021 (Thousands) † |
|---|---|---|---|---|
| Rwanda | AFR | | | 13,462 |
| Saint Kitts and Nevis | AMR | | | 48 |
| Saint Lucia | AMR | | | 180 |
| Saint Vincent and the Grenadines | AMR | | | 104 |
| Samoa | WPR | | | 219 |
| San Marino | EUR | | | 34 |
| Sao Tome and Principe | AFR | | | 223 |
| Saudi Arabia | EMR | | | 35,950 |
| Senegal | AFR | | | 16,877 |
| Serbia | EUR | | | 7297 |
| Seychelles | AFR | | | 106 |
| Sierra Leone | AFR | | | 8421 |
| Singapore | WPR | | | 5941 |
| Slovakia | EUR | | | 5448 |
| Slovenia | EUR | | | 2119 |
| Solomon Islands | WPR | | | 708 |
| Somalia | EMR | | | 17,066 |
| South Africa | AFR | | | 59,392 |
| South Sudan | AFR | | | 10,748 |
| Spain | EUR | | | 47,487 |
| Sri Lanka | SEAR | | | 21,773 |
| Sudan | EMR | | | 45,657 |
| Suriname | AMR | | | 613 |
| Sweden | EUR | | | 10,467 |
| Switzerland | EUR | | | 8691 |
| Syrian Arab Republic | EMR | | | 21,324 |
| Tajikistan | EUR | | | 9750 |
| Tanzania, United Republic of | AFR | | | 63,588 |
| Thailand | SEAR | | | 71,601 |
| Timor-Leste | SEAR | | | 1321 |
| Togo | AFR | | | 8645 |
| Tonga | WPR | | | 106 |
| Trinidad and Tobago | AMR | | | 1526 |
| Tunisia | EMR | | | 12,263 |
| Türkiye | EUR | | | 84,775 |
| Turkmenistan | EUR | | | 6342 |
| Tuvalu | WPR | | | 11 |
| Uganda | AFR | | | 45,854 |
| Ukraine | EUR | | | 43,531 |
| United Arab Emirates | EMR | | | 9365 |
| United Kingdom of Great Britain and Northern Ireland | EUR | | | 67,281 |
| United States of America | AMR | | | 336,998 |
| Uruguay | AMR | | | 3426 |

**Table 4.** *Cont.*

| WHO Member States | WHO Region | Measles Elimination Category 2022 * | Rubella Elimination Category 2022 * | Total Population 2021 (Thousands) † |
|---|---|---|---|---|
| Uzbekistan | EUR | | | 34,081 |
| Vanuatu | WPR | | | 319 |
| Venezuela ‡ | AMR | | | 28,200 |
| Vietnam | WPR | | | 97,468 |
| Yemen | EMR | | | 32,982 |
| Zambia | AFR | | | 19,473 |
| Zimbabwe | AFR | | | 15,994 |
| **Territory/Region** | **WHO Region** | **Measles Elimination Category 2022 *** | **Rubella Elimination Category 2022 *** | **Total, Population 2021 (Thousands), †** |
| American Samoa (US) | WPR | | | 45 |
| French Polynesia (France) | WPR | | | 304 |
| Guam (US) | WPR | | | 171 |
| Hong Kong SAR (China) | WPR | | | 7495 |
| Macao SAR (China) | WPR | | | 687 |
| New Caledonia (France) | WPR | | | 288 |
| Northern Mariana Islands (US) | WPR | | | 49 |
| Occupied Palestinian Territories | EMR | | | 5133 |
| Pitcairn Islands (UK) | WPR | | | 0,§ |
| Tokelau (New Zealand) | WPR | | | 2 |
| Wallis and Futuna (France) | WPR | | | 12 |

| Category * | Definition | Code |
|---|---|---|
| Endemic | Continuous transmission of measles and/or rubella that persists for ≥12 months in any defined geographical area and no previous verification of elimination. | |
| Eliminated | Absence of endemic transmission for a continuous period of ≥12 months in the presence of a high-quality surveillance system. | |
| Verified | Verification of elimination for a region requires that all countries in the region document interruption of endemic virus transmission for a period of ≥36 months. | |
| Re-established endemic transmission post-verification | Presence of a chain of transmission that continues uninterrupted for ≥12 months in a defined geographical area (region or country) after previous verification of elimination. | |
| No report | National Verification Committee annual report not provided to the Regional Verification Commission for review | |

Abbreviation: AFR = African Region; AMR = Region of Americas; EMR = Eastern Mediterranean Region; EUR = European Region, SAR = special administrative region SEAR = South-East Asia Region; UK = United Kingdom of Great Britain and Northern Ireland; US = United States of American, WPR = Western Pacific Region; WHO = World Health Organization. [* Categories for classifying the elimination status of countries and territories and definitions are derived from the Weekly Epidemiological Record (WER) 12 October 2018 (93): 544–552 [16]. Guidance for evaluating progress towards elimination of measles and rubella. https://iris.who.int/bitstream/handle/10665/275394/WER9341-544-552.pdf?sequence=1&isAllowed=y (accessed on 30 April 2024). † United Nations, Department of Economic and Social Affairs, Population Division (2022). World Population Prospect 2022, Online Edition. World Population Prospects—Population Division—United Nations. ‡ Re-verification of Venezuela at the Pan American Health Organization (PAHO)/World Health Organization (WHO) Region of the Americas, third annual meeting of the measles, rubella, and congenital rubella syndrome post-elimination Regional Monitoring and Re-Verification Commission held from 14–16 November 2023 and include a review of data from the first semester of 2023. § Only 50 permanent inhabitants—source: Government of The Pitcairn Islands http://www.government.pn/gpi-policies (accessed on 11 July 2024)].

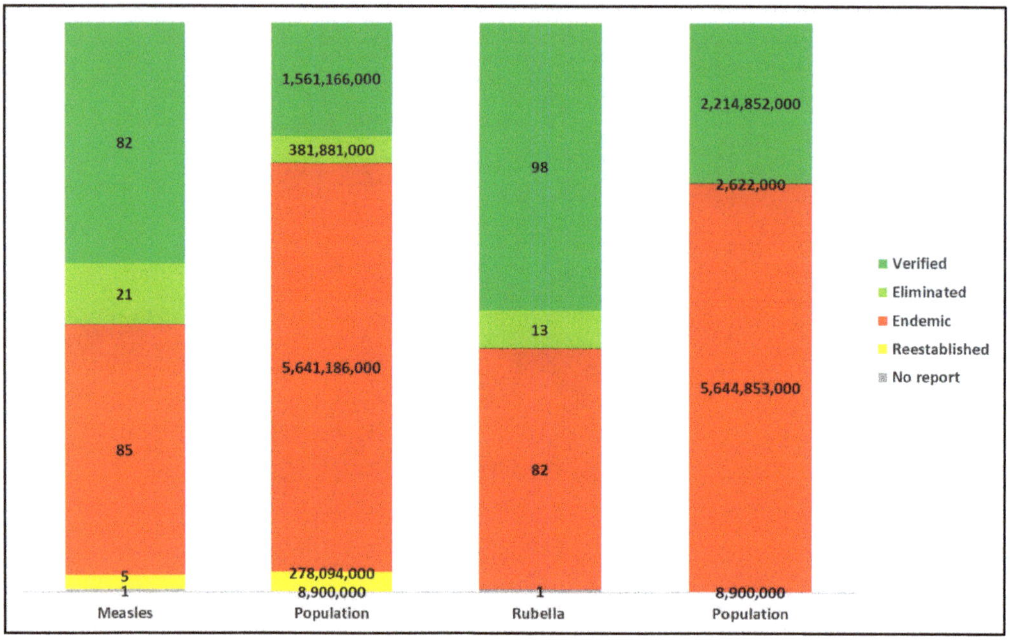


**Figure 1.** Measles and rubella elimination categories * by number of WHO Member States and total population †, 2022. Abbreviation: WHO = World Health Organization. [* Categories for classifying the elimination status of countries and territories and definitions are derived from the Weekly Epidemiological Record (WER) 12 October 2018 (93): 544–552 [16]. Guidance for evaluating progress towards elimination of measles and rubella. https://iris.who.int/bitstream/handle/10665/275394/WER9341-544-552.pdf?sequence=1&isAllowed=y (accessed on 30 April 2024). † United Nations, Department of Economic and Social Affairs, Population Division (2022). World Population Prospect 2022, Online Edition. World Population Prospects—Population Division—United Nations].

## 4. Discussion: Accelerating Verification of Measles and Rubella Elimination

While the regional measles and rubella elimination goals outlined in the GVAP and endorsed by the WHA were not fully achieved by 2020 [4], there has been progress toward achieving and maintaining elimination: 42% of Member States have been verified for measles elimination and 51% of Member States have been verified for rubella elimination. The challenges towards achieving measles and rubella elimination can be categorized into two main groups: (1) interrupting endemic transmission supported by a well-performing measles and rubella surveillance system, and (2) documenting elimination for verification.

First, interrupting endemic transmission of measles and rubella requires high, uniform, and equitable immunization coverage. Ensuring that all Member States have routine immunization programs with two doses of a measles and rubella vaccine is critical. As of the beginning of 2024, there are 19 Member States that need to fully introduce a rubella vaccine and four Member States that need to introduce a second measles vaccine into their national immunization program [23]. Completing this work is critical to establishing equitable conditions, ensuring that all eligible individuals have access to measles and rubella vaccines, and achieving high immunity to these viruses. Reaching 95% coverage with two routine doses of measles and rubella vaccines is a global challenge and when that target is not achieved in a single year or over many years, immunization gaps can emerge, resulting in an increasing risk of measles outbreaks.

Developing timely, regular opportunities to catch up and deliver doses missed by the routine program is critical to having population immunity high enough to stop endemic transmission and prevent the morbidity and mortality associated with measles and rubella infections. These opportunities may take different forms in different places: enhanced routine immunization sessions with record or immunization card review, call-back services, and defaulter tracing; mobile and outreach immunization services to communities with limited access; targeted immunization campaigns for specific geographic locations, age groups, or occupations; and large-scale, non-selective nationwide campaigns. Initiatives like the *Big Catch-up* and strategies to expand eligibility have been developed to support the post-COVID-19 pandemic recovery of immunization services and ensure that missed routine doses are received [24,25]. In addition to the doses provided by routine immunization programs and regular catch-up opportunities, robust outbreak preparedness and response will be necessary to interrupt chains of transmission and rapidly boost population immunity. Immunization activities need to be complemented by well-performing, sensitive, laboratory-supported measles and rubella surveillance systems.

Secondly, adequately documenting elimination for verification can be challenging and requires an in-depth analysis of current and historical data to develop a national report that follows the five lines of evidence for verifying elimination: (1) detailed description of the current and past epidemiology of measles, rubella, and congenital rubella syndrome (CRS); (2) analysis of molecular epidemiology to document viral transmission patterns and the duration of circulation of viruses of specific lineages; (3) quality of surveillance and monitoring systems for measles, rubella, and CRS; (4) population immunity presented as a birth cohort analysis, with subanalysis on adults, underserved communities, migrants, and refugee groups; and, (5) accountability, ownership, and political commitment [15].

The national-level report needs to be submitted to the RVC by an established, functioning NVC with a supporting secretariat. The initial documentation and subsequent analysis to demonstrate interruption of virus transmission can be time-consuming and has in many Member States been supported by global and regional measles and rubella partners. Even countries that may be far from achieving measles and rubella elimination can benefit from the process of preparing verification documents and having the NVC submit a report to the RVC for review. It is an opportunity for an annual review of the national immunization program, surveillance system, and outbreak response by a group of independent public health and immunization experts and should be leveraged as an important tool for accelerating elimination by national public health programs. Additionally, there are Member States with well-performing immunization programs, robust laboratory-supported vaccine-preventable disease surveillance systems, and rapid outbreak response mechanisms that have probably already interrupted endemic transmission but are missing an NVC and/or a report outlining progress. Additional technical support and advocacy may be needed to assist Member States in completing this required documentation.

The achievement in the Region of the Americas (AMR) of regional rubella elimination in 2015 and measles elimination in 2016 demonstrates that the tools for achieving elimination exist. While the use of innovations and new technologies such as measles–rubella rapid diagnostic tests and measle–rubella patch vaccines may help with accelerating progress, efforts to achieve and maintain the current elimination goals should not be delayed. The Region of the Americas also showed that maintaining regional measles elimination is difficult. Unfortunately, importations and ongoing chains of transmission ultimately resulted in the loss of the regional measles elimination status in 2018. It is important to recognize that measles and rubella elimination is a dynamic process [26]. Member States might find it challenging to interrupt endemic transmission for 12 months, or might achieve elimination and interrupt transmission for greater than 12 months but are unable to maintain it for 36 months to be verified, or might interrupt endemic transmission and are verified but re-establish transmission due to importations with transmission that lasts more than 12 months. The verification of measles and rubella elimination should not be seen as something to be achieved and forgotten, but as an ongoing process that requires high-level political and technical engagement and commitment.

The re-establishment of endemic transmission illustrates the need for a well-crafted national post-verification sustainability plan. While the WHO Regions and Member States are at different points on the pathway or stages towards measles and rubella elimination, maintaining focus on the ultimate goals of achieving a world free of measles and rubella should guide our current efforts towards improving routine immunization coverage, introducing a rubella vaccine and a second opportunity for a measles vaccine, planning regular supplementary activities to fill immunity gaps, and rapidly responding to outbreaks. The RVCs and NVCs are composed of independent public health and immunization experts who are well-placed to support accelerating measles and rubella elimination. RVCs and NVCs should be leveraged not only to develop and review elimination documents but also to advocate for and champion public health programming that supports all measles and rubella activities. The verification of elimination process is one of many tools that should be deployed to reinforce the efforts towards achieving a world free of measles and rubella.

**Author Contributions:** Writing—original draft, P.O.; Writing—review & editing, P.O., B.M., D.P., N.M., J.H., S.K., C.-W.L. and N.C. All authors have read and agreed to the published version of the manuscript.

**Funding:** This research received no external funding.

**Institutional Review Board Statement:** Not applicable.

**Informed Consent Statement:** Not applicable.

**Data Availability Statement:** The data presented in this study are available in this article.

**Conflicts of Interest:** The authors declare no conflicts of interest.

## References

1. World Health Organization. Proceedings of the global technical consultation to assess the feasibility of measles eradication, 28–30 July 2010. *J. Infect. Dis.* **2011**, *204* (Suppl. S1), S4–S13. [CrossRef] [PubMed]
2. World Health Organization. Meeting of the Strategic Advisory Group of Experts on Immunization, November 2010 Summary, Conclusions, and Recommendations. *Wkly. Epidemiol. Rec. (WER)* **2011**, *86*, 1–16. Available online: https://iris.who.int/bitstream/handle/10665/241695/WER8601_02_1-16.pdf?sequence=1 (accessed on 30 April 2024).
3. World Health Organization. *Sixty-Fifth World Health Assembly*; World Health Organization: Geneva, Switzerland, 2012. Available online: http://apps.who.int/gb/DGNP/pdf_files/A65_REC1-en.pdf (accessed on 30 April 2024).
4. World Health Organization. *Global Vaccine Action Plan 2011–2020*; World Health Organization: Geneva, Switzerland, 2013. Available online: https://www.who.int/publications/i/item/global-vaccine-action-plan-2011-2020 (accessed on 30 April 2024).
5. World Health Organization. *Global Vaccine Action Plan Monitoring, Evaluation & Accountability: Secretariat Annual Report 2020*; World Health Organization: Geneva, Switzerland, 2020. Available online: https://www.who.int/publications/i/item/global-vaccine-action-plan-monitoring-evaluation-accountability-secretariat-annual-report-2020 (accessed on 30 April 2024).
6. World Health Organization. *Immunization Agenda 2030: A Global Strategy to Leave No One Behind*; World Health Organization: Geneva, Switzerland, 2020. Available online: https://www.who.int/publications/m/item/immunization-agenda-2030-a-global-strategy-to-leave-no-one-behind (accessed on 30 April 2024).
7. World Health Organization. *Measles and Rubella Strategic Framework: 2021–2030*; World Health Organization: Geneva, Switzerland, 2020. Available online: https://www.who.int/publications/i/item/measles-and-rubella-strategic-framework-2021-2030 (accessed on 30 April 2024).
8. Carter, A.; Msemburi, W.; Sim, S.Y.; Gaythorpe, K.A.M.; Lambach, P.; Lindstrand, A.; Hutubessy, R. Modeling the impact of vaccination for the Immunization Agenda 2030: Deaths averted due to vaccination against 14 pathogens in 194 countries from 2021 to 2030. *Vaccine* **2023**, *42*, S28–S37. [CrossRef] [PubMed]
9. Vynnycky, E.; Knapp, J.K.; Papdopoulos, T.; Cutts, F.T.; Hachiya, M.; Miyano, S.; Reef, S.E. Estimates of the global burden of Congenital Rubella Syndrome, 1996–2019. *Int. J. Infect. Dis.* **2023**, *137*, 149–156. [CrossRef] [PubMed] [PubMed Central]
10. Pan American Health Organization. *24th Pan American Sanitary Conference*; CSP24. R16, CD38; Pan American Health Organization: Washington, DC, USA, 1994. Available online: http://iris.paho.org/bitstream/handle/10665.2/57514/CSP24-res_eng.pdf?sequence=1&isAllowed=y (accessed on 30 April 2024).
11. World Health Organization. *Sixty-First Session of the WHO Regional Committee for Africa*; AFR/RC6/R1; World Health Organization, Regional Office for Africa: Brazzaville, Congo, 2011. Available online: http://iris.who.int/bitstream/handle/10665/259610/AFR-RC61-R1-eng.pdf?sequence=1&isAllowed=y (accessed on 30 April 2024).

12. World Health Organization. *Sixty-Second Session of the Regional Committee for the Eastern Mediterranean*; EM/RC62/6; World Health Organization, Regional Office for Eastern Mediterranean: Cairo, Egypt, 2015. Available online: https://applications.emro.who.int/docs/RC_final_Rep_2015_16735_EN.pdf?ua=1 (accessed on 30 April 2024).
13. World Health Organization. *Sixty-Fourth Session of the WHO Regional Committee for Europe*; EUR/RC64/R5; World Health Organization, Regional Office for Europe: Copenhagen, Denmark, 2014. Available online: http://iris.who.int/bitstream/handle/10665/337451/64rp00e-Rep-140754.pdf?sequence=1&isAllowed=y (accessed on 30 April 2024).
14. World Health Organization. *Seventy-Second Session of the Regional Committee*; SEA/RC72/R3; World Health Organization, Regional Office for South-East Asia: New Delhi, India, 2019. Available online: http://iris.who.int/bitstream/handle/10665/327923/sea-rc72-r3-eng.pdf?sequence=1 (accessed on 30 April 2024).
15. World Health Organization. *Sixty-Eighth Session of the Regional Committee*; WPR/RC68.R1; World Health Organization, Regional Office for the Western Pacific: Manila, Philippines, 2017. Available online: http://iris.who.int/bitstream/handle/10665/361628/WPR-RC068-Res01-2017-en.pdf (accessed on 30 April 2024).
16. World Health Organization. Guidance for evaluating progress towards elimination of measles and rubella. *Wkly. Epidemiol. Rec. (WER)* **2018**, *93*, 541–552. Available online: https://iris.who.int/bitstream/handle/10665/275394/WER9341-544-552.pdf?sequence=1&isAllowed=y (accessed on 30 April 2024).
17. World Health Organization, Regional Office for Africa. *Proceedings of the 3rd Meeting of the African Regional Commission for the Verification of Measles Elimination (RVC)*; World Health Organization: Geneva, Switzerland, 2023.
18. World Health Organization, Regional Office for South-East Asia. *Eighth Meeting of the WHO South-East Asia Regional Verification Commission for Measles and Rubella*; World Health Organization: Geneva, Switzerland, 2023. Available online: http://iris.who.int/handle/10665/370787 (accessed on 24 June 2024).
19. World Health Organization, Regional Office for the Western Pacific. *Eleventh Annual Meeting of the Regional Verification Commission for Measles and Rubella Elimination in the Western Pacific*; World Health Organization: Geneva, Switzerland, 2023.
20. World Health Organization, Regional Office for Europe. *Twelfth Meeting of the European Regional Verification Commission for Measles and Rubella*; World Health Organization: Geneva, Switzerland, 2023. Available online: https://iris.who.int/bitstream/handle/10665/376606/WHO-EURO-2024-9722-49494-74055-eng.pdf?sequence=1 (accessed on 24 June 2024).
21. Pan American Health Organization; World Health Organization, Regional Office of the Americas. *Third Annual Meeting of the Measles and Rubella and Congenital Rubella Syndrome Post Elimination Regional Monitoring and Re-verification Commission (Virtual)*; Pan American Health Organization; World Health Organization, Regional Office of the Americas: Washington, DC, USA, 2023.
22. World Health Organization, Regional Office for the Eastern Mediterranean. *Sixth Meeting of the Regional Verification Commission of Measles and Rubella Elimination in the Eastern Mediterranean Region*; World Health Organization: Geneva, Switzerland, 2024. Available online: https://iris.who.int/bitstream/handle/10665/376390/WHOEMEPI363E-eng.pdf?sequence=1&isAllowed=y (accessed on 18 June 2024).
23. World Health Organization. *Vaccination Schedule for Measles, Vaccination Schedule for Rubella*; World Health Organization: Geneva, Switzerland, 2024. Available online: https://immunizationdata.who.int/global?topic=Vaccination-schedule&location= (accessed on 30 April 2024).
24. World Health Organization. *The Big Catch-Up: An Essential Immunization Recovery Plan for 2023 and Beyond*; World Health Organization: Geneva, Switzerland; The United Nations Children's Fund (UNICEF): New York, NY, USA, 2023. Available online: https://www.who.int/publications/i/item/9789240075511 (accessed on 13 May 2024).
25. World Health Organization. *Leave No One Behind: Guidance for Planning and Implementing Catch-Up Vaccination–Working Draft*; World Health Organization: Geneva, Switzerland, 2020. Available online: https://www.who.int/docs/default-source/immunization/catch-up/who-catch-up-guidance-working-draft-11-08-20.pdf?sfvrsn=6d65982a_4 (accessed on 13 May 2024).
26. Winter, A.K.; Lambert, B.; Klein, D.; Klepac, P.; Papadopoulos, T.; Truelove, S.; Burgess, C.; Santos, H.; Knapp, J.K.; Reef, S.E.; et al. Feasibility of measles and rubella vaccination programmes for disease elimination: A modelling study. *Lancet Glob. Health* **2022**, *10*, e1412–e1422. [CrossRef] [PubMed] [PubMed Central]

*vaccines*

MDPI

*Article*

# Tracking Measles and Rubella Elimination Progress—World Health Organization African Region, 2022–2023

**Balcha G. Masresha [1,*], Charles Shey Wiysonge [1], Reggis Katsande [1], Patrick Michael O'Connor [2], Emmaculate Lebo [3] and Robert T. Perry [3]**

[1] WHO Regional Office for Africa, Brazzaville P.O. Box 06, Congo; sheyc@who.int (C.S.W.)
[2] WHO Headquarters, 1211 Geneva, Switzerland; oconnorp@who.int
[3] US Centers for Disease Control, Atlanta, GA 30333, USA; rmp9@cdc.gov (R.T.P.)
* Correspondence: masreshab@who.int

**Abstract:** Measles or rubella elimination is verified when endemic transmission of the corresponding virus has been absent for over 36 months in a defined area, in the presence of a well-performing surveillance system. This report updates the progress by 47 countries in the WHO African Region towards the goal of attaining verification of measles and rubella elimination in at least 80% of the countries of the region by 2030. We reviewed the WHO-UNICEF vaccination coverage estimates for the first and second doses of measles- and measles-rubella-containing vaccines, as well as the available coverage data for measles supplementary immunization activities, during 2022–2023. We also reviewed the measles-surveillance performance and analyzed the epidemiological trends of measles and rubella as reported in the case-based surveillance database. The WHO-UNICEF estimates of first measles vaccine dose (MCV1) and second measles vaccine dose (MCV2) coverage for the African Region for 2022 were 69% and 45%, respectively. Rubella-containing vaccines have been introduced in the routine immunization program in 32 of 47 (68%) countries as of the end of 2022, with no introductions during 2023. In 2022 and 2023, a total of 144,767,764 children were vaccinated in the region with measles or MR vaccines in 24 countries through 32 mass vaccination campaigns. The administrative coverage target of 95% was reached in only 15 (49%) of the 32 vaccination campaigns. In 2023, a total of 125,957 suspected cases of measles were reported through the case-based surveillance system, and 73,625 cases (58%) were confirmed to be measles, either by laboratory testing, by epidemiological linkage, or based on clinical compatibility. A total of 4805 confirmed rubella cases were reported, though this total represents substantial under-ascertainment. The regional incidence of measles was 60.3 cases per million population. Twenty-six countries (55%) met the targets for the two principal surveillance system performance-monitoring indicators. No country in the region has attained the verification of measles or rubella elimination as of the end of 2023. Addressing systemic problems with routine immunization and using tailored approaches to reach unvaccinated children can contribute to progress towards measles and rubella elimination. In addition, periodic and timely high-quality preventive SIAs remain a critical programmatic strategy to reach unvaccinated children.

**Keywords:** measles; rubella; elimination; Africa; vaccination; coverage; surveillance

## 1. Introduction

In 2011, the 46 member states (South Sudan joined the WHO African Region in 2012) in the WHO African Region adopted the goal of measles elimination by 2020, with programmatic targets including ≥95% coverage with two doses of measles-containing vaccine (MCV) at national and district levels through routine immunization or supplementary immunization activities (SIAs); a confirmed annual measles incidence of less than one case per million population; and case-based measles-rubella surveillance performance that meets the performance targets [1]. Countries would be verified as having eliminated measles or rubella when endemic transmission of the corresponding virus has been absent for over 36 months, in the presence of a well-performing surveillance system [2]. However, by the end of 2020, none of the countries in the region had been verified for measles or rubella elimination.

In 2021, as part of the strategic framework of implementation of the Immunization Agenda 2030 (IA2030), the regional goal was revised to attaining verification of measles and rubella elimination in at least 80% of the countries of the region by 2030 [3].

In 2020 and 2021, during the COVID-19 pandemic, many countries in the African Region and beyond experienced a decline in immunization coverage and surveillance performance [4]. In addition, scheduled introduction of rubella vaccine and second dose of measles or measles-rubella (MR) vaccines were delayed in some countries, and scheduled measles and MR campaigns were postponed, leading to increasing immunity gaps among vulnerable populations [5].

Despite the efforts to strengthen the routine immunization, the regional coverage with the first MCV dose has remained stagnant over the last decade [6].

This report describes progress towards the regional measles- and rubella-elimination goals, updating an earlier report covering measles-elimination through 2021 [7].

## 2. Methods

We reviewed the WHO-UNICEF vaccination coverage estimates for the first and second doses of MCV, which were available at the time of this analysis only for the year 2022, as well as the available coverage data from 2022 and 2023 for supplementary immunization activities utilizing measles- and measles-rubella-containing vaccines. We also reviewed measles-surveillance performance and analyzed the epidemiological trends of measles as reported in the case-based surveillance database. In addition, we reviewed country progress to establish national verification committees and reports of meetings of the Regional Verification Commission to assess progress in countries towards achieving measles or rubella verification.

WHO and UNICEF generate country-specific annual estimates of vaccination coverage for all antigens, including for the first and second measles-containing vaccine doses (MCV1 and MCV2, respectively) delivered through routine immunization services [8].

Countries are recommended to conduct measles or measles-rubella SIAs (implemented through a mass vaccination campaign effort) before the estimated number of children under five years of age and susceptible to measles approaches the size of one birth cohort. Countries are requested to report the timing, target age range and geographic areas targeted (if not nationwide), and administrative coverage, defined as the number of doses delivered during the campaign divided by the estimated target population. Coverage should also be documented through a high-quality post-campaign coverage survey [9].

All 47 countries in the African Region implement case-based measles surveillance and are expected to provide data on suspected and confirmed cases to the WHO on a weekly basis. Suspected measles cases are investigated at district level, with the investigation including relevant epidemiological information using a standard case investigation form and the collection of serum specimens for serological testing [10]. Testing is done in one of the 52 serological laboratories in the 43 countries of the regional measles laboratory network. Laboratories are regularly accredited to meet performance standards by the WHO Global Measles and Rubella Laboratory Network (GMRLN) [11].

Case-based surveillance performance is regularly monitored using standard performance indicators against annual targets such as the number of discarded cases of non-measles febrile rash illness per 100,000 population annually (target: two or more per year), and the proportion of districts reporting at least one suspected case with the collection of a blood specimen (target: $\geq$80% of districts per year) [10].

A confirmed case of measles is a suspected case testing positive for measles-specific IgM antibody who had not received measles vaccination within 30 days before the specimen collection, or a suspected case with epidemiological linkage to a laboratory-confirmed case of measles during a confirmed outbreak period, or a suspected case clinically compatible but not investigated with a lab specimen or linked to an outbreak [10].

Some national serological laboratories conduct rubella IgM testing for all measles seronegative specimens, while others run the tests in parallel. Therefore, the measles-surveillance system also generates data on the epidemiology of rubella in the countries.

In addition to serum specimens for IgM testing, surveillance officers are expected to collect throat swab specimens from patients with acute cases of measles and rubella to send to designated virological laboratories to identify and characterize the circulating viral strains.

For some countries, we also reviewed data on measles cases from aggregate reporting systems. Reports give the number of reported suspected measles cases weekly and by health district. These countries, generally with large disease burdens, officially report aggregate numbers of suspected measles cases to WHO and UNICEF during the annual joint reporting process.

## 3. Results

### *3.1. Coverage through Routine Immunization*

The WHO UNICEF estimate of MCV1 coverage for the African Region for 2022 was 69% (increasing from 68% in 2021), while the estimate of MCV2 coverage was 45% (increasing from 41% in 2021). Five countries reported ≥95% MCV1 coverage in 2022 (Cabo Verde, Ghana, Mauritius, Rwanda, and Seychelles). Comparing the 2022 MCV1 coverage estimates against those for 2021, 18 countries documented increased coverage. The increase was >5 percentage points in six countries, Guinea Bissau, Liberia, Mauritania, Mauritius, Rwanda, and Tanzania, with Liberia increasing by 21 points, from 58% in 2021 to 79% in 2022. On the other hand, 13 countries had lower MCV1 coverage levels in 2022. The coverage decline was more than five percentage points in Botswana, Gabon, Lesotho, Malawi, Niger, and Senegal, with the biggest decline of 15% points documented in Niger. MCV1 coverage in 2022 remained the same as the estimates for 2021 in 16 countries (Table 1).

**Table 1.** Measles vaccination first dose and second dose coverage by country, and year of rubella vaccine introduction. African Region. WHO-UNICEF coverage estimates, 2022.

| Country | 2022 | | 2021 | | Year of Rubella Vaccine Introduction |
|---|---|---|---|---|---|
| | MCV1 | MCV2 | MCV1 | MCV2 | |
| Algeria | 79% | 71% | 79% | 73% | 2013 |
| Angola | 37% | 25% | 36% | 22% | 2017 |
| Benin | 68% | | 68% | | 2018 |
| Botswana | 90% | 77% | 97% | 70% | 2015 |
| Burkina Faso | 88% | 71% | 88% | 71% | 2014 |
| Burundi | 89% | 85% | 90% | 85% | 2016 |
| Cabo Verde | 95% | 86% | 95% | 86% | 2009 |
| Cameroon | 65% | 44% | 62% | 35% | 2014 |
| Central African Republic | 41% | | 41% | | |
| Chad | 56% | 2% | 55% | | |
| Comoros | 86% | 79% | 90% | 19% | 2021 |
| Congo | 65% | 34% | 68% | 31% | 2018 |
| Côte d'Ivoire | 65% | 20% | 68% | 1% | 2017 |
| DR Congo | 56% | | 55% | | |

**Table 1.** *Cont.*

| Country | 2022 | | 2021 | | Year of Rubella Vaccine Introduction |
|---|---|---|---|---|---|
| | MCV1 | MCV2 | MCV1 | MCV2 | |
| Eq Guinea | 53% | 13% | 53% | 17% | |
| Eritrea | 93% | 85% | 93% | 85% | 2017 |
| Eswatini | 83% | 77% | 80% | 69% | 2015 |
| Ethiopia | 56% | 48% | 54% | 46% | |
| Gabon | 52% | | 64% | | |
| Gambia | 74% | 52% | 79% | 61% | 2015 |
| Ghana | 95% | 84% | 94% | 83% | 2012 |
| Guinea | 47% | 3% | 47% | | |
| Guinea-Bissau | 75% | 1% | 63% | | |
| Kenya | 90% | 56% | 89% | 57% | 2016 |
| Lesotho | 81% | 75% | 90% | 82% | 2016 |
| Liberia | 79% | 59% | 58% | 35% | |
| Madagascar | 44% | 32% | 44% | 24% | |
| Malawi | 82% | 60% | 90% | 74% | 2016 |
| Mali | 70% | 44% | 70% | 33% | |
| Mauritania | 72% | | 63% | | 2017 |
| Mauritius | 98% | 93% | 87% | 83% | 1996 |
| Mozambique | 84% | 70% | 84% | 70% | 2017 |
| Namibia | 91% | 79% | 91% | 56% | 2015 |
| Niger | 65% | 42% | 80% | 66% | |
| Nigeria | 60% | 38% | 60% | 38% | |
| Rwanda | 96% | 82% | 87% | 85% | 2013 |
| Sao Tome and Principe | 77% | 69% | 77% | 69% | 2015 |
| Senegal | 80% | 66% | 87% | 75% | 2012 |
| Seychelles | 98% | 98% | 94% | 86% | 1980 |
| Sierra Leone | 90% | 73% | 87% | 67% | 2018 |
| South Africa | 86% | 86% | 87% | 82% | |
| South Sudan | 72% | | 74% | | |
| Tanzania | 86% | 76% | 77% | 62% | 2013 |
| Togo | 71% | 57% | 70% | 50% | 2017 |
| Uganda | 90% | 49% | 90% | | 2018 |
| Zambia | 90% | 81% | 90% | 81% | 2016 |
| Zimbabwe | 90% | 77% | 88% | 76% | 2014 |

Blank = not yet introduced.

The trends indicate an increase in MCV2 coverage since 2012, with an increasing number of countries introducing a second dose measles vaccine in the past decade. Out of the 41 countries which had WHO-UNICEF coverage estimates of MCV2 in 2022, only Seychelles attained >95% coverage. Amongst the countries that had had MCV2 in their routine immunization program for more than 3 years, the drop-out rate between MCV1 and MCV2 is 10% or more in 23 countries, while the dropout rate is 20% or more in 9 countries (Figure 1).

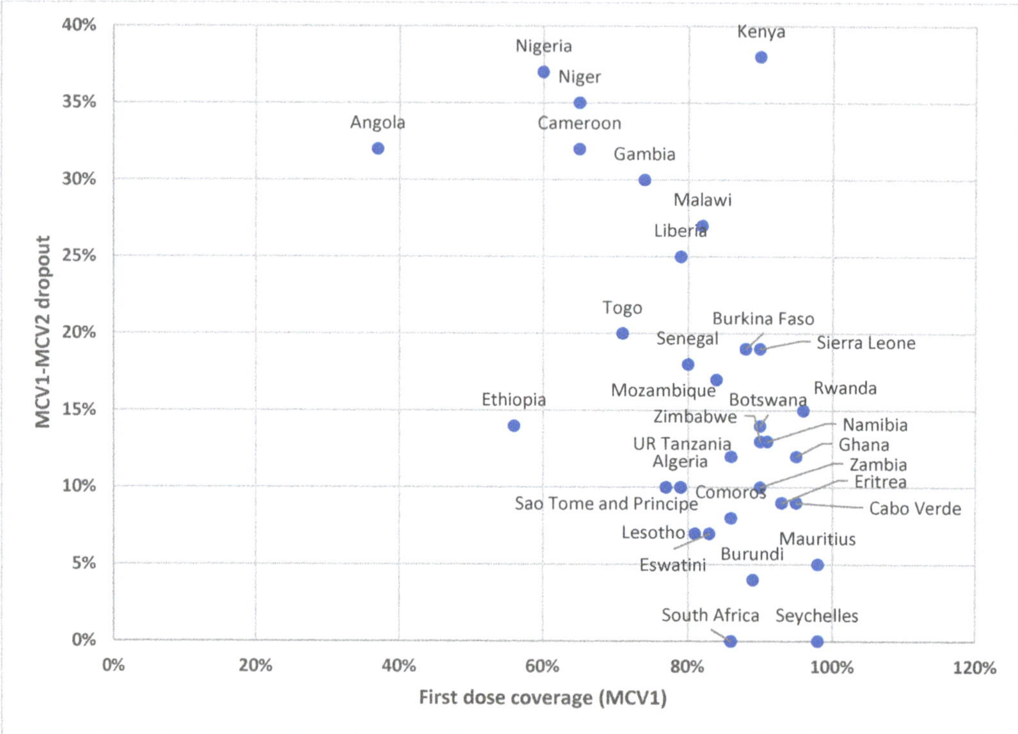


**Figure 1.** Measles first dose coverage and drop-out rates by country. African Region, 2022.

Rubella-containing vaccines (RCVs) had been introduced in the routine immunization program in 32 (68%) of 47 countries as of the end of 2022, with no country having introduced it in 2023. The remaining 15 countries include three countries not eligible for support from Gavi, the Vaccine Alliance (Equatorial Guinea, Gabon, and South Africa), and 12 Gavi-eligible countries that have yet to meet the requirements set by WHO of 80% measles vaccination coverage through SIAs or through the routine vaccination program before receiving Gavi support to introduce RCV (Central African Republic (CAR), Chad, Democratic Republic of Congo (DRC), Ethiopia, Guinea, Guinea Bissau, Liberia, Madagascar, Mali, Niger, Nigeria, and South Sudan). The WHO-UNICEF estimate of first dose rubella-containing vaccine coverage in 2022 was 36%, reflecting the large countries in the region not yet having introduced the vaccine.

As of December 2023, at least 12 countries had utilized measles-containing vaccines packaged in 5-dose or lesser dose vials for routine vaccination service. These are Botswana, Cabo Verde, Comoros, DRC, Equatorial Guinea, Eritrea, Eswatini, Lesotho, Mauritius, Niger, Seychelles, and Zimbabwe.

### *3.2. Supplementary Immunization Activities (SIAs)*

Countries in the African Region continue to implement periodic follow-up vaccination campaigns to reach unvaccinated children and close immunity gaps, especially in the youngest birth cohorts. These campaigns are scheduled at an interval based on the rate of accumulation of unprotected children within the under-five-years age group and based on the epidemiology of measles in the countries. In 2022 and 2023, a total of 24 countries implemented 32 preventive or outbreak-response vaccination campaigns, reaching a cumulative total of 144,763,470 children (Table 2).

**Table 2.** Measles supplemental immunization coverage by country. African Region, 2022–2023.

| Country | Year | Type of SIAs | Age Group of Children Targeted | Number of Children Targeted | Number of Children Vaccinated | Administrative Coverage (Percent of Target) |
|---|---|---|---|---|---|---|
| Angola | 2022 | MR Follow-up | 9–59 months | 1,636,915 | 1,533,568 | 93.70% |
| Angola | 2023 | MR Follow-up | 6–59 months | 2,990,813 | 2,575,131 | 86.10% |
| Cameroon | 2022 | outbreak response | 6 mo–7 years | 1,179,372 | 1,119,550 | 94.90% |
| Cameroon | 2023 | MR Follow-up | 9–59 months | 4,416,588 | 3,433,312 | 77.70% |
| Central African Republic | 2023 | Measles follow-up | 6–59 months | 1,240,480 | 1,307,023 | 105.40% |
| Chad | 2023 | Measles follow-up | 6–59 months | 1,999,072 | 2,238,730 | 112.00% |
| Congo | 2022 | MR Follow up | 6 mo–9 yrs | 1,600,115 | 1,726,547 | 107.90% |
| DR Congo | 2022 | outbreak response | 6–59 months | 3,368,775 | 3,372,997 | 100.10% |
| DR Congo | 2023 | Measles follow-up | 9–59 months | 18,226,531 | 18,520,710 | 101.60% |
| Ethiopia | 2022 | outbreak response | 6 mo–10 years | 649,065 | 686,381 | 105.70% |
| Ethiopia | 2022 | Measles Follow-up | 6–59 months | 15,471,740 | 14,579,818 | 94.20% |
| Ethiopia | 2023 | Measles Follow-up | 6–59 months | 830,535 | 690,668 | 83.20% |
| Gabon | 2022 | Measles Follow-up | 9–59 months | 292,147 | 102,132 | 35.00% |
| Gambia | 2022 | MR follow-up | 9–59 months | 341,446 | 180,506 | 52.90% |
| Guinea | 2022 | Measles Follow-up | 6–59 months | 2,529,539 | 2,551,234 | 100.90% |
| Lesotho | 2022 | MR Follow-up | 9–59 months | 189,643 | 85,582 | 45.10% |
| Liberia | 2022 | outbreak response | 9–59 months | 313,817 | 283,579 | 90.40% |
| Madagascar | 2022 | Measles Follow-up | 9–59 months | 4,355,433 | 4,142,296 | 95.10% |
| Malawi | 2023 | MR Follow-up | 9–59 months | 3,180,449 | 2,644,144 | 83.10% |
| Mozambique | 2023 | MR Follow-up | 9–59 months | 4,811,849 | 5,047,614 | 104.90% |
| Namibia | 2022 | MR Follow-up | 9–59 months | 309,916 | 293,705 | 94.80% |
| Niger | 2022 | outbreak response | 6–59 months | 992,259 | 990,839 | 99.80% |
| Niger | 2022 | Measles follow-up | 9–59 months | 5,098,682 | 5,329,865 | 104.50% |
| Nigeria | 2022 | Measles follow-up | 9–59 months | 5,736,063 | 6,281,891 | 119.50% |
| Nigeria | 2022 | Measles follow-up | 9–59 months | 27,393,635 | 26,837,536 | 98.00% |
| Nigeria | 2023 | Measles follow-up | 9–59 months | 15,181,695 | 15,824,218 | 104.20% |
| S Africa | 2023 | Measles Follow-up | 6 mo–14 yrs | 17,700,872 | 9,593,955 | 54.20% |
| S Sudan | 2023 | Measles follow-up | 6–59 months | 2,597,415 | 2,383,771 | 91.80% |
| Togo | 2022 | MR follow-up | 9–59 months | 1,480,161 | 1,400,154 | 94.60% |
| Uganda | 2022 | MR follow-up | 9–59 months | 7,015,156 | 6,608,277 | 94.20% |
| Zambia | 2023 | outbreak response | 6 mo–10 yrs | 1,219,787 | 1,418,453 | 116.30% |
| Zimbabwe | 2022 | MR follow up | 9–59 months | 2,292,989 | 1,970,123 | 85.90% |

The administrative coverage target of 95% was reached in 15 of these campaigns. Post-campaign coverage surveys were implemented after only 6 campaigns, and survey coverage showed that 95% coverage was not attained in any of the campaigns in the four countries where results are available (Madagascar, Malawi, Nigeria, and Zimbabwe). Official results are not yet available from the post-campaign surveys in Senegal or Ethiopia.

### *3.3. Measles and Rubella Surveillance and Incidence*

In 2022, a total 114,347 suspected cases of measles were reported in the African Region through the case-based surveillance system, of which 60,857 (53%) were confirmed by lab, epidemiological linkage, or clinical compatibility. The regional incidence of confirmed measles was 51.5 per million population. Nigeria, Ethiopia, Liberia, and Zimbabwe accounted for 37,815 (62%) of the confirmed measles cases. The highest incidence of confirmed measles was in Liberia (1162 cases per million population), followed by Gabon (489 cases per million) and Zimbabwe (289 cases per million), and Nigeria (103 cases per million). The annual detection rate of non-measles febrile rash illnesses (NMFRI) was 3.8 per 100,000 population, and 89% of districts reported at least one suspected measles case with a blood specimen. A total of 28 countries met the targets (NMFRI rate of at least 2 per 100,000 and at least 80% districts reporting) for these two performance indicators in 2022.

In 2023, a total 125,957 suspected cases of measles were reported through the case-based surveillance system. Blood specimens were collected from 77,998 cases (62%), of which 22,258 cases (29%) were confirmed to be IgM positive for measles. Of the cases without a specimen, 42,098 cases were confirmed by epidemiological linkage, and 9269 cases confirmed as clinically compatible measles. As of the end of March 2024, a total of

1163 cases reported in 2023 still had pending lab results or pending case classification in the surveillance database.

In 2023, the largest number of confirmed measles cases was reported in Ethiopia (16,505 cases), Nigeria (12,245 cases), DRC (10,662 cases), and Cameroon (6174 cases). The regional incidence of measles was 60.3 cases per million population (22% increase from 2022), while the highest national incidence rates of confirmed measles were documented in Liberia (831.6 cases per million population), Gabon (480.4), Equatorial Guinea (268), Central African Republic (240), Cameroon (217.1) and Ethiopia (154.1). Only 3 countries (Cabo Verde, Algeria, Seychelles) attained incidence of <1 per million population, while 6 countries reported measles incidence of 1–4.9 per million population, and 5 countries reported incidence of 5–9.9 per million (Table 3).

According to the case-based surveillance data, the annual detection rate of non-measles febrile rash illness for 2023 was 4.2 per 100,000 at the regional level with 34 (72%) countries meeting the target of at least 2 per 100,000. At the regional level, 87% of the districts investigated at least one suspected case with a blood specimen in 2023. Thirty-four (72%) countries met the target of at least 80% districts investigating one or more suspected cases with a blood specimen. Twenty-six countries (55%) met the targets for the two principal surveillance performance indicators in 2023, while three countries (6.4%) missed both targets.

Countries also receive weekly reports of suspected measles cases through aggregate reporting systems. Some countries have operational or other challenges that prevent them from reporting all suspected measles cases through the case-based surveillance system, such as DRC (311,500 suspected measles cases notified through aggregate reporting in 2023), Guinea (910 suspected cases in the aggregate reporting database for 2023), and South Sudan (7957 suspect cases in 2023). These countries are typically those with large outbreaks.

A total of 4805 lab-confirmed rubella cases were reported in the region for 2023, of which 933 (19%) were from Ethiopia, 746 (16%) from Nigeria, 591 (12%) from DRC, 440 (9%) from Tanzania, and 389 (8%) from Madagascar. The regional incidence of laboratory-confirmed rubella was 4.0 cases per million population. The highest rubella incidence was reported in Guinea Bissau, at 74 per million population, with 155 lab-confirmed rubella cases (Table 3).

In 2022, seven countries documented the genotype of circulating measles viruses, with D8 genotype viruses detected in South Africa and Zimbabwe, while B3 genotype viruses were documented in Algeria, Benin, South Africa, Tanzania, Uganda, and Zambia. In 2023, seven countries (Algeria, Cote d'Ivoire, DRC, South Sudan, Tanzania, Togo, and Uganda) reported B3 genotype measles viruses. No country reported D8 viruses in 2023.

**Table 3.** Measles and rubella case reporting by country. African Region, 2023.

| Country | Total Population (In Millions) | Total Reported Measles Cases | Blood Specimens Collected | Lab Confirmed (IgM Positive) Measles | Lab Confirmed Rubella Cases | Measles Cases Confirmed by Epidemiological Linkage | Clinically Compatible Measles Cases | Total Confirmed Measles | Cases with Pending Results/Pending Classification | Measles Incidence Rate per 1,000,000 Population | Rubella Incidence Rate per 1,000,000 Population |
|---|---|---|---|---|---|---|---|---|---|---|---|
| Algeria | 43.5 | 89 | 89 | 24 | 2 | 2 | 1 | 27 | 0 | 0.6 | 0.0 |
| Angola | 34.1 | 2960 | 1665 | 24 | 85 | 1905 | 18 | 1947 | 540 | 57.1 | 2.5 |
| Benin | 12.9 | 912 | 910 | 368 | 31 | 110 | 8 | 486 | 0 | 37.7 | 2.4 |
| Botswana | 2.5 | 1471 | 1434 | 50 | 62 | 0 | 1 | 51 | 0 | 20.5 | 24.9 |
| Burkina Faso | 22.9 | 1968 | 1568 | 596 | 10 | 968 | 32 | 1596 | 0 | 69.7 | 0.4 |
| Burundi | 13.1 | 1936 | 475 | 115 | 37 | 1460 | 120 | 1695 | 24 | 129.4 | 2.8 |
| Cameroon | 28.4 | 6812 | 1269 | 506 | 10 | 5612 | 56 | 6174 | 2 | 217.1 | 0.4 |
| Cabo Verde | 0.6 | 2 | 2 | 0 | 0 | 0 | 0 | 0 | 0 | 0.0 | 0.0 |
| Central African Republic | 6.4 | 1928 | 537 | 144 | 120 | 1388 | 4 | 1536 | 5 | 240.0 | 18.8 |
| Chad | 18.6 | 2853 | 2766 | 1130 | 186 | 87 | 289 | 1506 | 0 | 81.0 | 10.0 |
| Comoros | 0.8 | 48 | 48 | 1 | 2 | 0 | 0 | 1 | 10 | 1.2 | 2.4 |
| Congo | 6.1 | 598 | 399 | 184 | 5 | 199 | 9 | 392 | 0 | 64.7 | 0.8 |
| Cote d'Ivoire | 31.5 | 5687 | 5612 | 1286 | 114 | 75 | 0 | 1361 | 0 | 43.1 | 3.6 |
| D. R. Congo | 123.5 | 13,888 | 7304 | 4111 | 591 | 6426 | 125 | 10,662 | 108 | 86.4 | 4.8 |
| Equatorial Guinea | 0.9 | 393 | 264 | 94 | 4 | 131 | 13 | 238 | 36 | 267.9 | 4.5 |
| Eritrea | 3.8 | 105 | 105 | 18 | 5 | 0 | 1 | 19 | 0 | 5.0 | 1.3 |
| Eswatini | 1.2 | 120 | 120 | 3 | 1 | 0 | 0 | 3 | 1 | 2.6 | 0.9 |
| Ethiopia | 107.1 | 20,878 | 6673 | 2268 | 933 | 14,193 | 44 | 16,505 | 21 | 154.1 | 8.7 |
| Gabon | 2.5 | 1296 | 149 | 56 | 7 | 1145 | 0 | 1201 | 2 | 480.4 | 2.8 |
| Gambia | 1.7 | 241 | 239 | 33 | 13 | 2 | 2 | 37 | 0 | 21.2 | 7.5 |
| Ghana | 32.1 | 5588 | 5587 | 1348 | 92 | 924 | 41 | 2313 | 0 | 72.1 | 2.9 |
| Guinea | 13.6 | 533 | 532 | 28 | 63 | 177 | 0 | 205 | 0 | 15.0 | 4.6 |
| Guinea Bissau | 2.1 | 267 | 267 | 3 | 155 | 14 | 0 | 17 | 0 | 8.1 | 74.0 |
| Kenya | 52.3 | 2342 | 1997 | 580 | 50 | 247 | 3 | 830 | 50 | 15.9 | 1.0 |
| Lesotho | 2.1 | 868 | 868 | 14 | 9 | 0 | 1 | 15 | 0 | 7.2 | 4.3 |

**Table 3.** *Cont.*

| Country | Total Population (In Millions) | Total Reported Measles Cases | Blood Specimens Collected | Lab Confirmed (IgM Positive) Measles | Lab Confirmed Rubella Cases | Measles Cases Confirmed by Epidemiological Linkage | Clinically Compatible Measles Cases | Total Confirmed Measles | Cases with Pending Results/Pending Classification | Measles Incidence Rate per 1,000,000 Population | Rubella Incidence Rate per 1,000,000 Population |
|---|---|---|---|---|---|---|---|---|---|---|---|
| Liberia | 5.2 | 4525 | 43 | 43 | 0 | 4115 | 207 | 4365 | 0 | 831.6 | 0.0 |
| Madagascar | 29.0 | 2033 | 1775 | 81 | 389 | 0 | 9 | 90 | 269 | 3.1 | 13.4 |
| Malawi | 19.2 | 438 | 409 | 127 | 5 | 28 | 9 | 164 | 0 | 8.5 | 0.3 |
| Mali | 22.5 | 796 | 796 | 364 | 15 | 1 | 71 | 436 | 0 | 19.4 | 0.7 |
| Mauritania | 4.5 | 479 | 460 | 271 | 4 | 64 | 1 | 336 | 0 | 75.1 | 0.9 |
| Mauritius | 5.0 | 5 | 5 | 5 | 0 | 0 | 0 | 5 | 0 | 1.0 | 0.0 |
| Mozambique | 31.6 | 3630 | 3546 | 652 | 83 | 0 | 20 | 672 | -4 | 21.3 | 2.6 |
| Namibia | 2.7 | 406 | 406 | 20 | 10 | 0 | 21 | 41 | 1 | 15.4 | 3.8 |
| Niger | 25.4 | 1090 | 1087 | 608 | 61 | 26 | 52 | 686 | 0 | 27.0 | 2.4 |
| Nigeria | 240.1 | 20,036 | 10,391 | 2067 | 2209 | 2209 | 7969 | 12,245 | 0 | 51.0 | 9.2 |
| Rwanda | 13.1 | 1316 | 1315 | 44 | 12 | 0 | 0 | 44 | 0 | 3.4 | 0.9 |
| Saotome and Principe | 0.0 | 0 | 0 | 0 | 0 | 0 | 0 | 0 | 0 | 0.0 | 0.0 |
| Senegal | 18.3 | 1756 | 1756 | 561 | 30 | 0 | 60 | 621 | 0 | 34.0 | 1.6 |
| Seychelles | 0.0 | 0 | 0 | 0 | 0 | 0 | 0 | 0 | 0 | 0.0 | 0.0 |
| Sierra Leone | 8.7 | 207 | 207 | 119 | 5 | 21 | 0 | 140 | 0 | 16.1 | 0.6 |
| South Africa | 60.6 | 4950 | 4934 | 884 | 96 | 0 | 4 | 888 | 99 | 14.7 | 1.6 |
| South Sudan | 14.6 | 863 | 808 | 520 | 45 | 0 | 31 | 551 | 37 | 37.7 | 3.1 |
| Tanzania | 61.3 | 4456 | 4208 | 1124 | 440 | 131 | 0 | 1255 | 263 | 20.5 | 7.2 |
| Togo | 8.3 | 883 | 877 | 547 | 14 | 52 | 14 | 613 | 0 | 73.4 | 1.7 |
| Uganda | 42.9 | 1648 | 1444 | 188 | 77 | 216 | 2 | 406 | 47 | 9.5 | 1.8 |
| Zambia | 18.9 | 1552 | 1549 | 501 | 50 | 170 | 30 | 701 | 53 | 37.0 | 2.6 |
| Zimbabwe | 17.0 | 1105 | 1103 | 17 | 136 | 0 | 1 | 18 | 130 | 1.1 | 8.0 |
| **African Region** | **1213.0** | **125,957** | **77,998** | **21,727** | **6268** | **42,098** | **9269** | **73,094** | **1694** | **60.3** | **5.2** |

### 3.4. Verification of Measles and Rubella Elimination

By the end of 2023, a total of 18 countries (Botswana, Burundi, Cabo Verde, Cameroon, Eswatini, Gambia, Ghana, Kenya, Lesotho, Mauritius, Nigeria, Rwanda, Sao Tome e Principe, Senegal, Seychelles, Tanzania, Uganda, and Zimbabwe) had established national verification committees to support documentation of progress towards measles elimination. Sixteen of these national committees have been actively engaged in documenting the countries' progress. WHO provided training on the verification standards to the verification committee members as well as to the national immunization and disease-control program members. In addition, WHO supported the analysis of programmatic data to be used for developing the national progress document in preparation for the verification of measles and rubella elimination. The African Regional Commission for the Verification of measles and rubella elimination (RVC) met for a third time in May 2023. However, no country in the region has attained the verification of measles or rubella elimination.

## 4. Discussion

Following the well documented declines in vaccination coverage in 2020 and 2021 related to the COVID-19 pandemic, many countries implemented efforts to recover their vaccination coverage levels in 2022 and 2023 [12,13]. The African Region witnessed little overall gain in measles vaccination (MCV1 and MCV2) coverage in 2022. Instead, the WHO UNICEF coverage estimates show that 13 countries had further decreases in MCV1 coverage in 2022 as compared to 2021 estimates [14]. Several countries, including the populous countries of Nigeria, Ethiopia, and Angola, had MCV1 coverage levels less than 60%, contributing to large numbers of children who missed measles doses in the region.

During the years covered in this analysis, MCV1 and MCV2 coverage remained below the WHO-recommended level of 95% to attain elimination of measles.

A common barrier to raising measles-vaccination coverage is the reluctance of health workers to open a 10-dose vial when few children are present at the vaccination post. As a result of this concern about vaccine wastage, many vaccination posts provide measles vaccines on specific days of the week only or on appointed days of the month. In addition to adopting policies and practices to allow for vaccinating every child using every possible opportunity, switching from 10-dose to 5-dose measles-containing vaccine vials can lead to reducing missed opportunities for measles vaccination [15].

The high incidence of measles in many countries in the region reflects chronic immunity gaps as a result of low coverage with two doses of MCV, as well as suboptimal implementation of SIAs (which includes delaying the implementation of time-sensitive scheduled SIAs, lack of adequate funding resources for SIAs, poor preparation, and suboptimal coverage in SIAs). Some of the challenges to attaining and sustaining high vaccination coverage include weak health systems, civil unrest, population displacement, and multiple other program priorities including disease outbreaks (e.g., vaccine-derived poliomyelitis, diphtheria, cholera, meningitis, yellow fever, etc.) [16,17].

The civil conflict which erupted in the Sudan in early 2023 leading to an influx of refugees and returnees into Chad, Ethiopia, and South Sudan is an example of an unprecedented situation that contributed to the continued high incidence of measles in the host countries [18].

In 2023, Nigeria, Guinea, and Niger reported large diphtheria outbreaks, while many countries in the African Region experienced cholera outbreaks [16,19]. These outbreaks required extensive response measures which diverted the attention and resources of national immunization program away from measles- and rubella-elimination activities.

While there is some improvement in MCV2 coverage, the drop-out rate between the first and second doses remains high in many countries, indicating that the platform for vaccination in the second year of life has not been optimized to strengthen the routine immunization service and support measles elimination. A number of country-level studies have documented gaps in MCV2 coverage [20,21].

Addressing systemic problems with routine immunization can help countries attain measles elimination. As the contextual reasons for vaccination coverage gaps vary from country to country, countries would benefit from using tailored approaches to reach unvaccinated children. These may include improving access to vaccines through expanding fixed and/or outreach vaccination services, shifting to lower dose per measles-vaccine-containing vial formulations, conducting intensified immunization activities, and improving vaccine demand and confidence. Periodic and timely high-quality preventive SIAs remain a critical programmatic strategy to reach unvaccinated children.

The efforts to address immunization coverage gaps will benefit from addressing policy- and practice-level barriers to catching up on zero-dose or under-vaccinated children, especially those in the age group beyond two years of age who are often excluded from routine immunization services. One of these operational barriers is the fear of wasting doses in 10-dose vaccine vials. More and more countries have indicated interest to shift from 10-dose to 5-dose vials in the coming years. Using smaller dose vials ideally should create better conditions for readily opening measles-containing vaccine vials in every immunization session. In those countries that implement this shift in the doses of measles vials, there is a need to evaluate the impact of the shift from 10-dose to 5-dose vials in terms of frequency of measles vaccination service delivery, immunization coverage with MCV1 and MCV2, and in reducing missed opportunities. Data collection and monitoring systems for coverage now focus on doses delivered to children in the first year of life, and will need adaptations to capture doses of vaccines given in the second year of life or later.

WHO policy indicates that, in order to introduce rubella-containing vaccines, countries should be able to achieve 80% MCV1 coverage in routine immunization or during SIAs [22]. As of the end of 2023, 15 countries in the WHO African Region have yet to introduce rubella-containing vaccines. GAVI funding support is available for 12 of these 15 countries, provided they can demonstrate the required level of MCV1 vaccination. The 3 remaining countries (Equatorial Guinea, Gabon, and South Africa) must prioritize and self-finance the introduction of rubella vaccines, while observing the WHO rubella vaccine policy guidelines in terms of the recommended approach to introducing rubella vaccines.

Despite more than two decades of experience, SIA quality remains an issue. In 2022–2023, Gabon, Gambia, and Lesotho attained administrative SIA coverage of less than 60%. Each of these three campaigns had important contextual factors that adversely affected the coverage levels. Delayed and incomplete funding, poor level of preparations and vaccine hesitancy in the face of other concurrent events affected the coverage levels [23,24]. Overall, more than half of the SIAs in 2022 and 2023 failed to reach the 95% administrative coverage target at the national level. Only a small proportion of the countries implemented post-campaign coverage surveys to corroborate the administrative SIA coverage. Subnational level breakdown also indicates gaps which reflect the challenges with inadequate and delayed operational funding, as well as insufficient quality preparations for these mass campaigns, which are primarily organized to reach children who do not have the chance to receive routine doses of measles vaccine.

Measles and rubella case-based surveillance continues to suffer from significant underfunding, and this further exacerbates the performance gaps. As countries make progress towards the elimination goal, there is a need to increase the sensitivity of disease surveillance, including such elements as collecting specimens from all reported febrile rash illness cases, carrying out contact tracing and detailed investigation of each chain of transmission, as well as root cause analysis of outbreaks, all of which will require committed human and funding resources. Unfortunately, the current levels of local and donor financing are not yet adequate to support the implementation of elimination standard measles-rubella surveillance.

Attaining the elimination of measles and rubella in 80% of the countries in the region by 2030 will require significant financial investments as well as high-quality technical and political leadership to improve routine immunization and SIA coverage, as well as funding for high-quality disease surveillance. The available baseline data on circulating measles genotypes remains scant. Understanding current genotype distribution will be critical as more and more countries move closer to elimination.

Innovations to bring diagnosis and vaccination to hard to reach areas in countries of the African Region could be potentially transformative in reaching measles elimination in the region. Rapid diagnostic tests, already under field trials for measles and under development for rubella, would allow for more rapid detection and response to outbreaks [25]. The introduction of micro-array patches (MAPs) for the administration of measles and rubella vaccines would facilitate transportation of the vaccine outside of the cold chain and enable the provision of MR vaccines in areas hitherto unreached, administered by minimally trained persons, including vaccine administration on a house-to-house level [26].

Countries that have maintained high coverage and low incidence of measles may apply to be verified for the elimination of measles and/or rubella. Globally, as of April 2024, a total of 99 countries have been verified for eliminating rubella and 89 countries have been verified for eliminating measles [6]. In the African Region, countries like Botswana, Cabo Verde, Mauritius, and Seychelles have made significant progress towards eliminating measles and rubella and will need to finalize their progress documentation for review and verification by the Regional Commission for the verification of measles and rubella elimination (RVC).

This report provides valuable information on the status of measles and rubella elimination in Africa but has the following limitations. The case-based surveillance data and incidence levels do not include the data from aggregate reporting of suspected measles in countries with large outbreaks, and so represent an underestimation of the measles incidence in those countries. In countries with wide diversity in subnational level immunization coverage, the national level vaccination coverage estimates tend to mask these subnational gaps.

## 5. Conclusions

Following the COVID pandemic, the measles vaccination coverage in the African Region in 2022 remains below the targets for attaining elimination, with a large number of children who missed measles doses, and continued high incidence of measles. Countries need to provide the leadership and mobilise resources to address systemic problems with routine immunisation, and to improve the timeliness and quality of periodic SIAs to ensure reaching unvaccinated populations.

**Author Contributions:** Conceptualization, B.G.M. and R.T.P.; Methodology, B.G.M., C.S.W., R.K., P.M.O. and E.L.; Validation, E.L.; Formal analysis, B.G.M. and R.K.; Investigation, B.G.M., E.L. and R.K.; Data curation, R.K.; Writing—original draft, B.G.M. and R.T.P.; Writing—review & editing, B.G.M., C.S.W., P.M.O. and R.T.P.; Supervision, R.T.P. All authors have read and agreed to the published version of the manuscript.

**Funding:** This research received no external funding.

**Data Availability Statement:** The data presented in this study are available on request from the corresponding author.

**Conflicts of Interest:** The authors declare no conflict of interest.

## References

1. World Health Organization; Regional Committee for Africa. Measles Elimination by 2020: A Strategy for the African Region. Yamoussoukro: 2011. Available online: https://www.afro.who.int/sites/default/files/sessions/working_documents/AFR-RC61-8-Measles-elimination-by-2020---strategy-forthe-African-Region---with-Resolution.pdf (accessed on 12 March 2024).
2. World Health Organization. Guidance for evaluating progress towards elimination of measles and rubella. *Wkly. Epidemiol. Rec.* **2018**, *41*, 541–552.

3. WHO Regional Office for Africa. Framework for the Implementation of the Immunization Agenda 2030 in the WHO African Region: Report of the Secretariat. Brazzaville: 2021. Available online: https://apps.who.int/iris/handle/10665/345322 (accessed on 12 March 2024).
4. Rachlin, A.; Danovaro-Holliday, C.; Murphy, P.; Sodha, S.V.; Wallace, A.S. Routine Vaccination Coverage—Worldwide, 2021. *Wkly. Epidemiol. Rec.* **2022**, *97*, 567–574. Available online: https://iris.who.int/bitstream/handle/10665/364083/WER9744-eng-fre.pdf (accessed on 17 March 2024). [CrossRef] [PubMed]
5. Ho, L.L.; Gurung, S.; Mirza, I.; Nicolas, H.D.; Steulet, C.; Burman, A.L.; Danovaro-Holliday, M.C.; Sodha, S.V.; Kretsinger, K. Impact of the SARS-CoV-2 pandemic on vaccine-preventable disease campaigns. *Int. J. Infect. Dis.* **2022**, *119*, 201–209. [CrossRef] [PubMed]
6. Minta, A.A.; Ferrari, M.; Antoni, S.; Portnoy, A.; Sbarra, A.; Lambert, B.; Hatcher, C.; Hsu, C.H.; Ho, L.L.; Steulet, C.; et al. Crowcroft. Regional progress towards measles elimination globally up to 2022. *Wkly. Epidemiol. Rec.* **2023**, *98*, 587–598.
7. Masresha, B.G.; Hatcher, C.; Lebo, E.; Tanifum, P.; Bwaka, A.M.; Minta, A.A.; Antoni, S.; Grant, G.B.; Perry, R.T.; O'Connor, P. Progress towards measles elimination—African Region, 2017–2021. *Wkly. Epidemiol. Rec.* **2023**, *36*, 396–408. [CrossRef] [PubMed]
8. Burton, A.; Monasch, R.; Lautenbach, B.; Gacic-Dobo, M.; Neill, M.; Karimov, R.; Wolfson, L.; Jones, G.; Birmingham, M. WHO and UNICEF estimates of national infant immunization coverage: Methods and processes. *Bull. World Health Organ.* **2009**, *87*, 535–541. [CrossRef] [PubMed]
9. World Health Organization. Measles vaccines: WHO position paper—April 2017. *Wkly. Epidemiol. Rec.* **2017**, *92*, 205–228. Available online: https://www.who.int/publications/i/item/who-wer9217-205-227 (accessed on 22 April 2024).
10. World Health Organization; African Regional Office. African Regional Guidelines for Measles and Rubella Surveillance. 2015. Available online: https://www.afro.who.int/sites/default/files/2017-06/who-african-regional-measles-and-rubella-surveillance-guidelines_updated-draft-version-april-2015_1.pdf (accessed on 22 April 2024).
11. Mulders, M.N.; Rota, P.A.; Icenogle, J.P.; Brown, K.E.; Takeda, M.; Rey, G.J.; Ben Mamou, M.C.; Dosseh, A.R.G.A.; Byabamazima, C.R.; Ahmed, H.J.; et al. Global measles and rubella laboratory network support for elimination goals, 2010–2015. *Wkly. Epidemiol. Rec.* **2016**, *91*, 240–246. Available online: https://iris.who.int/bitstream/handle/10665/254439/WER9118.pdf (accessed on 12 April 2024). [CrossRef] [PubMed]
12. World Health Organization. The Big Catch-Up: An Essential Immunization Recovery Plan for 2023 and Beyond. Available online: https://www.who.int/publications/i/item/9789240075511 (accessed on 22 April 2024).
13. O'Brien, K.L.; Lemango, E. The big catch-up in immunisation coverage after the COVID-19 pandemic: Progress and challenges to achieving equitable recovery. *Lancet* **2023**, *402*, 510–512. [CrossRef] [PubMed]
14. Kaur, G.; Danovaro-Holliday, C.; Mwinnyaa, G.; Gacic-Dobo, M.; Francis, L.; Grevendonk, J.; Sodha, S.V.; Sugerman, C.; Wallace, A. Routine vaccination coverage—Worldwide, 2022. *Wkly. Epidemiol. Rec.* **2023**, *98*, 555–563. Available online: https://iris.who.int/bitstream/handle/10665/373831/WER9844-eng-fre.pdf (accessed on 12 March 2024). [CrossRef] [PubMed]
15. Kanagat, N.; Krudwig, K.; Wilkins, K.A.; Kaweme, S.; Phiri, G.; Mwansa, F.D.; Mvundura, M.; Robertson, J.; Kristensen, D.; Gueye, A.; et al. Health Care Worker Preferences and Perspectives on Doses per Container for 2 Lyophilized Vaccines in Senegal, Vietnam, and Zambia. *Glob. Health Sci. Pract.* **2020**, *8*, 4. [CrossRef] [PubMed]
16. World Health Organization. WHO's Health Emergencies Programme: Acute Emergencies Monthly Summary—August and September 2023. *Wkly. Epidemiol. Rec.* **2023**, *98*, 503–509. Available online: https://iris.who.int/bitstream/handle/10665/373475/WER9842-eng-fre.pdf (accessed on 22 April 2024).
17. Davlantes, E.; Jorba, J.; Henderson, E.; Bullard, K.; Deka, M.A.; Kfutwah, A.; Martin, J.; Bessaud, M.; Shulman, L.M.; Hawes, K.; et al. Notes from the Field: Circulating Vaccine-Derived Poliovirus Type 2 Emergences Linked to Novel Oral Poliovirus Vaccine Type 2 Use—Six African Countries, 2021–2023. *MMWR Morb. Mortal Wkly. Rep.* **2023**, *72*, 1041–1042. [CrossRef] [PubMed]
18. World Health Organization; Regional Office for Africa. Combatting Disease Threats among People Fleeing the Sudan Conflict. June 2023. Available online: https://www.afro.who.int/countries/south-sudan/news/combatting-disease-threats-among-people-fleeing-sudan-conflict (accessed on 12 March 2024).
19. WHO. African Region Health Emergency Situation Report. Multi-Country Outbreak of Diphtheria. Available online: https://iris.who.int/bitstream/handle/10665/376308/AFRO.Diphtheria.Sitrep007-20240225.pdf (accessed on 25 February 2024).
20. Adjei, M.R.; Longsignikuu, A.; Iddris, I.S.; Suuri, T.N.; Asamoah, B.; Okoye, M.; Baafi, J.V.; Kubio, C.; Ohene, S.A.; Grobusch, M.P. Trend of measles-rubella vaccination coverage and impact on measles epidemiology in the Savannah Region, Ghana; 2018–2022: A secondary data analysis. *Vaccine* **2024**, *42*, 1910–1917. [CrossRef] [PubMed]
21. Chilot, D.; Belay, D.G.; Shitu, K.; Gela, Y.Y.; Getnet, M.; Mulat, B.; Muluneh, A.G.; Merid, M.W.; Bitew, D.A.; Alem, A.Z. Measles second dose vaccine utilization and associated factors among children aged 24-35 months in Sub-Saharan Africa, a multi-level analysis from recent DHS surveys. *BMC Public Health* **2022**, *22*, 2070. [CrossRef] [PubMed]
22. World Health Organization. Rubella vaccines: WHO Position Paper—July 2020. *Weekly Epidemiol. Rec.* **2020**, *95*, 301–324.
23. Amadou Jallow, M.S.P.H.; Momodou Nyassi, M.D.; Jerry Thomas, M. Acute Kidney Injury among Children Likely Associated with Diethylene Glycol–Contaminated Medications—The Gambia, June–September 2022. *MMWR Morb. Mortal Wkly. Rep.* **2023**, *72*, 217–222. [CrossRef]
24. National measles and measles-rubella supplementary Immunisation Activity technical reports submitted to WHO Regional Office for Africa.

25. Brown, D.W.; Warrener, L.; Scobie, H.M.; Donadel, M.; Waku-Kouomou, D.; Mulders, M.N.; Rota, P.A. Rapid diagnostic tests to address challenges for global measles surveillance. *Curr. Opin. Virol.* **2020**, *41*, 77–84. [CrossRef] [PubMed]
26. Richardson, L.C.; Moss, W.J. Measles and rubella microarray array patches to increase vaccination coverage and achieve measles and rubella elimination in Africa. *Pan Afr. Med. J.* **2020**, *35* (Suppl. S1), 3. [CrossRef] [PubMed]

*vaccines*

MDPI

*Review*

# Sustaining the Elimination of Measles, Rubella and Congenital Rubella Syndrome in the Americas, 2019–2023: From Challenges to Opportunities

**Gloria Rey-Benito [1], Desirée Pastor [1,*], Alvaro Whittembury [1], Regina Durón [1], Carmelita Pacis-Tirso [1], Pamela Bravo-Alcántara [1], Claudia Ortiz [1] and Jon Andrus [2]**

1 Comprehensive Immunization Program, Pan American Health Organization, 525 23rd Street, NW, Washington, DC 20037, USA; reyglori@paho.org (G.R.-B.); whittemburya@paho.org (A.W.); duronreg@paho.org (R.D.); paciscar@paho.org (C.P.-T.); bravopam@paho.org (P.B.-A.); ortizcla@paho.org (C.O.)

2 Department of Global Health, Milken Institute School of Public Health, George Washington University, Washington, DC 20037, USA; andrusjonkim@yahoo.com

* Correspondence: dpastor@paho.org; Tel.: +1-240-277-1744

**Abstract:** This report reviews national data from all Member States on measles, rubella, and congenital rubella syndrome (CRS) elimination in the Region of the Americas during 2019–2023. It includes an analysis of compliance with vaccination coverage, surveillance indicators, and measles outbreaks, as well as an analysis of the response capacity of the laboratory network and a country case study that meets all indicators. The sources of information were the integrated epidemiological surveillance system for measles and rubella of the Pan American Health Organization (PAHO)/World Health Organization (WHO) and the Joint Reporting Form (eJRF), among others. From 2020 to 2022, regional coverage with first (MMR-1) and second doses (MMR-2) decreased to rates below 90%. The regional suspected case notification rate was maintained above the minimum expected 2.0 suspect cases per 100,000 population, except in 2021. During 2019 to 2023, 18 countries experienced outbreaks, with two of the outbreaks resulting in re-established endemic transmission. In conclusion, two countries in the Americas have not maintained measles elimination, but by the end of 2023 no country showed endemic measles transmission. One of the countries that lost its certification of elimination in 2018 managed to be reverified in 2023; the other is pending reverification. All countries maintained rubella elimination. Despite these challenges, the sustainability of the elimination of these diseases remains a health priority in the Region.

**Keywords:** measles; rubella; vaccination coverage; epidemiological factors; laboratories; Pan American Health Organization; Americas

## 1. Introduction

In 1994, the countries of the Region of the Americas, led by the Pan American Health Organization (PAHO), set the goal of interrupting endemic measles virus transmission by the year 2000 [1]. Between 1994 and 2014, these countries implemented two classic elimination strategies based on achieving high vaccination coverage (≥95%) and maintaining adequate epidemiological surveillance, including laboratory surveillance [2]. To date, the Region of the Americas has been the only region of the World Health Organization (WHO) to have achieved the elimination of endemic measles and rubella viruses, a process that was verified by an International Committee of Experts; it was also the first region to create an Action Plan to Verify the Elimination of Measles, Rubella and Congenital Rubella Syndrome (CRS), with essential criteria and basic principles to verify the elimination process [3]. This plan was implemented by all countries and territories in the Region between 2011 and 2016. Regional verification of the elimination of rubella and CRS occurred in April 2015, with verification of measles elimination occurring in September 2016 [4].

Following the verification of the elimination of both endemic diseases, the Ministers of Health of the Member States approved the implementation of the Action Plan for the Sustainability of Measles, Rubella and CRS Elimination 2018–2023 to set new strategic guidelines to maintain these two public health milestones [5]. Due to the resurgence of measles outbreaks globally which spread to the region between 2018 and 2019, the PAHO Technical Advisory Group on Vaccine-Preventable Diseases (TAG) recommended the creation of a new Regional Commission for the Monitoring and Re-verification of Measles, Rubella and CRS Elimination (RVC) in 2019 [6]. Two countries, Venezuela and Brazil, unfortunately experienced re-established endemic transmission in 2018 and 2019, respectively, from cases imported from other regions. During the Third RVC Annual Meeting held in November 2023, Venezuela was reverified as being free of measles and Brazil was classified as pending reverification. The United States came close to re-establishing endemic circulation, which fortunately was interrupted before 12 months [7].

However, four countries could not be verified as free of measles or rubella and must submit a new report to the RVC in 2024.

As with other parts of the world, in the Americas the COVID-19 pandemic had a substantial negative impact on vaccination coverage and the quality of epidemiological surveillance indicators between 2020 and 2021. A recent analysis of measles mortality in the six WHO regions between 2000 and 2022 estimated that for the Americas, 6.07 million deaths were averted, being the region with the lowest number of cases and deaths reported in these two decades [8].

An important factor highlighted in this report is the strengthening of the national response capacity of many countries and the contribution of the laboratory members of the regional measles–rubella laboratory network.

The regional measles laboratory network began in 1995 with a region-wide training plan implemented for measles IgM capture by Enzyme Immunoassay (EIA), targeting the biggest countries of the region and following the example of the Polio Laboratory Network. This activity was coordinated by the PAHO and facilitated by the US-CDC in Atlanta. In 1996, rubella IgM testing was implemented among specimens with negative IgM measles results. Since 1999 and following the TAG's recommendation to accelerate rubella and CRS prevention [9], rubella was integrated into the measles surveillance system. Sequential testing for both measles IgM and rubella IgM was implemented in the regional laboratory network [10]. Sequential testing for rubella occurs when measles serology is negative. In addition, viral isolation and molecular testing was realized in many laboratories.

Since 2003, IgM parallel testing for measles and rubella suspected cases was conducted in each laboratory member of the regional network. The implementation of this testing for both measles and rubella simultaneously was facilitated by IgM tests being readily available. The availability of commercial assays of the same manufacturer (Dade Behring Enzygnost) and same EIA type (indirect IgM assay) allowed for rapid response.

By 2011, the PAHO measles and rubella laboratory network had 138 members. The structure of the network comprised 1 global specialized laboratory, 2 regional reference laboratories, 21 national laboratories, and 114 subnational laboratories in eight countries: Argentina, Bolivia, Brazil, Colombia, Ecuador, Mexico, Paraguay, and Venezuela [11]. By 2023, there were 139 measles and rubella laboratories in the region, comprising 1 global specialized laboratory, 2 regional reference laboratories, 20 national laboratories, and 116 subnational laboratories in six countries: 27 in Argentina, 27 in Brazil, 26 in Canada, 3 in Colombia, 2 in Ecuador, and 31 in Mexico.

After the region achieved the verification of the elimination of rubella and measles, a reduction in the notification rate of measles and rubella suspected cases occurred. As a result, some countries unfortunately even reduced the number of subnational laboratories. However, during the last few years, in order to maintain a timely response to the surveillance system, some countries correctly decided to seize the opportunity to increase the number of subnational laboratories to provide a timely response to the program.

## 2. Materials and Methods

This review describes the main regional strategies and their impact on sustaining the elimination of rubella and CRS from 2019 to 2023 and on the recovery of measles-free status.

The sources of information consulted were the PAHO/WHO-ISIS Integrated Measles and Rubella Epidemiological Surveillance System [12], the Joint Reporting Form (eJRF) of the WHO/Unicef [13], Technical Advisory Group (TAG) reports [7], measles–rubella national reference laboratory reports, and national measles–rubella elimination sustainability reports to the Regional Measles–Rubella Elimination Monitoring and Re-verification Commission [14].

The analysis of vaccination coverage indicators and epidemiological surveillance indicators is presented in the tables and one figure. The qualitative analysis is presented with the description of the activities for strengthening the measles–rubella laboratory network, the best practices that the countries applied to improve vaccination coverage, and surveillance indicators.

## 3. Results

### 3.1. Vaccination Coverage in 2019–2022

Regional coverage with the measles, rubella, and mumps (MMR) vaccine has been declining since before the pandemic. In 2018, the coverages of the first (MMR-1) and second doses (MMR-2) were 91% and 84%, respectively. In 2019, they were 87% and 75%, respectively; in 2020, they were 87% and 65%; in 2021, they were 85% and 68%; and in 2022, they were 85% and 71%, respectively (Table 1).

During 2024, PAHO estimated that in 2019 there were 1.4 million 1-year-old children at the regional level that did not receive a timely first dose of MMR-1. In 2020, 1.8 million children did not receive a timely first dose; in 2021, 1.7 million did not, and in 2022, 1.6 million did not. Almost half of the children who did not receive MMR-1 lived in seven countries that accumulated 48% of the total cohort of children aged 12–23 months in the region [15].

Of the 35 PAHO/WHO Member States, in 2019, 16 of the 35 countries achieved 95% coverage with MMR-1 and 9 of 35 with MMR-2. In 2020, only 8 of 35 countries reached 95% coverage with MMR-1 and 5 of 35 with MMR-2. In 2021, only 6 of 35 countries reached 95% coverage with MMR-1 and 2 of 35 with MMR-2. In 2022, this coverage was reached in 9 of 35 countries with MMR-1 and f5 of 35 with MMR-2 (Table 1).

Given the limitations of the Member States in achieving adequate vaccination coverage with second doses of the MMR vaccine, in accordance with the PAHO TAG and RVC recommendations, the countries have taken the opportunity to implement national follow-up vaccination campaigns (VCs), which included vaccination of the entire target population against measles and rubella regardless of their vaccination history (indiscriminate vaccination). These campaigns were monitored for quality, coverage of the target population, efficiency, homogeneity, and timeliness of response. Between 2019 and 2023, 17 countries in Latin America and the Caribbean (LAC) conducted 17 VCs against measles and rubella, vaccinating 47,274,472 children aged 1 to 12 years with MMR and bivalent measles–rubella (MR) vaccines. Of these 16 VCs, seven achieved a coverage of ≥95% and six between 80 and 94%. During and after the COVID-19 pandemic, between 2021 and 2023, 12 countries conducted follow-up vaccination campaigns (VCs), vaccinating 37,479,561 million children in an age range of 1–12 years; five of them targeted the age group of 1–6 years and half of them applied the PAHO's high-quality criteria and microplanning process. One important fact is that at least seven of the twelve VCs had an impact on the recovery of MMR-1 and MMR-2 coverage. These VCs were conducted in Argentina, Brazil, Bolivia, Colombia, Dominican Republic, Ecuador, El Salvador, Honduras, Mexico, Nicaragua, Paraguay, and Venezuela (Table 2) [13].

**Table 1.** MMR vaccination schedule, estimated coverage with the first and second doses of measles-containing vaccines *, number of confirmed measles cases **, and confirmed measles incidence § by country or area—Pan American Health Organization/World Health Organization.

| | MMR Schedule ¶ | | 2019 | | | 2020 | | | 2021 | | | 2022 | | |
|---|---|---|---|---|---|---|---|---|---|---|---|---|---|---|
| | First Dose Age, mos | Second Dose Age, mos | Coverage, % | | No. of Measles Cases ** (Incidence) § | Coverage, % | | No. of Measles Cases ** (Incidence) § | Coverage, % | | No. of Measles Cases ** (Incidence) § | Coverage, % | | No. of Measles Cases ** (Incidence) § |
| Member States | | | MMR1 | MMR2 | | MMR1 | MMR2 | | MMR1 | MMR2 | | MMR1 | MMR2 | |
| **The Americas** | | | 87 | 75 | 24,079 ** (17.7) | 87 | 65 | 8321 (6.07) | 85 | 68 | 724 ** (0.53) | 85 | 71 | 168 (0.12) |
| **North America** | | | 90 | 94 | 1387 (3.78) | 91 | 83 | 14 (0.04) | 92 | 83 | 49 (0.13) | 92 | 79 | 124 (0.33) |
| Canada | 12 | | 90 | 87 | 113 (3.02) | 90 | 83 | 1 (0.03) | 90 | 83 | 0 (0) | 92 | 79 | 3 (0.08) |
| United States | 12 | 48 | 90 | 95 | 1274 (3.87) | 91 | | 13 (0.04) | 92 | | 49 (0.15) | 92 | | 121 (0.36) |
| **Mexico** | 12 | 18–72 | 73 | 73 | 20 (0.16) | 100 †† | 83 | 196 (1.52) | 100 †† | 97 | 0 (0) | 86 | 83 | 0 (0) |
| **Central America** | | | 91 | 86 | 10 (0.2) | 86 | 79 | 0 (0) | 86 | 75 | 0 (0) | 83 | 73 | 0 (0) |
| Costa Rica | 15 | 48 | 95 | 100 | 10 (1.98) | 95 | 81 | 0 (0) | 89 | 69 | 0 (0) | 90 | 75 | 0 (0) |
| Guatemala | 12 | 18 | 90 | 78 | 0 (0) | 88 | 79 | 0 (0) | 81 | 72 | 0 (0) | 83 | 69 | 0 (0) |
| El Salvador | 12 | 15–18 | 82 | 87 | 0 (0) | 71 | 56 | 0 (0) | 85 | 70 | 0 (0) | 65 | 59 | 0 (0) |
| Honduras | 12 | 18 | 89 | 85 | 0 (0) | 82 | 79 | 0 (0) | 81 | 75 | 0 (0) | 77 | 71 | 0 (0) |
| Nicaragua | 12 | 18 | 100 †† | 100 | 0 (0) | 100 †† | 100 †† | 0 (0) | 100 | 86 | 0 (0) | 100 †† | 100 †† | 0 (0) |
| Panama | 12 ¶ | 18 ¶ | 97 | 97 | 0 (0) | 80 | 74 | 0 (0) | 92 | 75 | 0 (0) | 87 | 75 | 0 (0) |
| **Latin Caribbean** | | | 85 | 59 | 1 (0.03) | 86 | 59 | 0 (0) | 83 | 60 | 0 (0.13) | 89 | 71 | 0 (0) |
| Cuba | 12 | 72 | 100 | 100 | 1 (0.09) | 98 | 99 | 0 (0) | 100 | 100 | 0 (0) | 100 | 100 | 0 (0) |
| Dominican Republic | 12 | 18 | 96 | 60 | 0 (0) | 82 | 55 | 0 (0) | 88 | 60 | 0 (0) | 100 †† | 87 | 0 (0) |
| Haiti | 9 * | 12–23 * | 70 | 41 | 0 (0) | 83 | 46 | 0 (0) | 73 | 44 | 0 (0) | 76 | 46 | 0 (0) |
| **Andean** | | | 89 | 62 | 802 (5.72) | 82 | 61 | 3 (0.02) | 77 | 63 | 0 (0) | 79 | 66 | 0 (0) |
| Bolivia (Plurinational State of) | 12 | 18–23 | 79 | 44 | 0 (0) | 74 | 46 | 2 (0.17) | 75 | 56 | 0 (0) | 69 | 49 | 0 (0) |
| Colombia | 12 | 60 | 95 | 89 | 252 (5.01) | 91 | 88 | 1 (0.02) | 86 | 86 | 0 (0) | 88 | 84 | 0 (0) |
| Ecuador | 12 | 18 | 83 | 76 | 0 (0) | 81 | 70 | 0 (0) | 65 | 58 | 0 (0) | 74 | 60 | 0 (0) |
| Peru | 12 | 18 | 85 | 66 | 2 (0.06) | 77 | 52 | 0 (0) | 78 | 60 | 0 (0) | 74 | 54 | 0 (0) |
| Venezuela (Bolivarian Republic of) | 12 ¶ | 18 ¶ | 93 | 13 | 548 (19.22) | 76 | 28 | 0 (0) | 68 | 38 | 0 (0) | | | 0 (0) |
| **Brazil** | 12 | | 91 | 54 | 21,704 (102.84) | 80 | 44 | 8035 (37.8) | 73 | 46 | 670 (3.13) | 81 | 58 | 41 (0.19) |
| **Southern Cone** | | | 87 | 84 | 150 (2.02) | 79 | 73 | 73 (0.97) | 84 | 79 | 0 (0) | 82 | 84 | 3 (0.04) |
| Argentina | 12 | 60 | 86 | 84 | 130 (2.9) | 77 | 71 | 69 (1.53) | 86 | 79 | 0 (0) | 85 | 94 | 2 (0.04) |
| Chile | 12 | 36 | 95 | 91 | 11 (0.58) | 91 | 83 | 2 (0.1) | 92 | 91 | 0 (0) | 94 | 81 | 0 (0) |
| Paraguay | 12 | 48 | 75 | 71 | 0 (0) | 68 | 60 | 0 (0) | 56 | 55 | 0 (0) | 42 | 41 | 1 (0.15) |
| Uruguay | 12 | 15 | 96 | 99 | 9 (2.6) | 96 | 92 | 2 (0.58) | 93 | 82 | 0 (0) | 96 | 92 | 0 (0) |
| **non-Latin Caribbean** | | | 94 | 87 | 4 (0.63) | 90 | 84 | 0 (0) | 87 | 80 | 0 (0) | 91 | 84 | 0 (0) |
| Antigua and Barbuda | 12 | 18 | 97 | 71 | 0 (0) | 89 | 80 | 0 (0) | 85 | 76 | 0 (0) | 100 | 100 | 0 (0) |
| Bahamas | 12 | 15 | 83 | 83 | 3 (7.7) | 87 | 83 | 0 (0) | 82 | 80 | 0 (0) | 80 | 65 | 0 (0) |
| Belize | 12 | 18 | 96 | 95 | 0 (0) | 82 | 87 | 0 (0) | 79 | 77 | 0 (0) | 81 | 77 | 0 (0) |
| Barbados | | | 100 †† | 85 | 0 (0) | 89 | 78 | 0 (0) | 77 | 70 | 0 (0) | 85 | 73 | 0 (0) |

**Table 1.** *Cont.*

| | MMR Schedule ¶ | | 2019 | | | 2020 | | | 2021 | | | 2022 | | |
|---|---|---|---|---|---|---|---|---|---|---|---|---|---|---|
| | First Dose Age, mos | Second Dose Age, mos | Coverage, % | | No. of Measles Cases ** (Incidence) § | Coverage, % | | No. of Measles Cases ** (Incidence) § | Coverage, % | | No. of Measles Cases ** (Incidence) § | Coverage, % | | No. of Measles Cases ** (Incidence) § |
| Member States | | | MMR1 | MMR2 | | MMR1 | MMR2 | | MMR1 | MMR2 | | MMR1 | MMR2 | |
| Dominica | 12 | 18 | 92 | 92 | 0 (0) | 92 | 90 | 0 (0) | 88 | 87 | 0 (0) | 87 | 87 | 0 (0) |
| Grenada | 12 | 18 | 94 | 82 | 0 (0) | 83 | 79 | 0 (0) | 70 | 55 | 0 (0) | 76 | 68 | 0 (0) |
| Guyana | 12 | 18 | 98 | 92 | 0 (0) | 100 †† | 97 | 0 (0) | 95 | 83 | 0 (0) | 100 †† | 100 †† | 0 (0) |
| Jamaica | 12 | 18 | 94 | 92 | 0 (0) | 93 | 89 | 0 (0) | 88 | 85 | 0 (0) | 91 | 83 | 0 (0) |
| Saint Kitts and Nevis | 12 | 18 | 97 | 98 | 0 (0) | 95 | 99 | 0 (0) | 96 | 94 | 0 (0) | 95 | 93 | 0 (0) |
| Saint Lucia | 12 | 18 | 96 | 75 | 1 (5.47) | 89 | 72 | 0 (0) | 77 | 66 | 0 (0) | 81 | 63 | 0 (0) |
| Saint Vincent and the Grenadines | 12 | 18 | 100 †† | 100 †† | 0 (0) | 100 †† | 100 †† | 0 (0) | 96 | 94 | 0 (0) | 99 | 100 | 0 (0) |
| Suriname | 12 | 18 | 85 | 43 | 0 (0) | 66 | 35 | 0 (0) | 79 | 58 | 0 (0) | 95 | 65 | 0 (0) |
| Trinidad and Tobago | 12 | 24 | 99 | 92 | 0 (0) | 91 | 90 | 0 (0) | 93 | 88 | 0 (0) | 92 | 92 | 0 (0) |

Abbreviations: MMR = measles-mumps and rubella vaccine; MMR1 = first MMR dose; MMR2 = second MMR dose; NA = not applicable; NR = not reported; WHO = World Health Organization. * According to OFFICIAL coverage reported. For MMR1, among children aged 1 year or, if MMR is given at age ≥1 year, among children aged 24 months. For MMR2, among children at the recommended age for administration of MMR2, per the national immunization schedule. Haiti administers MR vaccine. The data were last revised on 15 July 2023 at https://immunizationdata.who.int. ** Includes cases confirmed by laboratory testing or epidemiologic linkage and clinically compatible cases. Clinically compatible cases met the WHO measles clinical case definition, had no adequate specimen collected, and could not be epidemiologically linked to a laboratory-confirmed case of measles. Case totals based on country reports to CIM-PAHO weekly surveillance reports. WHO Non-member states Curaçao and French Guiana reported measles cases, 1 (2019) and 5 (2022) respectively. § Cases per 1 million population. ¶ MMR schedule is the 2022 schedule; Panama and Venezuela schedule from 2021. †† coverage data >100%. The data of each subregion have been bolded to highlight the average of all countries belonging to that subregion.

**Table 2.** Follow-up campaigns and impact on the administrative vaccination coverage with MMR-1 and MMR-2. Americas 2021–2023.

| Countries with Follow-up Campaigns 2021 | Age group | Vaccine | Target group | Vaccinated children | Coverage VC Follow-up | MMR-1 (%) 2020 | MMR-2 (%) 2020 | MMR-1 (%) 2021 | MMR-2 (%) 2021 | MMR-1 (%) change | MMR-2 (%) change | Use high-quality criteria (Y/N) | Applied micro planning (Y/N) |
|---|---|---|---|---|---|---|---|---|---|---|---|---|---|
| **Mexico** | 1–9 yo | MR/MMR | 11,662,394 | 11,202,785 | **96** | 100 | 83 | 100 | 97 | 0 | 14 | Yes | Yes |
| **Colombia** | 1–10 yo | MR/MMR | 7,552,514 | 7,208,981 | **95** | 91 | 88 | 86 | 86 | −5 | −2 | Yes | Yes |
| **Bolivia** | 1–6 yo | MR/MMR | 1,181,729 | 1,039,922 | 88 | 74 | 46 | 75 | 56 | 1 | 10 | No | No |
| **Paraguay** | 1–5 yo | MMR | 738,619 | 535,703 | 73 | 68 | 60 | 56 | 51 | −12 | −9 | No | No |
| **Total children vaccinated in 2022** | | | **21,135,256** | **19,987,391** | 95 | | | | | | | | |
| **Countries with Follow up Campaigns in 2022** | **Age group** | **Vaccine** | **Target group** | **Vaccinated children** | **Coverage VC Follow-up** | **MMR-1 (%) 2021** | **MMR-2 (%) 2021** | **MMR-1 (%) 2022** | **MMR-2 (%) 2022** | **MMR-1 (%) change** | **MMR-2 (%) change** | **Use high-quality criteria (Y/N)** | **Applied micro planning (Y/N)** |
| **Argentina** | 13–59 m | MMR | 2,315,692 | 1604631 | 69 | 86 | 79 | 85 | 94 | −1 | 15 | No | No |
| **Brazil** | 1–4 yo | MR/MMR | 12,927,057 | 6,552,277 | 51 | 73 | 46 | 81 | 58 | 8 | 12 | No | No |
| **Dominican Republic** | 1–5 yo | MR/MMR | 951,554 | 934,329 | **98** | 88 | 60 | 100 | 87 | 12 | 27 | Yes | Yes |
| **El Salvador** | 1–6 yo | MMR | 644,089 | 592,562 | 92 | 85 | 70 | 65 | 59 | −20 | −11 | No | No |
| **Honduras** | 1–6 yo | MMR | 1,669,999 | 1,386,099 | 83 | 81 | 75 | 77 | 71 | −4 | −6 | No | No |
| **Nicaragua** | 1–6 yo | MMR | 723,790 | 823,127 | **114** | 100 | 96 | 100 | 100 | 4 | 0 | Yes | Yes |
| **Venezuela** | 1–6 yo | MR/MMR | 2,811,860 | 2,479,675 | 88 | 68 | 38 | N/D | N/D | N/D | N/D | No | No |
| **Total children vaccinated in 2022** | | | **22,044,041** | **14,372,700** | 65 | | | | | | | | |

**Table 2.** *Cont.*

| Countries with Follow up in 2023 | Age group | Vaccine | Target group | Goal | Coverage | MMR-1 2022 | MMR-2 2022 | MMR-1 2023 * | MMR-2 2023 * | MMR-1 (%) change | MMR-2 (%) change | Use high-quality criteria (Y/N) | Applied micro planning (Y/N) |
|---|---|---|---|---|---|---|---|---|---|---|---|---|---|
| Ecuador * | 1–12 yo | MR/MMR | 3,189,901 | 3,119,470 | **98** | 74 | 60 | 97 | 81 | 23 | 21 | Yes | Yes |
| **Total children vaccinated in 2023** | | | **3,189,901** | **3,119,470** | 98 | | | | | | | | |
| **Total children targeted and vaccinated** | | | **46,369,198** | **37,479,561** | **81** | | | | | | | | |

* Preliminary data eJRF. Abbreviations: MR = measles-rubella vaccine; MMR = measles-mumps-rubella vaccine; MMR1 = first MMR dose; MMR2 = second MMR dose; VC = vaccination campaign; yo = years old; m = months. Source: Country reports through the electronic PAHO-WHO/UNICEF Joint Reporting Form (eJRF), 2020–2023 and country reports to the Measles Rubella Elimination Regional Commission. Bold numbers are those percentages ≥ 95% of vaccination coverage.

### *3.2. Measles Outbreaks in the Period 2019–2023*

Large global measles outbreaks between 2018 and 2019 facilitated the importation of the virus to countries in the region. In the Americas, from 2019 to 2023, eighteen countries reported 29,364 imported, import-related, or endemic measles cases, and in two of them, Brazil and Venezuela, endemic transmission was re-established as previously mentioned.

Brazil reported 30,450 confirmed endemic measles cases for this period. Venezuela had an outbreak that started in 2017 from an importation, and in 2019 reported 548 confirmed endemic measles cases. From 2019 to 2023, the United States reported 1515 confirmed measles cases, all imported or related to importation. These three countries accounted for 97.4% of the confirmed measles cases reported in the entire region. Other smaller, well-contained measles outbreaks occurred during this period without re-establishment of endemic transmission: Colombia reported 252 cases in 2019, Mexico reported 216 cases between 2019 and 2020, and Argentina reported a total of 201 confirmed measles cases in the period 2019 to 2022, none with chains of transmission of more than one year. In 2023, only 72 cases were reported in four countries: Canada (12), Chile (1), Costa Rica (1), and the United States (58). Indeed, the year 2023 had the lowest number of confirmed measles cases reported in the history of the region [16–19] (Figure 1).

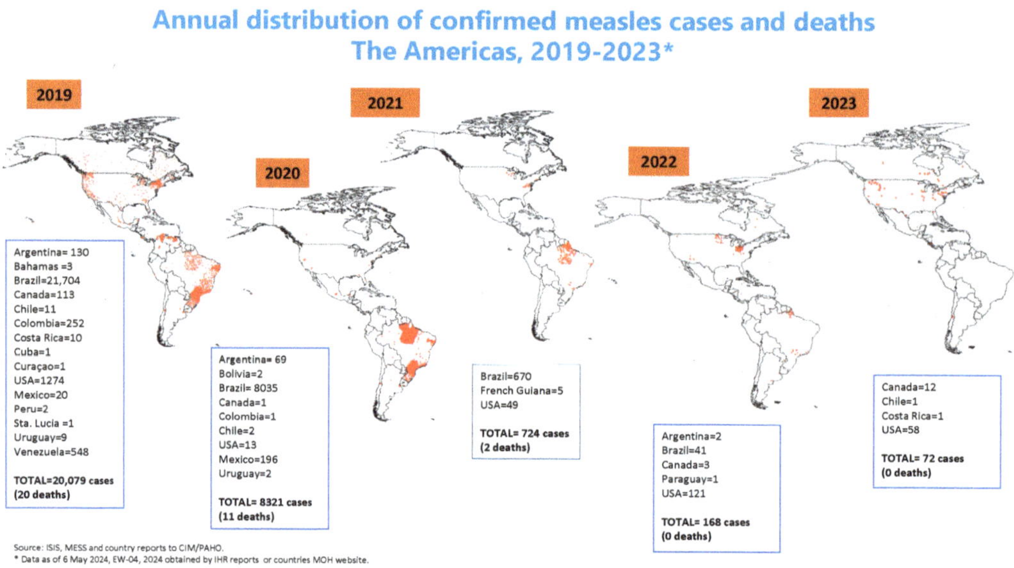


**Figure 1.** Annual distribution of confirmed measles cases and deaths The Americas, 2019–2023 *.

In December 2021, the PAHO/WHO conducted a Regional Risk Assessment on Vaccine-Preventable Diseases (VPDs) like Diphtheria, Measles, Yellow Fever, and Polio in the Context of COVID-19. This assessment alerted countries to the very-high-risk potential for other VPD outbreaks due to extremely the low vaccination coverage rates of all antigens, coupled with the weak surveillance performance indicators. This assessment also alerted countries to an increase in migration and population movement across borders during 2022 to 2023, and its potential negative impact on the healthcare systems across the region [16].

### *3.3. Epidemiological Surveillance Indicators between 2019 and 2023*

The PAHO/WHO regional measles–rubella surveillance system monitors weekly case-based active rash and fever surveillance in the 21 countries that report directly to the PAHO/WHO through ISIS. The PAHO uses these data to issue a biweekly bulletin to alert all countries to their surveillance compliance. Using data from 2019 to 2023, the PAHO conducted a intensive analysis of compliance with the four strategic lines related to vaccination coverage, epidemiological surveillance indicators, and preparedness for rapid response to outbreaks of these diseases. With gaps defined in surveillance performance defined, the PAHO targets support to countries whose surveillance performance is declining [20].

The notification rate of suspected cases should be of at least 2 cases per 100,000 habitants. In 2019, the rate was 14.13; in 2020 it was 3.93: in 2021 it was 1.44; in 2022 it was 2.32, and in 2023 it was 2.32. Fortunately, this indicator was achieved in all years except for 2021. Table 3 demonstrates a significant reduction in the countries that met each indicator in the study period during the pandemic years (Table 3).

**Table 3.** Measles and rubella surveillance indicators performance *.

| | Number and Percentage of Countries Meeting the Indicators | | | | |
|---|---|---|---|---|---|
| **MR ** Surveillance Indicators Quality** | **2019** | **2020** | **2021** | **2022** | **2023** |
| Annual suspected MR ** case rate per 100,000 population | 16 (76) | 7 (33) | 6 (29) | 10 (48) | 10 (48) |
| Percentage of MR ** suspected cases with adequate case investigation | 14 (67) | 13 (62) | 12 (57) | 14 (67) | 13 (62) |
| Percentage of suspected cases with adequate serum specimen collected, tested in a proficient laboratory | 19 (90) | 16 (76) | 16 (76) | 19 (90) | 14 (67) |
| Percentage of suspected cases with serum specimens sent to laboratory within 5 days | 11 (52) | 10 (48) | 10 (48) | 11 (52) | 13 (62) |
| Percentage of IgM laboratory results reported to national public health authorities within 4 days | 14 (67) | 11 (52) | 12 (57) | 15 (71) | 13 (62) |
| Regional rate of MR suspected cases by 100,000 habitants | 14.13 | 3.93 | 1.44 | 2.32 | 2.32 |

* Data from 21 countries and 13 countries of English Caribbean Subregion reporting to PAHO (except Canada and USA). ** MR = measles rubella.

### 3.4. *Best Practices for Strengthening the Laboratory Network*

Twenty-three measles and rubella laboratories (global specialized, regional reference, and national) participated annually in the Global Measles and Rubella Laboratory Network (GMRLN's) External Quality Assurance (EQA) exercises for IgM, real-time Reverse-Transcription–Polymerase Chain Reaction (rRT-PCR), and genotyping for both viruses. All the laboratories have IgM and IgG testing capacities, and in addition 13 have rRT-PCR and 9 have IgM, IgG, rRT-PCR, and sequencing capacities.

In the countries that have a subnational laboratory network, the national laboratory is responsible for providing training, quality control, and confirmatory testing, and in some countries it is also responsible for performing the genetic characterization of the virus identified in confirmed measles or rubella cases.

From 2019 to 2023, the PAHO conducted three regional meetings of the measles and rubella laboratory network to review the progress, achievements, and challenges of the network. The intent of these meetings was also to learn about the experiences of countries of the region related to laboratory surveillance, laboratory confirmation, and case classification, and to discuss the new assays available in the GMRLN and quality control.

Because the COVID-19 pandemic diverted all public health attention to the pandemic response, countries found it nearly impossible to advance any of the immunization activities planned. In 2021, the lab network re-started some virtual activities, and then transitioned back to face-to-face training and meetings.

During this period, the PAHO seized the opportunity to deliver a total of five on-site visits, three on-site training courses on rRT-PCR, one virtual training course on rRT-PCR, one hands-on genotyping training course, and one sequence analysis training course to laboratories of the regional network.

In elimination settings, when incidence declines the predictive positive value of IgM testing should be lower, and false positive results will increase. To face this challenge, the PAHO used this opportunity to help enhance laboratory performance. Critically, important additional sampling (second serum specimens, nasal swab, throat swab, urine) and additional testing (IgG seroconversion, IgG-avidity, rRT-PCR, sequencing) is required to improve the certainty of confirming or discarding suspected cases [21]. Countries have embraced this support. Laboratories of the regional network have used this support to improve their technical capacities and capabilities to perform these assays. This collective action among those responsible for epidemiological and laboratory surveillance advances a deeper analysis of special cases, mitigating the risk of reporting false positives.

In addition, the Regional Laboratory Network has contributed to expanding the genetic information of viruses related to confirmed measles cases. During 2019 to 2023, there was a steady uptrend in the proportion of measles sequences reported to the WHO's database for Measles Virus Nucleotide Surveillance (MeaNS), with a range between 4 and 64% and an average of 6%. Nevertheless, the number of confirmed measles cases substantially decreased, with 23,284 cases reported in 2019 and only 72 cases reported in 2023. Therefore, the uptrend observed in the proportion of measles genotypes could be explained by this significant reduction in confirmed measles cases. In addition, when countries are experiencing large-size outbreaks, such as in Brazil in 2019, the regional recommendation is to test a proportion of confirmed cases for virologic surveillance every two months to monitor if the same genotype and strain are still circulating, or a new importation or introduction has occurred [21]. The latter should be supported by sound epidemiological information.

### 3.5. Best Practices to Increase Vaccination Coverage

Due to the emergence of other public health priorities and an increasingly complex political, social, and epidemiological scenario, as with surveillance, countries are committed to revitalizing their national immunization programs in the post-pandemic period [22].

Colombia is a special example of a country that has maintained good vaccination coverage, outstanding performance related to surveillance indicators, and timely responses to outbreaks. Colombia reported the following progress to the RVC during the Third Annual Meeting in 2023: In the VC carried out in Colombia between 2021 and 2022 aimed at children between 1 and 10 years of age, the country reached a target of 95%, vaccinating 7,208,981 children. During the same period, 680,463 one-year-old children were vaccinated with an additional dose of MR and 335,920 children aged 2 to 11 years were vaccinated with a zero dose of MMR-1. The Ministry of Health continued the search for the susceptible population after the VC by conducting mop-up and active searches for the missing children to be vaccinated from 3 to 13 years of age, vaccinating 63,240 children.

The country also implemented a vaccination plan for migrants coming into the country and for Colombian travelers bound for Europe and other regions of the world. These efforts were intended to help increase population immunity and to prevent the spread of the virus in the event of importations.

## 4. Discussion

Between 2020 and 2023, the WHO declared a public health emergency of international concern (PHEIC) for COVID-19. The pandemic imposed immense challenges to global health. Undoubtedly, the COVID-19 pandemic had a negative impact on MRE strategies worldwide and specifically in the Americas, with a decline in MMR vaccination coverage and surveillance indicators. The decline in coverage was most notable with the first dose (MMR-1), which stagnated at 85% in 2022–2023. In contrast, there was a slow and sustained recovery in coverage with the second dose (MMR-2), with 68% and 70% rates in 2021 and 2022.

An opportunity to improve MMR coverage is conducting VCs when linked to essential immunization services. Together, these strategies with essential immunization taking the lead can potentially increase population immunity everywhere, which is needed to ultimately stop measles virus transmission. Those countries that applied the PAHO's high-quality criteria and microplanning in their VCs achieved the goal $\geq$ 95%. This confirms once again that VCs are a key intervention for sustaining measles and rubella elimination in our region when they have been organized with high-quality criteria and a good microplanning process.

The COVID-19 pandemic negatively impacted the notification of suspected cases, reducing the sensitivity of surveillance. The work force was directed to focus on the pandemic, so measles–rubella surveillance suffered. In 2020 and 2021, all indicators dropped, but the important thing is that the countries began to recover their suspect case notification rates from 2022 and 2023.

The performance of the surveillance indicators was relatively better in the Central American and Latin Caribbean countries, followed by the South American countries and finally the English-speaking Caribbean countries. From 2023 onwards, an increase in the number of countries complying with the suspect case notification rate occurred in all subregions.

In countries that had active outbreaks in 2020, a decrease in confirmed measles cases occurred, possibly due to the social and physical distancing measures that prevented virus circulation.

In terms of the lessons learned from the countries, Colombia implemented a high-quality follow-up vaccination campaign during 2021 and 2022 targeting children aged 1–11 years based on the available epidemiologic data. Colombia acted on the opportunity to strengthen and contain the decline in the coverage of the other biologics in the children's immunization schedule. Their approach raised awareness among parents to ensure their children's adherence to the national immunization schedule.

Increasingly important is the need to be able to document the viral genotypes and lineages associated with infection [23]. Molecular epidemiological data are of great value in documenting importations, especially when there are multiple importations of measles in a defined area, especially over a short period of time.

## 5. Conclusions

The countries of the region must concentrate their efforts on maintaining achievements in immunization, irrespective of the targeted disease. Failure to recover good vaccination coverage could have negative repercussions on the sustainability of regional MRE, given the active outbreaks in the countries of the other five regions of the world. Nevertheless, the countries of the Americas are clearly committed to sustaining MRE despite the challenges they face, as evidenced by the fact that currently no country has endemic virus circulation, and the region is once again moving towards regaining the status of a region free of endemic measles virus.

The countries must remain vigilant, improve the sensitivity of the surveillance system and be prepared for a rapid response due to the likelihood of importation of measles and rubella cases. For any suspect case, a serum specimen, nasopharyngeal swabs, and/or urine specimens should be collected for laboratory testing and ultimately for timely case confirmation.

**Author Contributions:** The following contributions were made by the authors: Conceptualization: all authors; methodology: all authors; validation: G.R.-B., D.P., C.P.-T. and C.O.; formal analysis, G.R.-B., D.P. and J.A.; writing—original draft preparation, D.P.; writing—review and editing, G.R.-B., D.P., A.W., J.A., R.D. and P.B.-A.; visualization, C.P.-T. and C.O. All authors have read and agreed to the published version of the manuscript.

**Funding:** PAHO is paying for the time of authors involved in this article, except for Dr. Jon Andrus who works at the University of George Washington.

**Conflicts of Interest:** The authors declare no conflicts of interest.

## References


1. Pan American Health Organization. Elimination of Measles in the Americas. In Proceedings of the XXIV Meeting of the Pan American Sanitary Conference, Washington, DC, USA, 26–30 September 1994. Available online: https://iris.paho.org/bitstream/handle/10665.2/57514/CSP24-res_eng.pdf?sequence=1&isAllowed=y (accessed on 30 April 2024).
2. Castillo, S.C.; Ruiz Matus, C.; Flannery, B. The Americas: Paving the Road Toward Global Measles Eradication. *J. Infect. Dis.* **2011**, *204* (Suppl. S1), 270–278. [CrossRef]
3. Pan American Health Organization. Plan of Action for Documentation and Verification of Measles, Rubella and Congenital Rubella Syndrome in the Region of the Americas. 2011. Available online: https://www3.paho.org/hq/dmdocuments/2012/PoA-Documentation-Verification-MRCRS-Elimination-s.pdf (accessed on 30 April 2024).
4. Pan American Health Organization. CD55/DIV/09 Special Report on Diverse Documents Remarks by Dr. Merceline Dahl-Regis President of the International Expert Committee for the Verification of Measles and Rubella Elimination. 55 Directing Council. In Proceedings of the 68th Session of the Regional of the World Health Organization, Washington, DC, USA, 26–30 September 2016. Available online: https://www3.paho.org/hq/dmdocuments/2016/CD55-DIV-9-s.pdf (accessed on 30 April 2024).
5. Pan American Health Organization. Resolution CSP29/8. Plan of Action for the Sustainability of Measles, Rubella, and Congenital Rubella Syndrome Elimination in the Americas 2018–2023. In Proceedings of the 29th Pan American Sanitary Conference at the 69th Session of the Regional Committee of the Americas, Washington, DC, USA, 25–29 September 2017. Available online: https://www3.paho.org/hq/index.php?option=com_docman&view=download&category_slug=29-en-9249&alias=41210-csp29-8-e-210&Itemid=270&lang=en (accessed on 30 April 2024).
6. Pan American Health Organization. Final Report of the XXV TAG Meeting, Held in Cartagena, Colombia, 9–11 July 2019. Cartagena (Colombia). Available online: https://www.paho.org/en/documents/25-tag-final-report-2019 (accessed on 30 April 2024).
7. Patel, M.; Lee, A.D.; Clemmons, N.S.; Redd, S.B.; Poser, S.; Blog, D.; Zucker, J.R.; Leung, J.; Link-Gelles, R.; Pham, H.; et al. National Update on Measles Cases and Outbreaks—United States, January 1–October 1, 2019. *Morb. Mortal. Wkly. Rep.* **2019**, *68*, 893–896. [CrossRef] [PubMed] [PubMed Central]
8. Minta, A.A.; Ferrari, M.; Antoni, S.; Portnoy, A.; Sbarra, A.; Lambert, B.; Hatcher, C.; Hsu, C.H.; Ho, L.L.; Steulet, C.; et al. Progress Toward Measles Elimination—Worldwide, 2000–2022. *Morb. Mortal. Wkly. Rep.* **2023**, *72*, 1262–1268. [CrossRef] [PubMed]
9. Pan American Health Organization. Division of Vaccines and Immunization. In *Conclusions and Recommendations from the Final Report of the 12th Meeting of the Technical Advisory Group on Vaccine-Preventable Diseases, Guatemala*; PAHO: Washington, DC, USA, 1997. Available online: https://www.paho.org/en/documents/12-tag-final-report-1997 (accessed on 30 April 2024).
10. Castillo-Solórzano, C.; Carrasco, P.; Tambini, G.; Reef, S.; Brana, M.; de Quadros, C.A. New horizons in the control of rubella and prevention of congenital rubella syndrome in the Americas. *J. Infect. Dis.* **2003**, *187*, S146–S152. Available online: https://pubmed.ncbi.nlm.nih.gov/12721906/ (accessed on 30 April 2024). [CrossRef]
11. Bispo de Filippis, A.M.; Icenogle, J.; Matus, C.R.; Andrus, J.K. Enhanced Laboratory Surveillance for the Elimination of Rubella and Congenital Rubella Syndrome in the Americas. *J. Infect. Dis.* **2011**, *204* (Suppl. S2), S652–S658. [CrossRef]
12. Pan American Health Organization. Measles and Rubella Bi-Weekly Bulletin. Available online: https://www.paho.org/en/measles-rubella-weekly-bulletin (accessed on 30 April 2024).
13. World Health Organization. *WHO/UNICEF Joint Reporting Process*; World Health Organization: Geneva, Switzerland, 2021. Available online: https://www.who.int/teams/immunization-vaccines-and-biologicals/immunization-analysis-and-insights/global-monitoring/who-unicef-joint-reporting-process (accessed on 30 April 2024).
14. Pan American Health Organization. *Proceedings of the Third Meeting of the Regional Commission for Monitroing and Re-verification of Measles, Rubella and Congenita Syndrome Elimination, Brasilia, Brazil, 14–16 November 2023*; Pan American Health Organization: Washington, DC, USA, 2023.
15. World Health Organization. PAHO's Regional presentation to the Strategic Advisory Group of Expert on Immunization (SAGE). In Proceedings of the Meeting of the Strategic Advisory Group of Experts (SAGE) on Immunization, Geneva, Switzerland, 11–14 March 2024. Available online: https://cdn.who.int/media/docs/default-source/agenda-sage/sage_agenda-final.pdf?sfvrsn=36bd91a5_1 (accessed on 2 May 2024).
16. Pan American Health Organization. Regional Risk Assessment on Vaccine-Preventable-Diseases (Diphtheria, Measles, Yellow Fever, and Polio) in the Context of the COVID-19 Pandemic: Implications for the Region of the Americas (15 December 2021). Available online: https://iris.paho.org/handle/10665.2/55636 (accessed on 2 May 2024).
17. Pan American Health Organization. *Epidemiological Update on Measles*; PAHO: Washington, DC, USA, 2020. Available online: https://iris.paho.org/bitstream/handle/10665.2/53110/EpiUpdate16November2020_eng.pdf?sequence=1&isAllowed=y (accessed on 2 May 2024).
18. Pan American Health Organization. *Epidemiological Update on Measles*; PAHO: Washington, DC, USA, 2024. Available online: https://www.paho.org/en/documents/epidemiological-alert-measles-region-americas-29-january-2024 (accessed on 2 May 2024).
19. Pan American Health Organization. *Measles Cases in the Americas*; PAHO: Washington, DC, USA. Available online: https://www.paho.org/en/topics/measles (accessed on 2 May 2024).

20. Pan American Health Organization. *Plan of Action for the Sustainability of Measles, Rubella, and Congenital Rubella Syndrome Elimination in the Americas 2018–2023: Progress Report*; PAHO: Washington, DC, USA, 2021. Available online: https://www.paho.org/en/documents/cd59inf16-e-plan-action-sustainability-measles-rubella-and-congenital-rubella-syndrome (accessed on 30 April 2024).
21. Pan American Health Organization. *Guidance for Testing of Measles and Rubella in the Laboratory Network of the Region of the Americas*; PAHO: Washington, DC, USA, 2019. Available online: https://iris.paho.org/handle/10665.2/34932 (accessed on 30 April 2024).
22. Pan American Health Organization. *CD59.R13—Reinvigorating Immunization as a Public Good for Universal Health*; PAHO: Washington, DC, USA, 2021. Available online: https://iris.paho.org/handle/10665.2/5830He8 (accessed on 30 April 2024).
23. Williams, D.; Penedos, A.; Bankamp, B.; Anderson, R.; Hübschen, J.; Mamou, M.B.; Beck, A.; Brown, D.; Rey-Benito, G.; Evans, R.; et al. Update: Circulation of active genotypes of measles virus and recommendations for use of sequence analysis to monitor viral transmission. *Wkly. Epidemiol. Rec.* **2022**, *97*, 481–492. Available online: https://iris.who.int/handle/10665/363330 (accessed on 30 April 2024).

*vaccines*

MDPI

*Article*

# Progress of Measles and Rubella Surveillance in the Context of Measles Elimination in the WHO Eastern Mediterranean Region, 2019–2022

**Muhammad Farid [1,*], Kamal Fahmy [1], Amany Ghoniem [1], Md Sharifuzzaman [1], Quamrul Hasan [1], Natasha Crowcroft [2] and Patrick O'Connor [2]**

1 Immunization Vaccine Preventable Disease and Polio Transition Unit, Department of Communicable Diseases, WHO Regional Office of the Eastern Mediterranean Region, Cairo 11371, Egypt
2 Department of Immunization, Vaccines and Biologicals, World Health Organization, 1202 Geneva, Switzerland; oconnorp@who.int (P.O.)
* Correspondence: faridmu@who.int

**Abstract:** In 2015, the 62nd session of the Regional Committee [RC] of the Eastern Mediterranean Region [EMR] endorsed the Eastern Mediterranean Vaccine Action Plan 2016–2020 (EMVAP) that included postponement of the measles elimination target to before 2020. However, the EMR does not have a regional rubella control or elimination goal. We reviewed the progress of measles and rubella surveillance in context of measles elimination in the Eastern Mediterranean Region during 2019–2022. We compiled data on coverage, reported cases, surveillance indicators, incidence, and genotypes. We conducted an age-cohort analysis to estimate the size of the susceptible population using coverage and SIAs coverage data. We reviewed the dossiers of countries that applied to the Regional Verification Commission [RVC] for the verification of measles and rubella elimination. Between 2019 and 2022, the regional coverage of the vaccine against measles and rubella was stable at 83% for the first dose [MCV1] and increased from 75% to 78% for the second dose [MCV2] after a dip during COVID-19. In the EMRO, eighteen countries are using MR (measles–rubella) and/or measles–mumps–rubella (MMR) vaccines and four are using measles vaccines. The reported regional measles incidence per 1,000,000 was 23.3 in 2019, decreased to 7.4 in 2020, and re-increased to 50 in 2022, with two main genotypes–D8 and B3–in circulation. Both genotypes are considered to be actively circulating in eighteen countries, with different circulating variants of each genotype. There were no genotyping data available from four countries. Measles and rubella surveillance indicators deteriorated in the region. The number of susceptible individuals exceeded one birth cohort in nine of the 22 countries. In 2019–2022, Bahrain, Egypt, Iran, and Oman were verified to have eliminated measles and rubella. While four countries eliminated measles and rubella and another five progressed toward measles and rubella elimination, however, immunity gaps and reported incidence increased in eleven countries. Countries approaching elimination need to prepare verification dossiers, while others need to increase their routine coverage, conduct follow-up campaigns, and improve surveillance. Submission of progress reports to the RVC will measure progress toward the goal.

**Keywords:** measles and rubella elimination in EMR; measles and rubella surveillance; disease surveillance; epidemiology; disease incidence; immunization coverage; WHO Eastern Mediterranean region and vaccine preventable disease

## 1. Research in Context

### 1.1. What Is Already Known about This Topic?

The annual reported regional measles incidence increased from 33.5 per million population in 2013 to 91.2 in 2018, primarily because of large outbreaks in Pakistan, Somalia, and Yemen, before decreasing to 23.3 in 2019.

### 1.2. *What Is Added by This Report?*

In 2015, the member states of the Eastern Mediterranean Region adopted the postponement of the measles elimination goal, setting up a new timeline for measles elimination by the year 2020. Between 2019 to 2022, four countries were verified for measles and rubella (MR) elimination, and another five have been progressing toward achieving MR elimination. Other countries had large immunity gaps for measles and rubella with surveillance deteriorating for various reasons, including the COVID-19 pandemic.

### 1.3. *What Are the Implications for Public Health Practice?*

Collaborative efforts are needed to mobilize resources to increase routine measles coverage, implement timely high-quality preventive campaigns, and strengthen measles case-based surveillance.

All countries are encouraged to submit early dossiers to the Regional Verification Commission (RVC) for verification.

## 2. Introduction

In August 2020, in resolution WHA 72/90, the Seventy-Third session of the World Health Assembly endorsed The Immunization Agenda 2030: A Global Strategy to Leave No One Behind (IA2030) [1]. The IA2030 outlines goals for reducing morbidity and mortality from vaccine-preventable diseases throughout the course of life, leaving no one behind by increasing equitable access to vaccines for all children [2]. The IA 2030 agenda has identified measles incidence and measles vaccination coverage as an important tracer of inadequate coverage and gaps in immunization for every country, which may also signal people's inadequate access to primary health care services [3]. This highlights the importance of having a rigorous measles surveillance program to detect immunity gaps and achieve an adequate uptake of at least 95% coverage with two timely doses of a measles-containing vaccine (MCV) among children. The Global Measles–Rubella Strategic Framework 2021–2030 [4], and the Global Measles Outbreaks Strategic Response Plan 2021–2023 [5] align with the IA2030 to achieve measles and rubella elimination by strengthening surveillance for measles and rubella and using effective elimination standard measles surveillance as a critical indicator of the effectiveness of the immunization program.

Between 2000 and 2022, global efforts to strengthen immunization systems across all countries were accelerated, which increased measles vaccination coverage globally until the time of COVID-19 pandemic, when the progress witnessed a backslide. Among the 194 WHO countries, the number of countries that included a rubella-containing vaccine (RCV) in their immunization schedules increased from 132 (68%) in 2012 to 170 (88%) in 2019, and further increased to 175 (90%) in 2022. Between 2000 and 2021, the estimated global coverage with a first MCV dose (MCV1) increased from 72% in 2000, peaked at 86% in 2019, then decreased to 83% in 2020 and 81% in 2021 during the COVID-19 pandemic, the lowest estimated coverage since 2008. Similarly, the global coverage of the rubella-containing vaccine decreased from 69% in 2019 to 68% in 2020 and 66% in 2021, then slightly increased in 2022 to 68%. While surveillance for measles and rubella remained key to achieving the elimination goals, in 2021, only 47 out of the 135 countries reporting (35%), such information achieved the sensitivity indicator target of two or more non-measles, non-rubella discarded rate cases per 100,000 population, pointing to the underperformance and inadequacies of the surveillance system monitoring measles and rubella in many countries. Globally, annual reported measles rates dropped by 88% from 145 to 18 cases per million population during the period 2000–2016, rebounded to 120 in 2019, then declined to 21 in 2020 and 17 in 2021, then increased to 29 in 2022. Between 2000 and 2021, the annual number of estimated measles deaths decreased by 83%, from 761,000 to 128,000 [3], but then increased to 136,000 in 2022 [6]. Globally, reported rubella cases have decreased from 49,180 in 2019 to 17,082 in 2022.

In 2015, the 62nd session of the Regional Committee [RC] of the Eastern Mediterranean Region [EMR] endorsed the Eastern Mediterranean Vaccine Action Plan 2016–2020

(EMVAP) [7]. EMVAP included a postponement of the measles elimination target that had been endorsed by the RC in 1997, which stated that elimination should be achieved at the earliest possible date and before 2020. To achieve elimination, the EMVAP proposed four strategies: First, every district must achieve a high population immunity by achieving at least 95% coverage of two doses of a measles-containing vaccine through routine vaccination and supplementary immunization activities (SIAs) whenever needed. Second, all countries must establish high-quality case-based surveillance with the support of proficient laboratories. Third, countries need to prepare for measles outbreaks and create response plans to detect them and respond with optimal measles case management, including dietary supplementation with vitamin A. Fourth, national immunization programs must communicate effectively to engage communities and build public confidence and demand for immunization. Since the endorsement of the elimination target in 1997, the member states have committed to implementing these regional strategies with various levels of quality.

In February 2018, the WHO Eastern Mediterranean Regional Office (EMRO) established a regional committee for the verification of measles and rubella elimination [8]. This system included establishing a national verification committee in every country and a Regional Verification Commission for Measles and Rubella (RVC-MR) to monitor and verify the status of countries' measles and rubella elimination. EMRO published a series of reports to document progress toward measles elimination. The last one, published in 2024, indicated that the annual regional measles incidence decreased from 29.8 cases per 1 million population in 2019 to 7.4 in 2020, but then increased 68% to 50.0 in 2022 because of the challenges of providing immunization services and conducting surveillance during the COVID-19 pandemic. In recent times, the molecular characterization data of the measles virus, such as on the circulating genotypes and sequence variants, have formed an integral component of measles surveillance. The identification of the genotypes of confirmed measles cases is an important performance indicator for viral surveillance, which is strongly recommended in support of achieving the national and global goals of measles and rubella elimination. The accurate description of the distribution of measles genotypes in a country or region can provide valuable data on the source of the transmission pathway of the virus, detect imported cases, and can provide evidence of the interruption of the endemic transmission of measles in any country or region. Such data can therefore be used to verify elimination. Conversely, documenting any change in the circulating genotypes can also serve as a valuable tool for measuring the effectiveness of a measles control and elimination program in the countries of the WHO Eastern Mediterranean Region.

By integrating measles genomic surveillance into the epidemiological surveillance of measles, the countries of the WHO Eastern Mediterranean Region can track the circulating genotypes and document the progress of programs to eliminate the transmission of the endemic virus [9,10].

To achieve measles elimination, the report recommended efforts to (a) improve surveillance including laboratory component especially genotyping, (b) increase MCV1 and MCV2 coverage and conduct high-quality supplementary immunization activities, and (c) reach populations at high risk of not accessing immunization services, including those living in areas of civil strife. This report describes the progress of measles and rubella surveillance in the context of measles elimination in the WHO Eastern Mediterranean Region during 2019–2022. The WHO Eastern Mediterranean comprises 21 member states (Afghanistan, Bahrain, Djibouti, Egypt, Iran, Iraq, Jordan, Kuwait, Lebanon, Libya, Morocco, Oman, Pakistan, Qatar, Saudi Arabia, Somalia, Sudan, Syria, Tunisia, the United Arab Emirates, and Yemen) and the occupied Palestinian territory (including East Jerusalem), with a population of nearly 745 million people.

## 3. Methods

We extracted and reviewed the WHO-UNICEF vaccination coverage estimates for the first and second doses of MCV for all of the 21 countries and the occupied Palestinian territory (including East Jerusalem) of the WHO Eastern Mediterranean Region that were available at the time of this analysis, up to the year 2022. These data were shared by the countries with WHO and UNICEF using the Joint Reporting Form. We estimated the coverage using both the routine and supplementary immunization activities carried out in the 21 countries and the occupied Palestinian territory of the WHO Eastern Mediterranean Region from 2019 to 2022. We also reviewed measles surveillance performance and analyzed the epidemiological trends of measles as reported in the case-based surveillance database. Additionally, we reviewed the laboratory surveillance data, including information on the genotyping of the measles virus, from the measles and rubella laboratory network of the WHO Eastern Mediterranean Region, which is a part of the WHO's global measles and rubella laboratory network.

### 3.1. Immunization

As of 2022, all of the Member States in the region have a routine immunization schedule that include two doses of a measles-containing vaccine, eighteen countries are providing rubella-containing vaccines with measles vaccines. and four countries (Afghanistan, Djibouti, Somalia, and Sudan) are providing only measles-containing vaccines. The WHO's and UNICEF's national coverage estimates review the data that WHO and UNICEF receive from all member states through the Joint Reporting Form [JRF] [11], which is submitted to WHO and the United Nations Children's Fund (UNICEF) on a yearly basis, and available survey results to generate annual estimates of vaccination coverage. Vaccinations against measles and rubella are offered free in the region, and the private sector's participation in delivering routine immunization services is very limited or marginal.

### 3.2. Immunity Profile

Based on data related to routine immunization coverage including age at administration, SIAs type, age group targeted, and coverage data as well as the anticipated efficacy of the vaccine by the age of administration (85% at 9 months, 95% at 12 months, and 97% at 18 months), we used an age-cohort analysis to estimate the proportion of children remaining susceptible for measles in each age cohort and expressed it as a ratio of the birth cohort [9].

### 3.3. Surveillance System Performance Indicators

All EMR countries except one have established a case-based measles and rubella surveillance system including laboratory testing of all identified suspected cases. Given the disease burden and field constraints, Somalia has implemented aggregate surveillance with limited laboratory testing. All countries use the definition of fever and rash to identify suspected cases and report measles data monthly using a standardized EMRO reporting template. Countries confirm suspected measles cases based on laboratory findings, epidemiologic linkages, and clinical criteria. Measles and rubella laboratory surveillance is based on the serological confirmation of suspected cases and virological characterization of circulating viruses. If a suspected case turns out to be negative for measles by serology, then it is tested for a confirmation of rubella. Countries report viral sequence data to the WHO global measles nucleotide surveillance database [12]. The EMRO monitors case-based measles and rubella in countries using selected surveillance performance indicators. Those include (1) the annualized rate of non-measles non-rubella discarded cases (target rate equal to or exceeding 2/100,000 population), (2) $\geq$80% of suspected measles and rubella cases meeting the criteria for timeliness and completeness of investigation, (3) $\geq$80% of suspected cases with adequate specimens collected and tested in a proficient laboratory, (4) $\geq$80% IgM results reported to national public health authorities by the laboratory within 4 days, (5) $\geq$80% of specimens received at a laboratory within 5 days of collection. We used the reported incidence rate of rubella and measles cases per 1,000,000 population, the WUENIC estimated coverage of the two MCV doses [13], and the sensitivity of the surveillance system represented by the annual non-measles non-rubella discarded rate equal to or exceeding 2/100,000 population to classify the countries' progress toward elimination (i.e., eliminated, approaching elimination, or endemic).

### 3.4. Laboratory Methods

EMRO hosts a measles and rubella laboratory network, which is part of the WHO global measles and rubella laboratory network. Each country hosts a national measles and rubella laboratory, while Pakistan hosts a subregional reference laboratory and Oman and Tunisia host regional reference laboratories (RRLs). All of the 22 national laboratories can perform tests of human blood serum samples for the detection of measles and/or rubella specific Immunoglobulin M (IgM) antibody using an Enzyme Linked Immunosorbent Assay (ELISA) In addition, sixteen of the 22 countries established virus detection by Real Time Polymerase Chain Reaction (RT-PCR) or virus isolation in cell culture using a blood sample. Sequencing and genotyping at national or reference laboratories further characterizes viruses. Countries who only have serology capacity can access RRLs for genotyping and sequencing. All of the national measles/rubella laboratories and the RRLs are subjected to regular WHO accreditation to confirm that they are adequate to perform the laboratory surveillance and document progress toward elimination. The molecular surveillance of the measles and rubella virus epidemiology documents the impact of immunization programs, assesses the sensitivity of the surveillance system to detect imported cases, and measures progress toward elimination goals through the identification of the genotypes of confirmed cases. We described each outbreak in terms of sequence diversity, which tracks multiple transmission pathways and monitors the elimination of virus strains and the interruption of endemic virus circulation.

The members of the EMR measles laboratory network submit most of the measles sequence data generated to the measles and rubella nucleotide surveillance sequence database [12], which is a web-accessible and quality-controlled nucleotide database used by the WHO Measles and Rubella Laboratory Network that allow the comparison of identified viruses with viruses in other countries [11].

### 3.5. Regional Verification

The National Verification Committees (NVCs) of countries approaching elimination submit their initial verification reports for the review of the RVC. The EMRO shares the RVC's comments with the NVCs to finalize their reports. During RVC meetings, the RVC reviews and discusses the dossiers to decide on the elimination status.

The RVC-MR met four times between 2019 and 2022 (including the initial orientation and establishment). In 2019, six countries submitted applications, and three of them were verified for measles and rubella: Iran, Bahrain, and Oman. In 2022, the three countries verified in 2019 were confirmed for sustained elimination status. One additional country (Egypt) was verified for measles and rubella elimination.

## 4. Results

### 4.1. Immunization

In 2019–2022, the estimated regional MCV1 coverage remained stable at 83%, while the estimated MCV2 coverage increased from 76% to 78%. The number of countries that reached the target of 95% coverage for two doses at the national level remained stable at eight from 2019 to 2022. (Table 1). Eighteen countries of the Eastern Mediterranean Region used an MR vaccine in their routine immunization program.

**Table 1.** MCV1 and MCV2 coverage, number of confirmed measles and rubella cases by country—WHO Eastern Mediterranean Region, 2019–2022.

| | 2019 | | | | 2020 | | | | 2021 | | | | 2022 | | | |
|---|---|---|---|---|---|---|---|---|---|---|---|---|---|---|---|---|
| | Coverage (%) | | Cases (*n*) | | Coverage (%) | | Cases (*n*) | | Coverage (%) | | Cases (*n*) | | Coverage (%) | | Cases (*n*) | |
| Country | MCV1 | MCV2 | No. of Measles Cases | No. of Rubella Cases | MCV 1 | MCV2 | No. of Measles Cases | No. of Rubella Cases | MCV 1 | MCV2 | No. of Measles Cases | No. of Rubella Cases | MCV1 | MCV2 | No. of Measles Cases | No. of Rubella Cases |
| Afghanistan *** | 64 | 41 | 212 | 59 | 66 | 43 | 452 | 12 | 63 | 44 | 2916 | 43 | 68 | 49 | 5090 | 197 |
| Bahrain | 99 | 99 | - | - | 99 | 99 | - | - | 99 | 99 | - | - | 99 | 99 | - | - |
| Djibouti *** | 83 | 81 | NR | NR | 62 | 60 | NR | NR | 50 | 48 | NR | NR | 50 | 48 | 182 | 21 |
| Egypt | 95 | 94 | - | - | 94 | 94 | - | - | 96 | 96 | - | - | 96 | 96 | - | 5 |
| Iran | 99 | 98 | - | 16 | 99 | 98 | 1 | 2 | 99 | 98 | 104 | 28 | 99 | 98 | - | 90 |
| Iraq | 82 | 86 | 1177 | 19 | 76 | 94 | 312 | - | 75 | 83 | 15 | 3 | 88 | 97 | 36 | 27 |
| Jordan | 87 | 93 | 45 | 2 | 76 | 90 | - | - | 76 | 90 | 2 | - | 76 | 90 | 21 | 1 |
| Kuwait | 97 | 94 | 12 | 2 | 95 | 94 | - | - | 94 | 94 | 4 | 1 | 99 | 94 | 7 | - |
| Lebanon | 82 | 63 | 1046 | 19 | 74 | 64 | 15 | - | 67 | 59 | 5 | - | 67 | 59 | 86 | 2 |
| Libya | 73 | 72 | 188 | 31 | 73 | 72 | 20 | 3 | 73 | 72 | 5 | 9 | 73 | 72 | 13 | 32 |
| Morocco | 99 | 99 | 12 | 8 | 99 | 99 | 5 | 3 | 99 | 99 | - | 1 | 99 | 99 | 2 | 18 |
| Oman | 99 | 99 | - | - | 99 | 99 | - | - | 99 | 99 | - | - | 97 | 98 | - | - |
| Pakistan | 81 | 74 | 2066 | 1370 | 83 | 77 | 2747 | 99 | 81 | 79 | 7040 | 98 | 82 | 79 | 7068 | 309 |
| Palestine | 99 | 99 | 228 | - | 99 | 99 | 833 | - | 98 | 99 | - | - | 97 | 93 | - | - |
| Qatar | 99 | 98 | 5 | 1 | 90 | 88 | 3 | - | 99 | 99 | - | 1 | 99 | 99 | 4 | - |
| Saudi Arabia | 95 | 96 | 1035 | 52 | 96 | 96 | 30 | 24 | 98 | 97 | 13 | 4 | 98 | 98 | 149 | 40 |
| Somalia *** | 46 | NA ¶ | 4482 | - | 46 | NA ¶ | 2518 | - | 46 | 4 | 746 | 2 | 46 | 8 | 805 | - |
| Sudan *** | 90 | 74 | 3555 | 280 | 86 | 68 | 354 | 243 | 81 | 63 | 627 | 251 | 81 | 63 | 1272 | 694 |
| Syria | 65 | 54 | 27 | 4 | 59 | 53 | 15 | 4 | 59 | 53 | 11 | 7 | 41 | 38 | 217 | 23 |
| Tunisia | 98 | 97 | 4669 | 162 | 98 | 96 | 11 | 26 | 95 | 98 | 2 | 5 | 95 | 98 | 10 | 16 |
| United Arab Emirates | 99 | 94 | 186 | 102 | 99 | 92 | 50 | 11 | 99 | 96 | 29 | 1 | 98 | 91 | 98 | 4 |
| Yemen | 67 | 46 | 1162 | 268 | 68 | 46 | 222 | 88 | 71 | 52 | 5341 | 530 | 73 | 56 | 23,924 | 1654 |
| EMR | 83 | 76 | 20,107 | 2395 | 83 | 77 | 7588 | 515 | 82 | 77 | 16,860 | 984 | 83 | 78 | 38,984 | 3133 |

Source: EMR measles and rubella surveillance database. WHO and United Nations Children's Fund Estimates of National Immunization Coverage (WUENIC). Color scale: Red color is for lower coverage and green is high coverage. *** Countries providing only measles-containing vaccines in their routine immunization schedule. ¶ Dose was not included in the vaccination schedule for that year.

During 2019–2022, 5 countries (Bahrain, Iran, Morocco, Oman, and Qatar) were able to maintain a high coverage of 99% with both doses of both measles and rubella vaccines, seven countries were able to improve their coverage. In seven countries, coverage decreased from 2019 to 2022, and in Somalia coverage remained stable at 46% for MCV1. (Table 1).

### 4.2. *Immunity Profile*

The ratio of the estimated proportion of susceptible children under five years old to the birth cohort size ranged from 0.4 in Morocco to 2.5 in Somalia, with nine countries having a ratio equal to or exceeding 1.

Surveillance: The key indicators deteriorated from 2019 to 2022. The number of countries that achieved the target of ≥80% of suspected cases having adequate specimens collected and tested in a proficient laboratory decreased from 21 countries in 2019 to 18 in 2022. The regional reported incidence rates of measles reached 23.3 per million in 2019, decreased to 7.4 per million in 2020, re-increased to 9.6 per million in 2021, then jumped to 50 per million in 2022. During 2019, the regional incidence rate of rubella was 3.2 per million, decreased to 0.7 in 2020, then increased to 1.3 in 2021 and 4 per million in 2022 (Table 2). The number of countries achieving 80% timeliness and completeness of investigations decreased from 7 in 2019 to 6 in 2022. The number of countries with a non-measles non-rubella discarded rate ≥2/100,000 population decreased from 14 in 2019 to 11 in 2022 (which might indicate that the reduction in reported cases in 2020–2021 might be false) and the number of countries with ≥80% IgM results reported to national public health authorities by the laboratory within 4 days decreased from 12 in 2019 to 9 in 2022 (Table 2). The number of countries with ≥80% of specimens received at the laboratory within 5 days of collection decreased from 13 in 2019 to 12 in 2022.

**Table 2.** Key surveillance indicators, WHO Eastern Mediterranean Region, 2019–2022.

| Indicator | Target | No. (%) of Countries | | | |
|---|---|---|---|---|---|
| | | 2019 | 2020 | 2021 | 2022 |
| Surveillance quality | | | | | |
| Timeliness and Completeness of Suspected Measles and Rubella Case Investigation | ≥80% | 7 (32) | 5 (23) | 3 (14) | 6 (27) |
| Percentage of Specimens Received at the Laboratory within 5 Days of Collection | ≥80% | 13 (59) | 13 (59) | 12 (55) | 12 (55) |
| Percentage of Suspected Cases with Adequate Specimens Collected and Tested in a Proficient Laboratory | ≥80% | 21 (95) | 21 (95) | 14 (64) | 18 (82) |
| Percentage of IgM Laboratory Results Reported to National Public Health Authorities within 4 days | ≥80% | 12 (55) | 12 (55) | 11 (50) | 9 (41) |
| Discarded (Non-Measles and Non-Rubella) Case Rate per 100,000 Population | ≥2 | 14 (64) | 9 (41) | 8 (36) | 11 (50) |
| Number of Countries Eliminated Measles | 22 | 3 (14) | 3 (14) | 3 (14) | 4 (18) |
| Number of Countries Eliminated Rubella | 22 | 3 (14) | 3 (14) | 3 (14) | 4 (18) |
| **Measles incidence *** | 0 | 29.8 | 7.4 | 9.6 | 50 |
| **Rubella incidence *** | 0 | 3.2 | 0.7 | 1.3 | 4.0 |

IgM = Immunoglobulin M. * Cases per 1 million Population.

From 2019 to 2022 in the WHO EMR, six countries (Afghanistan, Iraq, Pakistan, Sudan, Somalia, and Yemen) reported high number of measles cases compared to other countries in the region. Measles had two peak seasons during the years 2019 to 2022; one peak appeared from January to April in all years, decreased from May to October, then increased again from November to the end of the year, except for 2022, when cases increased from January to March, decreased in April, then increased in May and June, decreased in July, and increased from August to December (Figure 1). While rubella cases had a peak season from March to May of all years except 2022, when high number of cases was reported from March to May and again in October and November. Rubella cases were reported mainly by Pakistan, Sudan, and Yemen. (Figure 2). There was a drop in reported cases of both measles and rubella during 2020, most probably because of COVID-19.

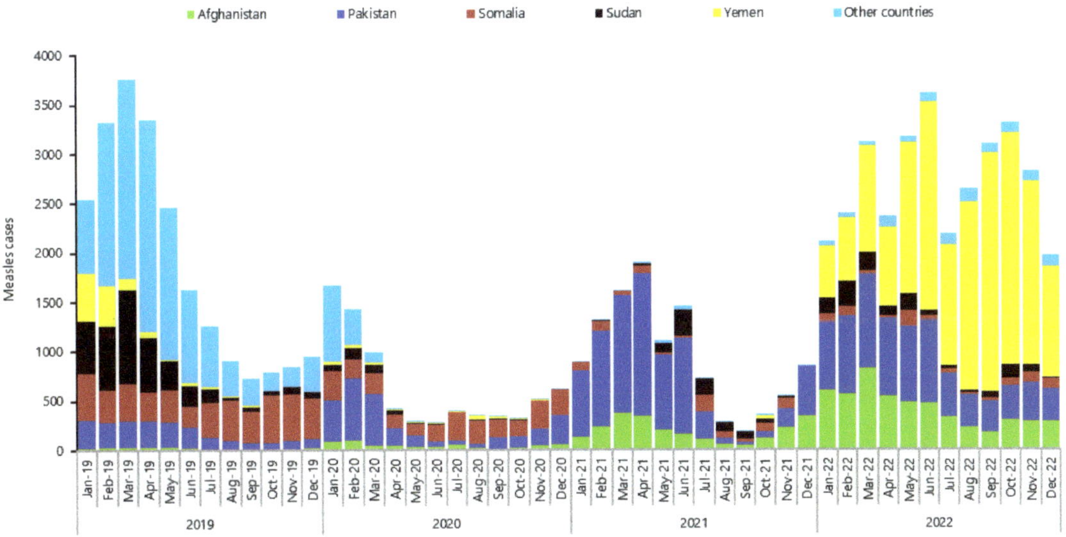


**Figure 1.** Confirmed measles cases by month of rash onset, WHO Eastern Mediterranean Region, 2019–2022.

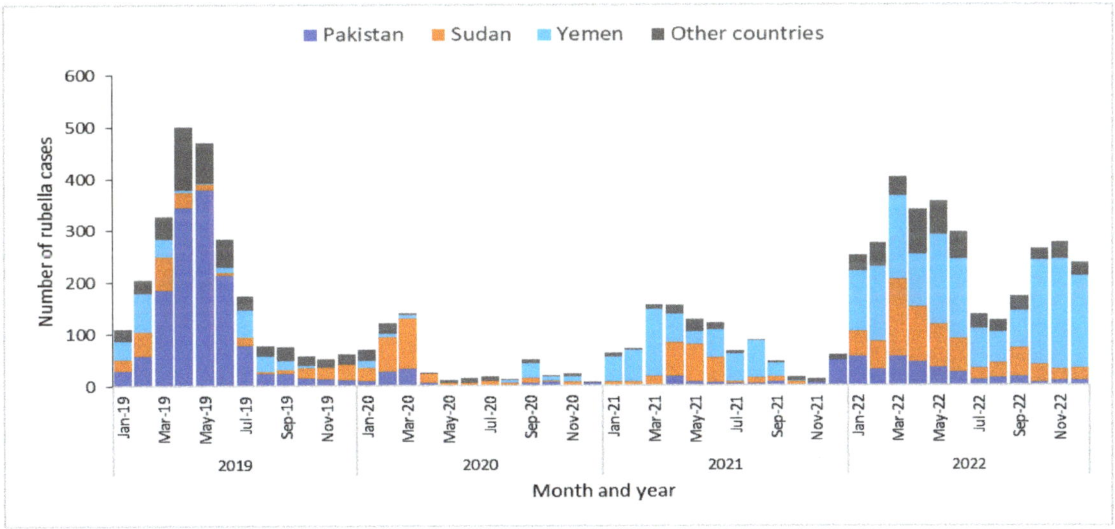


**Figure 2.** Confirmed rubella cases by month of rash onset, WHO Eastern Mediterranean Region, 2019–2022.

During 2019, 8 countries reported 95% of the year's measles cases, compared to 96% of the annual measles cases reported by four countries (Afghanistan, Pakistan, Sudan, and Yemen) in 2022. (Table 1). While 96% of the cases were reported by seven countries in 2019, the majority (57%) of cases were reported from Pakistan, compared to 95% of the cases being reported by six countries in 2022; the majority (53%) of these cases were reported from Yemen.

### 4.3. Genotypes

Table 3 shows that measles genotype B3 and D8 are considered to be actively circulating in eighteen countries, with different circulating variants of both genotypes. The B3 types were more dominant, with 1273 sequences submitted to MeaNS, while the D8 types had 51 sequences submitted. There were no genotyping data available from four countries. During period of 2019 to 2022, rubella genotype 2B was circulating in three countries, (Egypt, Iran, and Oman) of the WHO EMR. Data from other countries on rubella genotyping are not available.

**Table 3.** Measles Genotyping, circulating variants in the WHO Eastern Mediterranean Region 2019–2022 *.

| Country | 2019 | 2020 | 2021 | 2022 |
|---|---|---|---|---|
| Afghanistan | B3 | | | B3 |
| Bahrain | B3, D8 | | | B3 |
| Djibouti ** | | | | |
| Egypt | B3 | | | D8 |
| Iran | B3, D8 | | B3 | B3 |
| Iraq | B3, D8 | | | |
| Jordan | B3 | | | |
| Kuwait ** | | | | |
| Lebanon | D8 | | | B3 |
| Libya | B3 | | | |
| Morocco ** | | | | |
| Palestine | D8 | | | |
| Oman | B3, D8 | B3 | | B3 |
| Pakistan | B3 | B3 | B3 | B3 |
| Qatar | | | | B3, D8 |
| Saudi Arabia | B3 | B3 | B3 | |
| Somalia | B3 | | | |
| Sudan | B3 | B3 | | |
| Syria | | | | D8 |
| Tunisia | B3 | B3 | | B3 |
| United Arab Emirates | B3 | B3, D8 | B3 | B3, D8 |
| Yemen ** | | | | |

* Based on global surveillance for measles viruses and data reported to MeaNS, which may be incomplete

B3 D8

Genotype B3 and D8 are considered to be actively circulating in 18 countries, with different circulating variants of both genotypes

** Measles genotype data not available in 4 countries

Fifty percent of the circulating B3 sequences were related to thirteen named strains, and most of them related to MVs/Kabul.AFG/20.14/3 ($n$ = 231) in 2019–2022, and MVs/Quetta. PAK/44.20 ($n$ = 209) 2020–2022, followed by MVs/Kohistan.PAK/51.20 ($n$ = 53) 2020–2022, MVs/Bradford.GBR/13.18 ($n$ = 44) 2019–2022, MVs/Alburaimi.OMN/15.20 ($n$ = 32) 2020–2022, MVi/Harare.ZWE/38.09 ($n$ = 21) 2019, MVs/Ohio.USA/37.22 ($n$ = 16) 2022, MVs/Salalah.OMN/23.18 ($n$ = 10) 2020–2022, MVs/Kansas.USA/1.12 ($n$ = 8) 2019–2020, MVs/Islamabad.PAK/1.13 ($n$ = 6) 2019, 2021,2022, and MVs/Oslo.NOR/16.18 ($n$ = 4) 2019–2022, and two cases reported in 2019 matching MVs/Minnesota. USA/15.17 and MVs/Niger.NGA/8.13.

The remaining 50% of circulating B3 variants ($n$ = 637) detected in 2019–2022 are still unnamed.

The reported named strains of the D8 genotype accounted for 86.3% of cases. They were MVs/Gir Somnath.IND/42.16 (20) 2019, MVs/Gaziantep.TUR/13.17 (12) 2019, MVs/ Frankfurt Main.DEU/17.11 (10) 2019, 2022, and two cases reported in 2022 matching

MVs/Patan.IND/16.19 and MVs/Rudaki.TJK/49.21. The remaining 13.7% were unnamed D8 variants (7) 2019–2022.

**5. Discussion**

The WHO EMR has made substantial progress in reducing measles and rubella cases and deaths since 2000 [8]. The regional MCV1 coverage increased steadily, although it remained below the level of ≥95% necessary to achieve and sustain measles elimination. The WHO Eastern Mediterranean Region, as a whole, did not attain the measles elimination goal. The member states faced challenges, including complex operating environments and the COVID-19 pandemic. Despite the COVID-19 pandemic, NVCs continued to report, the RVC continued to meet and to verify the elimination statuses of the countries in the region, and some progress continued to be made toward measles and rubella elimination.

Eleven Member States of the WHO EMR are in a better situation in the region. Among them, four countries (Bahrain, Egypt, Iran, and Oman) have achieved measles and rubella elimination. Key aspects of the successful member states include sustained high immunization coverage (≥95%) with the two routine doses of measles- and rubella-containing vaccines, supplemented by national or subnational SIAs where required and a strong surveillance system that includes strong laboratory support. This led to zero endemic measles and rubella cases, which was well documented in their dossiers. In these countries, high political commitment and strong health systems were important contributing factors. Seven other countries (Kuwait, Morocco, Palestine, Qatar, Saudi Arabia, Tunisia, and the United Arab Emirates) also have these systems and commitments, but technical issues persist, including gaps in subnational coverage and surveillance indicators that must be addressed.

Unfortunately, the eleven other countries of the region (Afghanistan, Djibouti, Lebanon, Libya, Iraq, Jordan, Pakistan, Somalia, Sudan, Syria, and Yemen) are in crises situations that prevent or hamper system strengthening and the prioritization of elimination. Some of them faced economic crises, armed conflicts, and unpredictable mass population displacements and resettlements. All of these challenges resulted in underperformance of the immunization program and hence measles and/or rubella immunity gaps with a high ratio of susceptible children to the size of one birth cohort. Such immunity gaps lead to an increased risk of frequent large-scale measles and rubella outbreaks that cause a substantial disease burden. Therefore, frequent and/or regular preventive SIAs will be needed in the short term to build immunity and prevent measles mortality. Conducting SIAs in areas with complex humanitarian emergencies requires strong partnerships and local communities' engagement, the availability of adequate human resources, funds for vaccines and supplies, and the operational costs to achieve high coverage and quality campaigns. In such countries, weak health systems have also prevented the establishment of effective surveillance systems. Moreover, the logistics constraints and limited human resources prevent case identification and investigation, including specimen collection for serology, genotyping, and transport. This is particularly true where the large number of cases increases the need for laboratory supplies and specimen management logistics. In 2020 and 2022, the supply chain disruption secondary to the COVID-19 pandemic led to a global shortage/stockout of measles/rubella laboratory kits. Unfortunately, four countries have not reported measles genotypes for the period 2019–2022. For Djibouti and Kuwait, the program was not collecting clinical specimens. In Morocco, despite collecting many types of specimens for molecular testing, they were unable to genotype. In Yemen, they are collecting some clinical specimens. However, they are not doing genetic analysis or sending specimens to an RRL for genotyping.

Countries that have verified elimination have been able to provide molecular and epidemiological evidence for interrupted measles and rubella viral transmission with no endemic circulation.

From 2019 to 2022, 6 countries (Afghanistan, Iraq, Pakistan, Sudan, Somalia, and Yemen) reported high numbers of cases compared to other countries in the region. Rubella cases were reported mainly by Pakistan, Sudan, and Yemen.

Genotypes B3 and D8 are actively circulating in eighteen countries, with different circulating variants of both genotypes. The B3 types were more dominant, with 1273 sequences submitted to MeaNS, while the D8 types had 51 sequences submitted. There were no genotyping data available from four countries. During period of 2019 to 2022, rubella genotype 2B was circulating in three countries (Egypt, Iran and Oman) of the WHO EMR. Data from other countries on rubella genotyping are not available.

Surveillance activities are challenging, especially in areas with insecure and complex operating environments. As a result, the absence of a strong data system prevents the reporting, analysis, and use of data for action. Poor surveillance leads to delays in notifications of outbreaks and ineffective responses. Many countries have extremely heterogeneous access to immunization and surveillance quality and large populations, and hence also require subnational data to guide public health action tailored to local contexts. In addition, poor data quality of routine immunization coverage and/or campaign coverage assessed by post campaign coverage surveys hampers an accurate assessment of immunity gaps, which makes it challenging to plan timely national campaigns to prevent outbreaks.

Globally, by the end of 2022, no WHO region had achieved and sustained measles and/or rubella elimination [14]. Globally, measles incidence declined during 2020 and 2021, presumably as a result of decreased virus transmission related to COVID-19 mitigation measures and immunity acquired through high rates of infection during the global measles resurgence during 2017–2019 [14]. However, from 2021 to 2022, reported measles cases increased by 67% globally as COVID-19 mitigation measures were lifted and the routine immunization program faced a backslide. We have seen a similar situation in the WHO Eastern Mediterranean Region, where the reported regional incidence rates of measles decreased from 23.3 per million in 2019 to 7.4 per million in 2020 but increased to 9.6 per million in 2021 and 50 per million population in 2022. Similar to the WHO Eastern Mediterranean Region, none of the 47 countries of the WHO Africa region has attained the verification of measles or rubella elimination at the end of 2023, with a total of 125,957 suspected cases of measles being reported through the case-based surveillance system in the countries of WHO Africa region and a regional incidence rate of measles being reported as 60.3 cases per million population, an increase of 22% when compared to the incidence in 2022 (18). Among the other low resourced countries of Africa, the highest national incidence rates of confirmed measles per million population were documented in Liberia (831.6), Gabon (480.4), Equatorial Guinea (268), Central African Republic (240), Cameroon (217.1), and Ethiopia (154.1) [15].

Based on our analysis, we can conclude that the region has experienced heterogeneity concerning progress toward measles and rubella elimination. Eleven of the EMR countries (50%) are doing better, with four countries (Bahrein, Egypt, Iran, and Oman) verified for measles and rubella elimination between 2019 and 2022. The seven countries (Kuwait, Morocco, Palestine, Qatar, Saudi Arabia, Tunisia, and the United Arab Emirates) have coverage, incidence, and surveillance profiles suggesting that they are approaching elimination. The other half of the countries face a widening immunity gap, exposing them to measles and rubella outbreaks. Furthermore, the quality of surveillance is deteriorating in most of the countries in the region. Based on these findings, we can propose three main recommendations. First, countries approaching elimination should prepare and fill dossiers and submit them to the RVC through the NVCs. This will help them understand the requirements for elimination and to practice self-assessment. Second, countries with immunity gaps need to increase routine measles and rubella vaccine coverage and implement preventive campaigns. Third, countries struggling with surveillance performance indicators need to resume efforts, including timely case-based surveillance with complete investigations, laboratory testing, and genotyping so that they can meet key surveillance performance indicators. Along the same lines, countries reporting measles and rubella cases are encouraged to monitor circulating viruses through improved collection of clinical specimens (throat swab, urine, or oral fluid) for virus detection and genotyping. At the regional level, as countries are integrating measles and rubella surveillance, it is time to consider setting a rubella elimination goal to bring the EMR into line with the global MR strategies.

## 6. Conclusions

During 2019–2022, surveillance indicators deteriorated. In 2019, 21 countries achieved the target of ≥80% of suspected cases having adequate specimens collected and tested in a proficient laboratory, compared to eighteen countries in 2022. Fourteen countries achieved ≥2 discarded (non-measles and non-rubella) case rate per 100,000 population in 2019, compared to eleven countries in 2022. The regional reported incidence rate for measles increased from 23.3 per million population in 2019 to 50 per million population in 2022. The regional incidence rate for rubella also increased from 3.2 per million population in 2019 to 4 per million population in 2022. Eighteen countries reported the circulation of the measles genotypes B3 and D8, with different circulating variants of both genotypes. There were no measles genotyping data available from four countries. During the period of 2019 to 2022, rubella genotype 2B was circulating in three countries (Egypt, Iran, and Oman) of the WHO EMR. Data from other countries on rubella genotyping are not available.

All 21 countries and the occupied Palestinian territory of the WHO Eastern Mediterranean Region need to strengthen their measles and rubella surveillance, including obtaining appropriate specimens for genotyping and improving genotyping testing capacity for both measles and rubella.

**Author Contributions:** Conceptualization, M.F. and K.F.; Methodology, M.F., K.F. and A.G.; Validation, Q.H., P.O. and N.C.; Formal analysis, M.F. and K.F.; Data curation, M.S. and K.F.; Writing—original draft preparation, M.F.; Writing—review and editing, Q.H., M.F., N.C. and P.O. All authors have read and agreed to the published version of the manuscript.

**Funding:** This research received no external funding.

**Institutional Review Board Statement:** Not applicable.

**Informed Consent Statement:** Not applicable.

**Data Availability Statement:** The data presented in this study are available on request from the corresponding author.

**Conflicts of Interest:** The authors declare no conflict of interest.

## References

1. Immunization Agenda 2030. Available online: https://www.who.int/teams/immunization-vaccines-and-biologicals/strategies/ia2030 (accessed on 10 November 2022).
2. Release of the Global Vaccine Action Plan Review and Lessons Learned Report. Available online: https://www.who.int/news/item/10-12-2019-release-of-the-global-vaccine-action-plan-review-and-lessons-learned-report (accessed on 21 September 2023).
3. Minta, A.A.; Ferrari, M.; Antoni, S.; Portnoy, A.; Sbarra, A.; Lambert, B.; Hauryski, S.; Hatcher, C.; Nedelec, Y.; Datta, D.; et al. Progress Toward Regional Measles Elimination—Worldwide, 2000–2021. *MMWR Morb. Mortal. Wkly. Rep.* **2022**, *71*, 1489–1495. [CrossRef]
4. Measles and Rubella Strategic Framework: 2021–2030. Available online: https://www.who.int/publications/i/item/measles-and-rubella-strategic-framework-2021-2030 (accessed on 21 September 2023).
5. Measles Outbreaks Strategic Response Plan: 2021–2023: Measles Outbreak Prevention, Preparedness, Response and Recovery. Available online: https://apps.who.int/iris/handle/10665/340657 (accessed on 17 September 2023).
6. Measles-World Health Organization Factsheet. Available online: https://www.who.int/news-room/fact-sheets/detail/measles (accessed on 10 November 2022).
7. World Health Organization. Regional Office for the Eastern Mediterranean. Eastern Mediterranean Vaccine Action Plan 2016–2020: A Framework for Im-plementation of the Global Vaccine Action Plan. World Health Organization, Regional Office for the Eastern Mediterranean, 2019; p. 28. Available online: https://apps.who.int/iris/handle/10665/311578 (accessed on 17 September 2023).

8. Goodson, J.L.; Teleb, N.; Ashmony, H.; Musa, N.; Ghoniem, A.; Hassan, Q.; Waciqi, A.S.; Mere, M.O.; Farid, M.; Mukhtar, H.E.A.; et al. Progress Toward Measles Elimination—Eastern Mediterranean Region, 2013–2019. *MMWR Morb. Mortal. Wkly. Rep.* **2020**, *69*, 439–445. Available online: http://www.cdc.gov/mmwr/volumes/69/wr/mm6915a2.htm?s_cid=mm6915a2_w (accessed on 10 November 2022).
9. Guide to the Documentation and Verification of Measles and Rubella Elimination in the WHO Eastern Mediterranean Region. Available online: https://apps.who.int/iris/handle/10665/351519 (accessed on 16 December 2022).
10. Mulders, M. Manual for the Laboratory-Based Surveillance of Measles, Rubella, and Congenital Rubella Syndrome—TechNet-21. Available online: https://www.technet-21.org/en/hot-topics-items/15272-manual-for-the-laboratory-based-surveillance-of-measles-rubella-and-congenital-rubella-syndrome (accessed on 21 September 2022).
11. WHO/UNICEF Joint Reporting Process. Available online: https://www.who.int/teams/immunization-vaccines-and-biologicals/immunization-analysis-and-insights/global-monitoring/who-unicef-joint-reporting-process (accessed on 17 September 2023).
12. MeaNS2. Available online: https://who-gmrln.org/means2 (accessed on 17 September 2023).
13. WHO/UNICEF Estimates of National Immunization Coverage. Available online: https://www.who.int/teams/immunization-vaccines-and-biologicals/immunization-analysis-and-insights/global-monitoring/immunization-coverage/who-unicef-estimates-of-national-immunization-coverage (accessed on 10 November 2022).
14. Minta, A.A.; Ferrari, M.; Antoni, S.; Portnoy, A.; Sbarra, A.; Lambert, B.; Hatcher, C.; Hsu, C.H.; Ho, L.L.; Steulet, C.; et al. Progress Toward Measles Elimination—Worldwide, 2000–2022. *MMWR Morb Mortal Wkly Rep.* **2023**, *72*, 1262–1268. [CrossRef]
15. Masresha, B.G.; Wiysonge, C.S.; Katsande, R.; O'Connor, P.M.; Lebo, E.; Perry, R.T. Tracking Measles and Rubella Elimination Progress—World Health Organization African Region, 2022–2023. *Vaccines* **2024**, *12*, 949. [CrossRef]

*vaccines*

MDPI

*Article*

# Progress and Challenges in Measles and Rubella Elimination in the WHO European Region

**Mark Muscat *, Myriam Ben Mamou, Catharina Reynen-de Kat, Dragan Jankovic, José Hagan, Simarjit Singh and Siddhartha Sankar Datta**

Vaccine-Preventable Diseases and Immunization Programme, World Health Organization Regional Office for Europe, DK-2100 Copenhagen, Denmark; benmamoum@who.int (M.B.M.); reynendekatc@who.int (C.R.-d.K.); jankovicd@who.int (D.J.); haganj@who.int (J.H.); singhsi@who.int (S.S.); dattas@who.int (S.S.D.)

* Correspondence: muscatm@who.int

**Abstract:** The elimination of both measles and rubella remains a priority for all 53 Member States of the World Health Organization (WHO) European Region. To provide an update on the epidemiological status of measles and rubella in the Region, we reviewed surveillance data on both diseases for 2023 submitted monthly by national surveillance institutions. We analyzed the cases of measles and rubella for 2023 by age group, case classification, vaccination, hospitalization, and importation status and report on measles-related deaths. In 2023, 60,860 measles cases, including 13 fatal cases, were reported in 41 countries. Most cases (95%; n = 57,584) were reported by six countries: Azerbaijan, Kazakhstan, Kyrgyzstan, Romania, the Russian Federation, and Türkiye. Of the 60,848 cases with data on age, 19,137 (31%) were 1–4 years old and 12,838 (21%) were 5–9 years old. A total of 10,412 (17%) were 20 years and older. The genotypes identified in the Region were largely dominated by D8 variants (n = 1357) and the remainder were B3 variants (n = 221). In 2023, 345 rubella cases were reported by 17 countries, mostly from Poland, Kyrgyzstan, Tajikistan, Türkiye, and Ukraine. A total of 262 cases (76%) were classified as clinically compatible and 79 (23%) were laboratory-confirmed. To achieve the elimination of measles and rubella in the Region, political commitment needs to be revived to enable urgent efforts to increase vaccination coverage, improve surveillance and outbreak preparedness, and respond immediately to outbreaks.

**Keywords:** disease elimination; disease outbreaks; epidemiology; European region; measles; public health surveillance; rubella; vaccines; verification

## 1. Introduction

Measles and rubella incidence in the World Health Organization (WHO) European Region declined significantly in recent decades because of the widespread use and increasing coverage of measles- and rubella-containing vaccines (MRCVs) [1]. This success enabled its 53 Member States, all of which include two doses of MRCVs in their routine immunization schedules to jointly establish the ambitious goal of eliminating endemic measles and rubella transmission from the entire Region. In this context, disease elimination is defined as the interruption of endemic measles or rubella transmission in a defined geographical area such as a country or WHO Region for a period of at least 12 months in the presence of a well-performing surveillance system.

The Health for All policy framework for the WHO European Region (Health21), approved by the WHO Regional Committee for Europe in 1998, identified targets for nine vaccine-preventable diseases, including measles elimination by 2007 and the incidence of congenital rubella syndrome (CRS) of <1 case per 100,000 live births by 2010 [2]. The strategic plan for measles and congenital rubella infection in the WHO European Region targeted both the interruption of the endemic transmission of measles and the prevention of congenital rubella infection by 2010 [3]. In 2005, the inclusion of rubella elimination into the strategy was approved at the fifty-fifth session of the WHO Regional Committee for Europe as part of the resolution on strengthening national immunization systems through the elimination of measles and rubella and the prevention of congenital rubella infection [4]. In 2010, all of the Region's 53 Member States reaffirmed their commitment to achieving this goal [5], which was subsequently included as a priority in the European Vaccine Action Plan 2015–2020 (EVAP) [6,7] and is an important component of the European Immunization Agenda 2030 (EIA2030) [8].

In this article, we provide an update on the epidemiological status of measles and rubella in the Region based on a review of surveillance data on both diseases for 2023. We also discussed the challenges and actions needed to reach the elimination goal for both diseases.

## 2. Materials and Methods

We present an analysis of preliminary measles and rubella surveillance data for 2023 and report on the number of cases of these diseases in the Region for 2013–2023 and by country for 2022. All surveillance data are as of 6 March 2024. We report on vaccination coverage with the first and second doses of MRCV (MRCV1 and MRCV2, respectively) for 2013 up to 2022, the last year for which coverage data were available at the time of submission of this article. We also report on measles and rubella virus sequence data as submitted by the national and regional reference laboratories of the WHO European Region for 2023 in the Measles Nucleotide Surveillance database (MeaNS) [9] and Rubella Nucleotide Surveillance database (RubeNS) [10], respectively, by 29 April 2024.

Surveillance data were submitted monthly by national surveillance institutions and incorporated in the WHO Immunization Information System (WIISE) [11]. Data from the 27 Member States of the European Union, Iceland, and Norway were entered into WIISE after collection and processing by The European Surveillance System—TESSy, of the European Centre for Disease Prevention and Control [12]. MRCV1 and MRCV2 coverage data were obtained from WHO/United Nations Children's Fund Estimates of National Immunization Coverage (WUENIC) (as of 26 June 2023) [1]. We refer to the elimination status of measles and rubella as of 2022 as concluded by the European Regional Verification Commission for Measles and Rubella Elimination (RVC) at its most recent meeting held in 2023 [13].

The analyses of the surveillance data were performed on the cases with disease onset dates during 2022 and 2023. Where these dates were unavailable, the cases with the date of notification reported during these years, respectively, were included. The reported cases of measles and rubella for 2023 were analyzed by age group, case classification (laboratory-confirmed, epidemiologically linked, and clinically compatible [14]), vaccination, and importation status. The cases were categorized by age groups: younger than 1 year, 1–4 years, 5–9 years, 10–14 years, 15–19 years, 20–29 years, and 30 years and older. In addition, we report on hospitalization and measles-related deaths among the cases that occurred in 2023.

The incidence of disease was calculated with the number of cases of reported measles as the numerator and the country population obtained from the Population Division of the United Nations Organization [15] as the denominator. We expressed disease incidence as cases per million inhabitants per specified timeframe (2022 and 2023) and case–fatality rate as the total number of deaths per 1000 measles cases. All the reported cases (including endemic cases, imported cases, importation-related cases, and cases with unknown importation status) were included when calculating incidences. Percentages were rounded to the nearest whole number.

## 3. Results

### 3.1. Measles

#### 3.1.1. Incidence—Notifications and Laboratory Data

Except for 2018 and 2019, there was an overall declining trend in measles cases in the WHO European Region from 2013 to 2021, when the number of measles cases was the lowest ever recorded. Thereafter, the number of cases increased significantly in 2022 and 2023 (Figure 1).

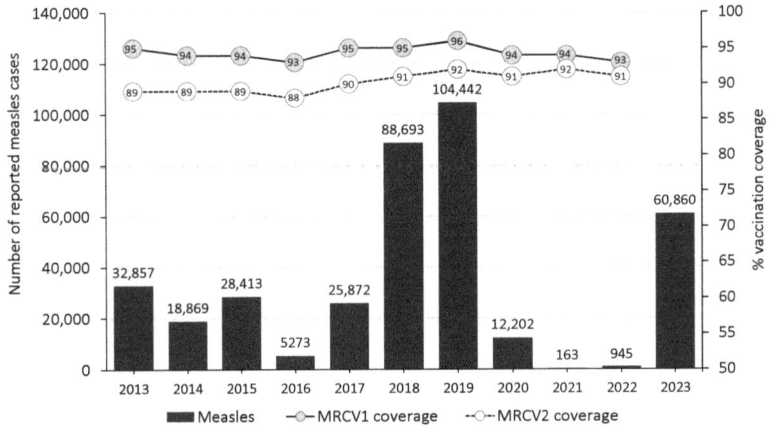


**Figure 1.** Reported measles cases and MRCV1 and MRCV2 coverage by year, WHO European Region, 2013–2023. MRCV1: first dose of measles- and rubella-containing vaccine; MRCV2: second dose of measles- and rubella-containing vaccine.

In 2023, 60,860 measles cases were reported in 41 countries compared to 945 measles cases for 2022 reported in 27 countries (Table 1). Of the total cases for 2023, 31,173 cases (51%) were reported by the nine countries that, as concluded by the RVC, were considered endemic for 2022, and 1477 cases (2%) by two countries that were considered to have re-established endemicity in 2022. A total of 13,129 cases (22%) were reported by eight countries that as of the end of 2022 had interrupted measles transmission for at least the previous 12 months. A total of 15,063 cases (25%) were reported by the 33 countries considered as previously having eliminated measles. The remaining 18 cases were reported by one country whose review was pending.

Most cases in 2023 (95%; n = 57,584) were reported by six countries: Azerbaijan (13,735; 23%), Kazakhstan (15,111; 25%), Kyrgyzstan (7463; 12%), Romania (3419; 6%), the Russian Federation (12,872; 21%), and Türkiye (4984; 8%). The remaining 3276 cases (5%) were reported by 35 countries. The highest incidence per million population for 2023 was in Azerbaijan (1319) followed by Kyrgyzstan (1108).

Of the total cases for 2023, 41,209 (68%) were laboratory-confirmed and 10,088 (17%) were epidemiologically linked to other measles cases. The remaining 9563 cases (16%) were classified as clinically compatible. In 2023, 32 (78%) of the countries reporting measles cases submitted genomic sequence information for 1578 cases (as of 29 April 2024) to the Measles Nucleotide Surveillance database (MeaNS) [9] through WHO-accredited laboratories. The genotypes identified in the Region were largely dominated by D8 variants (n = 1357) and the remainder were B3 variants (221). As in recent years, no other genotype was reported. The reported named strains for the D8 genotype were MVs/Rudaki.TJK/49.21 (n = 444), MVs/Patan.IND/16.19 (331), MVs/Victoria.AUS/6.11 (29), and (MVs/Frankfurt Main.DEU/17.11 (12). The other dominant D8 variants that are still unnamed include MeaNS Distinct Sequence Identifier 8350, which was reported in 123 cases. For the B3 genotype, MVs/Quetta.PAK/44.20 accounted for the majority of the B3 sequences (n = 132).

The other named strains of the B3 genotype were MVs/Alburaimi.OMN/15.20 (n = 1) and MVs/Ohio.USA/37.22 (1). Of the 1578 cases that had sequences reported, 1412 cases (89%) had information on the date of disease onset (Figure 2).

**Table 1.** Incidence of measles per million population in the WHO European Region, 2022 and 2023.

| Country | Number of Measles Cases | | Incidence per Million Inhabitants * | | Number of Measles Cases 2023 | | | |
|---|---|---|---|---|---|---|---|---|
| | 2022 | 2023 | 2022 | 2023 | Laboratory-confirmed | Epidemiologically Linked | Clinically Compatible | Imported |
| Albania | 1 | 3 | 0.4 | 1.1 | 3 | 0 | 0 | 0 |
| Andorra | 0 | 0 | 0 | 0 | 0 | 0 | 0 | - |
| Armenia | 0 | 556 | 0 | 200.1 | 547 | 9 | 0 | 38 |
| Austria | 1 | 186 | 0.1 | 20.8 | 186 | 0 | 0 | 8 |
| Azerbaijan | 1 | 13,735 | 0.1 | 1319.1 | 1429 | 5466 | 6840 | 57 |
| Belarus | 0 | 188 | 0 | 19.8 | 188 | 0 | 0 | 0 |
| Belgium | 17 | 68 | 1.5 | 5.8 | 52 | 12 | 4 | - |
| Bosnia and Herzegovina | 6 | 10 | 1.9 | 3.1 | 8 | 0 | 2 | 0 |
| Bulgaria | 1 | 0 | 0.1 | 0 | 0 | 0 | 0 | - |
| Croatia | 0 | 3 | 0 | 0.7 | 3 | 0 | 0 | 3 |
| Cyprus | 0 | 0 | 0 | 0 | 0 | 0 | 0 | - |
| Czechia | 0 | 1 | 0 | 0.1 | 1 | 0 | 0 | 0 |
| Denmark | 0 | 9 | 0 | 1.5 | 5 | 4 | 0 | 3 |
| Estonia | 0 | 4 | 0 | 3.0 | 4 | 0 | 0 | 4 |
| Finland | 1 | 1 | 0.2 | 0.2 | 1 | 0 | 0 | 1 |
| France | 19 | 117 | 0.3 | 1.8 | 102 | 7 | 8 | 31 |
| Georgia | 12 | 39 | 3.2 | 10.5 | 37 | 0 | 2 | 13 |
| Germany | 15 | 83 | 0.2 | 1.0 | 75 | 3 | 5 | 30 |
| Greece | 0 | 0 | 0 | 0 | 0 | 0 | 0 | - |
| Hungary | 0 | 1 | 0 | 0.1 | 1 | 0 | 0 | 1 |
| Iceland | 0 | 0 | 0 | 0 | 0 | 0 | 0 | - |
| Ireland | 2 | 4 | 0.4 | 0.8 | 1 | 3 | 0 | 2 |
| Israel | 0 | 18 | 0 | 2.0 | 15 | 1 | 2 | 3 |
| Italy | 15 | 44 | 0.3 | 0.7 | 39 | 1 | 4 | 17 |
| Kazakhstan | 4 | 15,111 | 0.2 | 770.7 | 14,087 | 688 | 336 | - |
| Kyrgyzstan | 23 | 7463 | 3.5 | 1108.0 | 2023 | 3373 | 2067 | 4 |
| Latvia | 0 | 1 | 0 | 0.5 | 1 | 0 | 0 | 1 |
| Lithuania | 0 | 4 | 0 | 1.5 | 4 | 0 | 0 | 1 |
| Luxembourg | 0 | 0 | 0 | 0 | 0 | 0 | 0 | |
| Malta | 0 | 0 | 0 | 0 | 0 | 0 | 0 | - |
| Monaco | 0 | 0 | 0 | 0 | 0 | 0 | 0 | - |
| Montenegro | 0 | 0 | 0 | 0 | 0 | 0 | 0 | - |
| Netherlands (Kingdom of the) | 6 | 7 | 0.3 | 0.4 | 6 | 1 | 0 | 3 |
| North Macedonia | 0 | 1 | 0 | 0.5 | 1 | 0 | 0 | 0 |
| Norway | 1 | 2 | 0.2 | 0.4 | 2 | 0 | 0 | 1 |
| Poland | 41 | 29 | 1.0 | 0.7 | 16 | 0 | 13 | 1 |
| Portugal | 0 | 1 | 0 | 0.1 | 0 | 0 | 1 | 0 |
| Republic of Moldova | 0 | 3 | 0 | 0.9 | 3 | 0 | 0 | 2 |
| Romania | 9 | 3419 | 0.5 | 171.9 | 3018 | 281 | 120 | 17 |
| Russian Federation | 117 | 12,872 | 0.8 | 89.1 | 12,570 | 189 | 113 | 292 |
| San Marino | 0 | 0 | 0 | 0 | 0 | 0 | 0 | - |
| Serbia | 0 | 52 | 0 | 7.3 | 47 | 1 | 4 | 0 |
| Slovakia | 0 | 6 | 0 | 1.0 | 6 | 0 | 0 | 2 |
| Slovenia | 0 | 0 | 0 | 0 | 0 | 0 | 0 | - |
| Spain | 1 | 13 | 0.02 | 0.3 | 10 | 0 | 3 | 6 |
| Sweden | 4 | 11 | 0.4 | 1.0 | 11 | 0 | 0 | 6 |
| Switzerland | 1 | 37 | 0.1 | 4.2 | 34 | 3 | 0 | 13 |
| Tajikistan | 451 | 294 | 45.3 | 29.0 | 250 | 44 | 0 | 0 |
| Türkiye | 127 | 4984 | 1.5 | 58.1 | 4969 | 2 | 13 | 66 |
| Turkmenistan | 0 | 0 | 0 | 0 | 0 | 0 | 0 | - |
| Ukraine | 11 | 66 | 0.3 | 1.8 | 57 | 0 | 9 | 0 |
| United Kingdom | 50 | 231 | 0.7 | 3.4 | 231 | 0 | 0 | 30 |
| Uzbekistan | 8 | 1183 | 0.2 | 33.6 | 1166 | 0 | 17 | 3 |
| WHO European Region | 945 | 60,860 | 1.0 | 65.3 | 41,209 | 10,088 | 9563 | 659 |

* based on estimated 2022 and 2023 population data, respectively. There may be differences in the numbers documented in the reports based on the data derived from the WHO/UNICEF Joint Reporting Form—the data we present for 2022 include updated numbers reported by some countries and for 2023, the data may be updated following the publication of this article. Discrepancies might also arise with nationally reported data if these include cases by the year of notification rather than the year of disease onset.

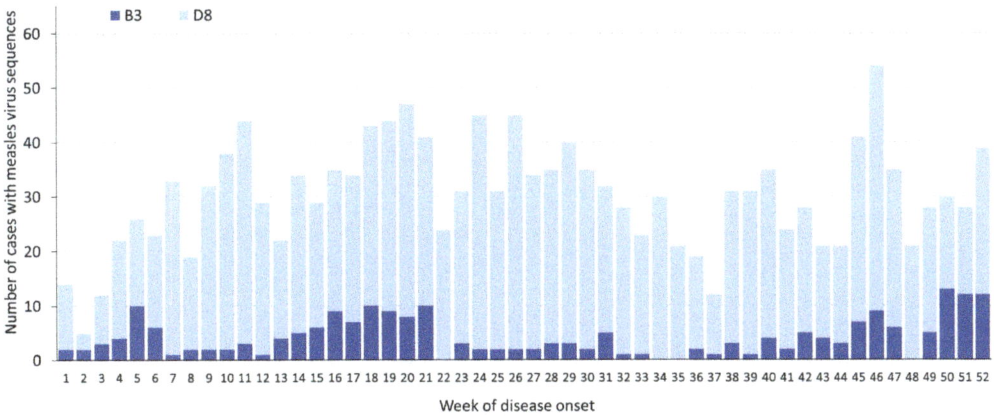


**Figure 2.** Number of cases with measles virus sequences in the WHO European Region reported to MeaNS by the genotype and week of disease onset, 2023 (as of 29 April 2024) *. * For 166 cases, the date of disease onset was missing. They were categorized by the week of specimen collection or the week when the clinical specimen was received at the laboratory, according to which date came first.

### 3.1.2. Age Distribution

Of the total cases for 2023, age was known for 60,848 cases: 7597 (12%) were <1 year old, 19,137 (31%) were 1–4 years old, 12,838 (21%) were 5–9 years old, 10,864 (18%) were 10–19 years old, and 10,412 (17%) were 20 years and older (Figure 3). Figure 4 shows the age distribution of measles cases in the six countries reporting the highest numbers of cases in the Region: Azerbaijan, Kazakhstan, Kyrgyzstan, Romania, the Russian Federation, and Türkiye by proportion and age-specific incidence. Among these six countries, the largest proportion of cases in children 1–4 years old was reported in Kazakhstan (45%; n = 6738) followed by Kyrgyzstan (43%; 3216). The largest proportion of cases in adults aged 20 years and older was reported in the Russian Federation (29%; 3717) and Türkiye (21%; 1057).

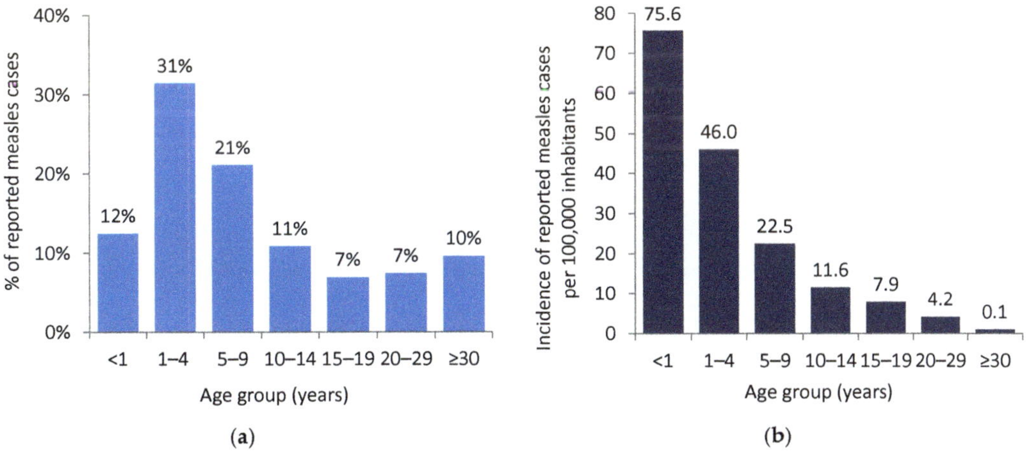


**Figure 3.** Age distribution of measles cases by proportion (**a**) and incidence per 100,000 inhabitants (**b**) in the WHO European Region, 2023 (n = 60,848) *. * For 12 cases, the age group was not reported. These are excluded from the graph.

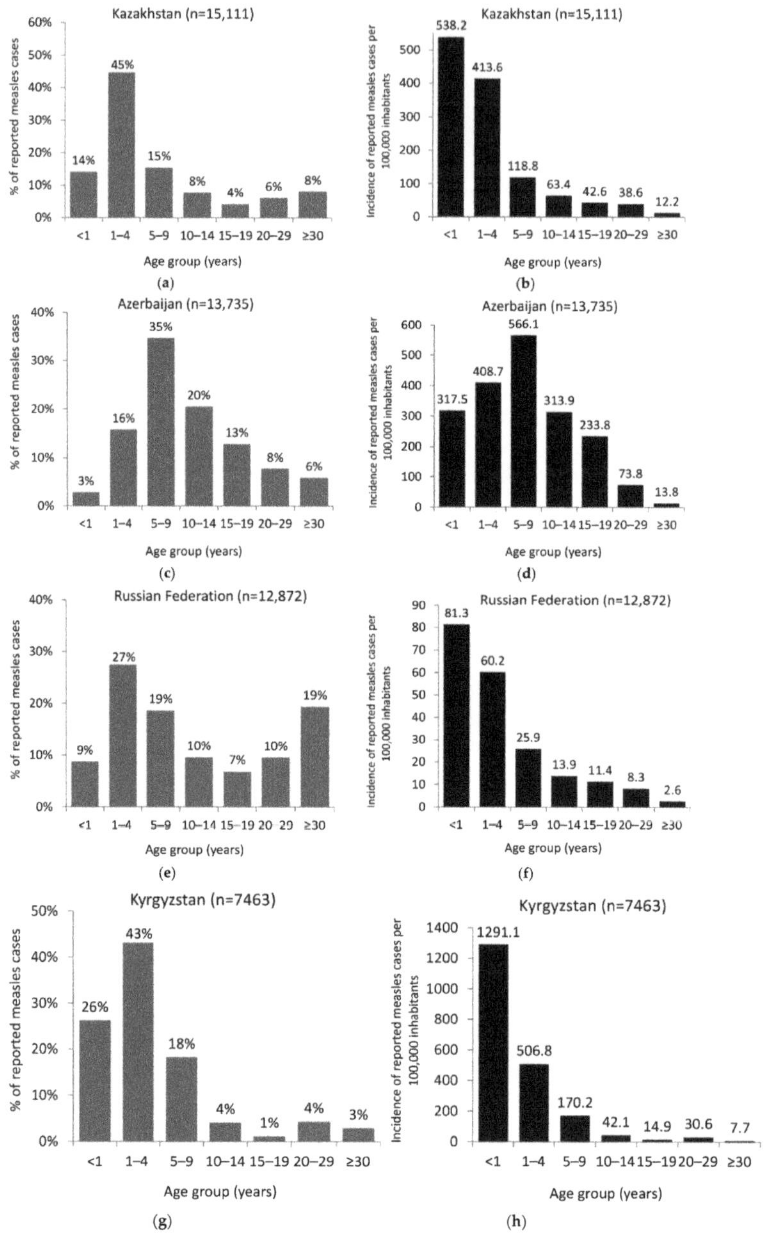


**Figure 4.** *Cont.*

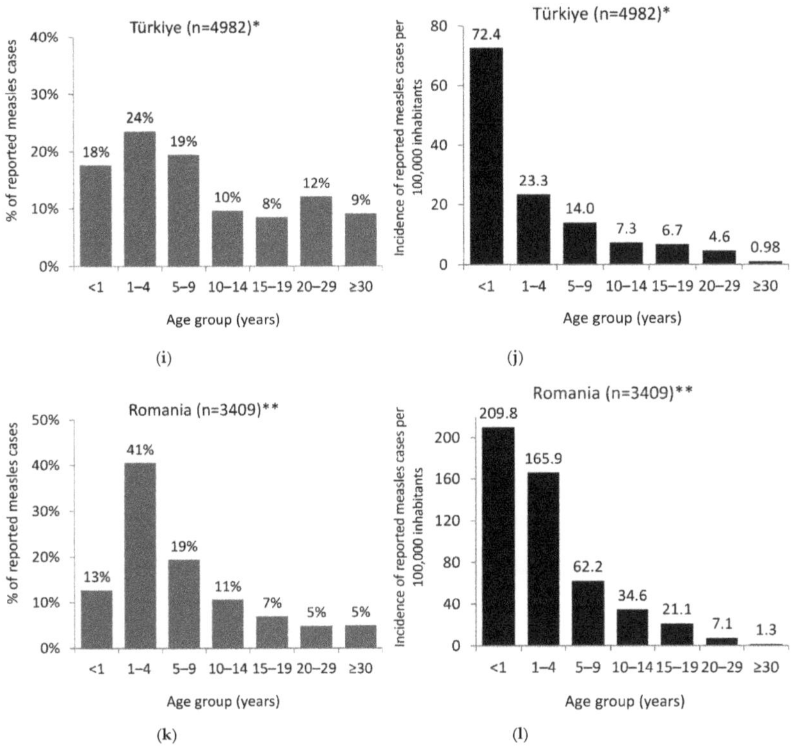


**Figure 4.** Age distribution of measles cases by proportion (**a**,**c**,**e**,**g**,**i**,**k**) and incidence per 100,000 inhabitants (**b**,**d**,**f**,**h**,**j**,**l**) in the six countries with the largest numbers of cases in the WHO European Region for 2023. * For 2 cases, the age group was not reported. These are excluded from the graph. ** For 10 cases, the age group was not reported. These are excluded from the graph.

### 3.1.3. Vaccination Status

Of the total cases for 2023, the vaccination status was known for 47,413 cases (78%). Of these, 39,045 cases (64%) were unvaccinated: 6804 (17%) were <1 year old, 14,652 (38%) were 1–4 years old, 7945 (20%) were 5–9 years old, 5574 (14%) were 10–19 years old, and 4062 (10%) were 20 years and older, and for 8 cases the age was unknown. The remaining 8368 cases (14%) were reportedly vaccinated with at least one dose of a measles-containing vaccine. The number of reported measles cases by vaccination status and age group is shown in Table 2.

### 3.1.4. Measles-Rrelated Deaths

In 2023, there were 13 reported measles-related deaths in three countries: Kyrgyzstan (9 deaths), Romania (3), and Armenia (1). This corresponds to a case–fatality rate per 1000 measles cases of 0.21. Two fatal cases were reported in infants: one in a 5-month-old and another in a 6-month-old. Eight cases were in the 1–4-year-old age group, one case occurred in a 12-year-old, one case was in an 18-year-old, and another case was in a 35-year-old. Five fatal cases were laboratory-confirmed, five cases were epidemiologically linked to another case of measles, and three cases were classified as clinically compatible. Eleven fatal cases were unvaccinated, and one case was reportedly vaccinated with two doses of a measles-containing vaccine. In the remaining case, the vaccination status was unknown.

**Table 2.** Measles cases by vaccination status and age group in the WHO European Region, 2023 (n = 60,860).

| | <1 Years | | 1–4 Years | | 5–9 Years | | 10–14 Years | | 15–19 Years | | 20–29 Years | | ≥30 Years | | Unknown Age | | Total | |
|---|---|---|---|---|---|---|---|---|---|---|---|---|---|---|---|---|---|---|
| Unvaccinated | 6804 | 90% | 14,652 | 77% | 7945 | 62% | 3515 | 53% | 2059 | 49% | 1848 | 41% | 2214 | 38% | 8 | 67% | 39,045 | 64% |
| Vaccinated with a single dose | 88 | 1% | 2220 | 12% | 1288 | 10% | 621 | 9% | 300 | 7% | 204 | 4% | 221 | 4% | 1 | 8% | 4943 | 8% |
| Vaccinated with at least two doses | 6 | 0% | 148 | 1% | 917 | 7% | 881 | 13% | 591 | 14% | 441 | 10% | 440 | 7% | 1 | 8% | 3425 | 6% |
| Unknown status | 699 | 9% | 2117 | 11% | 2688 | 21% | 1609 | 24% | 1288 | 30% | 2051 | 45% | 2993 | 51% | 2 | 17% | 13,447 | 22% |
| Total | 7597 | 100% | 19,137 | 100% | 12,838 | 100% | 6626 | 100% | 4238 | 100% | 4544 | 100% | 5868 | 100% | 12 | 100% | 60,860 | 100% |

3.1.5. Hospitalization

For 2023, data on hospitalization status were available for 52,259 cases (86%). Of these, 33,505 cases (64%) were hospitalized. The largest proportion of hospitalized cases were reported from Kazakhstan (39%; n = 13,149) followed by the Russian Federation (21%; 7104) and Kyrgyzstan (18%, 6133). In Kazakhstan, where the hospitalization status was known in all the reported cases (n = 15,111), 87% (13,149) were hospitalized.

3.1.6. Imported Cases

For 2023, the status of measles virus importation was known for 50% (n = 30,608) of the cases. Of these, 659 were reported as imported cases, amounting to 2.2% of the cases with a known importation status. The largest proportion of imported cases by country was reported by the Russian Federation (44%; n = 292) followed by Türkiye (10%; 66) and Azerbaijan (9%; 57).

*3.2. Rubella*

3.2.1. Incidence—Notifications and Laboratory Data

There has been an overall steady declining trend in rubella cases in the WHO European Region from 2013 to 2021, when the number of rubella cases was the lowest ever recorded. Thereafter, the number of cases increased in 2022 and 2023 (Figure 5). In 2023, 345 rubella cases were reported by 17 (33%) of the 51 countries that submitted rubella data (including zero reporting) (Table 3). Most (76%; n = 263) of the cases were reported by Poland followed by Türkiye (6%; 20), Kyrgyzstan (3%; 11), and Ukraine (3%; 11).

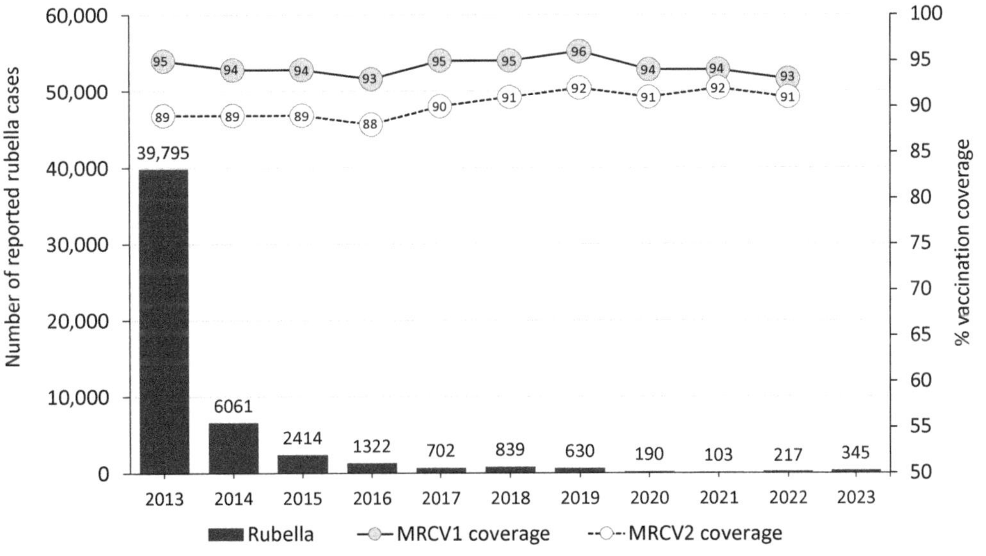


**Figure 5.** Reported rubella cases and MRCV1 and MRCV2 coverage by year, WHO European Region, 2013–2023. MRCV1: first dose of measles- and rubella-containing vaccine; MRCV2: second dose of measles- and rubella-containing vaccine.

**Table 3.** Incidence of rubella per million population in the WHO European Region, 2022 and 2023.

| Country | Number of Rubella Cases | | Incidence per Million Inhabitants * | | Number of Rubella Cases 2023 | | | |
|---|---|---|---|---|---|---|---|---|
| | 2022 | 2023 | 2022 | 2023 | Laboratory-confirmed | Epidemiologically Linked | Clinically Compatible | Imported |
| Albania | 0 | 1 | 0 | 0.4 | 1 | 0 | 0 | 0 |
| Andorra | 0 | 0 | 0 | 0 | 0 | 0 | 0 | - |
| Armenia | 0 | 0 | 0 | 0 | 0 | 0 | 0 | - |
| Austria | 0 | 0 | 0 | 0 | 0 | 0 | 0 | - |
| Azerbaijan | 4 | 0 | 0.4 | 0 | 0 | 0 | 0 | - |
| Belarus | - | 0 | - | 0 | 0 | 0 | 0 | - |
| Belgium [1] | - | - | - | - | - | - | - | - |
| Bosnia and Herzegovina | 0 | 2 | 0 | 0.6 | 1 | 0 | 1 | - |
| Bulgaria | 0 | 0 | 0 | 0 | 0 | 0 | 0 | - |
| Croatia | 0 | 0 | 0 | 0 | 0 | 0 | 0 | - |
| Cyprus | 0 | 0 | 0 | 0 | 0 | 0 | 0 | - |
| Czechia | 0 | 0 | 0 | 0 | 0 | 0 | 0 | - |
| Denmark [2] | - | - | - | - | - | - | - | - |
| Estonia | 0 | 0 | 0 | 0 | 0 | 0 | 0 | - |
| Finland | 1 | 1 | 0.2 | 0.2 | 1 | 0 | 0 | 0 |
| France | 0 | 0 | 0 | 0 | 0 | 0 | 0 | - |
| Georgia | 0 | 0 | 0 | 0 | 0 | 0 | 0 | - |
| Germany | 8 | 8 | 0.1 | 0.1 | 5 | 0 | 3 | 0 |
| Greece | 0 | 0 | 0 | 0 | 0 | 0 | 0 | - |
| Hungary | 0 | 0 | 0 | 0 | 0 | 0 | 0 | - |
| Iceland | 0 | 0 | 0 | 0 | 0 | 0 | 0 | - |
| Ireland | 0 | 0 | 0 | 0 | 0 | 0 | 0 | - |
| Israel | 0 | 1 | 0 | 0.1 | 1 | 0 | 0 | 0 |
| Italy | 4 | 2 | 0.1 | 0.03 | 1 | 0 | 1 | 0 |
| Kazakhstan | 0 | 7 | 0 | 0.4 | 6 | 1 | 0 | - |
| Kyrgyzstan | 2 | 11 | 0.3 | 1.6 | 11 | 0 | 0 | 1 |
| Latvia | 1 | 0 | 0.5 | 0 | 0 | 0 | 0 | - |
| Lithuania | 1 | 1 | 0.4 | 0.4 | 1 | 0 | 0 | 0 |
| Luxembourg | 0 | 0 | 0 | 0 | 0 | 0 | 0 | - |
| Malta | 0 | 0 | 0 | 0 | 0 | 0 | 0 | - |
| Monaco | 0 | 0 | 0 | 0 | 0 | 0 | 0 | - |
| Montenegro | 0 | 0 | 0 | 0 | 0 | 0 | 0 | - |
| Netherlands (Kingdom of the) | 0 | 0 | 0 | 0 | 0 | 0 | 0 | - |
| North Macedonia | 0 | 0 | 0 | 0 | 0 | 0 | 0 | - |
| Norway | 0 | 0 | 0 | 0 | 0 | 0 | 0 | - |
| Poland | 147 | 263 | 3.7 | 6.4 | 10 | 3 | 250 | - |
| Portugal | 0 | 0 | 0 | 0 | 0 | 0 | 0 | - |
| Republic of Moldova | 0 | 0 | 0 | 0 | 0 | 0 | 0 | - |
| Romania | 0 | 1 | 0 | 0.1 | 1 | 0 | 0 | 1 |
| Russian Federation | 0 | 3 | 0 | 0.02 | 3 | 0 | 0 | 0 |
| San Marino | 0 | 0 | 0 | 0 | 0 | 0 | 0 | - |
| Serbia | - | 0 | - | 0 | 0 | 0 | 0 | - |
| Slovakia | 0 | 0 | 0 | 0 | 0 | 0 | 0 | - |
| Slovenia | 0 | 0 | 0 | 0 | 0 | 0 | 0 | - |
| Spain | 0 | 0 | 0 | 0 | 0 | 0 | 0 | - |
| Sweden | 0 | 0 | 0 | 0 | 0 | 0 | 0 | - |
| Switzerland | 0 | 1 | 0 | 0.1 | 0 | 0 | 1 | 0 |
| Tajikistan | 0 | 10 | 0 | 1.0 | 10 | 0 | 0 | 0 |
| Türkiye | 40 | 20 | 0.5 | 0.2 | 20 | 0 | 0 | 0 |
| Turkmenistan | 0 | 0 | 0 | 0 | 0 | 0 | 0 | - |
| Ukraine | 9 | 11 | 0.2 | 0.3 | 5 | 0 | 6 | 0 |
| United Kingdom | 0 | 0 | 0 | 0 | 0 | 0 | 0 | - |
| Uzbekistan | 0 | 2 | 0 | 0.1 | 2 | 0 | 0 | 0 |
| WHO European Region | 217 | 345 | 0.2 | 0.4 | 79 | 4 | 262 | 2 |

* based on estimated 2022 and 2023 population data, respectively. [1] country does not have a comprehensive rubella surveillance system. [2] comprehensive rubella surveillance system for all ages became effective on 1 November 2023. There may be differences in the numbers documented in the reports based on the data derived from the WHO/UNICEF Joint Reporting Form—the data we present for 2022 include updated numbers reported by some countries and for 2023, the data may be updated following the publication of this article. Discrepancies might also arise with nationally reported data if these include cases by the year of notification rather than the year of disease onset.

Of the total cases for 2023, 262 (76%) were classified as clinically compatible. These were largely reported by Poland (n = 250, 95%). Seventy-nine cases (23%) were laboratory-confirmed and were mostly reported by Türkiye (20) followed by Kyrgyzstan (11), Poland (10), and Tajikistan (10). Four cases were classified as epidemiologically linked to another rubella case. In 2023, no rubella virus sequences were submitted to the Rubella Nucleotide Surveillance database (RubeNS) [10] (as of 29 April 2024).

### 3.2.2. Age Distribution

Of the total cases for 2023, age was known for 82 cases: 13 (16%) were <1 year old, 24 (29%) were 1–4 years old, 10 (12%) were 5–9 years old, 11 (13%) were 10–19 years old, and 24 (29%) were 20 years and older (Figure 6). Of the 24 cases 20 years and older, 18 cases were laboratory-confirmed. Of these, data on sex were known for 15 cases. Eight cases were males and seven cases were females of whom two were 20–29 years old and five were 30 years and older.

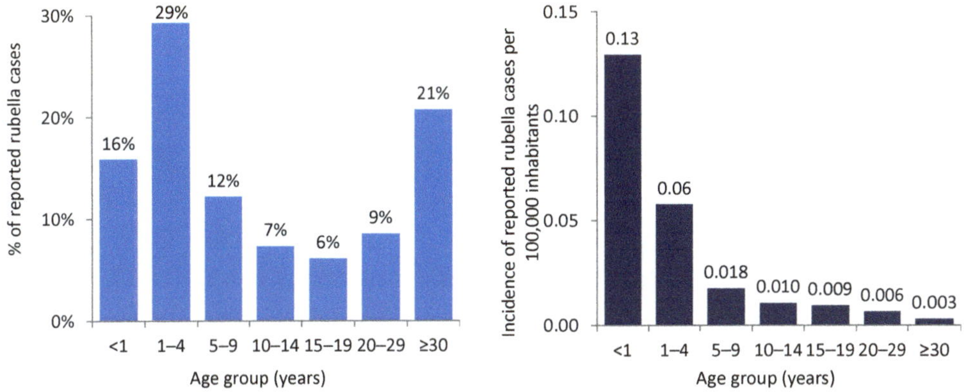


**Figure 6.** Age distribution of rubella cases by proportion (**left**) and incidence per 100,000 inhabitants (**right**) in the WHO European Region, 2023 (n = 82) *. * For 263 cases, the age group was not reported. These are excluded from the graph.

### 3.2.3. Vaccination Status

Of the total cases for 2023, the vaccination status was known for 33 cases (10%). Of these, ten cases were unvaccinated: seven cases were <1 year old, two cases were 1–4 years old, and for one case the age was unknown. The remaining 23 cases were reportedly vaccinated with at least one dose of rubella-containing vaccine. The number of reported rubella cases by vaccination status and age is shown in Table 4.

### 3.2.4. Imported Cases

The status of rubella virus importation was known in 54 (16%) rubella cases. Two were imported cases.

**Table 4.** Rubella cases by vaccination status and age group in the WHO European Region, 2023 (n = 345).

| | <1 Years | | 1–4 Years | | 5–9 Years | | 10–14 Years | | 15–19 Years | | 20–29 Years | | ≥30 Years | | Unknown Age | | Total | |
|---|---|---|---|---|---|---|---|---|---|---|---|---|---|---|---|---|---|---|
| Unvaccinated | 7 | 54% | 2 | 8% | 0 | 0% | 0 | 0% | 0 | 0% | 0 | 0% | 1 | 6% | 0 | 0% | 10 | 3% |
| Vaccinated with a single dose | 0 | 0% | 13 | 54% | 2 | 20% | 0 | 0% | 0 | 0% | 0 | 0% | 1 | 6% | 0 | 0% | 16 | 5% |
| Vaccinated with at least two doses | 0 | 0% | 1 | 4% | 3 | 30% | 2 | 33% | 0 | 0% | 1 | 14% | 0 | 0% | 0 | 0% | 7 | 2% |
| Unknown status | 6 | 46% | 8 | 33% | 5 | 50% | 4 | 67% | 5 | 100% | 6 | 86% | 15 | 88% | 263 | 100% | 312 | 90% |
| Total | 13 | 100% | 24 | 100% | 10 | 100% | 6 | 100% | 5 | 100% | 7 | 100% | 17 | 100% | 263 | 100% | 345 | 100% |

## 4. Discussion

### 4.1. Measles

The WHO European Region experienced a declining trend in measles cases from 2013 to 2022, except for the years 2018 and 2019, when cases spiked due to large outbreaks in just a few countries [16]. Cases for the Region as a whole began to increase again at the start of 2022, and this increasing trend has continued into 2024 [17]. The marked drop in reported measles cases in 2020 and 2021 is at least partly due to diminished virus transmission resulting from the non-pharmaceutical interventions, particularly lockdowns, implemented to contain the COVID-19 pandemic. These interventions were implemented throughout the Region starting in the spring of 2020 and continued throughout most of 2021. However, the under-reporting of cases was also very likely as fewer cases of measles could be detected due to disruptions in the usual disease surveillance activities and the diversion of resources to focus on COVID-19-related work. Furthermore, people were less likely to seek medical attention in healthcare facilities for mild illnesses during full or partial lockdowns resulting in mild cases of measles being undetected and thus not reported. It is plausible that the high coverage of measles-containing vaccines in the years preceding the pandemic also contributed to preventing large-scale measles outbreaks in the Region. Between 2016 and 2019, regional coverage with the first dose increased from 93% to 96%, while coverage with the second dose increased from 88% to 92%.

Following the evaluation of the submitted annual reports for 2022 from 52 of the 53 Member States of the Region, the RVC verified in 2023 that 33 countries sustained interruption for $\geq$36 months and are therefore considered to have eliminated endemic measles. Furthermore, one country had interrupted endemic measles transmission for 24 months and 7 countries had interrupted endemic measles transmission for 12 months by the end of 2022 [13]. The overall declining trend observed from 2013 to 2021, together with the verification of elimination status in 33 countries by the end of 2022, indicates that progress has been made towards interrupting endemic transmission of measles viruses in the Region. Despite this progress, the number of reported measles cases in the Region for 2023 (n = 60,860) increased 64-fold compared with that reported for 2022 (945). The number of cases for 2023 is probably even higher based on preliminary data reported in WIISE, as the delayed reporting of cases often occurs in countries with large-scale outbreaks. The number of countries reporting measles also increased from 27 in 2022 to 41 in 2023. The marked increase in the incidence of measles in many countries in 2023 compared to 2022 threatens the progress made so far and puts the Region at risk of delaying the achievement of the measles elimination goal.

Several countries have experienced challenges in achieving and sustaining optimal routine immunization coverage rates, particularly in 2020–2021, at the height of the COVID-19 pandemic, and in 2022. Among them, hesitancy to vaccinations and anti-vaccination sentiment has been reported to contribute to suboptimal vaccination rates in some countries [18,19]. Overall, coverage with the first MRCV dose for the Region decreased by two percentage points to 94% in 2020 compared with 2019 [1]. It remained at 94% in 2021 but decreased again by one percentage point to 93% in 2022. Coverage with the second dose showed less of a change in 2020–2022 and remained at 91–92%, similar to the coverage in 2018–2019.

Although coverage with the first MRCV dose may be considered as having declined only minimally at the regional level, at the national level, the decline in coverage varied widely. From 2019 to 2022, a decline in coverage, ranging between 1% and 62%, was observed in 28 countries for the first MRCV dose and between 1% and 23% for the second MRCV dose in 28 countries. Although the recommended ages for the first and second doses of MRCV vary between countries [1], it is probably the decline in first-dose coverage that had the largest impact on the observed increase in measles cases since 2022. This decline implies a widening of immunity gaps in the population large enough to allow the emergence of outbreaks, with over a third (31%) of the measles cases in 2023 occurring among children aged 1–4 years. Children in this age group would have been mostly affected by the observed decline in routine immunization coverage rates particularly in 2020–2021. In addition, the persistence of cases among adults aged 20 years and older (17%) suggests lingering immunity gaps in the adult population. Modeling studies have shown that to ensure measles elimination, 95% immunity would have to be achieved by the age of five years and that it is important not to have immunity gaps in older age groups [20].

The data we present for hospitalization due to measles should be interpreted with caution in the absence of a definition of hospitalization. Although hospitalization generally implies inpatient admission to a hospital, the term could also be interpreted to include outpatient ambulatory care at a healthcare facility. Across the Region, there is a diversity in the national regulations on the hospitalization of patients with measles. The high rate of hospitalized cases in the Region for 2023 was mostly caused by the large number of cases reported from Kazakhstan, Kyrgyzstan, and the Russian Federation, where the hospital admission of measles cases is a legal requirement. Further studies will be required for a better understanding of the number of cases with serious disease and to describe the burden of measles on hospitals.

The reported number of deaths is probably an underestimate and is therefore unlikely to indicate the true extent of mortality from measles. Surveillance systems do not necessarily collect outcome data systematically and measles might not be recorded on death certificates. Indeed, death certification errors are well recognized [21,22]. Moreover, death from complications, such as subacute sclerosing panencephalitis, can occur long after disease onset [23]. This means that the death rate per 1000 cases for 2023 is likely to be even higher than 0.21.

### 4.2. Rubella

The progress made towards rubella elimination is encouraging. The steady decline in the number of rubella cases and of countries reporting the disease suggests that the Region is close to eliminating rubella. The RVC verified in 2023 that 49 countries had interrupted endemic rubella transmission by the end of 2022 [13]. Thirty-three countries have achieved the elimination of both measles and rubella. Despite the observed increase in rubella cases in 2023, the low number of cases reported from the Member States of the Region at least since 2017 and low number of congenital rubella syndrome cases (45 cases for 2017–2022) [1] suggest that rubella elimination is an imminently achievable goal for the Region. Indeed, only four countries in the Region have not yet been verified as having eliminated rubella. Bosnia and Herzegovina, Poland, and Ukraine have not yet produced adequate documentation, including information on surveillance performance, to satisfy the RVC criteria to verify the absence of ongoing rubella transmission, while the submitted data from Israel are pending review. The next step to attaining the rubella elimination goal for the Region is to retrospectively review these remaining countries' surveillance and vaccination data and any other alternative and supporting data in depth. The analysis of these data may also be coupled with an overall epidemiological assessment of rubella transmission in the Region as a whole.

The number of reported rubella cases in the Region increased for 2023 compared with 2022, with 128 more cases, a rise of 59%. The number of countries reporting rubella also increased between 2022 and 2023 from 10 to 17. These increases should be interpreted in light of the concurrent measles outbreaks in many countries since more clinical specimens from suspected measles cases that test negative would be tested for rubella, as is required. In both years, fewer countries reported rubella cases (including zero reporting) than measles cases.

As in previous years, most (76%) reported rubella cases for 2023 continue to be classified as clinically compatible, with Poland reporting 95% of such cases in the Region. With such a high proportion of clinically compatible cases, an accurate epidemiological assessment to identify the true incidence of rubella in the country cannot be made. Countries with a high number of suspected rubella cases need to make efforts to increase specimen collection to allow laboratory testing. Without laboratory confirmatory tests for rubella, other rash-producing viral infections such as those caused by human herpes viruses and parvovirus B19 are easily misdiagnosed as rubella. Nevertheless, the observed rare occurrence of the laboratory-confirmed cases of rubella among females of childbearing age signals a persisting potential risk for congenital rubella syndrome (CRS) and underlines the important role of rubella vaccination to prevent CRS.

### 4.3. Limitations of Surveillance Data

We did not evaluate the surveillance systems for measles and rubella and the extent of the implementation of case definitions used for reporting these diseases by each country. Not all countries may conduct disease surveillance with the needed sensitivity appropriate for diseases targeted for elimination. Therefore, our evaluation could only permit the identification of regional and country-specific trends over time. Moreover, the under-reporting of cases and incompleteness of data reporting are notorious with routine communicable disease surveillance systems based on passive reporting. Consequently, making accurate comparisons between countries may be challenging. Despite these limitations, the surveillance data we presented are the best possible data that national surveillance agencies could provide and are likely to be at least consistent over time, reflecting the general trends in each country. Differences in the quality of surveillance systems between countries are not expected to affect the observed general trends for both diseases.

### 4.4. Measles and Rubella Elimination Strategies

The elimination of both measles and rubella remains a priority goal for all the countries of the WHO European Region. Countries are urged to review their vaccination programs, surveillance systems, and outbreak response capacities and adhere to the core strategies for achieving this goal. These strategies are reiterated in the recently published integrated guidance on surveillance, outbreak response, and the verification of elimination [14] and are discussed under the headings below.

#### 4.4.1. Achieving and Sustaining High Vaccination Coverage

High vaccination coverage of at least 95% with two doses of MRCVs administered through high-quality routine immunization services is needed to prevent outbreaks and attain the measles and rubella elimination goal. Tailored approaches to achieve high coverage at the subnational level and in every community are essential to prevent the accumulation of susceptible individuals even within countries and areas that otherwise report high overall coverage rates.

Countries are urged to closely monitor vaccination coverage, preferably using electronic registers, to identify disparities at the local level and among various population groups that could point to inequities in immunization service delivery. Measles outbreaks have often affected ethnic, religious, and philosophical population groups [24] with low vaccination coverage. Therefore, countries should implement tailored approaches to achieve equitable immunization coverage across all geographic and demographic segments. To inform such approaches, behavioral insights research may be conducted to improve the understanding of whether low coverage in a particular area or community is related to factors such as the lack of convenient access to immunization services, lack of awareness, or loss of public confidence in the benefits of vaccines. The WHO Regional Office for Europe has just producedguidance for countries on how to identify and address inequities [25].

Where disruption in routine immunization service delivery has occurred for any length of time, such as at the height of the COVID-19 pandemic [26], countries are urged to undertake tailored immunization catch-up campaigns to close resulting population immunity gaps not only among children but also adults. This requires identifying the birth cohorts and any special populations or risk groups that have missed their vaccine doses and offering them the opportunity to be vaccinated. The WHO Regional Office for Europe published guidance to support countries in planning and implementing catch-up immunization using a structured algorithm [27].

#### 4.4.2. Improving the Availability and Use of High-Quality, Evidence-based Information on Immunization

To enhance acceptance and demand for immunization, health authorities are urged to improve the availability and use of high-quality, evidence-based information for healthcare professionals and the public on the benefits and risks associated with immunization. Indeed, pre- and in-service training of the health workforce on vaccines and the diseases they prevent is essential if they are to confidently recommend and communicate about vaccination. The WHO Regional Office for Europe has developed various training packages [28–30] for health workers to increase their knowledge about vaccines and help them answer questions from their clients and patients, as well as guidance for health authorities to ensure the timely and effective investigation of any adverse events following vaccination and the transparent communication of the results to sustain public trust [31].

Health literacy can be strengthened from a young age to promote positive health-seeking behavior throughout a person's life. Adding health topics to school curricula has been demonstrated to improve students' knowledge on these topics [32,33], with positive spillover effects benefiting caregivers and communities alike [34]. Health education that includes information on vaccines and the diseases they prevent can create positive attitudes toward vaccines, thereby increasing children's resilience to misinformation, empowering them to make informed health-related choices related to vaccination [35]. The possibility of increasing vaccination coverage among adolescents using a website-based educational program with tailored information has been described [36]. To increase health literacy among 10–12-year-olds, the WHO Regional Office for Europe has developed a game-based learning platform to teach them about vaccines, the immune system, and online source criticism [37]. This educational tool called "Immune Patrol" is currently being rolled out in schools in several countries in the Region.

Joint initiatives such as European Immunization Week (EIW) [38], which takes place every April, provide national authorities, international partners, and civil society organizations a platform through which to raise awareness and engagement at the local level. From social media campaigns to national conferences, lectures, talk shows, interviews, and public events, many channels and opportunities are used to make accurate information about the role of vaccines in protecting health available and accessible. Since its inception in 2007, EIW has helped keep the measles and rubella elimination goals, and the broader implementation of EVAP and now EIA2030, high on the political agenda. At the same time, it serves to promote innovation, highlight challenges, and encourage actions needed to achieve measles and rubella elimination and other immunization targets and goals.

#### 4.4.3. Strengthening Surveillance

Surveillance systems for measles and rubella need to be sensitive and specific enough to detect, confirm, and classify all suspected cases. This involves rigorous case investigation and the laboratory confirmation of suspected sporadic cases and outbreaks. To confirm the occurrence or absence of disease, efforts need to be made to increase specimen collection to allow the laboratory testing of suspected measles and rubella cases, including virus characterization. Supported with epidemiological information, this will facilitate the monitoring of regional patterns of circulation and the tracking of transmission pathways, and will help distinguish between new importations and ongoing disease transmission, as well as the different chains of transmission. Countries are also reminded to report their sequence data to the WHO global sequence databases (MeaNs and RubeNS) to allow the in-depth analyses of the molecular epidemiology of measles and rubella viruses.

In 2023, the importation status of measles cases in the Region was reported in only 50% of the cases and the importation status of rubella cases in only 16% of the cases. This low proportion of cases with known importation status poses challenges for determining whether prolonged periods of virus transmission were the result of prolonged uninterrupted transmission chains or multiple unrelated importations, with important potential implications for the verification of elimination status. The WHO Regional Office for Europe has recently published updated guidance on how to conduct elimination-standard surveillance [14].

#### 4.4.4. Ensuring Adequate Outbreak Preparedness and Response

As the Region works towards attaining elimination, timely outbreak investigation and response become crucial. Timely response to outbreaks is indeed a core strategy for measles and rubella elimination and is also embedded in EIA2030. Not all countries in the Region have responded timeously and adequately to measles outbreaks, allowing prolonged virus transmission and the associated increase in morbidity and hospitalization, burdening healthcare systems and increasing healthcare costs [39].

An adequate outbreak response requires a thorough field investigation including enhanced laboratory surveillance, active case finding, and contact tracing for the vaccination of any susceptible individuals. The most important immediate response measure after the detection of measles cases is to identify and provide vaccination to the susceptible individuals and population groups at risk of exposure. Rapid immunization efforts in an outbreak setting are aimed at interrupting disease transmission without delay in order to reduce the extent and duration of outbreaks and associated morbidity and mortality. Achieving sufficient vaccination coverage to prevent an outbreak and convincing those at risk to be vaccinated during an outbreak require tailored efforts to sustain or gain public trust in health authorities and vaccination.

Health authorities are encouraged to collect comprehensive and timely surveillance data using sophisticated technologies, if feasible, such as real-time data collection and analysis tools. Data generated from thorough outbreak investigations should be used to identify and address inequities in vaccine service delivery. Indeed, the root cause analysis of outbreaks should be conducted to better inform improvements in programmatic interventions to prevent future outbreaks [40].

Nosocomial transmission of the virus contributes to measles outbreaks. Apart from the risk of the amplification of outbreaks by virus transmission between patients, and between healthcare workers and patients in healthcare settings [41], increased mortality can result from serious complications in hospitalized infants and adults who may already be weakened by other medical conditions. For 2023, the relatively large proportion (64%) of measles cases that were hospitalized highlights the importance of ensuring that all the necessary precautions are taken to prevent nosocomial transmission by implementing effective infection control practices.

Apart from having national plans of action for the elimination of measles and rubella in place and regularly updated, every country should have a national outbreak preparedness and response plan that particularly addresses measles outbreaks. WHO guidance for the early detection of outbreaks describes how to conduct a rapid and appropriate response [14] and can be used to structure response plans.

## 5. Conclusions

The resurgence of measles in the Region reflects ongoing challenges in endemic countries and countries experiencing large-scale outbreaks that may slow progress to achieve the elimination goal in the Region. It also reflects the need for sustained efforts to protect gains in countries that are considered to have interrupted or eliminated endemic measles. At the same time, efforts made to eliminate rubella need to be sustained. The high cost of these diseases in terms of morbidity, hospitalizations, and mortality continues to undeniably justify the efforts to eliminate these diseases in the Region.

To attain the elimination goal for the Region, all the countries need to ensure that the immunization coverage of at least 95% is reached and maintained in all districts, and immunity gaps in the population are identified and closed. Furthermore, high-quality surveillance is necessary to monitor disease occurrence and detect outbreaks so that appropriate and timely response measures can be taken. Accurate surveillance data are also needed to adequately ascertain the status of measles and rubella transmission as part of the elimination verification process. The goal will not be met unless all the Member States of the Region translate their political commitment into adequate investment and concrete programmatic actions that address identified challenges.

**Author Contributions:** Conceptualization of the article, methodology, data validation, data analysis, data visualization, and writing—original draft preparation, M.M.; data curation, S.S.; data validation and writing—review and editing, M.B.M.; writing—review and editing, C.R.-d.K., D.J., J.H., and S.S.D. All authors have read and agreed to the published version of the manuscript.

**Funding:** This research received no external funding.

**Institutional Review Board Statement:** Not applicable.

**Informed Consent Statement:** Not applicable.

**Data Availability Statement:** Data sources supporting the results have already been indicated by the references.

**Acknowledgments:** We thank all the countries of the WHO European Region for providing epidemiological and laboratory surveillance data. We are also grateful to Belete Gebrie for assisting with data collection and curation, and Brett Craig, Shahin Huseynov, and Siff Malue Nielsen for their contributions to the article.

**Conflicts of Interest:** The authors affiliated with the World Health Organization (WHO) are alone responsible for the views expressed in this publication and they do not necessarily represent the decisions or policies of the WHO. The authors declare no conflicts of interest.

## References

1. World Health Organization. Immunization Data Portal. Available online: https://immunizationdata.who.int/ (accessed on 9 April 2024).
2. World Health Organization. Regional Office for Europe. *HEALTH21—Health for All in the 21st Century: An Introduction*; WHO Regional Office for Europe: Copenhagen, Denmark, 1998. Available online: https://iris.who.int/handle/10665/107327 (accessed on 16 April 2024).
3. World Health Organization. Regional Office for Europe. *Strategic Plan for Measles and Congenital Rubella Infection in the European Region of WHO*; WHO Regional Office for Europe: Copenhagen, Denmark, 2003. Available online: https://iris.who.int/handle/10665/107526 (accessed on 16 April 2024).
4. World Health Organization. Regional Office for Europe. *Fifty-Fifth Regional Committee for Europe: Bucharest, 12–15 September 2005: Draft Resolution: Strengthening National Immunization Systems through Measles and Rubella Elimination and Prevention of Congenital Rubella Infection in WHO's European Region*; WHO Regional Office for Europe: Copenhagen, Denmark, 2005. Available online: https://iris.who.int/handle/10665/365068 (accessed on 16 April 2024).
5. World Health Organization. Regional Office for Europe. *Sixtieth Regional Committee for Europe: Moscow, 13–16 September 2010: Resolution: Renewed Commitment to Elimination of Measles and Rubella and Prevention of Congenital Rubella Syndrome by 2015 and Sustained Support for Polio-Free Status in the WHO European Region*; WHO Regional Office for Europe: Copenhagen, Denmark, 2010. Available online: https://apps.who.int/iris/handle/10665/333436 (accessed on 29 September 2022).
6. World Health Organization. Regional Office for Europe. *Sixty-Fourth Regional Committee for Europe: Copenhagen, 15–18 September 2014: Resolution: European Vaccine Action Plan 2015–2020*; WHO Regional Office for Europe: Copenhagen, Denmark, 2014. Available online: https://apps.who.int/iris/handle/10665/337429 (accessed on 1 August 2022).
7. World Health Organization. Regional Office for Europe. *European Vaccine Action Plan 2015–2020*; WHO Regional Office for Europe: Copenhagen, Denmark, 2014. Available online: https://apps.who.int/iris/handle/10665/340400 (accessed on 29 September 2022).
8. World Health Organization. Regional Office for Europe. *The European Immunization Agenda 2030*; WHO Regional Office for Europe: Copenhagen, Denmark, 2021. Available online: https://www.who.int/europe/initiatives/the-european-immunization-agenda-2030 (accessed on 24 January 2024).
9. Measles Nucleotide Surveillance Database (MeaNs). Available online: https://who-gmrln.org/means2 (accessed on 5 March 2024).
10. Rubella Nucleotide Surveillance database (RubeNS). Available online: https://who-gmrln.org/rubens2 (accessed on 5 March 2024).
11. World Health Organization. Regional Office for Europe. *Monitoring and Reporting of Routine Immunization-Related Data*; WHO Regional Office for Europe: Copenhagen, Denmark, 2023. Available online: https://www.who.int/europe/activities/monitoring-and-reporting-of-routine-immunization-related-data (accessed on 30 April 2024).

12. European Centre for Disease Prevention and Control. The European Surveillance System (TESSy). European Centre for Disease Prevention and Control: Stockholm, Sweden, 2017. Available online: https://www.ecdc.europa.eu/en/publications-data/european-surveillance-system-tessy (accessed on 5 March 2024).
13. World Health Organization. Regional Office for Europe. *Twelfth Meeting of the European Regional Verification Commission for Measles and Rubella Elimination: 8–11 September 2023 Copenhagen, Denmark: Meeting Report*; Licence: CC BY-NC-SA 3.0 IGO; WHO Regional Office for Europe: Copenhagen, Denmark, 2024. Available online: https://www.who.int/europe/publications/i/item/WHO-EURO-2024-9722-49494-74055 (accessed on 30 April 2024).
14. World Health Organization. Regional Office for Europe. *Eliminating Measles and Rubella in the WHO European Region: Integrated Guidance for Surveillance, Outbreak Response and Verification of Elimination*; WHO Regional Office for Europe: Copenhagen, Denmark, 2024. Available online: https://iris.who.int/handle/10665/375923 (accessed on 11 April 2024).
15. United Nations, Department of Economic and Social Affairs, Population Division. *World Population Prospects: The 2022 Revision*; Online edition; Population Division: New York, NY, USA, 2022. Available online: https://population.un.org/wpp/ (accessed on 1 February 2024).
16. World Health Organization. Regional Office for Europe. *WHO EpiBrief no. 1/2020: A Report on the Epidemiology of Selected Vaccine-preventable Diseases in the European Region*; WHO Regional Office for Europe: Copenhagen, Denmark, 2020. Available online: https://iris.who.int/handle/10665/360803 (accessed on 30 April 2024).
17. World Health Organization. Regional Office for Europe. *WHO EpiData 4/2024*; WHO Regional Office for Europe: Copenhagen, Denmark, 2024. Available online: https://www.who.int/europe/publications/m/item/epidata-4-2024 (accessed on 30 April 2024).
18. Akilbekova, D.; Yerdessov, S.; Gaipov, A. Urgent health update: Rising measles cases in Kazakhstan. *Lancet Reg. Health* **2024**, *37*, 1–2. [CrossRef] [PubMed]
19. Dubé, E.; Laberge, C.; Guay, M.; Bramadat, P.; Roy, R.; Bettinger, J.A. Vaccine hesitancy: An overview. *Human Vaccin. Immunother.* **2013**, *9*, 1763–1773. [CrossRef] [PubMed]
20. Funk, S.; Knapp, J.K.; Lebo, E.; Reef, S.E.; Dabbagh, A.J.; Kretsinger, K.; Jit, M.; Edmunds, W.J.; Strebel, P.M. Combining serological and contact data to derive target immunity levels for achieving and maintaining measles elimination. *BMC Med.* **2019**, *17*, 180. [CrossRef] [PubMed]
21. Pritt, B.S.; Hardin, N.J.; Richmond, J.A.; Shapiro, S.L. Death certification errors at an academic institution. *Arch. Pathol. Lab. Med.* **2005**, *129*, 1476–1479. [CrossRef] [PubMed]
22. Armour, A.; Bharucha, H. Nosological inaccuracies in death certification in Northern Ireland. *Ulster Med. J.* **1997**, *66*, 13–17. [PubMed] [PubMed Central]
23. Wendorf, K.A.; Winter, K.; Zipprich, J.; Schechter, R.; Hacker, J.K.; Preas, C.; Cherry, J.D.; Glaser, C.; Harriman, K. Subacute sclerosing panencephalitis: The devastating measles complication is more common than we think. *Clin. Infect. Dis.* **2017**, *65*, 226–232. [CrossRef] [PubMed]
24. Muscat, M. Who gets measles in Europe? *J. Infect. Dis.* **2011**, *204*, S353–S365. [CrossRef] [PubMed]
25. World Health Organization. Regional Office for Europe. *A practical guide to identifying, addressing and tracking inequities in immunization*; WHO Regional Office for Europe: Copenhagen, Denmark, 2024; In Press.
26. Shet, A.; Carr, K.; Danovaro-Holliday, M.C.; Sodha, S.V.; Prosperi, C.; Wunderlich, J.; Wonodi, C.; Reynolds, H.W.; Mirza, I.; Gacic-Dobo, M.; et al. Impact of the SARS-CoV-2 pandemic on routine immunisation services: Evidence of disruption and recovery from 170 countries and territories. *Lancet Glob. Health* **2022**, *10*, e186–e194. [CrossRef] [PubMed]
27. World Health Organization. Regional Office for Europe. *Operational Considerations for Planning and Implementing Catch-Up Vaccination in the WHO European Region*; WHO Regional Office for Europe: Copenhagen, Denmark, 2023. Available online: https://apps.who.int/iris/handle/10665/351183 (accessed on 12 April 2024).
28. World Health Organization. Regional Office for Europe. *Communicating with Health Workers about COVID-19 Vaccination*; WHO Regional Office for Europe: Copenhagen, Denmark, 2021. Available online: https://iris.who.int/handle/10665/343962 (accessed on 25 April 2024).
29. World Health Organization. Regional Office for Europe. *Communicating with Patients about COVID-19 Vaccination: Evidence-Based Guidance for Effective Conversations to Promote COVID-19 Vaccine Uptake*; WHO Regional Office for Europe: Copenhagen, Denmark, 2021. Available online: https://iris.who.int/handle/10665/340751 (accessed on 25 April 2024).
30. World Health Organization. Regional Office for Europe. *Communicating about Vaccination with Caregivers and Patients: A Communication Training Module for Health Workers*; WHO Regional Office for Europe: Copenhagen, Denmark, 2023. Available online: https://iris.who.int/handle/10665/375090 (accessed on 25 April 2024).
31. World Health Organization. Regional Office for Europe. *Vaccination and Trust: How Concerns Arise and the Role of Communication in Mitigating Crises*; WHO Regional Office for Europe: Copenhagen, Denmark, 2017. Available online: https://iris.who.int/handle/10665/343299 (accessed on 26 April 2024).
32. Lahti, A.; Rosengren, B.E.; Nilsson, J.Å.; Karlsson, C.; Karlsson, M.K. Long-term effects of daily physical education throughout compulsory school on duration of physical activity in young adulthood: An 11-year prospective controlled study. *BMJ Open Sport Exerc. Med.* **2018**, *4*, e000360. [CrossRef] [PubMed] [PubMed Central]
33. Goldfarb, E.S.; Lieberman, L.D. Three decades of research: The case for comprehensive sex education. *J. Adolesc. Health* **2021**, *68*, 13–27. [CrossRef] [PubMed]

34. Berniell, L.; de la Mata, D.; Valdés, N. Spillovers of health education at school on parents' physical activity. *Health Econ.* **2013**, *22*, 1004–1020. [CrossRef] [PubMed]
35. Maisonneuve, A.R.; Witteman, H.O.; Brehaut, J.; Dubé, È.; Wilson, K. Educating children and adolescents about vaccines: A review of current literature. *Expert Rev. Vaccines* **2018**, *17*, 311–321. [CrossRef] [PubMed]
36. Esposito, S.; Bianchini, S.; Tagliabue, C.; Umbrello, G.; Madini, B.; Di Pietro, G.; Principi, N. Impact of a website based educational program for increasing vaccination coverage among adolescents. *Human Vaccin. Immunother.* **2018**, *14*, 961–968. [CrossRef] [PubMed]
37. World Health Organization. Regional Office for Europe. Immune Patrol. 2022. Available online: https://www.who.int/europe/multi-media/item/immune-patrol---overview# (accessed on 25 April 2024).
38. World Health Organization. Regional Office for Europe. European Immunization Week. Available online: https://www.who.int/europe/campaigns/european-immunization-week (accessed on 25 April 2024).
39. Filia, A.; Brenna, A.; Panà, A.; Maggio Cavallaro, G.; Massari, M.; Ciofi degli Atti, M.L. Health burden and economic impact of measles-related hospitalizations in Italy in 2002–2003. *BMC Public Health* **2007**, *7*, 169. [CrossRef] [PubMed]
40. World Health Organization. *Measles Outbreak Guide*; WHO: Geneva, Switzerland, 2022. Available online: https://apps.who.int/iris/handle/10665/360891 (accessed on 30 April 2024).
41. Botelho-Nevers, E.; Cassir, N.; Minodier, P.; Laporte, R.; Gautret, P.; Badiaga, S.; Thiberville, D.J.; Ninove, L.; Charrel, R.; Brouqui, P. Measles among healthcare workers: A potential for nosocomial outbreaks. *Euro Surveill.* **2011**, *16*, 19764. [CrossRef] [PubMed]

*vaccines*

MDPI

*Review*

# Progress towards Measles and Rubella Elimination in the South-East Asia Region—2013–2023

**Sudhir Khanal [1,*], Vinod Bura [1], Lucky Sangal [1], Raman Sethi [1], Deepak Dhongde [1] and Sunil Kumar Bahl [2]**

1 WHO Regional Office for South-East Asia, New Delhi 110002, India; burav@who.int (V.B.); sanagllu@who.int (L.S.); sethir@who.int (R.S.); dhongded@who.int (D.D.)

2 Public Health Expert (Formerly with WHO Regional Office for South-East Asia), New Delhi 110002, India; bahlsk@gmail.com

* Correspondence: khanals@who.int; Tel.: +91-9650197391

**Abstract:** The South-East Asia (SEA) Region of the World Health Organization (WHO), through a Regional Committee resolution in 2013, adopted the goal of "measles elimination and rubella control by 2020". The goal was revised in 2019 to "measles and rubella elimination by 2023". Countries of the Region have made significant efforts to achieve the goal. Progress has been made in the Region, with five of the 11 countries of the Region having been verified for having eliminated measles and rubella. Surveillance and immunization program performance for measles and rubella has shown an improvement since 2013. This progress has been possible due to a high level of political and programmatic commitment in the countries of the Region, as well as due to the alliances and infrastructures established for disease elimination initiatives in the past, notably for polio, being utilized effectively to implement strategies for measles and rubella elimination. The unforeseen COVID-19 pandemic had a detrimental effect on the immunization and surveillance efforts, leading to a delay in the achievement of measles and rubella elimination in the Region. Challenges to achieve the goal remain; however, efforts are ongoing in countries to not only protect the gains made so far but also to make further progress towards the goal of measles and rubella elimination.

**Keywords:** measles; rubella; vaccination; elimination; vaccine preventable diseases; SEA Region

## 1. Introduction

The WHO South-East Asia Region (WHO South-East Asia Region has eleven countries —Bangladesh, Bhutan, DPR Korea, India, Indonesia, the Maldives, Myanmar, Nepal, Sri Lanka, Thailand, and Timor-Leste) adopted the goal of measles elimination (absence of endemic measles cases for a period of ≥12 months) and rubella and congenital rubella syndrome control (ninety-five percent reduction in disease incidence from the 2013 level) by 2020 through a Regional Committee resolution in 2013 [1,2]. An independent review of the progress towards rubella control in the Region was conducted in 2019, which recommended countries of the Region take advantage of the opportunity provided by measles elimination activities to revise the goal to include rubella elimination [2]. Following the recommendation, in the subsequent regional committee meeting of the South-East Asia Region held in September 2019, countries resolved to eliminate both measles and rubella by 2023 [3]. The strategies adopted by countries of the Region to eliminate measles and rubella included: (a) achieving high population immunity with more than 95% coverage of two doses of measles and rubella-containing vaccine through routine immunization, periodic intensification or supplementary immunization campaigns; (b) ensuring a sensitive laboratory supported case-based fever and rash surveillance system; (c) maintaining an accredited laboratory network to support fever and rash surveillance; (d) identifying, investigating and responding to measles and rubella outbreaks in a timely manner; and (e) linking these initiatives with other public health interventions to ensure optimal implementation of the four strategies listed above [4].

This article presents a review of progress towards measles and rubella elimination and the changes in epidemiology of the diseases over time in the WHO South-East Asia Region, the factors determining the progress, and the remaining challenges.

## 2. Methods and Materials

The progress towards measles and rubella elimination was measured between 2013 and 2023.

Cessation of transmission, disease incidence, reported cases, mortality information (only for measles), surveillance performance across various indicators (for the last 3 years), and epidemiological analysis were used to measure progress.

Published data from the WHO-UNICEF estimates of national immunization coverage were used to review progress towards vaccination coverage, while the estimated number of measles fatalities and cases prevented over this time was taken from WHO published articles on global progress towards measles and rubella elimination [5].

The change in epidemiology of measles and rubella during the last 3 years was reviewed for changes in age distribution and vaccination status using the data from case-based surveillance for suspected measles and rubella submitted by countries of the Region to WHO through the joint reporting form as well as weekly reports [6,7].

Data on the changing genotype of measles and rubella since last 10 years are also presented using the measles and rubella nucleotide surveillance database—MeaNS and RubeNS, respectively [8,9].

The reports from the Regional Verification Commission for Measles and Rubella Elimination (SEA-RVC) [10–13] and the reports from the Regional Immunization Technical Advisory Group (SEAR-ITAG) [14–17] were reviewed for information needed to identify the timelines and the challenges related to program implementation.

## 3. Results

### 3.1. Cessation of Transmission

In 2013, all the countries in the South-East Asia Region of WHO were endemic to measles and rubella. As of 2023, five of the eleven countries in the Region—Bhutan, DPR Korea, the Maldives, Sri Lanka, and Timor-Leste—have been verified by the SEA-RVC to have eliminated measles and rubella, based on the verification guidelines developed by WHO [18,19].

### 3.2. Disease Incidence, Reported Cases and Mortality

The reported incidence for measles cases in the SEA Region increased from 16.2 per million population in 2013 to 40.9 per million in 2023. Only four countries experienced a decline in incidence, with significant increases in incidence reported in India and Indonesia. The reported incidence of rubella cases in the Region decreased from 5.5 per million population in 2013 to 1.4 per million population in 2023. All countries in the Region reported a decline [7]. The variations in the incidence in different countries are depicted in Table 1.

While the reported incidence has increased, deaths due to measles are estimated to have decreased by 96% (from 255,133 to 9542) from 2013 to 2022. The significant enhancement in surveillance performance resulting in better reporting could be partly attributed to this observed phenomenon, as well as the shift in the age range of measles cases, which may have resulted in decreased number of deaths due to measles in the older age groups. In 2013, the Region contributed 26% of estimated global measles deaths [20]. This percentage declined to 7% (9542 of total 136,216) in 2022 [21–23].

**Table 1.** Reported cases and incidence of measles and rubella in WHO South-East Asia Region, by country, 2013 and 2023.

| | 2013 | | | | 2023 | | | | % Change in Incidence | |
|---|---|---|---|---|---|---|---|---|---|---|
| | No. Reported Measles Cases (JRF †) | Measles Incidence § | No. Reported Rubella Cases (JRF †) | Rubella Incidence § | No. Reported Measles Cases (JRF †) | Measles Incidence § | No. Reported Rubella Cases (JRF †) | Rubella Incidence § | Measles | Rubella |
| Bangladesh | 237 | 1.5 | 3034 | 19.7 | 281 | 1.6 | 182 | 1.1 | 6.7% | −94.0% |
| Bhutan | 0 | 0.0 | 6 | 8.2 | 10 | 12.7 | 4 | 5.1 | 0.0% | −33.3% |
| DPR Korea | 0 | 0.0 | 0 | 0.0 | 0 | 0.0 | 0 | 0.0 | 0.0% | 0.0% |
| India | 13,822 | 11.1 | 3698 | 2.9 | 65,150 | 45.6 | 2952 | 2.1 | 310.8% | −20.2% |
| Indonesia | 8419 | 33.9 | 2355 | 9.3 | 18,063 | 65.1 | 584 | 2.1 | 92.0% | −75.2% |
| Maldives | 0 | 0.0 | 0 | 0.0 | 5 | 9.6 | 0 | 0.0 | 0.0% | 0.0% |
| Myanmar | 1010 | 16.2 | 23 | 0.5 | 15 | 0.3 | 2 | 0.0 | −98.1% | −91.3% |
| Nepal | 1861 | 68.3 | 755 | 27.6 | 963 | 31.2 | 34 | 1.1 | −54.3% | −95.5% |
| Sri Lanka | 2107 | 102.9 | 24 | 1.1 | 810 | 37.0 | 0 | 0.0 | −64.0% | −100.0% |
| Thailand | 2641 | 40.7 | 539 | 7.7 | 64 | 0.9 | 12 | 0.2 | −97.8% | −97.8% |
| Timor-Leste | 4 | 3.4 | 0 | 0.0 | 7 | 5.1 | 3 | 2.2 | 50.0% | 0.0% |
| Region Overall | 30,101 | 16.2 | 10,434 | 5.5 | 49,201 | 40.9 | 3773 | 1.8 | 152.5% | −63.8% |

Abbreviations: JRF = Joint Reporting Form; Data source: Data are from WHO and UNICEF estimates, 2023 revision (as of June 2024). Data available at http://immunizationdata.who.int (accessed on 18 July 2024); † JRF was submitted to WHO and UNICEF by member states with the official immunization data and the number of measles cases in the country for the year. § Incidence is calculated based on the reported cases and population by member states through WHO/UNICEF JRF.

### 3.3. Immunization Coverage

In 2013, all eleven countries in the Region had introduced a dose of measles-containing vaccine, while nine countries had introduced two doses in their routine childhood immunization program. Five countries had introduced one dose of rubella-containing vaccine, and three countries had introduced two doses of rubella-containing vaccines in 2013. By 2023, all countries in the Region had introduced two doses of a measles and rubella-containing vaccine in routine immunization [20] (Table 2).

The WHO-UNICEF estimated regional coverage for MCV1 increased from 85% in 2013 to an all-time high of 94% in 2019 [19] Similarly, the estimated regional coverage for MCV2 was 83% in 2019 compared to 59% in 2013, while the regional coverage of RCV1 was estimated at 93% in 2019 compared to 12% in 2013 [19] In 2020–2021, after the COVID-19 pandemic, the region observed a significant decline in coverages of measles and rubella-containing vaccines (Figures 1 and 2). An estimated decline of 8% in MCV1 coverage, 11% in MCV2 coverage, and 7% in RCV1 coverage was witnessed in 2021 compared with 2019 levels. However, intensive efforts to catch-up, restore, and strengthen immunization in all countries ensured that coverage with MCV and RCV improved in 2022, achieving an estimated 92% coverage for MCV1, 85% for MCV2, and 92% for RCV1. Catch-up, restore, and strengthen efforts to improve coverage through routine immunization conducted by all countries resulted in an increase in routine coverage and have continued through 2023 and 2024.

**Table 2.** Date of introduction of measles and rubella-containing vaccines in countries of WHO South-East Asia Region (SEAR).

| Country | MCV1 † | MCV2 † | RCV1 † | RCV2 † |
|---|---|---|---|---|
| Bangladesh | 1979 | 2012 | 2012 | 2015 |
| Bhutan | 1979 | 2006 | 2006 | 2006 |
| DPR Korea | 1997 | 2008 | 2019 | 2019 |
| India | 1985 | 2010 | 2017 | 2017 |
| Indonesia | 1982 | 2003 | 2017 | 2017 |
| Maldives | 1983 | 2007 | 2007 | 2017 |
| Myanmar | 1987 | 2012 | 2015 | 2017 |
| Nepal | 1988 | 2015 | 2013 end | 2015 |
| Sri Lanka | 1984 | 2001 | 1996 | 2001 |
| Thailand | 1984 | 1996 | 1986 | 1997 |
| Timor-Leste | 1982 | 2016 | 2016 | 2016 |

† Abbreviations: MCV1—first dose of measles-containing vaccine; MCV2—second dose of measles-containing vaccine; RCV1—first dose of rubella-containing vaccine and RCV2—second dose of rubella-containing vaccine. Data Source: Immunizaitondata.who.int.

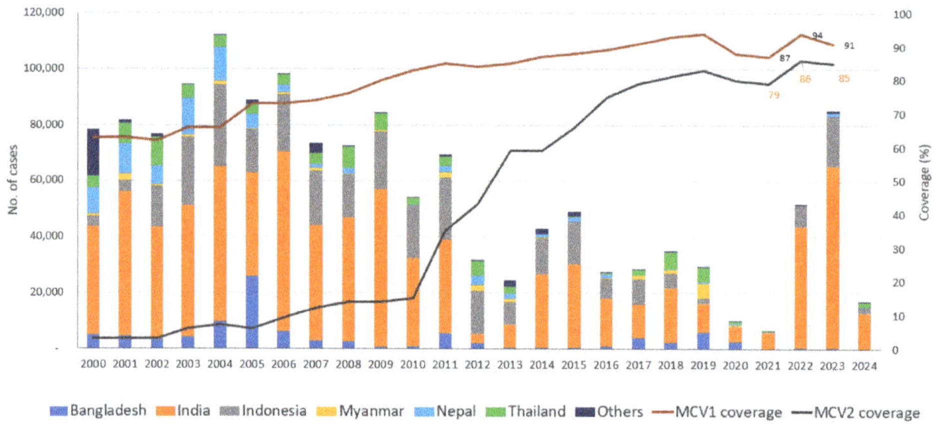


Source: WHO/UNICEF coverage estimates , July 2024 and WHO /UNICEF JRF; Measles cases from JRF 2000-2024

**Figure 1.** Number of reported measles cases * and estimated percentage of children who received their first and second dose of measles-containing vaccine (MCV), † by country—World Health Organization (WHO) South-East Asia Region (SEAR), 2000–2023. Abbreviations: MCV1 = first dose of MCV in routine immunization; MCV2 = second dose of MCV in routine immunization. * Cases of measles reported to WHO and the United Nations Children's Fund (UNICEF) through the Joint Reporting Form from WHO-SEAR. † Data are from WHO and UNICEF estimates for SEAR, available at http://immunizationdata.who.int. Adapted from [24].

There remain some variations in the timing of administration of MCV2 and RCV1 as well as of the coverage of MCV1, MCV2, and RCV in countries of the Region, as depicted in Table 3 below.

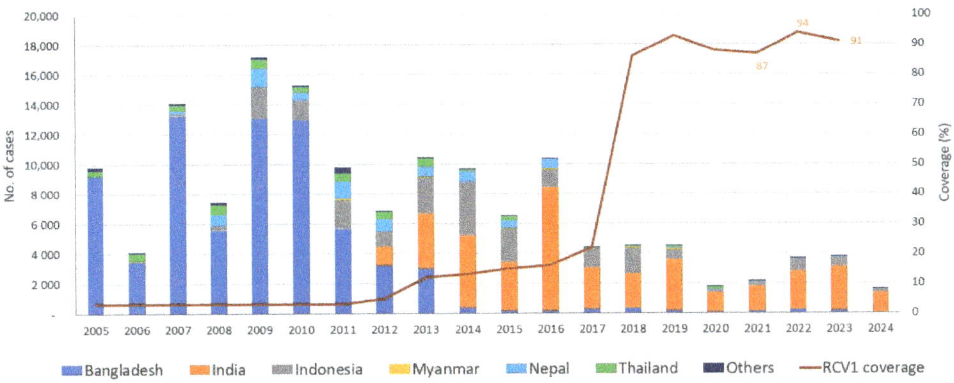


Source: WHO/UNICEF coverage estimates , July 2024 and WHO /UNICEF JRF; Rubella cases from JRF 2000-2024

**Figure 2.** Number of reported rubella cases * and estimated percentage of children who received their first dose of rubella vaccine (RCV), † by country—World Health Organization (WHO) South-East Asia Region (SEAR), 2005–2023. Abbreviations: MCV1 = first dose of MCV in routine immunization; MCV2 = second dose of MCV in routine immunization. * Cases of measles reported to WHO and the United Nations Children's Fund (UNICEF) through the Joint Reporting Form from WHO-SEAR. † Data are from WHO and UNICEF estimates for SEAR, available at http://immunizationdata.who.int. Adapted from [24].

**Table 3.** Estimated coverage with the first and second dose of measles-containing vaccine (MCV) and one dose of rubella-containing vaccine, vaccination schedule, by country—World Health Organization South-East Asia Region, 2013 and 2022.

| Country | 2013 | | | | | 2023 | | | | | % Change, 2013–2023 | | |
|---|---|---|---|---|---|---|---|---|---|---|---|---|---|
| | WHO/UNICEF Estimated Coverage * (%) | | | MCV Schedule † | | WHO/UNICEF Estimated Coverage * (%) | | | MCV Schedule † | | MCV1 Coverage | MCV2 Coverage | RCV1 Coverage |
| | MCV1 | MCV2 | RCV1 | MCV1 | MCV2 | MCV1 | MCV2 | RCV1 | MCV1 | MCV2 | | | |
| Bangladesh | 91 | 82 | 91 | MR-9 m | M-15 m | 97 | 93 | 97 | MR-9 m | MR-15 m | 7 | 13 | 7 |
| Bhutan | 94 | 89 | 94 | MR-9 m | M-24 m | 99 | 97 | 99 | MMR-9 m | MMR-24 m | 5 | 9.0 | 5 |
| DPR Korea | 99 | 76 | § | M-9 m | M-15 m | 28 | 16 | 28 | MR-9 m | MR-15 m | −72 | −79 | 280 |
| India | 83 | 51 | § | M-9 m | M-16-24 m | 93 | 90 | 93 | MR-9 m | MR-16–24 m | 12 | 76 | 930.0 |
| Indonesia | 87 | 76 | § | M-9 m | M-6 years | 82 | 62 | 82 | MR-9 m | MR-18 m | −6 | −18 | 820.0 |
| Maldives | 99 | 99 | 99 | M-9 m | MMR-18 m | 99 | 99 | 99 | MR-9 m | MMR-18 m | 0 | 0 | 0 |
| Myanmar | 86 | 80 | § | M-9 m | M-18 m | 74 | 65 | 74 | MR-9 m | MR-18 m | −14 | −19 | 740 |
| Nepal | 88 | 0 | 88 | MR-9 m | § | 93 | 89 | 93 | MR-9 m | MR-15 m | 6 | 100.0 | 6 |

**Table 3.** *Cont.*

| Country | 2013 | | | | | 2023 | | | | | % Change, 2013–2023 | | |
|---|---|---|---|---|---|---|---|---|---|---|---|---|---|
| | WHO/UNICEF Estimated Coverage * (%) | | | MCV Schedule † | | WHO/UNICEF Estimated Coverage * (%) | | | MCV Schedule † | | MCV1 Coverage | MCV2 Coverage | RCV1 Coverage |
| | MCV1 | MCV2 | RCV1 | MCV1 | MCV2 | MCV1 | MCV2 | RCV1 | MCV1 | MCV2 | | | |
| Sri Lanka | 99 | 99 | 99 | MMR-12 m | MMR 3 years | 99 | 99 | 99 | MMR-1 y | MMR-3 y | 0.0 | 0 | 0.0 |
| Thailand | 99 | 94 | 99 | MMR-9 m | MMR-7 y | 93 | 87 | 93 | MMR-9 m | MMR-2.5 y | -6 | -7 | -6 |
| Timor-Leste | 70 | 0 | § | M-9 m | § | 72 | 72 | 72 | MR-9 m | MR-18 m | 3 | 100.0 | 720 |
| SEA Region | 78 | 53 | 12 | | | 91 | 85 | 91 | | | 17 | 60 | 658 |

Abbreviations: m = months; M = measles; MCV = measles-containing vaccine; MR = measles-rubella; MMR = measles-mumps-rubella; UNICEF = United Nations Children's Fund; y = years. * Data are from WHO and UNICEF estimates, 2023 revision (as of 15 July 2024). Data available at http://immunizationdata.who.int. † As reported to WHO/UNICEF on JRFs for the year. § vaccine was not introduced into routine immunization.

Based on reports received by national programs through the joint reporting mechanism [7], 322 million children were reported to have received MCV1, around 273 million MCV2, and 196 million children were reported to have received RCV1 as part of routine immunization activities between 2013 and 2023 [7]. More than 789 million children of various age groups received at least one additional dose of measles and rubella-containing vaccine through supplementary immunization activities (SIAs) during 2013–2022 [25].

### 3.4. Surveillance Performance

In 2013, following a regional resolution to eliminate measles and control rubella [26], all countries adopted laboratory-supported acute fever and rash surveillance and gradually moved away from outbreak-based surveillance; this transition was complete by 2022. This transition was also supported by an expansion of the laboratory network, increasing the number of WHO-proficient laboratories for measles and rubella surveillance from 23 in 2013 to 58 in 2023. Of these, 26 laboratories conduct both serology and viral detection for measles and rubella, and four laboratories also conduct viral genome sequencing. The sensitivity of fever and rash surveillance for measles and rubella, as measured by the key indicator of non-measles non-rubella discarded cases (A suspected case of measles/rubella that has been investigated and discarded as not being measles or rubella is termed a non-measles, nonrubella case if any of the following is true: An adequate specimen collected during the proper time period after the onset of rash has tested negative in a proficient laboratory; there is an epidemiological linkage to another communicable disease outbreak that is not measles or rubella; another etiology has been confirmed, regardless of whether it meets the definition of an epidemiological linkage; and the case does not match the definition of a clinically compatible measles/rubella case.) rate per 100,000 population increased from less than 0.5 per 100,000 population in 2013 to 5.13 per 100,000 population in 2023 [27]—a more than ten-fold increase in the sensitivity of surveillance [28]. Similarly, other surveillance performance indicators were maintained at high levels in 2023, although variations exist within countries and between countries (Table 4). A total of 207,155 suspected measles cases were reported in the Region in 2023, compared to 31,091 in 2020 [7].

**Table 4.** Key surveillance performance indicators in SEAR countries, 2023.

| 2023 | Number of Suspected Measles Cases | % Suspected Cases with Adequate Investigation-Initiated w/in 48 h of Notification | % Suspected Cases with Serum Specimens Collected | Number of Serum Specimens Received in Laboratory | % Serum Specimens Received at Laboratory w/in 5 Days of Collection | % Specimens Tested for Serology of Specimens Received in the Laboratory | % Serology Results Reported w/in 4 Days of Specimen Received at Laboratory | Non Measles, Non-Rubella Discard Rate per 100,000 Population | % Districts with Non-Measles Non Rubella Discard Rate of 2/100,000 Population |
|---|---|---|---|---|---|---|---|---|---|
| Bangladesh | 7346 | 97.2 | 89.4 | 6529 | 99.5 | 100.0 | 97.5 | 3.92 | 100 |
| Bhutan | 229 | 94.0 | 94.8 | 181 | 85.4 | 100.0 | 65.4 | 28.43 | 80 |
| DPR Korea | 491 | 100.0 | 100.0 | 491 | 100.0 | 100.0 | 100.0 | 1.99 | No data |
| India | 154,475 | 73.4 | 77.0 | 116,105 | 100.0 | 100.0 | 82.9 | 5.75 | 94 |
| Indonesia | 39,140 | 77.8 | 75.8 | 21,508 | 97.6 | 100.0 | 12.9 | 4.84 | 55 |
| Maldives | 177 | 73.4 | 85.3 | 149 | 100.0 | 100.0 | 84.7 | 28.97 | 62 |
| Myanmar | 180 | 100.0 | 98.9 | 174 | 100.0 | 100.0 | 100.0 | 0.3 | 5 |
| Nepal | 3030 | 98.9 | 81.7 | 2469 | 100.0 | 100.0 | 76.6 | 6.94 | 90 |
| Sri Lanka | 1217 | 76.5 | 80.4 | 1159 | 99.3 | 100.0 | 62.3 | 1.7 | 19 |
| Thailand | 668 | 54.3 | 90.4 | 569 | 93.1 | 100.0 | 95.8 | 0.94 | No data |
| Timor-Leste | 202 | 100.0 | 97.8 | 198 | 100.0 | 100.0 | 37.3 | 13.99 | 62 |
| SEAR | 207,155 | 75.6 | 77.5 | 149,532 | 99.6 | 100.0 | 73.7 | 5.13 | |

### 3.5. Genotypes of Measles and Rubella Viruses

During 2013–2023, the laboratories in the Region reported B3, D4, D8, D9, and H1 genotypes of the measles virus, which are now on a decline. The transmission of D9 and H1 genotypes has not been reported since 2019 and of D4 since 2020. The only genotypes of measles reported from the Region in 2022 and 2023 are B3 and D8. For rubella, the genotype data are sparse, and there has been no reporting of any genotypes of rubella since 2021.The last reported rubella genotype was 1E from Thailand in 2020 (presented to the WHO South-East Asia Regional Immunization Technical Advisory Group meeting in August 2023).

To assist countries in establishing and implementing elimination standard surveillance for measles and rubella, a surveillance guide for measles, rubella, and congenital rubella syndrome was developed in 2017 [29] and revised in 2022 [30].

### 3.6. Epidemiological Analysis of Measles and Rubella Cases

The vaccination history of suspected cases of measles from surveillance data for various age groups shows the challenge in collecting accurate information on vaccination history, with many cases being reported as having unknown vaccination history.

The reported cases over the last five years indicate a shift in age group towards older age for measles but not for rubella (Figure 3).

Surveillance data of the last five years continue to show a significant number of reported cases of measles with unknown vaccination status, not only in the adult population but also in younger age groups, indicating challenges with recording and reporting. However, the number of zero-dose children over the last five years has decreased in younger age groups, indicating the effect of better routine vaccination as well as SIAs and catch-up vaccination efforts (Figure 4).

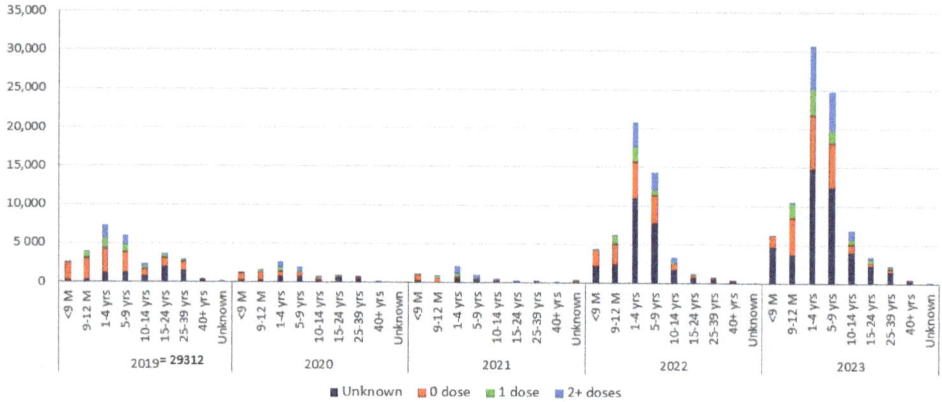


**Figure 3.** Reported cases of measles with vaccination status, WHO South-East Asia Region, 2019 to 2023.

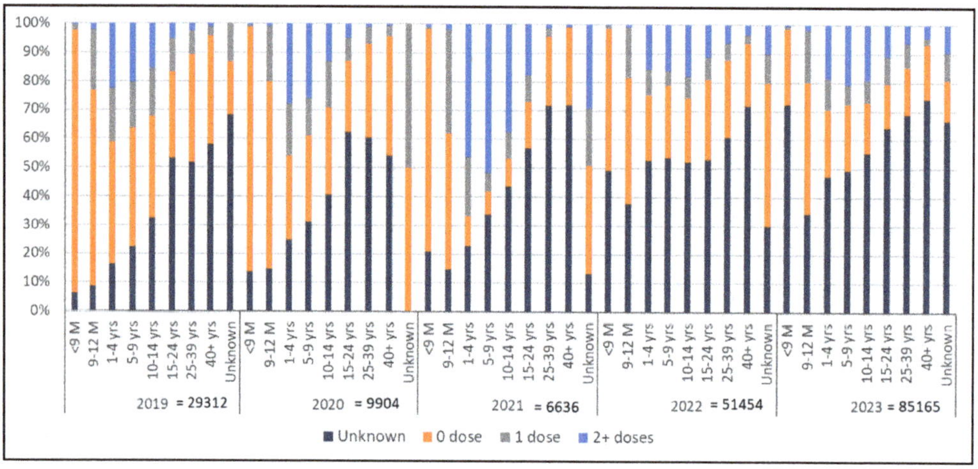


**Figure 4.** Proportion of measles cases, their vaccination status and age distribution, WHO Regional Office for South-East Asia, 2019 to 2023.

## 4. Discussion

The WHO South-East Asia Region has made significant strides toward elimination of measles and rubella [13]. Measles and rubella elimination was prioritized as a regional flagship program to support the countries to pursue the goal [31,32].

The region is home to almost a quarter of world population and a review of Demographic and Health Surveys from countries in the Region was conducted by WHO has shown that measles and rubella vaccinations are positively influenced by the education of mother (17.9 percentage point difference between children born to a mother with no education and higher education), education of father (16.6 percentage point difference between children born to a father with no education and higher education), place of delivery (14.7 percentage point difference between children born in health facility and elsewhere), birth order (14.1 percentage point difference between first-born children and 4+ birth order), household wealth quintile (14.7 percentage point difference between lowest and highest quintile) and number of antenatal care (ANC) visits (12.1 difference for measles between mother having 4+ visits and less than four visits). The region has been able to make progress in these social determinants, as demonstrated by the WHO study on review of the trends of demographic and health surveys over years [33].

This improvement in sociodemographic determinants may have enhanced access to vaccination with two doses of measles and rubella vaccine over the past decade, in addition to the introduction of MCV2, periodic SIAs, and catch-up vaccination conducted in the Region. These factors will need further enhancement to achieve very high coverage of two doses of measles and rubella-containing vaccine.

The surveillance performance in the Region as a whole has significantly improved, with all countries reporting immunization and surveillance data consistently at high rates despite diverse economic and social status.

While the reported number of cases has increased over the decade, the estimated deaths have decreased. This could possibly be due to better reporting due to enhanced surveillance performance as well as better case management, which could not be assessed in the article.

The reported genotypic information from the past several years indicates a decrease in the transmission of the number of genotypes of measles and rubella.

The implementation of strategies to eliminate measles and rubella had a jumpstart. The Region's successes against polio and maternal and neonatal tetanus laid the foundations for building confidence to establish the goal of elimination of measles and rubella [34,35]. The infrastructure and capacity built previously for other vaccine preventable disease elimination, notably polio elimination, were re-purposed to focus on measles and rubella elimination [36–38].

The political commitment of countries of the Region to protect their populations from these deadly preventable diseases was evident by the regional resolutions [2], especially in the context where there is no global-level goal to guide the program and no concrete global partner support to pursue the goal further [39,40]. Identifying and declaring measles and rubella elimination as a flagship program by the South-East Asia Region underscored the commitment and gave additional impetus to accelerate progress [30,31]. The Region successfully rode on polio elimination initiatives to eliminate measles, as well as used the platform of measles elimination to eliminate rubella due to its programmatic feasibility [34,41].

The strategic plan for measles elimination and rubella and congenital rubella syndrome control in the South-East Asia Region for the period 2014-2020 [42] had a focus to develop the platform and systems required for measles and rubella elimination, while the strategic plan for measles and rubella elimination for the period 2020–2024 [4] provided the strategic framework to the program focused more on innovative approaches to accelerating progress.

The progress was built on a consultative process backed by evidence. Prior to each goal being set or rescheduled, an independent assessment was conducted, and countries and experts were consulted to ensure technical, programmatic, and political support [43,44]. Periodic evaluations at both the regional and national levels were prioritized in order to facilitate prompt course corrections [39,45,46]. This included the regular review of progress by the SEA-RVC and National Verification Committees (NVCs) for the elimination of measles and rubella [10–13].

The advocacy and the evaluations resulted in periodic vaccine introductions, along with improved routine services, supplemental immunization activities, and periodic intensification of routine immunization activities, considerably expanding access to MCV1, MCV2, and RCV1 between 2013 and 2022.

The SEA Region has made some progress towards measles and rubella elimination, some of it is attributed to the power of collaborations that brought together a remarkable spectrum of stakeholders at the national and subnational levels, including those beyond the health sector, to implement the strategies targeted towards achieving the goal [32–34,47]. The subnational accountability mechanisms created for the polio program in larger countries were critical collaborators to ensure implementation of strategies for measles and rubella elimination and were re-energized and given the responsibility to enhance implementation of the strategies to eliminate measles and rubella [48,49].

The contributions of the Regional and National Immunization Technical Advisory Groups to support acceleration of progress through overall technical leadership to the elimination program have remained noteworthy [15,16]. Similarly, the national verification committee (NVC) in each country collaborated with the relevant governments to oversee advancements made toward elimination of measles and rubella and provided annual reports to SEA-RVC and guided the program forward [10–13].

*Challenges*

All WHO Regions have a regional mandate from Member States to pursue measles elimination, while the global program remains muted and does not have a global goal for measles and rubella eradication. As a result, the program is not able to harness the power of donors and partners to generate adequate resources to support optimal implementation of the strategies to eliminate measles and rubella.

The COVID-19 pandemic posed serious obstacles to achieving the target by 2023 and had a detrimental effect on vaccination and surveillance efforts. Despite the challenges brought on by the pandemic, Bhutan, DPR Korea, the Maldives, Sri Lanka, and Timor-Leste achieved and managed to sustain their measles and rubella elimination status. These countries will need continued efforts to sustain the elimination status as long as the measles and rubella viruses are circulating in neighboring countries and globally, by developing and effectively implementing the post-elimination sustainability plans. Larger countries like India and Indonesia have shown an increase in the number of measles cases, which may be partly because of the immunity gap added to the chronic gap during the pandemic and partly due to enhanced surveillance. These immunity gaps will need to be urgently addressed through tailored subnational targeted supplementary immunization activities to ensure these countries are back on track to achieve the measles and rubella elimination target.

There are several other challenges, the most significant of which is to achieve more than 95% coverage with two doses of measles and rubella-containing vaccine [50]. The subnational heterogeneity in coverage in several countries remains a substantial challenge and has resulted in outbreaks of measles in pockets of low coverage during recent years. The sensitivity of the surveillance for measles and rubella continued to remain sub-par in a large number of subnational areas in endemic countries, resulting in under-reporting and underestimating the disease burden as well as delaying a response to outbreaks. Adequate resources to optimally implement the strategies, coupled with national commitment not trickling down to the local level for optimal implementation of key strategies, have been identified as some of the other challenges to achieving measles and rubella elimination [51].

The delay in closing the immunity gap in children through high vaccination coverage has resulted in children escaping childhood without immunity to measles, which has led to a shift in the age group of the measles cases, making the elimination process more complex as this will require closing immunity gaps in other non-conventional age groups, increasing the cost of elimination.

## 5. Conclusions

While significant progress has been made across the Region on measles and rubella elimination, the region continues to be off track to achieve the elimination target by 2023 [44].

The year 2026 was considered to be the next feasible target date for the elimination of measles and rubella following a regional consultation with countries and experts that was held in 2023 [51]. The consultation considered the current momentum for measles and rubella elimination in the Region, the strengths, and enablers currently available across countries in the Region, the results from a modeling exercise, and factored in the loss of

2–3 years in program performance due to the COVID-19 pandemic for the achievement of the current target of measles and rubella elimination [50].

Measles and rubella elimination is feasible; however, this will require an optimal implementation of strategies within a very short period of time to achieve the target, which in turn is possible through significant public support and political will as well as sufficient financial resources mobilized for the program.

The year 2026 is an ambitious target to achieve measles and rubella in the WHO South-East Asia Region, which has a quarter of the world's population. The WHO South-East Asia Region has gained the required momentum and has established the necessary framework to eliminate measles and rubella. It will remain critical for the Region to ensure broad public support, political will, and adequate resources and mechanisms to rapidly accelerate implementation of strategies over the next few years to achieve the goal of eliminating both measles and rubella.

**Author Contributions:** Conceptualization, S.K., S.K.B. and V.B.; methodology, S.K.; software, D.D. and R.S.; validation, D.D. and R.S.; formal analysis, S.K., L.S., S.K.B. and V.B.; writing—original draft preparation, S.K.; writing—review and editing, S.K., S.K.B., V.B., L.S., D.D. and R.S.; visualization, D.D.; supervision, V.B. and S.K.B. All authors have read and agreed to the published version of the manuscript.

**Funding:** This research received no external funding.

**Institutional Review Board Statement:** Not applicable.

**Informed Consent Statement:** Not applicable.

**Data Availability Statement:** The data presented in the study are openly available at https://immunizationdata.who.int/ and https://www.who.int/southeastasia/health-topics/immunization/vaccine-preventable-disease-(vpd)-surveillance-data (accessed on 18 July 2024).

**Acknowledgments:** The authors would like to acknowledge the role of national immunization programs from WHO South-East Asia Member States, respective WHO country offices of the South-East Asia Region, UNICEF Regional and country offices for South-Asia and East-Asia and Pacific, donors, partners, civil society organizations, families and communities in ensuring progress towards measles and rubella elimination and directly and indirectly contributing to the program.

**Conflicts of Interest:** The views expressed are of the authors and do not reflect official position of the institution to which they are affiliated to. The authors declare no conflict of interest.

## References

1. Khanal, S.; Bahl, S.; Sangal, L.; Dhongde, D.; O'connor, P.M.; Crowcroft, N.S.; Morales, M. Progress Toward Rubella Elimination—World Health Organization South-East Asia Region, 2013-2021. *MMWR. Morb. Mortal. Wkly. Rep.* **2023**, *72*, 678–682. [CrossRef] [PubMed]
2. World Health Organization. Regional Office for South-East Asia. *Measles Elimination and Rubella/Congential Rubella Syndrome Control*; Report No.: SEA/RC66/R5; World Health Organization. Regional Office for South-East Asia: New Delhi, India, 2013. Available online: https://apps.who.int/iris/handle/10665/128273 (accessed on 14 December 2022).
3. World Health Organization. Regional Office for South-East Asia. Measles and Rubella Elimination by 2023; Report No.: SEA/RC72/R3. 2019. Available online: https://apps.who.int/iris/handle/10665/327923 (accessed on 14 December 2022).
4. World Health Organization. Regional Office for South-East Asia. Strategic Plan for Measles and Rubella Elimination in WHO South-East Asia Region: 2020–2024. 2019. Available online: https://apps.who.int/iris/handle/10665/330356 (accessed on 14 December 2022).
5. Eilertson, K.E.; Fricks, J.; Ferrari, M.J. Estimation and prediction for a mechanistic model of measles transmission using particle filtering and maximum likelihood estimation. *Stat. Med.* **2019**, *38*, 4146–4158. [CrossRef] [PubMed]
6. World Health Organization. Regional Office for South-East Asia. SEA Region Measles and Rubella Quarterly update October–December 2021. 2021. Available online: https://apps.who.int/iris/handle/10665/364212 (accessed on 14 June 2024).
7. World Health Organization. Measles Nucleotide Surveillance Database (MeaNs). Available online: https://who-gmrln.org/means2 (accessed on 24 June 2024).
8. WHO. Immunization Data Portal. Available online: https://immunizationdata.who.int/ (accessed on 14 June 2024).
9. World Health Organization. Rubella Nucleotide Surveillance Database (RubeNS). Available online: https://who-gmrln.org/rubens2 (accessed on 24 June 2024).

10. World Health Organization. Regional Office for South-East Asia. Fifth Meeting of the WHO South-East Asia Regional Verification Commission for Measles and Rubella, Virtual, 6–7 July 2020. Available online: https://apps.who.int/iris/handle/10665/338265 (accessed on 14 December 2022).
11. World Health Organization. Regional Office for South-East Asia. Sixth Meeting of the WHO South-East Asia Regional Verification Commission for Measles and Rubella; Report No.: SEA-Immun-124, Virtual, 27–29 September 2021. Available online: https://apps.who.int/iris/handle/10665/350119 (accessed on 14 December 2022).
12. World Health Organization. Regional Office for South-East Asia. Seventh Meeting of the WHO South-East Asia Regional Verification Commission for Measles and Rubella, Bali, Indonesia, 21–23 June 2022. Report No.: SEA-Immun-136. Available online: https://apps.who.int/iris/handle/10665/360441 (accessed on 14 December 2022).
13. World Health Organization. Regional Office for South-East Asia. Eighth Meeting of the WHO South-East Asia Regional Verification Commission for Measles and Rubella 2023, Bangkok, Thailand, 21–23 June 2023. Available online: https://iris.who.int/handle/10665/370787 (accessed on 14 December 2022).
14. World Health Organization. Regional Office for South-East Asia. Eleventh Meeting of the WHO South-East Asia Regional Immunization Technical Advisory Group, New Delhi, India, 21–22 July 2020. Available online: https://iris.who.int/handle/10665/335831 (accessed on 14 December 2022).
15. World Health Organization. Regional Office for South-East Asia. Twelfth Meeting of the WHO South-East Asia Regional Immunization Technical Advisory Group, New Delhi, India, 9–11 August 2021. Available online: https://iris.who.int/handle/10665/349583 (accessed on 14 December 2022).
16. World Health Organization. Regional Office for South-East Asia. Thirteenth Meeting of the WHO South-East Asia Regional Immunization Technical Advisory Group, New Delhi, India, 17–19 August 2022. Available online: https://apps.who.int/iris/handle/10665/364534 (accessed on 14 December 2022).
17. World Health Organization. Regional Office for South-East Asia. Fourteenth Meeting of the WHO South-East Asia Regional Immunization Technical Advisory Group, New Delhi, India, 29 August–1 September 2023. Available online: https://iris.who.int/handle/10665/375007 (accessed on 14 December 2022).
18. World Health Organization. Regional Office for South-East Asia. Framework for Verification of Measles and Rubella Elimination in the WHO South-East Asia Region. 2020. Available online: https://apps.who.int/iris/handle/10665/332737 (accessed on 14 December 2022).
19. World Health Organization. Regional Office for South-East Asia. Guidelines on Verification of Measles Elimination and Rubella/Congenital Rubella Syndrome Control in the South-East Asia Region. 2016. Available online: https://apps.who.int/iris/handle/10665/255875 (accessed on 14 December 2022).
20. Khanal, S.; Kassem, A.M.; Bahl, S.; Jayantha, L.; Sangal, L.; Sharfuzzaman, M.; Bose, A.S.; Antoni, S.; Datta, D.; Alexander, J.P. Progress Toward Measles Elimination—South-East Asia Region, 2003–2020. *MMWR. Morb. Mortal. Wkly. Rep.* **2022**, *71*, 1042–1046. [CrossRef] [PubMed]
21. Minta, A.A.; Ferrari, M.; Antoni, S.; Portnoy, A.; Sbarra, A.; Lambert, B.; Hatcher, C.; Hsu, C.H.; Ho, L.L.; Steulet, C.; et al. Progress Toward Measles Elimination—Worldwide, 2000–2022. *MMWR. Morb. Mortal. Wkly. Rep.* **2023**, *72*, 1262–1268. [CrossRef] [PubMed]
22. Perry, R.T.; Gacic-Dobo, M.; Dabbagh, A.; Mulders, M.N.; Strebel, P.M.; Okwo-Bele, J.M.; Rota, P.A.; Goodson, J.L. Centers for Disease Control and Prevention (CDC). Progress toward regional measles elimination—Worldwide, 2000–2013. *MMWR. Morb. Mortal. Wkly. Rep.* **2014**, *63*, 1034–1038. [PubMed] [PubMed Central]
23. World Health Organization = Organisation Mondiale de la Santé. Progress Towards Regional Measles Elimination, Worldwide, 2000–2014 = Progrès Accomplis Dans le Monde en Vue de L'élimination Régionale de la Rougeole, 2000–2014. *Wkly. Epidemiol. Rec. Relev. Épidémiologique Hebd.* **2015**, *90*, 623–631. Available online: https://apps.who.int/iris/handle/10665/254526 (accessed on 14 December 2022).
24. Bahl, S.; Khanal, S.; Sangal, L.; Tabassum, S.; Ungchusak, K.; Andrus, J. Measles and rubella elimination: Protecting children through immunization in South-East Asia Region (SEAR). *Lancet Reg. Health Southeast Asia* **2023**, *18*, 100303. [CrossRef] [PubMed] [PubMed Central]
25. Thapa, A.; Khanal, S.; Sharapov, U.; Swezy, V.; Sedai, T.; Dabbagh, A.; Rota, P.; Goodson, J.L.; McFarland, J. Progress Toward Measles Elimination—South-East Asia Region, 2003–2013. *MMWR. Morb. Mortal. Wkly. Rep.* **2015**, *64*, 613–617. [PubMed]
26. World Health Organization. Regional Office for South-East Asia. SEA/RC66/R5—Measles Elimination and Rubella/Congential Rubella Syndrome Control. 2013. Available online: https://iris.who.int/handle/10665/128273 (accessed on 14 December 2022).
27. World Health Organization. Regional Office for South-East Asia. Expanded Programme on Immunization9EPI) Factsheet 2023:SEAR. 2023. Available online: https://www.who.int/southeastasia/health-topics/vaccines-and-immunization/vaccine-preventable-disease-(vpd)-surveillance-data (accessed on 28 August 2024).
28. World Health Organization. Regional Office for South-East Asia. SEA Region Measles and Rubella Quarterly Update July–September 2022. 2022. Available online: https://apps.who.int/iris/handle/10665/364213 (accessed on 14 December 2022).
29. World Health Organization. Regional Office for South-East Asia. Surveillance Guide for Vaccine-Preventable Diseases in the WHO South-East Asia Region. 2017. Available online: https://iris.who.int/handle/10665/277459 (accessed on 14 December 2022).

30. World Health Organization. Regional Office for South-East Asia. Surveillance Guide for Vaccine-Preventable Diseases in the WHO South-East Asia Region (Strategic Guidance on VPD Surveillance in the WHO South-East Asia Region). Available online: https://iris.who.int/handle/10665/373606 (accessed on 14 December 2022).
31. World Health Organization. Regional Office for South-East Asia. Sustain Accelerate Innovate—South-East Asia: Flagship Priority Programmes Driving Impact in Countries for the Health of Billions. 2022. Available online: https://apps.who.int/iris/handle/10665/362030 (accessed on 14 December 2022).
32. World Health Organization. Regional Office for South-East Asia. Evaluation of Implementation of Regional Flagship Areas in the WHO South-East Asia Region 2014–2018. 2020. Available online: https://apps.who.int/iris/handle/10665/338722 (accessed on 14 December 2022).
33. World Health Organization. Regional Office for South-East Asia. Trend and Factors Affecting Zero-Vaccination Status of Children for Measles-Containing Vaccine in the WHO South-East Asia Region: Analysis from Two Recent Demographic and Health Surveys of the Countries (Bangladesh, India, Indonesia, Maldives, Myanmar, Nepal and Timor-Leste). 2021. Available online: https://iris.who.int/handle/10665/345264 (accessed on 14 December 2022).
34. Bahl, S.; Kumar, R.; Menabde, N.; Thapa, A.; McFarland, J.; Swezy, V.; Tangermann, R.H.; Jafari, H.S.; Elsner, L.; Wassilak, S.G.; et al. Polio-free certification and lessons learned—South-East Asia region, March 2014. *MMWR. Morb. Mortal. Wkly. Rep.* **2014**, *63*, 941 946. [PubMcd]
35. Kanu, F.A.; Yusuf, N.; Kassogue, M.; Ahmed, B.; Tohme, R.A. Progress Toward Achieving and Sustaining Maternal and Neonatal Tetanus Elimination—Worldwide, 2000–2020. *MMWR. Morb. Mortal. Wkly. Rep.* **2022**, *71*, 406–411. [CrossRef] [PubMed]
36. World Health Organization. Regional Office for South-East Asia. Immunization Achievements in South-East Asia: The Platform for Measles Elimination. 2017. Available online: https://apps.who.int/iris/handle/10665/258759 (accessed on 14 December 2022).
37. Paudel, K.P.; Hampton, L.M.; Gurung, S.; Bohara, R.; Rai, I.K.; Anaokar, S.; Swift, R.D.; Cochi, S. Adapting Nepal's polio eradication programme. *Bull. World Health Organ.* **2017**, *95*, 227–232. [CrossRef]
38. Rodriguez, D.C.; Neel, A.H.; Mahendradhata, Y.; Deressa, W.; Owoaje, E.; Akinyemi, O.; Sarker, M.; Mafuta, E.; Gupta, S.D.; Salehi, A.S.; et al. The effects of polio eradication efforts on health systems: A cross-country analysis using the Develop-Distort Dilemma. *Health Policy Plan.* **2021**, *36*, 707–719. [CrossRef] [PubMed]
39. Meeting of the International Task Force for Disease Eradication. 2015. Available online: https://www.who.int/publications-detail-redirect/WER9106 (accessed on 14 December 2022).
40. World Health Organization. Proceedings of the Global Technical Consultation to assess the feasibility of measles eradication, 28–30 July 2010. *J. Infect. Dis.* **2011**, *204* (Suppl. 1), S4–S13. [CrossRef] [PubMed]
41. World Health Organization. Regional Office for South-East Asia. Joint National and International Measles, Rubella and Congenital Rubella Syndrome Programme Review, Nepal 2019. Available online: https://iris.who.int/handle/10665/332883. (accessed on 14 December 2022).
42. World Health Organization. Regional Office for South-East Asia. Strategic Plan for Measles Elimination and Rubella and Congenital Rubella Syndrome Control in the South-East Asia Region, 2014–2020. 2015. Available online: https://iris.who.int/handle/10665/205923 (accessed on 14 December 2022).
43. World Health Organization. Regional Office for South-East Asia. WHO South-East Asia Regional High-Level Consultation on Adopting the Revised Goal of Measles and Rubella Elimination, New Delhi, India, 14–15 March 2019. Available online: https://iris.who.int/handle/10665/330566 (accessed on 14 December 2022).
44. World Health Organization. Regional Office for South-East Asia. Regional Consultation on Resetting the Target Date for Achieving the Goal of Measles and Rubella Elimination in the WHO South-East Asia Region, New Delhi, India, 14–16 March 2023. Available online: https://iris.who.int/handle/10665/368018 (accessed on 14 December 2022).
45. World Health Organization. Regional Office for South-East Asia. Midterm Review of the "Strategic Plan for Measles Elimination and Rubella and Congenital Rubella Syndrome Control in the South-East Asia Region: 2014–2020". Available online: https://iris.who.int/handle/10665/279993 (accessed on 14 December 2022).
46. World Health Organization. Regional Office for South-East Asia. Review of Progress and Way Forward on Measles and Rubella Elimination Activities in the WHO South-East Asia Region. Available online: https://iris.who.int/handle/10665/352255 (accessed on 14 December 2022).
47. World Health Organization. Regional Office for South-East Asia. *Lessons from the Big Six—Closing the Immunity Gap for Measles Elimination and Rubella/CRS Control: New Delhi, India 31 January–2 February 2018*; Report No.: SEA-IMMUN-120; World Health Organization. Regional Office for South-East Asia: New Delhi, India, 2017. Available online: https://apps.who.int/iris/handle/10665/277429 (accessed on 14 December 2022).
48. Cintyamena, U.; Azizatunnisa', L.; Ahmad, R.A.; Mahendradhata, Y. Scaling up public health interventions: Case study of the polio immunization program in Indonesia. *BMC Public Health.* **2021**, *21*, 614. [CrossRef] [PubMed]
49. Thacker, N.; Vashishtha, V.M.; Thacker, D. Polio Eradication in India: The Lessons Learned. *Pediatrics* **2016**, *138*, e20160461. [CrossRef] [PubMed]
50. Moss, W.J.; Shendale, S.; Lindstrand, A.; O'Brien, K.L.; Turner, N.; Goodman, T.; Kretsinger, K. Feasibility assessment of measles and rubella eradication. *Vaccine* **2021**, *39*, 3544–3559. [CrossRef]

51. World Health Organization. Regional Office for South-East Asia. *WHO Regional Committee for South-East Asia: Report of the Seventy-Fourth Session, Nepal (Virtual), 6–10 September 2021*; Report No.: SEA/RC74/21; World Health Organization. Regional Office for South-East Asia: New Delhi, India, 2021. Available online: https://apps.who.int/iris/handle/10665/355974 (accessed on 14 December 2022).

vaccines

MDPI

*Review*

# Measles and Rubella Elimination in the Western Pacific Region in 2013–2022: Lessons Learned from Progress and Achievements Made during Regional and Global Measles Resurgences

**Yoshihiro Takashima [1,*,†], Syeda Kanwal Aslam [1], Roger Evans [1], Kayla Mae Mariano [1], Chung-won Lee [1], Xiaojun Wang [1], Varja Grabovac [1] and David N. Durrheim [2]**

1 World Health Organization Regional Office for the Western Pacific, Manila 1000, Philippines; saslam@who.int (S.K.A.); revans@who.int (R.E.); marianok@who.int (K.M.M.); wangxia@who.int (X.W.); grabovacv@who.int (V.G.)
2 School of Medicine and Public Health, University of Newcastle, Callaghan, NSW 2308, Australia; david.durrheim@health.nsw.gov.au
* Correspondence: yoshi_takashima@cider.osaka-u.ac.jp
† Current address: Center for Infectious Disease Education and Research, Osaka University, Osaka 565-0871, Japan.

**Abstract:** Measles is the most contagious communicable disease, causing an estimated 5.5 million cases and more than 30,000 deaths in the Western Pacific Region (WPR) during 2000. Rubella infection in a pregnant woman can be devastating for the foetus, resulting in congenital rubella syndrome (CRS) in 90% of rubella infections in early pregnancy. It was estimated that approximately 9000 CRS cases occurred in the WPR in 2010. World Health Organization (WHO) Member States in the WPR decided in 2003 to eliminate measles and in 2014 to eliminate rubella from the region. While the WPR successfully attained historically low measles incidence in 2012, it experienced a region-wide measles resurgence in 2013–2016. During the regional resurgence, WHO and Member States accumulated greater knowledge on the epidemiology of measles and rubella in the WPR and strategies to maintain gains. The implementation of the resulting new regional strategy and plan of action from 2018 has proven that measles and rubella elimination is achievable and sustainable under the pressure of multiple importations of measles virus during the world-wide measles resurgences in 2018–2019. This article discusses this progress and achievements towards achieving the global eradication of measles and rubella.

**Keywords:** measles elimination; rubella elimination; sustainability of elimination; regional resurgence of measles; global resurgence of measles; import-related outbreak; global synchronization of elimination effort

## 1. Background

Measles is a highly contagious and serious disease caused by the measles virus. It was estimated that 5.5 million measles cases and 31,200 to 34,000 deaths occurred in 2000 in the Western Pacific Region (WPR) [1,2]. While rubella is usually a mild viral disease in children, infection in a pregnant woman can be devastating for the foetus. Congenital rubella syndrome (CRS) occurs in 90% of maternal rubella infections in early pregnancy. The estimated CRS incidence was 11,541 cases in 1996, 11,084 in 2000 and 8889 in 2010 in the Western Pacific Region [3].

In 2003, the World Health Organization (WHO) Regional Committee (RC) for the Western Pacific confirmed that measles elimination should be a regional goal, endorsed the Western Pacific Regional Plan of Action for Measles Elimination and urged Member States to offer all children two doses of measles-containing vaccine (MCV) to achieve and maintain a 95% population immunity of each birth cohort in every district and use measles elimination to strengthen routine immunization and other public health programmes, such as the prevention of CRS (WPR/RC54.R3) [4]. In 2005, the RC decided that the WPR should aim to eliminate measles by 2012 and urged Member States to develop or strengthen national plans for measles elimination as part of comprehensive multi-year plans for immunization services (WPR/RC56.R8) [5].

In 2010, the RC reaffirmed the 2012 measles elimination goal, requested WHO to establish regional verification mechanisms for measles elimination and urged Member States to commit the human and financial resources necessary to achieve and sustain measles elimination, accelerate the control of rubella and the prevention of CRS and establish an independent verification process for measles elimination (WPR/RC61.R7) [6].

Countries and areas in the WPR have progressively strengthened their national immunization programmes and significantly reduced measles transmission, morbidity and mortality. In 2012, the region recorded the lowest number of measles cases in its history—10,794 cases, or 5.9 cases per 1 million population, compared with 177,052 cases, or 105.1 cases per 1 million population, in 2000 (Figure 1).

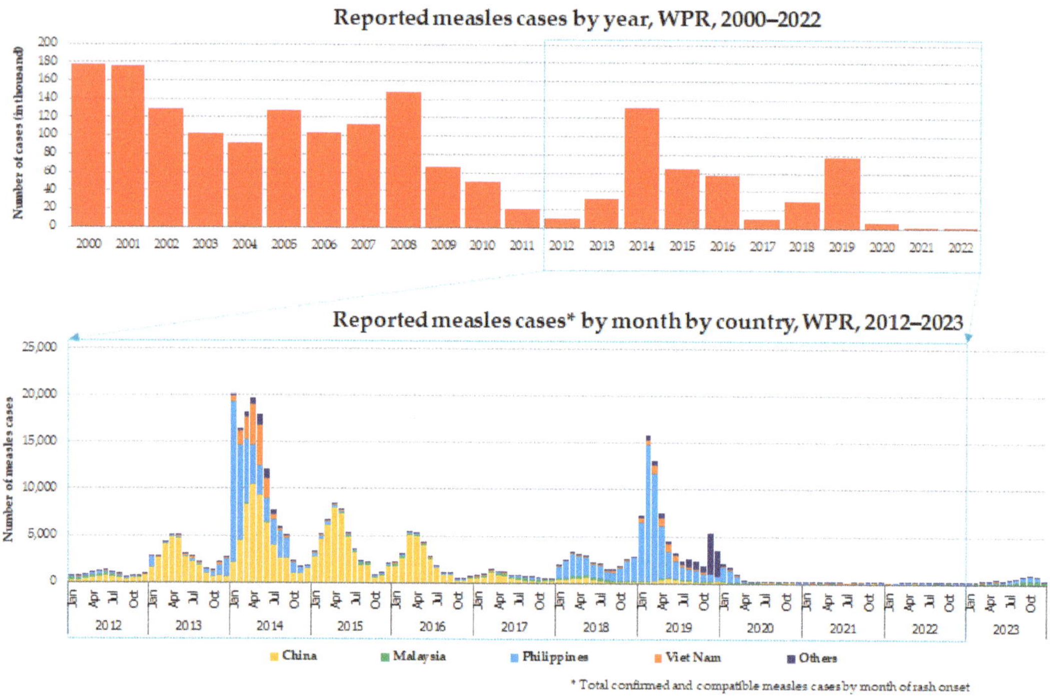


**Figure 1.** Measles cases by year 2000–2022 and by month 2012–2023 in the Western Pacific Region Source: [7].

In 2012, the RC reaffirmed its commitment to eliminate measles and accelerate rubella control in the WPR, and urged Member States to implement effective immunization strategies to identify and reach all vulnerable underserved communities in both rural and urban settings, interrupt all residual endemic measles virus transmission as rapidly as possible and establish national verification committees (NVCs) to develop regular progress reports for submission to the Regional Verification Commission for Measles Elimination in the Western Pacific (RVC) (WPR/RC63.R5) [8]. In 2014, the RC endorsed a regional rubella elimination goal as one of eight regional immunization goals in the Regional Framework for Implementation of the Global Vaccine Action Plan in the Western Pacific (WPR/RC65.R5) [9].

## 2. Regional Measles Resurgence in the Western Pacific 2013–2016

After the low number of measles cases in 2012, the Western Pacific experienced a region-wide measles resurgence from 2013 to 2016. The regional measles incidence rate per 1 million population increased from 5.9 in 2012 to 19.4 in 2013, 69.2 in 2014, 36.2 in 2015 and 30.2 in 2016 (Figure 1).

### *2.1. Resurgence of Measles Virus Transmission in Endemic Countries*

There were large national resurgences of measles virus transmission in endemic countries. In China, the ongoing transmission of the genotype H1 measles virus, which has been the only endemic genotype detected in China since surveillance began in 1993 [10], significantly decreased as a result of multiple province-wide measles supplementary immunization activities (SIAs) between 2003 and 2009 and a nation-wide measles SIA in 2010, resulting in the lowest measles incidence ever reported in China in 2012. However, transmission then increased and there was a nation-wide measles resurgence in China which lasted until 2016 [11]. In the Philippines, the measles genotype D9 was endemic and caused two large outbreaks in 2010 and 2011, but the genotype B3 virus became endemic in early 2013 [12,13]. A nation-wide measles rubella-containing vaccine SIA (MRCV-SIA) rolled out in September 2014 had sub-optimal coverage with measles virus transmission continuing, particularly in the middle and southern parts of the Philippines (Visayas and Mindanao) [14], and the nation-wide measles resurgence lasted until 2015. Malaysia, where the genotype D8 measles virus has continued to be detected since 2013 and the genotype D9 virus was identified in 2015–2017, experienced increased measles virus transmission between 2015 and 2018.

### *2.2. Importation of Measles Virus from Countries with Increased Endemic Transmission or Import-Related Large-Scale Outbreaks*

The multiple importations of the measles virus from countries with resurgences of endemic transmission or import-related large-scale outbreaks led to multiple small-scale outbreaks between 2013 and 2015 in Australia, Hong Kong SAR (China), Japan, the Republic of Korea, Singapore and Vanuatu [15–17].

### *2.3. Nation-Wide Measles Outbreaks after Importation*

Several countries experienced large-scale outbreaks following importation after a period of low or no documented transmission: New Zealand (genotype B3 virus in 2013–2014), Viet Nam (genotype H1, B3 and D8 viruses in 2013–2014), Papua New Guinea (genotype D8 virus imported from Indonesia in 2013 and genotype B3 virus in 2014) [18], the Federated States of Micronesia (genotype B3 virus in 2014), Solomon Islands (genotype B3 virus imported from Papua New Guinea in 2014) [19], Lao PDR (genotype H1 virus in 2014) and Mongolia (genotype H1 virus in 2015–2016) [20]. These importations resulted in large-scale measles outbreaks in 2013–2016, revealing important population immunity gaps [20].

### *2.4. Re-Established Measles Virus Transmission after Elimination*

In Mongolia, which was verified by the RVC in March 2014 to have achieved and sustained the interruption of endemic measles virus transmission for more than three years, a prolonged nation-wide measles outbreak began in March 2015 due to the imported genotype H1 virus [20], leading to classification by the RVC as having re-established endemic transmission as of September 2017 [21].

### *2.5. Response to the Regional Resurgence*

In response to the regional resurgence, the Technical Advisory Group (TAG) for Immunization and Vaccine-Preventable Diseases in the Western Pacific Region recommended WHO develop a new strategy and plan of action for measles elimination in the WPR [22], which was submitted to and endorsed by the RC in 2017 as the Regional Strategy and Plan of Action for Measles and Rubella Elimination in the Western Pacific (WPR/RC68.R1) [23].

The Regional Strategy and Plan of Action proposed Operational Targets for 2020 as milestones to attain the regional goal, which was not only to achieve but also sustain the elimination of measles and rubella in all countries and areas of the WPR. The targets included: (i) sustain the interruption of measles virus transmission in countries and areas that have reached measles elimination; (ii) prevent the resurgence of endemic measles virus transmission (genotypes B3, D8, D9 and H1); (iii) interrupt all ongoing measles transmission in endemic countries; and (iv) prevent large-scale outbreaks after importation for measles elimination; (v) set a national target year for rubella elimination in all countries; and (vi) establish CRS surveillance in all countries for rubella elimination [24].

## 3. Progress in Achieving and Sustaining Measles and Rubella Elimination in the Western Pacific Region after the 2013–2016 Regional Resurgence

### *3.1. Elimination of Measles and Rubella Verified by RVC from 2014 to 2023*

The Regional Verification Commission (RVC) was established in January 2012. In line with the resolution WPR/RC63.R5 in 2012, all 14 countries and 2 areas in the Western Pacific Region established National Verification Committees (NVCs) and the Pacific Island countries and areas (PICs), consisting of 21 countries and areas in the Pacific (which are considered one epidemiological block for the purpose of the verification of measles and rubella elimination), established a Sub-Regional Verification Committee (SRVC). NVCs and SRVC started the submission of annual progress reports towards measles and rubella elimination in the second half of 2013 and an annual meeting of the RVC has occurred since May 2014 to monitor progress towards elimination attainment.

The verification of measles and rubella elimination in the WPR requires the documentation of the interruption of endemic measles and rubella virus transmission for a period of at least 36 months from the last known endemic case [25]. From 2014 to 2023, eight countries and two areas in the region were verified to have achieved measles elimination and, among them, six countries and two areas were verified in 2023 to have sustained measles elimination. Since 2017, a total of five countries and two areas in the region were verified to have achieved and sustained rubella elimination (Figure 2).

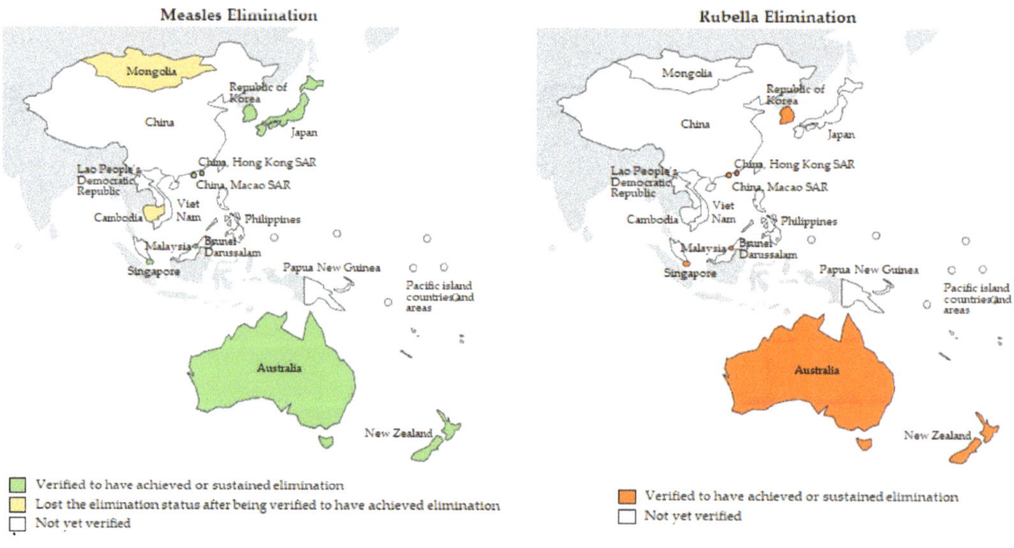


**Figure 2.** Status of verification on measles and rubella elimination in the Western Pacific Region in 2023.

Scheme 1 shows the status of measles and rubella elimination in countries, areas and the Pacific sub-region from 2014 to 2023 by (i) the status of measles elimination in 2023; (ii) sustainability of measles elimination; and (iii) the size of total population.

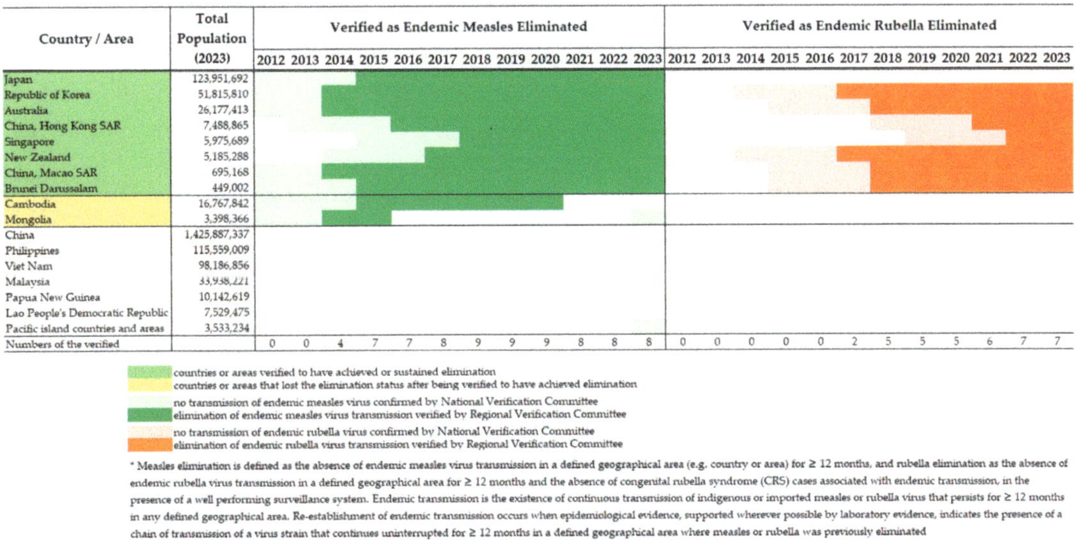


**Scheme 1.** Status of verification on measles and rubella elimination* in the Western Pacific Region by country, 2012–2023. Source: [25].

### 3.2. Measles Incidence

While Singapore, New Zealand, Macao SAR (China), Cambodia, Lao PDR, Samoa, Tonga and American Samoa experienced significant increases in measles incidence during the global measles resurgence in 2018 to 2019 [26–28], all six countries and two areas that had been verified by RVC to have achieved measles elimination, China, Papua New Guinea, Lao PDR and the Pacific sub-region have continued to achieve decrease in measles incidence (i.e., confirmed measles cases per million population) since 2019 and many of them have maintained a measles incidence of <1 per million population from 2021 to 2023 (Scheme 2).

### 3.3. Routine Immunization Programmes and Supplementary Immunization Activities (SIA)

All countries and areas which were verified by the RVC to have achieved and sustained measles elimination maintained >90% annual coverage of measles and rubella containing vaccine first dose (MRCV-1) from 2013 to 2022, and most countries maintained a >90% coverage of MRCV-2 from 2013 to 2022 (except Macao SAR (China) in 2013 (89.2%), New Zealand from 2013 to 2022 (82.3–90.7%) and Singapore in 2016 (87.9%) and 2018 (84.0%)) (Scheme 3). Of these countries, only New Zealand experienced notable declines in MRCV-2 coverage during the COVID-19 pandemic in 2021–2022.

Among countries which have not yet been verified to have achieved measles elimination, China and Malaysia sustained > 90% annual coverage with both MRCV-1 and MRCV-2 in each year from 2013 to 2022 (except MRCV-2 coverage in 2019 (87.0%) and 2020 (84.0%) in Malaysia). Viet Nam, which reported a >90% coverage of both MRCV-1 and MRCV-2 in each year from 2014 to 2020, experienced a marked decline in coverage with both MRCV-1 and MRCV-2 during the COVID-19 pandemic response in 2021 and 2022. The routine coverage of both MRCV-1 and MRCV-2 never reached 80% in the Philippines and Papua New Guinea from 2013 to 2022, and the Philippines had decreasing coverage for both MRCV-1 and MRCV-2 during the COVID-19 pandemic in 2021 and 2022.

| Country / Area (non-PIC) | Total Population (2023) | Measles — Cases (confirmed) 2012 | 2013 | 2014 | 2015 | 2016 | 2017 | 2018 | 2019 | 2020 | 2021 | 2022 | 2023 |
|---|---|---|---|---|---|---|---|---|---|---|---|---|---|
| Japan | 123,951,692 | 228 | 207 | 454 | 35 | 163 | 188 | 284 | 763 | 12 | 6 | 5 | 28 |
| Republic of Korea | 51,815,810 | 2 | 107 | 442 | 7 | 18 | 7 | 19 | 191 | 6 | 0 | 1 | 7 |
| Australia | 26,177,413 | 199 | 154 | 340 | 74 | 99 | 81 | 101 | 285 | 25 | 0 | 7 | 26 |
| China, Hong Kong SAR | 7,488,865 | 8 | 38 | 50 | 18 | 9 | 4 | 16 | 90 | 1 | 1 | 3 | 4 |
| Singapore | 5,975,689 | 40 | 66 | 171 | 45 | 157 | 81 | 37 | 162 | 14 | 1 | 6 | 11 |
| New Zealand | 5,185,288 | 55 | 13 | 274 | 12 | 104 | 15 | 36 | 2,229 | 7 | 0 | 0 | 14 |
| China, Macao SAR | 695,168 | 1 | 3 | 1 | 0 | 0 | 2 | 3 | 37 | 0 | 0 | 0 | 0 |
| Brunei Darussalam | 449,002 | 1 | 0 | 0 | 4 | 1 | 0 | 1 | 1 | 0 | 0 | 0 | 1 |
| Cambodia | 16,767,842 | 0 | 0 | 0 | 0 | 56 | 10 | 3 | 676 | 379 | 5 | 13 | 11 |
| Mongolia | 3,398,366 | 0 | 0 | 0 | 20,373 | 28,813 | 9 | 1 | 2 | 0 | 0 | 0 | 0 |
| China | 1,425,887,337 | 6,183 | 27,825 | 52,485 | 42,864 | 24,839 | 5,993 | 3,975 | 3,098 | 867 | 554 | 562 | 648 |
| Philippines | 115,559,009 | 1,536 | 5,798 | 54,669 | 2,003 | 641 | 2,432 | 22,869 | 48,521 | 3,723 | 218 | 589 | 2,442 |
| Viet Nam | 98,186,856 | 637 | 1,232 | 16,741 | 884 | 368 | 592 | 1,247 | 5,723 | 713 | 163 | 27 | 103 |
| Malaysia | 33,938,221 | 1,868 | 182 | 222 | 1,318 | 1,587 | 1,693 | 1,958 | 1,077 | 478 | 128 | 209 | 1,799 |
| Papua New Guinea | 10,142,619 | 0 | 7 | 2,589 | 53 | 0 | 7 | 15 | 1 | 4 | 0 | 0 | 12 |
| Lao People's Democratic Republic | 7,529,475 | 36 | 68 | 70 | 56 | 8 | 3 | 10 | 1,290 | 135 | 2 | 0 | 2 |

| Country / Area (non-PIC) | Measles — Incidence (confirmed cases per million population) 2012 | 2013 | 2014 | 2015 | 2016 | 2017 | 2018 | 2019 | 2020 | 2021 | 2022 | 2023 |
|---|---|---|---|---|---|---|---|---|---|---|---|---|
| Japan | 1.8 | 1.6 | 3.6 | 0.3 | 1.3 | 1.5 | 2.2 | 6.1 | 0.1 | 0.0 | 0.0 | 0.2 |
| Republic of Korea | 0.0 | 2.1 | 8.7 | 0.1 | 0.4 | 0.1 | 0.4 | 3.7 | 0.1 | 0.0 | 0.0 | 0.1 |
| Australia | 8.8 | 6.7 | 14.5 | 3.1 | 4.1 | 3.3 | 4.0 | 11.2 | 1.0 | 0.0 | 0.3 | 1.0 |
| China, Hong Kong SAR | 1.1 | 5.2 | 6.8 | 2.4 | 1.2 | 0.5 | 2.1 | 12.0 | 0.1 | 0.1 | 0.4 | 0.5 |
| Singapore | 7.4 | 12.0 | 30.7 | 8.0 | 27.5 | 14.1 | 6.4 | 27.6 | 2.4 | 0.2 | 1.0 | 1.8 |
| New Zealand | 12.5 | 2.9 | 60.7 | 2.6 | 22.3 | 3.2 | 7.4 | 449.5 | 1.4 | 0.0 | 0.0 | 2.8 |
| China, Macao SAR | 1.7 | 5.1 | 1.7 | 0.0 | 0.0 | 3.1 | 4.6 | 55.8 | 0.0 | 0.0 | 0.0 | 0.0 |
| Brunei Darussalam | 2.5 | 0.0 | 0.0 | 9.5 | 2.3 | 0.0 | 2.3 | 2.3 | 0.0 | 0.0 | 0.0 | 2.2 |
| Cambodia | 0.0 | 0.0 | 0.0 | 0.0 | 3.6 | 0.6 | 0.2 | 41.7 | 23.1 | 0.3 | 0.8 | 0.6 |
| Mongolia | 0.0 | 0.0 | 0.0 | 6,871.7 | 9,510.6 | 2.9 | 0.3 | 0.6 | 0.0 | 0.0 | 0.0 | 0.0 |
| China | 4.5 | 20.2 | 37.9 | 30.8 | 17.7 | 4.2 | 2.8 | 2.2 | 0.6 | 0.4 | 0.4 | 0.4 |
| Philippines | 15.7 | 58.2 | 539.5 | 19.4 | 6.1 | 22.8 | 210.6 | 439.6 | 33.2 | 1.9 | 5.2 | 21.4 |
| Viet Nam | 7.1 | 13.6 | 183.5 | 9.6 | 4.0 | 6.3 | 13.1 | 59.8 | 7.4 | 1.7 | 0.3 | 1.0 |
| Malaysia | 63.0 | 6.0 | 7.3 | 42.4 | 50.3 | 52.9 | 60.4 | 32.8 | 14.4 | 3.8 | 6.3 | 53.6 |
| Papua New Guinea | 0.0 | 0.8 | 305.9 | 6.1 | 0.0 | 0.8 | 1.6 | 0.1 | 0.4 | 0.0 | 0.0 | 1.3 |
| Lao People's Democratic Republic | 5.5 | 10.3 | 10.5 | 8.3 | 1.2 | 0.4 | 1.4 | 178.9 | 18.4 | 0.3 | 0.0 | 0.3 |

| Country / Area (PIC) | Total Population (2023) | Measles — Cases (confirmed) 2012 | 2013 | 2014 | 2015 | 2016 | 2017 | 2018 | 2019 | 2020 | 2021 | 2022 | 2023 |
|---|---|---|---|---|---|---|---|---|---|---|---|---|---|
| Fiji | 929,766 | 0 | 0 | 1 | 1 | 5 | 1 | 0 | 31 | 3 | 2 | 0 | 0 |
| Solomon Islands | 724,273 | 0 | 0 | 15 | 0 | 1 | 0 | 0 | 0 | 0 | 0 | 0 | 0 |
| Vanuatu | 326,740 | 0 | 0 | 5 | 19 | 0 | 0 | 0 | 0 | 0 | 0 | 0 | 0 |
| French Polynesia | 306,279 | 0 | 0 | 0 | 0 | 0 | 0 | 0 | 0 | 0 | 0 | 0 | 0 |
| New Caledonia | 289,950 | 0 | 0 | 0 | 1 | 0 | 1 | 0 | 0 | 0 | 0 | 0 | 0 |
| Samoa | 222,382 | 0 | 0 | 0 | 0 | 0 | 0 | 0 | 5,689 | 18 | 0 | 0 | 0 |
| Guam | 171,774 | 0 | 0 | 1 | 0 | 0 | 0 | 0 | 0 | 0 | 0 | 0 | 0 |
| Kiribati | 131,232 | 0 | 0 | 0 | 0 | 0 | 0 | 0 | 0 | 1 | 0 | 0 | 0 |
| Micronesia (Fed. States of) | 114,164 | 0 | 0 | 257 | 0 | 0 | 0 | 0 | 0 | 0 | 0 | 0 | 0 |
| Tonga | 106,858 | 0 | 0 | 0 | 0 | 0 | 0 | 0 | 608 | 51 | 0 | 0 | 0 |
| Northern Mariana Islands | 49,551 | 0 | 0 | 0 | 0 | 0 | 0 | 0 | 0 | 0 | 0 | 0 | 0 |
| American Samoa | 44,273 | 0 | 0 | 0 | 0 | 0 | 0 | 0 | 31 | 2 | 0 | 0 | 0 |
| Marshall Islands | 41,569 | 0 | 0 | 0 | 0 | 0 | 0 | 0 | 0 | 0 | 0 | 0 | 0 |
| Palau | 18,055 | 0 | 0 | 0 | 0 | 0 | 0 | 0 | 0 | 0 | 0 | 0 | 0 |
| Cook Islands | 17,011 | 0 | 0 | 0 | 0 | 0 | 0 | 0 | 0 | 0 | 0 | 0 | 0 |
| Nauru | 12,668 | 0 | 0 | 0 | 0 | 0 | 0 | 0 | 0 | 0 | 0 | 0 | 0 |
| Wallis and Futuna Islands | 11,572 | 0 | 0 | 0 | 0 | 0 | 0 | 0 | 0 | 0 | 0 | 0 | 0 |
| Tuvalu | 11,312 | 0 | 0 | 0 | 0 | 0 | 0 | 0 | 0 | 0 | 0 | 0 | 0 |
| Niue | 1,934 | 0 | 0 | 0 | 0 | 0 | 0 | 0 | 0 | 0 | 0 | 0 | 0 |
| Tokelau | 1,871 | 0 | 0 | 0 | 0 | 0 | 0 | 0 | 0 | 0 | 0 | 0 | 0 |

| Country / Area (PIC) | Measles — Incidence (confirmed cases per million population) 2012 | 2013 | 2014 | 2015 | 2016 | 2017 | 2018 | 2019 | 2020 | 2021 | 2022 | 2023 |
|---|---|---|---|---|---|---|---|---|---|---|---|---|
| Fiji | 0.0 | 0.0 | 1.1 | 1.1 | 5.4 | 1.1 | 0.0 | 33.8 | 3.3 | 2.2 | 0.0 | 0.0 |
| Solomon Islands | 0.0 | 0.0 | 25.1 | 0.0 | 1.6 | 0.0 | 0.0 | 0.0 | 0.0 | 0.0 | 0.0 | 0.0 |
| Vanuatu | 0.0 | 0.0 | 18.5 | 68.7 | 0.0 | 0.0 | 0.0 | 0.0 | 0.0 | 0.0 | 0.0 | 0.0 |
| French Polynesia | 0.0 | 0.0 | 0.0 | 0.0 | 0.0 | 0.0 | 0.0 | 0.0 | 0.0 | 0.0 | 0.0 | 0.0 |
| New Caledonia | 0.0 | 0.0 | 0.0 | 3.5 | 0.0 | 3.5 | 0.0 | 0.0 | 0.0 | 0.0 | 0.0 | 0.0 |
| Samoa | 0.0 | 0.0 | 0.0 | 0.0 | 0.0 | 0.0 | 0.0 | 26,846.9 | 83.7 | 0.0 | 0.0 | 0.0 |
| Guam | 0.0 | 0.0 | 6.0 | 0.0 | 0.0 | 0.0 | 0.0 | 0.0 | 0.0 | 0.0 | 0.0 | 0.0 |
| Kiribati | 0.0 | 0.0 | 0.0 | 0.0 | 0.0 | 0.0 | 0.0 | 0.0 | 7.9 | 0.0 | 0.0 | 0.0 |
| Micronesia (Fed. States of) | 0.0 | 0.0 | 2,357.3 | 0.0 | 0.0 | 0.0 | 0.0 | 0.0 | 0.0 | 0.0 | 0.0 | 0.0 |
| Tonga | 0.0 | 0.0 | 0.0 | 0.0 | 0.0 | 0.0 | 0.0 | 5,793.2 | 484.5 | 0.0 | 0.0 | 0.0 |
| Northern Mariana Islands | 0.0 | 0.0 | 0.0 | 0.0 | 0.0 | 0.0 | 0.0 | 0.0 | 0.0 | 0.0 | 0.0 | 0.0 |
| American Samoa | 0.0 | 0.0 | 0.0 | 0.0 | 0.0 | 0.0 | 0.0 | 655.1 | 43.3 | 0.0 | 0.0 | 0.0 |
| Marshall Islands | 0.0 | 0.0 | 0.0 | 0.0 | 0.0 | 0.0 | 0.0 | 0.0 | 0.0 | 0.0 | 0.0 | 0.0 |
| Palau | 0.0 | 0.0 | 0.0 | 0.0 | 0.0 | 0.0 | 0.0 | 0.0 | 0.0 | 0.0 | 0.0 | 0.0 |
| Cook Islands | 0.0 | 0.0 | 0.0 | 0.0 | 0.0 | 0.0 | 0.0 | 0.0 | 0.0 | 0.0 | 0.0 | 0.0 |
| Nauru | 0.0 | 0.0 | 0.0 | 0.0 | 0.0 | 0.0 | 0.0 | 0.0 | 0.0 | 0.0 | 0.0 | 0.0 |
| Wallis and Futuna Islands | 0.0 | 0.0 | 0.0 | 0.0 | 0.0 | 0.0 | 0.0 | 0.0 | 0.0 | 0.0 | 0.0 | 0.0 |
| Tuvalu | 0.0 | 0.0 | 0.0 | 0.0 | 0.0 | 0.0 | 0.0 | 0.0 | 0.0 | 0.0 | 0.0 | 0.0 |
| Niue | 0.0 | 0.0 | 0.0 | 0.0 | 0.0 | 0.0 | 0.0 | 0.0 | 0.0 | 0.0 | 0.0 | 0.0 |
| Tokelau | 0.0 | 0.0 | 0.0 | 0.0 | 0.0 | 0.0 | 0.0 | 0.0 | 0.0 | 0.0 | 0.0 | 0.0 |

(green) countries or areas verified to have achieved or sustained elimination
(yellow) countries or areas that lost the elimination status after being verified to have achieved elimination

**Scheme 2.** Confirmed cases and incidence of measles in the Western Pacific Region by country, 2012–2023. Source: [29,30].

| Country / Area (non-PIC) | Total Population (2023) | <1 year old | MRCV-1 type of vaccine | vaccination schedule* | Coverage** 2012 | 2013 | 2014 | 2015 | 2016 | 2017 | 2018 | 2019 | 2020 | 2021 | 2022 |
|---|---|---|---|---|---|---|---|---|---|---|---|---|---|---|---|
| Japan | 123,951,692 | 813,334 | MR | Y1 | 95.7 | 95.3 | 97.5 | 95.5 | 96.4 | 102.5 | 97.2 | 96.0 | 98.5 | 95.4 | 98.5 |
| Republic of Korea | 51,815,810 | 285,031 | MMR | M12-15 | 99.4 | 99.6 | 99.6 | 97.7 | 98.0 | 97.4 | 97.8 | 97.9 | 98.0 | 98.0 | 97.0 |
| Australia | 26,177,413 | 299,402 | MMR | M12 | 94.0 | 93.7 | 94.0 | 95.0 | 95.0 | 94.0 | 94.0 | 94.0 | 93.0 | 92.7 | 96.0 |
| China, Hong Kong SAR | 7,488,865 | 41,865 | MMR | M12 | | | | | | 95.0 | | 95.0 | 95.0 | 95.0 | 95.0 |
| Singapore | 5,975,689 | 42,263 | MMR | M12 | 95.0 | 95.0 | 95.0 | 95.0 | 94.6 | 95.4 | 95.0 | 96.3 | 96.8 | 96.0 | 96.2 |
| New Zealand | 5,185,288 | 63,879 | MMR | M12 | 92.4 | 92.4 | 92.6 | 93.0 | 92.0 | 93.3 | 91.9 | 91.8 | 91.5 | 91.1 | 90.0 |
| China, Macao SAR | 695,168 | 6,941 | MMR | M12 | 92.7 | 92.7 | 93.3 | 93.1 | 93.5 | 93.6 | 94.9 | 98.0 | 97.6 | 96.1 | 97.4 |
| Brunei Darussalam | 449,002 | 6,002 | MMR | M12 | 94.6 | 96.0 | 97.0 | 96.0 | 98.0 | 97.0 | 99.0 | 97.0 | 99.0 | 99.4 | 97.3 |
| Cambodia | 16,767,842 | 311,777 | MR | M9 | 93.4 | 90.2 | 94.0 | 95.0 | 122.7 | 101.1 | 103.8 | 103.8 | 107.0 | 102.7 | 102.0 |
| Mongolia | 3,398,366 | 68,865 | MMR | M9 | 98.8 | 97.1 | 98.3 | 98.1 | 98.5 | 99.5 | 98.7 | 98.0 | 97.2 | 95.2 | 94.5 |
| China | 1,425,887,337 | 10,694,436 | MMR | M8 | 99.0 | 99.6 | 99.0 | 99.5 | 99.5 | 99.6 | 98.6 | 98.8 | 99.2 | 99.4 | 99.1 |
| Philippines | 115,559,009 | 2,445,164 | MMR | M9 | 80.0 | 77.0 | 75.0 | 79.0 | 75.0 | 70.0 | 67.0 | 75.0 | 77.0 | 57.1 | 68.9 |
| Viet Nam | 98,186,856 | 1,421,158 | M | M9 | 96.4 | 97.7 | 97.4 | 97.5 | 98.6 | 97.4 | 97.2 | 95.4 | 97.3 | 89.0 | 87.7 |
| Malaysia | 33,938,221 | 506,221 | MMR | M9 | 95.0 | 95.3 | 92.1 | 93.0 | 95.8 | 96.2 | 97.6 | 97.0 | 95.0 | 96.0 | 103.4 |
| Papua New Guinea | 10,142,619 | 246,099 | MR | M9 | 67.0 | 70.0 | 65.0 | 60.0 | 51.0 | 43.0 | 42.0 | 32.7 | 43.6 | 35.1 | 40.9 |
| Lao People's Democratic Republic | 7,529,475 | 156,737 | MR | M9 | 71.7 | 82.0 | 87.0 | 99.0 | 87.0 | 92.0 | 92.0 | 88.8 | 85.5 | 79.2 | 81.6 |

| Country / Area (non-PIC) | MRCV-2 type of vaccine | vaccination schedule | Coverage** 2012 | 2013 | 2014 | 2015 | 2016 | 2017 | 2018 | 2019 | 2020 | 2021 | 2022 |
|---|---|---|---|---|---|---|---|---|---|---|---|---|---|
| Japan | MR | Y5 | 92.2 | 92.8 | 93.7 | 93.0 | 93.3 | 94.9 | 93.1 | 93.4 | 94.6 | 94.1 | 94.7 |
| Republic of Korea | MMR | Y4-6 | 97.0 | 95.0 | 96.3 | 97.0 | 97.3 | 96.8 | 96.8 | 96.3 | 95.0 | 95.0 | 95.0 |
| Australia | MMRV | M18 | 91.2 | 92.2 | 92.6 | 93.0 | 94.0 | 93.5 | 93.5 | 93.6 | 94.2 | 93.9 | 91.4 |
| China, Hong Kong SAR | MMRV | M18/Y6 | 98.7 | 98.7 | 98.5 | 98.6 | 97.1 | 95.0 | 98.1 | 95.0 | 91.4 | 95.0 | 95.4 |
| Singapore | MMR | M15-18 | 95.4 | 90.0 | 90.0 | 90.0 | 87.9 | 90.0 | 84.0 | 92.2 | 93.7 | 92.9 | 92.3 |
| New Zealand | MMR | M15 | 85.5 | 85.8 | 86.3 | 87.0 | 89.0 | 90.1 | 89.7 | 89.9 | 90.7 | 82.3 | 82.8 |
| China, Macao SAR | MMRV | M18 | 89.2 | 89.2 | 90.6 | 90.9 | 91.5 | 91.4 | 93.5 | 96.0 | 95.5 | 95.0 | 96.0 |
| Brunei Darussalam | MMR | M18 | 96.0 | 92.0 | 96.0 | 97.0 | 97.0 | 98.0 | 98.0 | 98.0 | 96.9 | 98.6 | 98.5 |
| Cambodia | MR | M18 | 81.8 | 63.5 | 73.0 | 72.0 | 105.0 | 83.3 | 81.4 | 92.5 | 90.5 | 82.5 | 88.2 |
| Mongolia | MMR | Y2 | 98.3 | 96.7 | 98.1 | 97.7 | 89.7 | 98.1 | 98.4 | 98.5 | 95.5 | 93.9 | 93.3 |
| China | MMR | M18 | 99.0 | 99.6 | 99.0 | 99.4 | 99.4 | 99.4 | 99.2 | 98.5 | 99.0 | 99.3 | 99.1 |
| Philippines | MMR | M12-15 | 42.0 | 54.0 | 53.0 | 84.0 | 61.0 | 61.0 | 59.0 | 69.0 | 73.0 | 55.0 | 63.7 |
| Viet Nam | MR | M18 | 83.2 | 85.8 | 93.8 | 91.8 | 94.6 | 92.7 | 90.4 | 92.4 | 92.9 | 84.9 | 80.7 |
| Malaysia | MMR | M12 | 98.6 | 99.1 | 98.9 | 99.0 | 99.1 | 98.9 | 90.1 | 87.0 | 84.0 | 97.5 | 96.3 |
| Papua New Guinea | MR | M18 | | | | | | | | 19.6 | 27.5 | 19.9 | 24.9 |
| Lao People's Democratic Republic | MR | M12 | 9.2 | | | | | 1.0 | 76.0 | 66.5 | 70.1 | 55.6 | 61.3 |

| Country / Area (PIC) | Total Population (2023) | <1 year old | MRCV-1 type of vaccine | vaccination schedule* | Coverage** 2012 | 2013 | 2014 | 2015 | 2016 | 2017 | 2018 | 2019 | 2020 | 2021 | 2022 |
|---|---|---|---|---|---|---|---|---|---|---|---|---|---|---|---|
| Fiji | 929,766 | 17,501 | MMR | M12 | 90 | 96 | 91 | 95 | 95 | 96.0 | 81.0 | 82.5 | 82.2 | 99.0 | 85 |
| Solomon Islands | 724,273 | 20,931 | MR | M12 | 84.8 | 75.89 | 75.88 | 75.25 | 82 | 84.3 | 93.0 | 81.0 | 81.0 | 67.3 | 90.31 |
| Vanuatu | 326,740 | 9,288 | MR | M12 | 94.15 | 64.658 | 90 | 76 | 84 | 80.0 | 75.0 | 80.0 | 78.0 | 50.0 | 70 |
| French Polynesia | 306,279 | 3,823 | MMR | M12 | | | 99 | 98 | | 97.5 | 97.0 | 97.0 | | | 98.4 |
| New Caledonia | 289,950 | 4,057 | MMR | M12 | 96.4 | 96.4 | 96.4 | 96.0 | 96.0 | 96.0 | 97.4 | | | | 97.0 |
| Samoa | 222,382 | 5,933 | MMR | M9 | 84.6 | 98.7 | 91.0 | 78.0 | 77.0 | 80.0 | 40.0 | 96.0 | 65.5 | 62.0 | 81.6 |
| Guam | 171,774 | 2,790 | MMR | M12 | 51.0 | 51.0 | | 84.9 | 91.7 | 90.0 | 82.5 | | | | |
| Kiribati | 131,232 | 3,381 | MR | M12 | 91.0 | 91.0 | 88.0 | 84.0 | 80.2 | 81.0 | 84.0 | 94.1 | 81.8 | 80.2 | 84.6 |
| Micronesia (Fed. States of) | 114,164 | 2,323 | MMR | M12 | 90.9 | 91.3 | 93.9 | 74.0 | 70.0 | 76.0 | 73.0 | 78.0 | 78.6 | 64.5 | 71.8 |
| Tonga | 106,858 | 2,433 | MR | M12 | 95.0 | 99.6 | 95.0 | 99.0 | 98.0 | 99.0 | 99.0 | 99.0 | 99.6 | 99.5 | 99.5 |
| Northern Mariana Islands | 49,551 | 600 | MMR | M12 | | | | | 62.0 | 64.8 | 73.0 | 75.3 | 78.9 | 85.6 | 85.3 |
| American Samoa | 44,273 | 760 | MMR | M15 | | | | | | | | | | | |
| Marshall Islands | 41,569 | 751 | MMR | M12 | 78.0 | 70.3 | 79.0 | 75.0 | 74.9 | 83.5 | 83.0 | 85.0 | 89.0 | 84.7 | 81.0 |
| Palau | 18,055 | 266 | MMR | M12 | 91.0 | 98.7 | 83.0 | 95.0 | 96.0 | 84.7 | 90.0 | 97.0 | 93.2 | 92.9 | 96.0 |
| Cook Islands | 17,011 | 273 | MMR | M12 | 97.0 | 97.0 | 98.0 | 99.0 | 90.0 | 98.0 | 100.0 | 100.0 | | | 61.3 |
| Nauru | 12,668 | 336 | MR | M12 | 96.0 | 97.0 | 65.0 | 98.0 | 98.0 | 95.0 | 100.0 | 95.0 | 98.2 | 101.8 | 98.0 |
| Wallis and Futuna Islands | 11,572 | 134 | MMR | M12 | 120.0 | 120.0 | | 79.0 | 155.0 | | | | | | |
| Tuvalu | 11,312 | 260 | MR | M12 | 97.6 | 96.0 | 93.6 | 94.0 | 96.0 | 94.6 | 88.2 | 96.3 | 92.8 | 93.3 | 90.0 |
| Niue | 1,934 | 26 | MMR | M12 | 100.0 | 100.0 | 99.0 | 100.0 | 100.0 | 100.0 | 100.0 | 100.0 | 99.0 | 99.0 | 100.0 |
| Tokelau | 1,871 | 35 | MMR | M12 | | 100.0 | 100.0 | 100.0 | | | 100.0 | 98.0 | 94.0 | 95.0 | 100.0 |

| Country / Area (PIC) | MRCV-2 type of vaccine | vaccination schedule | Coverage** 2012 | 2013 | 2014 | 2015 | 2016 | 2017 | 2018 | 2019 | 2020 | 2021 | 2022 |
|---|---|---|---|---|---|---|---|---|---|---|---|---|---|
| Fiji | MMR | M18 | 92 | 98.0 | 92.0 | 100.0 | 95.0 | 105.0 | 95.0 | 72.3 | 71.5 | | 76.0 |
| Solomon Islands | MR | M18 | 101.6 | | | | | | 54.0 | 54.0 | 51.0 | 39.7 | 90.3 |
| Vanuatu | - | - | | | | | | | | | | | |
| French Polynesia | MMR | M18 | | | 99.0 | 98.0 | | 97.5 | 97.0 | 97.0 | | | 99.3 |
| New Caledonia | MMR | M16 | 85.6 | 85.6 | 85.6 | 86.0 | 86.0 | 86.0 | 91.6 | | | | 92.0 |
| Samoa | MMR | M15 | 67.4 | 87.0 | 78.0 | 63.0 | 59.0 | 78.0 | 28.0 | 59.0 | 59.4 | 50.0 | 45.3 |
| Guam | MMR | Y4-6 | | | | | | 90.0 | 85.0 | | | | |
| Kiribati | MR | Y4 | 9.3 | 84.0 | 80.0 | 76.0 | 78.9 | 79.0 | 99.0 | 91.4 | 56.8 | 58.2 | 68.0 |
| Micronesia (Fed. States of) | MMR | M13 | 69.8 | 74.6 | 78.0 | 74.0 | 45.0 | 52.0 | 48.0 | 52.0 | 62.1 | 37.8 | 42.9 |
| Tonga | MR | M18 | 95.0 | 99.6 | 95.0 | 99.0 | 99.0 | 99.0 | 99.0 | 99.0 | 99.7 | 99.3 | 99.3 |
| Northern Mariana Islands | MMR | Y4-6 | | | | | 72.0 | 76.8 | 92.0 | 90.4 | 76.7 | 95.7 | 90.4 |
| American Samoa | MMR | Y4 | | | | | | | | | | | |
| Marshall Islands | MMR | M13 | 58.0 | 42.3 | 53.0 | 70.0 | 48.7 | 61.7 | 61.0 | 63.6 | 67.9 | 58.5 | 53.6 |
| Palau | MMR | M15 | 86.0 | 98.2 | 81.0 | 82.0 | 95.0 | 77.2 | 75.0 | 88.0 | 83.5 | 83.9 | 85.0 |
| Cook Islands | MMR | M18 | 98.0 | 95.0 | 98.0 | 95.0 | 90.0 | 95.0 | 100.0 | 98.0 | 82.0 | 67.0 | 50.7 |
| Nauru | MR | M15 | 81.0 | 88.0 | 49.0 | 96.0 | 97.0 | 94.0 | 94.0 | 95.0 | 97.0 | 100.9 | 99.7 |
| Wallis and Futuna Islands | MMR | M16 | 107.3 | 107.3 | | 80.0 | 121.0 | | | | | | |
| Tuvalu | MR | M18 | 93.1 | 84.0 | 91.2 | 86.0 | 92.0 | 93.5 | 80.9 | 92.3 | 85.5 | 84.1 | 89.2 |
| Niue | MMR | M15 | 98.0 | 100.0 | 99.0 | 100.0 | 100.0 | 100.0 | 100.0 | 100.0 | 99.0 | 99.0 | 100.0 |
| Tokelau | MMR | M15 | | 100.0 | 100.0 | 100.0 | | | 100.0 | 98.0 | 95.0 | 95.0 | 100.0 |

(green) countries or areas verified to have achieved or sustained elimination
(yellow) countries or areas that lost the elimination status after being verified to have achieved elimination

* vaccination schedule may have been changed in some countries during the period under review.
** If official coverage is not available, administrative coverage is used, if also not available, WUENIC is used.

MRCV-1 first dose of measles- and rubella-containing vaccine
MRCV-2 second dose of measles- and rubella-containing vaccine
M measles vaccine
MR measles-rubella vaccine
MMR measles, mumps and rubella vaccine
MMRV measles, mumps, rubella and varicella vaccine
M9 9 months of age
M12-15 12 to 15 months of age
Y1 one year of age
Y4-6 4 to 6 years of age

**Scheme 3.** Coverage of MRCV-1 and MRCV-2 (routine immunization with 1st and 2nd doses of measles- and rubella-containing vaccines) in the Western Pacific Region by country, 2012–2022. Source: [31].

Japan, the Republic of Korea, Australia, Hong Kong SAR (China), Singapore, New Zealand, Macao SAR (China) and Brunei Darussalam were verified by the RVC to have achieved and then verified to have sustained measles elimination without an implementation of nation-wide MCV-SIAs between 2013 and 2023.

Mongolia conducted a nation-wide MCV-SIA, targeting children aged 6 months to 6 years, in May and June 2015, and another nation-wide MCV-SIA, targeting young adults aged 18 to 30 years, in May 2016, in response to the largest measles outbreak since the introduction of MCV into the national immunization programme in 1973 (Scheme 4) [32]. This import-related outbreak in Mongolia predominantly affected young people aged 15 to 29 years followed by children aged 0 to 8 months (accounting for 59% and 12% of cases, respectively). Cambodia conducted a nation-wide MR-SIA targeting children aged 6 to 59 months in 2017 in response to an import-related measles outbreak in 2016.

| Country / Area | Total Population (2023) | <1 year old | | 2012 | 2013 | 2014 | 2015 | 2016 | 2017 | 2018 | 2019 | 2020 | 2021 | 2022 | 2023 |
|---|---|---|---|---|---|---|---|---|---|---|---|---|---|---|---|
| Cambodia | 16,767,842 | 311,777 | Type of<br>age group<br>targeted<br>vaccinated<br>coverage | | MR<br>9 M-14 Y<br>4,345,392<br>4,576,633<br>105.3% | | | | MR<br>6-59m<br>1,613,925<br>1,452,821<br>90% | | | | | | |
| Mongolia | 3,398,366 | 68,865 | Type of<br>age group<br>targeted<br>vaccinated<br>coverage | MR<br>3-14 Y<br>560,592<br>522,429<br>93.2% | | | M<br>6 M-6 Y<br>368,102<br>347,685<br>94.5% | MR<br>18-30 Y<br>624,000<br>549,846<br>88.1% | | | | | | | MR<br>10 M-8 Y<br>639,183<br>309,310<br>48.4% |
| Philippines | 115,559,009 | 2,445,164 | Type of<br>age group<br>targeted<br>vaccinated<br>coverage | | | MR<br>9-59 M<br>11,485,540<br>10,402,490<br>90.6% | | | | | | MR<br>9-59 M<br>9,463,434<br>8,549,093<br>90.3% | | | MR<br>9-59 M<br>9,704,231<br>8,184,944<br>84.30% |
| Viet Nam | 98,186,856 | 1,421,158 | Type of<br>age group<br>targeted<br>vaccinated<br>coverage | | | MR<br>1-14 Y<br>20,095,950<br>19,735,750<br>98.2% | | MR<br>16-17 Y<br>1,883,406<br>1,787,588<br>94.9% | | | | | | | |
| Papua New Guinea | 10,142,619 | 246,099 | Type of<br>age group<br>targeted<br>vaccinated<br>coverage | M<br>6-35 M<br>631,747<br>552,872<br>87.5% | | | MR<br>9 M-14 Y<br>1,286,410<br>801,436<br>62.3% | | | | MR<br>6-59 M<br>1,167,516<br>1,180,422<br>101.1% | | | | MR<br>6-59 M<br>1,223,284<br>871,429<br>71.2% |
| Lao People's Democratic Republic | 7,529,475 | 156,737 | Type of<br>age group<br>targeted<br>vaccinated<br>coverage | | | MR<br>9 M-9 Y<br>1,560,136<br>1,569,224<br>100.6% | | | MR<br>9m-<5y<br>702,756<br>703,924<br>100.2% | | | | | | |
| Fiji | 929,766 | 17,501 | Type of<br>age group<br>targeted<br>vaccinated<br>coverage | | | | | | MR<br>12m-11y<br>187,668<br>178,069<br>94.9% | | MR<br>6 M-39 Y<br><br>328,000<br>95.0% | | | | |
| Solomon Islands | 724,273 | 20,931 | Type of<br>age group<br>targeted<br>vaccinated<br>coverage | MR<br>12-59 M<br>67,160<br>67,832<br>101.0% | | MR<br>6 M-29 Y<br>376,286<br>394,584<br>104.9% | | | | | MR<br>6-71 M<br>88,916<br>88,138<br>99.1% | | | | |
| Vanuatu | 326,740 | 9,288 | Type of<br>age group<br>targeted<br>vaccinated<br>coverage | | MR<br>12-59 M<br>33,096<br>33,604<br>101.5% | | MR<br>1-15 Y<br>100,317<br>103,676<br>103.3% | | | | | | | | |
| Samoa | 222,382 | 5,933 | Type of<br>age group<br>targeted<br>vaccinated<br>coverage | | | | | | MR<br>1-12y<br>59,931<br>57,229<br>95.5% | | MR<br>6/12-50 Y<br>200,879<br>187,369<br>93.3% | | | | |
| Kiribati | 131,232 | 3,381 | Type of<br>age group<br>targeted<br>vaccinated<br>coverage | | | | | | | | MR<br>1-14 Y<br>40,564<br>39,035<br>96.2% | | | | |
| Micronesia (Fed. States of) | 114,164 | 2,323 | Type of<br>age group<br>targeted<br>vaccinated<br>coverage | | | MMR<br>6 M-49/57 Y<br>82,472<br>71,388<br>86.6% | | | | | | | | | |
| Tonga | 106,858 | 2,433 | Type of<br>age group<br>targeted<br>vaccinated<br>coverage | | | | | | | | MR<br>6 M-24 Y<br>58,067<br>54,590<br>94.0% | | | | |

| | |
|---|---|
| (highlighted) | countries or areas that lost the elimination status after being verified to have achieved elimination |
| MRCV-1 | first dose of measles- and rubella-containing vaccine |
| MRCV-2 | second dose of measles- and rubella-containing vaccine |
| M | measles vaccine |
| MR | measles-rubella vaccine |
| MMR | measles, mumps and rubella vaccine |
| MMRV | measles, mumps, rubella and varicella vaccine |
| M9 | 9 months of age |
| M12-15 | 12 to 15 months of age |
| Y1 | one year of age |
| Y4-6 | 4 to 6 years of age |

**Scheme 4.** Implementation of supplementary immunization activities with measles and rubella containing vaccines in the Western Pacific Region by country, 2012–2023. Source: [31].

The Philippines carried out nation-wide MR-SIAs targeting children aged 6 to 59 months in 2014 and 2020. Both SIAs followed periods of major resurgence in endemic transmission in 2013–2014 and 2018–2019. Fiji, Samoa and Tonga carried out nation-wide MR-SIAs targeting adults as well as children and adolescents during the latter periods of large-scale import-related measles outbreaks in 2019 in response to the global measles resurgence and importations from New Zealand.

While most MRCV-SIAs carried out in the WPR attained high vaccination coverage (>90%), their impact could have been substantially greater if they had targeted the specific groups with large immunity gaps and if they had been implemented before or very soon after the detection of resurgences or import-related outbreaks.

## 3.4. *Surveillance*

Several countries or areas verified by the RVC as having achieved measles elimination (e.g., Macao SAR (China), Brunei Darussalam, Cambodia and Mongolia) and some countries which have not yet achieved measles elimination (e.g., China, Malaysia, Lao PDR and the Pacific sub-region) have maintained highly sensitive measles and rubella surveillance measured by "discarded non-measles rate per 100,000 population" from 2013 to 2023 (Scheme 5).

| Country / Area | Total Population (2023) | Discarded non-measles rate per 100,000 pop ≥ 2 | | | | | | | | | | | |
|---|---|---|---|---|---|---|---|---|---|---|---|---|---|
| | | 2012 | 2013 | 2014 | 2015 | 2016 | 2017 | 2018 | 2019 | 2020 | 2021 | 2022 | 2023 |
| Japan | 123,951,692 | 0.1 | 0.7 | 0.5 | 0.2 | 0.7 | 0.4 | 1.1 | 2.2 | 0.2 | 0.1 | 0.1 | 0.4 |
| Republic of Korea | 51,815,810 | 0.3 | 0.8 | 2.3 | 0.6 | 0.6 | 0.5 | 1.2 | 8.6 | 0.5 | 0.4 | 0.3 | 0.5 |
| Australia[3] | 26,177,413 | ID | ID | ID | ID | ID | ID | ID | ID | ID | ID | ID | ID |
| China, Hong Kong SAR | 7,488,865 | 2.5 | 2.5 | 2.1 | 2.1 | 2.5 | 0.1 | 0.2 | 0.1 | 0.1 | 0.0 | 0.0 | 0.0 |
| Singapore | 5,975,689 | ID | 1.3 | 1.5 | 1.0 | 1.6 | 1.4 | 1.3 | 1.8 | 0.3 | 0.1 | 0.2 | 0.1 |
| New Zealand | 5,185,288 | ID | ID | 1.0 | 0.5 | 1.1 | 0.4 | 0.3 | 1.9 | 4.8 | 1.4 | 2.3 | 8.9 |
| China, Macao SAR | 695,168 | 3.9 | 2.9 | 2.7 | 1.6 | 1.9 | 2.5 | 4.5 | 14.3 | 1.5 | 3.4 | 1.6 | 2.3 |
| Brunei Darussalam | 449,002 | 1.5 | 3.9 | 3.6 | 4.8 | 2.8 | 4.2 | 5.3 | 4.6 | 4.3 | 4.1 | 4.5 | 5.3 |
| Cambodia | 16,767,842 | 6.8 | 3.6 | 4.2 | 4.7 | 4.3 | 5.5 | 6.8 | 9.5 | 15.2 | 2.1 | 5.6 | 5.7 |
| Mongolia | 3,398,366 | 22.0 | 7.6 | 4.8 | 51.1 | 46.6 | 4.7 | 8.4 | 10.5 | 3.0 | 0.2 | 1.1 | 3.2 |
| China | 1,425,887,337 | 2.3 | 3.7 | 4.3 | 4.5 | 3.2 | 2.1 | 2.2 | 5.3 | 1.99 | 2.0 | 1.8 | 2.3 |
| Philippines | 115,559,009 | 2.1 | 3.3 | 4.5 | 1.4 | 1.4 | 2.0 | 1.0 | 1.8 | 1.0 | 0.6 | 1.6 | 1.9 |
| Viet Nam | 98,186,856 | 0.9 | 1.2 | 5.0 | 2.1 | 1.3 | 1.7 | 1.1 | 0.9 | 0.4 | 0.2 | 0.6 | 0.4 |
| Malaysia | 33,938,221 | 22.7 | 22.5 | 14.2 | 12.6 | 15.8 | 20.6 | 26.7 | 28.1 | 14.9 | 6.1 | 12.1 | 25.2 |
| Papua New Guinea | 10,142,619 | 0.6 | 1.3 | 24.7 | 1.2 | 0.6 | 0.5 | 0.8 | 1.0 | 1.3 | 0.1 | 0.4 | 1.5 |
| Lao People's Democratic Republic | 7,529,475 | 7.6 | 7.4 | 4.0 | 8.6 | 7.4 | 7.1 | 11.3 | 18.6 | 4.7 | 7.0 | 5.5 | 2.6 |
| Pacific island countries and areas[4] | 3,533,234 | 5.7 | 2.0 | 4.1 | 6.5 | 7.6 | 2.7 | 2.7 | 13.2 | 5.0 | 2.5 | 9.0 | 5.4 |
| Western Pacific Region | | 2.4 | 3.5 | 4.2 | 4.0 | 3.0 | 2.2 | 2.4 | 5.2 | 2.0 | 1.7 | 1.7 | 2.4 |

| Country / Area | Second level units with ≥ 2 discarded cases per 100,000 pop[1] ≥ 80% | | | | | | | | | | | |
|---|---|---|---|---|---|---|---|---|---|---|---|---|
| | 2012 | 2013 | 2014 | 2015 | 2016 | 2017 | 2018 | 2019 | 2020 | 2021 | 2022 | 2023 |
| Japan | 0.0% | 4.3% | 0.0% | 0.0% | 4.3% | 0.0% | 6.4% | 23.4% | 0.0% | 0.0% | 0.0% | 0.0% |
| Republic of Korea | 0.0% | 5.9% | 41.2% | 0.0% | 0.0% | 0.0% | 5.9% | 100.0% | 0.0% | 0.0% | 0.0% | 5.9% |
| Australia[3] | ID | ID | ID | ID | ID | ID | ID | ID | ID | ID | ID | ID |
| China, Hong Kong SAR | NA | NA | NA | NA | NA | NA | NA | NA | NA | NA | NA | NA |
| Singapore | NA | NA | NA | NA | NA | NA | NA | NA | NA | NA | NA | NA |
| New Zealand | ID | ID | ID | ID | ID | ID | ID | ID | 60.0% | 15.0% | 40.0% | 85.0% |
| China, Macao SAR | NA | NA | NA | NA | NA | NA | NA | NA | NA | NA | NA | NA |
| Brunei Darussalam | NA | NA | NA | NA | NA | NA | NA | NA | NA | NA | NA | NA |
| Cambodia | 62.5% | 45.8% | 83.3% | 91.7% | 72.0% | 80.0% | 84.0% | 96.0% | 100.0% | 24.0% | 64.0% | 84.0% |
| Mongolia | 31.8% | 36.4% | 31.8% | 81.8% | 95.5% | 13.6% | 50.0% | 50.0% | 22.7% | 4.5% | 4.5% | 45.5% |
| China | 71.0% | 64.5% | 71.0% | 83.9% | 77.4% | 64.5% | 64.5% | 77.4% | 32.3% | 0.0% | 35.5% | 74.2% |
| Philippines | 64.7% | 64.7% | 58.8% | 29.4% | 17.6% | 29.4% | 5.6% | 27.8% | 11.1% | 0.0% | 38.9% | 44.4% |
| Viet Nam | 12.5% | 21.9% | 40.6% | 15.6% | 22.2% | 49.2% | 22.2% | 14.3% | 6.3% | 1.6% | 11.1% | 9.5% |
| Malaysia | 93.8% | 100.0% | 93.8% | 87.5% | 93.8% | 93.8% | 93.8% | 93.8% | 87.5% | 62.5% | 87.5% | 87.5% |
| Papua New Guinea | 10.0% | 25.0% | 75.0% | 20.0% | 10.0% | 10.0% | 5.0% | 15.0% | 20.0% | 0.0% | 5.0% | 25.0% |
| Lao People's Democratic Republic | 64.7% | 58.8% | 58.8% | 88.2% | 70.6% | 64.7% | 88.2% | 100.0% | 61.1% | 5.6% | 50.0% | 55.6% |
| Pacific island countries and areas[4] | ID | ID | 21.7% | 8.7% | 13.0% | 13.0% | 5.0% | 10.0% | 5.0% | 5.0% | 10.0% | 10.0% |
| Western Pacific Region | 35.1% | 40.9% | 52.0% | 39.0% | 38.9% | 36.2% | 34.8% | 46.8% | 27.8% | 7.3% | 24.0% | 36.9% |

| Country / Area | Total Population (2023) | Suspected cases with adequate investigation ≥ 80% | | | | | | | | | | | |
|---|---|---|---|---|---|---|---|---|---|---|---|---|---|
| | | 2012 | 2013 | 2014 | 2015 | 2016 | 2017 | 2018 | 2019 | 2020 | 2021 | 2022 | 2023 |
| Japan | 123,951,692 | ID | ID | ID | ID | ID | ID | ID | ID | ID | ID | ID | ID |
| Republic of Korea | 51,815,810 | 84.0% | 63.7% | 95.6% | 68.8% | 92.1% | 71.2% | 78.1% | 87.2% | 61.5% | 92.9% | 65.8% | 95.8% |
| Australia[3] | 26,177,413 | ID | ID | ID | ID | ID | ID | ID | ID | ID | ID | ID | ID |
| China, Hong Kong SAR | 7,488,865 | 92.0% | 94.2% | 99.0% | 98.8% | 97.9% | 100.0% | 93.9% | 100.0% | 100.0% | 100.0% | 80.0% | 100.0% |
| Singapore | 5,975,689 | ID | 75.4% | 82.5% | 92.0% | 85.1% | 65.8% | 67.6% | 73.1% | 61.8% | 25.0% | 26.3% | 100.0% |
| New Zealand | 5,185,288 | ID | ID | ID | ID | ID | ID | ID | ID | ID | ID | ID | ID |
| China, Macao SAR | 695,168 | 95.7% | 95.0% | 100.0% | 100.0% | 100.0% | 83.3% | 78.1% | 99.2% | 100.0% | 91.3% | 100.0% | 100.0% |
| Brunei Darussalam | 449,002 | 71.4% | 100.0% | 93.8% | 100.0% | 100.0% | 100.0% | 100.0% | 100.0% | 94.7% | 100.0% | 100.0% | 100.0% |
| Cambodia | 16,767,842 | 56.1% | 68.5% | 68.9% | 80.5% | 88.3% | 81.9% | 83.2% | 91.3% | 93.2% | 96.3% | 90.3% | 93.4% |
| Mongolia | 3,398,366 | 64.2% | 100.0% | 100.0% | 7.7% | 8.0% | 88.3% | 98.1% | 94.4% | 100.0% | 100.0% | 97.4% | 100.0% |
| China | 1,425,887,337 | 99.0% | 99.4% | 91.0% | 95.0% | 97.1% | 97.8% | 97.7% | 96.8% | 100.0% | 98.8% | 98.5% | 99.3% |
| Philippines | 115,559,009 | 56.5% | 45.9% | 61.7% | 57.0% | 57.3% | 39.2% | 59.4% | 29.6% | 43.8% | 70.3% | 67.7% | 44.4% |
| Viet Nam | 98,186,856 | 44.3% | 73.3% | 41.0% | 39.8% | 55.6% | 45.2% | 68.2% | 25.2% | 30.1% | 38.9% | 0.0% | 3.3% |
| Malaysia | 33,938,221 | 74.4% | 82.3% | 73.2% | 72.8% | 79.6% | 83.8% | 92.1% | 84.8% | 88.0% | 80.3% | 87.6% | 86.2% |
| Papua New Guinea | 10,142,619 | 61.9% | 0.0% | 0.0% | 60.8% | 65.3% | 70.6% | 62.0% | 77.4% | 83.3% | 100.0% | 81.0% | 69.2% |
| Lao People's Democratic Republic | 7,529,475 | 49.3% | 36.1% | 74.5% | 85.1% | 98.6% | 82.2% | 89.1% | 64.3% | 68.6% | 46.7% | 3.7% | 18.6% |
| Pacific island countries and areas[4] | 3,533,234 | 0.0% | 0.0% | 0.0% | 39.7% | 90.1% | 86.6% | 45.7% | 0.9% | 42.7% | 45.7% | 98.8% | 92.9% |
| Western Pacific Region | | 88.8% | 92.1% | 22.7% | 78.3% | 70.9% | 88.2% | 84.0% | 66.1% | 87.5% | 94.8% | 91.1% | 88.0% |

| Country / Area | Suspected cases with adequate specimens for laboratory confirmation[2] ≥ 80% | | | | | | | | | | | |
|---|---|---|---|---|---|---|---|---|---|---|---|---|
| | 2012 | 2013 | 2014 | 2015 | 2016 | 2017 | 2018 | 2019 | 2020 | 2021 | 2022 | 2023 |
| Japan | ID | ID | ID | ID | ID | ID | ID | ID | ID | ID | ID | ID |
| Republic of Korea | 90.4% | 72.9% | 63.3% | 74.5% | 79.9% | 84.9% | 95.0% | 97.2% | 95.7% | 94.8% | 94.6% | 96.2% |
| Australia[3] | ID | ID | ID | ID | ID | ID | ID | ID | ID | ID | ID | ID |
| China, Hong Kong SAR | 97.3% | 91.1% | 92.8% | 97.7% | 99.5% | 100.0% | 97.0% | 90.8% | 85.7% | 100.0% | 80.0% | 83.3% |
| Singapore | ID | 18.1% | 25.3% | 19.0% | 51.8% | 67.1% | 78.4% | 73.1% | 76.5% | 25.0% | 42.1% | 68.8% |
| New Zealand | ID | ID | ID | ID | ID | ID | ID | ID | ID | ID | ID | ID |
| China, Macao SAR | 100.0% | 100.0% | 100.0% | 100.0% | 100.0% | 100.0% | 100.0% | 99.2% | 100.0% | 100.0% | 100.0% | 100.0% |
| Brunei Darussalam | 85.7% | 100.0% | 100.0% | 95.8% | 100.0% | 100.0% | 100.0% | 95.2% | 68.4% | 100.0% | 95.0% | 100.0% |
| Cambodia | 99.2% | 98.0% | 99.4% | 98.7% | 99.0% | 78.8% | 99.5% | 96.4% | 98.5% | 99.7% | 99.6% | 99.7% |
| Mongolia | 100.0% | 100.0% | 100.0% | 13.6% | 14.4% | 93.5% | 96.2% | 95.2% | 100.0% | 100.0% | 60.5% | 100.0% |
| China | 97.9% | 94.6% | 87.6% | 85.7% | 87.9% | 91.5% | 93.0% | 79.7% | 96.1% | 97.9% | 97.3% | 98.5% |
| Philippines | 79.5% | 62.9% | 83.6% | 69.7% | 70.2% | 59.1% | 52.7% | 38.6% | 49.8% | 72.8% | 72.2% | 45.4% |
| Viet Nam | 55.0% | 74.3% | 70.1% | 62.5% | 76.4% | 66.5% | 80.4% | 35.5% | 43.1% | 39.2% | 35.8% | 31.5% |
| Malaysia | 83.3% | 81.1% | 91.1% | 83.6% | 88.6% | 90.7% | 90.0% | 91.7% | 96.7% | 96.8% | 99.0% | 97.9% |
| Papua New Guinea | 81.0% | 76.3% | 63.5% | 91.1% | 89.8% | 84.3% | 91.3% | 88.2% | 94.7% | 87.5% | 87.3% | 74.0% |
| Lao People's Democratic Republic | 76.6% | 66.5% | 74.9% | 85.4% | 47.6% | 85.3% | 89.0% | 64.5% | 70.1% | 77.8% | 3.7% | 17.5% |
| Pacific island countries and areas[4] | ID | ID | 10.7% | 68.6% | 89.7% | 81.4% | 77.2% | 87.0% | 75.0% | 95.7% | 99.4% | 90.9% |
| Western Pacific Region | 93.1% | 90.1% | 83.5% | 73.7% | 67.7% | 87.8% | 81.9% | 62.5% | 87.2% | 95.4% | 92.9% | 90.3% |

countries or areas verified to have achieved or sustained elimination
countries or areas that lost the elimination status after being verified to have achieved elimination

Reached or surpassed target
Nearly reached target: 1.00–1.99 for non-measles suspected case rate: 10.1–25% for percent clinically confirmed cases; 60–79% for other indicators
Substantially below target
ID insufficient data
NA not applicable

[1] This indicator is not applicable for countries which have no second-level administrative units
[2] Adequate specimen defined as blood specimen collected within 28 days of rash onset or other specimen (throat swab, nasopharyngeal swab, cerebrospinal fluid, urine) collected within 5 days of rash onset: excludes epidemiologically-linked cases
[3] Reports only confirmed cases
[4] Surveillance performance indicators refer to all the Pacific island countries and areas as one epidemiological bloc; each country is considered as second level unit

**Scheme 5.** Performance of measles surveillance in the Western Pacific Region by country, 2012–2023. Source: [29,30].

The Republic of Korea, Hong Kong SAR (China), Macao SAR (China), Brunei Darussalam, Cambodia and Mongolia (countries or areas verified by RVC to have achieved measles elimination) and China, Malaysia, Papua New Guinea and the Pacific sub-region (countries or sub-region which have not yet achieved measles elimination) have improved or sustained high case investigation performance, measured by "suspected cases with adequate investigation" (>80%), and sample collection, as reflected by "suspected cases with adequate specimens for laboratory confirmation" (>80%), from 2018 to 2023.

### *3.5. Genotypes of Measles Virus Detected in the Western Pacific Region*

Genotype D9, which was considered endemic in Malaysia until the end of 2017 and detected frequently as imported by Japan, Australia, Hong Kong SAR (China) and China from 2013 to the middle of 2015 and by Singapore from 2013 to late 2017, has not been detected and reported in the region since January 2018 (Scheme 6).

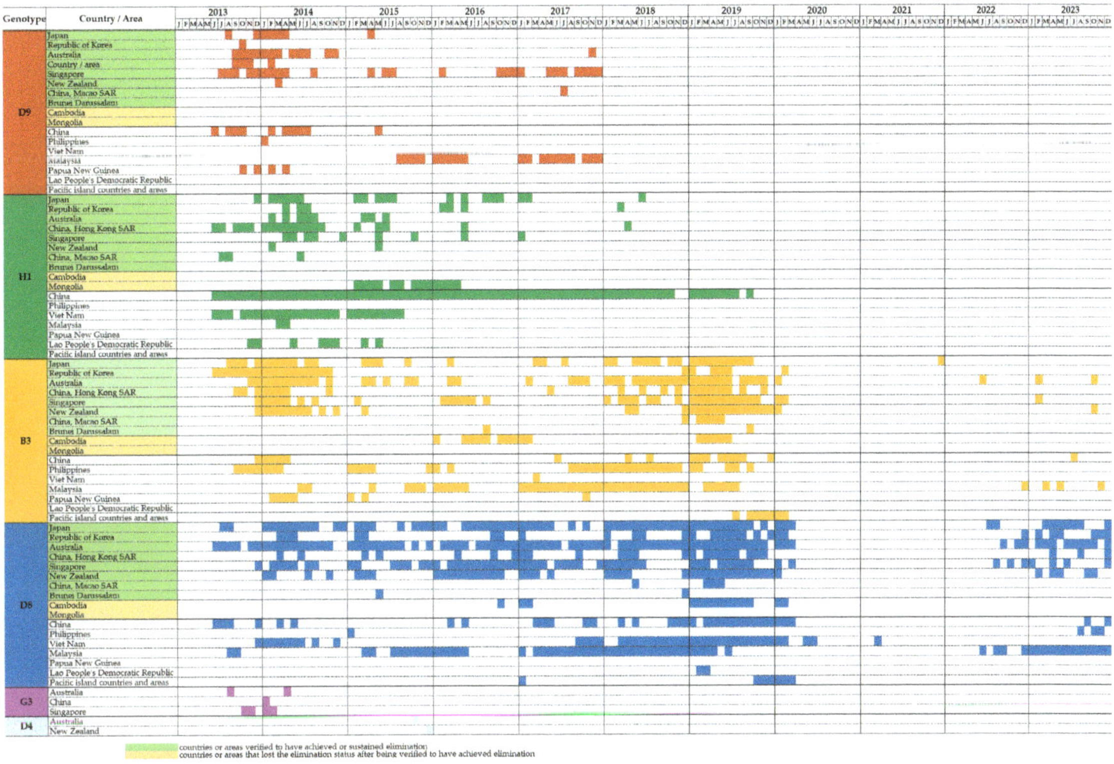


**Scheme 6.** Genotypes of measles virus detected in the Western Pacific Region by country, 2013–2023. Source: [30].

Genotype H1 has been the only endemic genotype detected in China since surveillance began in 1993 and was widely distributed throughout China from 1993 to 2010 [10,11]. It became endemic in Viet Nam in 2013–2015 and in Mongolia from 2015 to 2016 due to importation and was detected frequently as imported in Japan, the Republic of Korea, Australia, Hong Kong SAR (China), Macao SAR (China) and Lao PDR between 2013 and 2016. It has not been detected or reported in the WPR and globally since September 2019. Globally, the number of measles cases of genotype H1 declined from 2625 in 2016 to 333 in 2018 (87% decline), 28 in 2019 (99% decline) and 0 from 2020 onwards.

Genotype B3, which has been endemic in the Philippines since 2013 [14], continued to be detected as imported in all countries and areas of the region verified to have achieved measles elimination, except Mongolia, from 2013 to early 2020, particularly during the resurgences in the Philippines in 2013 to 2014 and in 2017 to 2019. Genotype B3 continued to be reported by Malaysia from 2022 to 2023 and was detected as imported in Australia, Singapore, New Zealand and China in 2023.

Genotype D8, which was considered endemic in Malaysia since 2015 and in Viet Nam in 2017–2020, continued to be detected as imported in all countries and areas of the region verified to have achieved measles elimination, except Mongolia, from 2013 to early 2020. Genotype D8 continued to be reported by Malaysia from 2022 to 2023 and as imported in several countries and areas of the region which were verified to have achieved measles elimination during this same period.

Since 2000, ten different measles virus genotypes have been detected in the WPR (B3, D3, D4, D5, D8, D9, D11, G3, H1 and H2). Currently only two genotypes, B3 and D8, continue to be detected and, although none of the remaining eight genotypes have been detected in the last four years, it is interesting to note that D5 "disappeared" in 2008 from China and Japan only to re-appear briefly in China in 2015, which has implications for when to consider a genotype as being finally eliminated.

### *3.6. Prevention of Endemic Measles Virus Transmission Resurgence*

The increased transmission of the genotype H1 measles virus was one of major causes of the regional resurgence of measles in the Western Pacific from 2013 to 2016 but has steadily declined in China from 2014 to 2019 and not been detected since September 2019 either by China or any other country or area in the region. This reflects China's commitment to achieve a very high two-dose routine MCV coverage in all sub-populations and for provinces to implement targeted annual SIAs in lower coverage areas. With the delayed nation-wide MCV-SIA conducted in the Philippines in 2020, the resurgence of the genotype B3 measles virus in 2018 to 2019 could not be prevented in the country and there was the international seeding of virus again. The endemic measles transmission of genotype D8 continues in Malaysia with cyclic resurgences in 2012, 2015–2018 and 2023 onwards, with specific sub-populations continuing to miss out on routine immunizations.

### *3.7. Prevention of Large-Scale Import-Related Measles Outbreaks*

During the 2018–2019 global measles resurgence, large-scale outbreaks were prevented after importation of measles cases in several countries in the WPR (e.g., Australia, Brunei Darussalam, Japan and the Republic of Korea). Hong Kong SAR (China), Macao SAR (China) and Singapore experienced import-related measles outbreaks, but their elimination status was maintained due to excellent outbreak response and existing high population immunity. New Zealand was able to maintain its elimination status despite experiencing a large-scale import-related measles outbreak from January 2019 to July 2020 [28] but remains under threat for resurgences due to falling immunization rates, particularly in the Māori and Pacific population.

Cambodia experienced multiple outbreaks in 2019 to 2020 due to measles virus importations from neighbouring countries with the increased endemic transmission of genotype D8 measles virus in 2018–2019. This resulted in the loss of measles elimination status for the country, which had been verified in 2015. Samoa and Tonga experienced large-scale import-related measles outbreaks from 2019 to 2020 [28] but the Tongan outbreak was rapidly extinguished due to prevailing high routine MCV coverage.

### *3.8. Interruption of Ongoing Transmission of Endemic Measles Virus*

The genotype D9 measles virus, which was endemic in Malaysia and reported as imported from some countries in the region where measles elimination was verified, has not been detected by either Malaysia or any other country since January 2018.

Genotype H1 measles virus, which was endemic in and reported by China until the third quarter of 2019 and detected as imported by countries verified to have achieved measles elimination, has not been detected by either China or any other country in the region since September 2019.

Mongolia and Cambodia, which the RVC concluded in 2016 and 2021, respectively, had re-established endemic measles virus transmission, and the Pacific sub-region, in which Samoa and Tonga experienced import-related large-scale measles outbreaks in 2019, have achieved and sustained very low measles incidence (<1 per one million population) for at least three years (since 2018 in Mongolia and since 2021 in Cambodia and the Pacific sub-region).

### 3.9. Rubella Elimination

Since the verification process for rubella elimination started in 2017, seven countries and areas in the WPR (the Republic of Korea, Australia, Hong Kong SAR (China), Singapore, New Zealand, Macao SAR (China) and Brunei Darussalam) have been verified to have achieved and sustained rubella elimination as of September 2023. Malaysia, Mongolia and the Pacific sub-region have established 2025 as their target year for rubella elimination. But several countries (e.g., Cambodia, China, Lao PDR, PNG, and the Philippines) are yet to establish an elimination target year.

In recent years, a higher proportion of rubella cases occurred among people > 14 years of age in the WPR. China experienced a resurgence of rubella virus transmission in 2018 to 2019, with most cases being individuals aged 15 to 25 years, reflecting immunity gaps among birth cohorts that were born prior to and around the time of rubella-containing vaccine introduction into the routine immunization schedule [33]. Japan had large outbreaks of rubella during 2012–2013 and 2018–2019 with most cases occurring among unvaccinated male adults, reflecting immunity gaps among the male birth cohorts from 1962 to 1979 that were historically not targeted for rubella-containing vaccine administration in routine immunization. A one-dose catch-up vaccination campaign was launched in 2019, targeting male birth cohorts [34]. The Philippines have consistently reported a high number of rubella cases over the past decade. There were large-scale rubella outbreaks in 2017, 2019 and 2020 and a significant proportion of rubella cases were reported among women of child-bearing age. The vaccination status for these groups was either undocumented or not vaccinated [35].

Several countries in the region, including China and the Philippines, have not yet established nation-wide CRS surveillance.

### 3.10. Expanding Laboratory Capacity in the Western Pacific Region

The measles and rubella laboratory network in the WPR has played a very significant role in its successes in eliminating these diseases. As other countries move towards elimination, this role will increase, particularly molecular detection and genotyping. During nation-wide measles resurgences in the Philippines, a single national laboratory for VPDs could not manage the huge increase in sample testing. To address this challenge, seven WHO accredited sub-national (referral) laboratories were established in the country. The establishment of more national VPD laboratories in countries of the Pacific Islands, which require in-country testing due to their remoteness, would greatly decrease the turnaround times inherent in the referral system. Six countries (Cook Islands, Kiribati, Solomon Islands, Tonga, Vanuatu and Western Samoa) have been identified for expansion and training is underway in their laboratories. Testing is intended to be operational by 2025.

The implementation of molecular detection methods is required in Cambodia, Lao PDR, Mongolia and Papua New Guinea. Therefore, Labshot 2030 was devised as a two-stage strategy: an assessment of priority countries (Cambodia, Fiji, Lao PDR, Malaysia, Mongolia, Papua New Guinea, Philippines and Viet Nam) and a road map drafted to integrate surveillance expertise and infrastructure leading to independent and sustainable laboratories within these countries. Reverse transcription polymerase chain reaction (RT-PCR) is important for detecting the measles or rubella viruses. However, it is possible to detect the vaccine strain (genotype A) post vaccination by this method, too. Epidemiological data are essential to suggest whether detection is vaccine-related, and confirmation is possible by vaccine-specific RT-PCR or genotyping. Once genotyping is established, it will provide faster results and more effective surveillance.

## 4. Conclusions

Notable progress towards measles and rubella elimination has been made in the WPR in the last 10 years, despite the region-wide measles resurgence in 2013–2016, the global measles resurgence in 2018–2019 and the COVID-19 pandemic in 2020–2023. This has provided empiric evidence that: (1) measles and rubella elimination are not only achievable but also sustainable even in countries with large populations (e.g., Japan and the Republic of Korea) under the pressure of multiple importations of measles virus from countries with endemic transmission or large-scale import-related outbreaks during region-wide and world-wide resurgences of measles virus transmission; (2) the interruption of endemic measles virus, including in one of the most populous countries in the world (China), appears feasible, as demonstrated through strong epidemiologic and virologic surveillance systems within the country and evidence throughout the WPR [36]; (3) the prevention of resurgence and large-scale import-related outbreaks is achieved where strong routine immunization programmes are maintained for extended periods (at least 10 years) with two doses of MRCV and high vaccination coverage (at least 90% for both with reliable coverage denominators), even in countries with large populations (e.g., China and Japan); and (4) many countries and areas in the WPR have established strong and resilient immunization programmes, including sensitive case-based surveillance systems with the strong support of public health laboratories across the region, that demonstrated sustained high routine immunization coverage during the COVID-19 pandemic.

This steady progress and considerable achievement have been made possible by the political commitments of the governments of the WHO's Member States and strong advocacy by the WHO's Regional Committee. The intensive sharing of lessons learned by countries' National Immunization Programmes during regular regional meetings organized by WHO has resulted in the translation of success across vast geographic regions and populations. Technical recommendations by regional immunization experts through the annual Technical Advisory Group (TAG) for Immunization and Vaccine-Preventable Diseases in the Western Pacific Region and the annual review and recommendations provided by the Regional Verification Commission for Measles and Rubella Elimination in the Western Pacific to each National or Sub-Regional Verification Committee for Measles and Rubella Elimination have been instrumental in bolstering these achievements. The proactive updating and active implementation of the regional and national operational targets and strategies for elimination with full consideration of country-specific situations and local disease epidemiology is indispensable for accelerating progress and sustaining gains at both national and regional levels.

Major challenges to achieving and sustaining measles and rubella elimination are: (1) the resurgence of virus transmission still occurring in many countries globally with the increased risk of virus importation into countries which have already achieved elimination or are approaching elimination; (2) weak routine immunization programmes (e.g., low vaccination coverage not yet reached >80%, target population underestimated or not included in the coverage denominator, etc.) in a few priority countries; (3) the delayed implementation of proactive and preventive supplementary immunization activities to fill residual or emerging immunity gaps before the accumulation of susceptibles that are found by imported virus; and (4) a growing proportion of adult populations susceptible to rubella infection and transmission in countries with large populations.

To overcome those challenges, a stronger global commitment to coordinating and synchronizing elimination efforts and progress across the world is essential. Countries should continue strengthening their health systems, particularly their immunization programmes. Not addressing, detecting and filling immunity gaps with the transmission of vaccine-preventable diseases among older age groups (i.e., adolescents and young adults) and high-risk groups with low vaccination coverage (e.g., ethnic minorities, migrants) will continue to threaten the achievement and maintenance of elimination.

**Author Contributions:** Conceptualization, Y.T.; methodology, Y.T. and S.K.A.; software, K.M.M.; validation, Y.T., S.K.A., R.E., C.-w.L., X.W., V.G. and D.N.D.; formal analysis, Y.T., K.M.M., S.K.A. and R.E.; investigation, Y.T., S.K.A., R.E., K.M.M. and D.N.D.; data curation, Y.T., K.M.M., S.K.A. and R.E.; writing—original draft preparation, Y.T. and S.K.A.; writing—review, Y.T., S.K.A., R.E., K.M.M., C.-w.L., X.W., V.G. and D.N.D.; writing—editing, Y.T., S.K.A., R.E., C.-w.L., X.W., V.G. and D.N.D.; visualization, Y.T., K.M.M., S.K.A. and R.E.; supervision, D.N.D. All authors have read and agreed to the published version of the manuscript.

**Funding:** This research received no external funding.

**Conflicts of Interest:** The authors declare no conflicts of interest.

## Abbreviations

The following abbreviations are used in this manuscript:

| | |
|---|---|
| CRS | Congenital Rubella Syndrome |
| MCV | Measles-Containing Vaccine |
| MMR | Measles–Mumps–Rubella (vaccine) |
| MR | Measles–Rubella (vaccine) |
| MRCV | Measles–Rubella-Containing Vaccine |
| MRCV-1 | Measles–Rubella-Containing Vaccine, First Dose |
| MRCV-2 | Measles–Rubella-Containing Vaccine, Second Dose |
| NIP | National Immunization Program |
| NVC | National Verification Committee |
| PICs | Pacific Island Countries and Areas |
| RC | Regional Committee |
| RT-PCR | Reverse Transcription–Polymerase Chain Reaction |
| RVC | Regional Verification Commission |
| SAR | Special Administrative Region |
| SIA | Supplementary Immunization Activities |
| SRVC | Sub-Regional Verification Committee |
| TAG | Technical Advisory Group |
| VPD | Vaccine-Preventable Disease |
| WHO | World Health Organization |
| WPR | Western Pacific Region |
| WUENIC | WHO and UNICEF estimates of national immunization coverage |

## References

1. Miller, M.A. Introducing a novel model to estimate national and global measles disease burden. *Int. J. Infect. Dis.* **2000**, *4*, 14–20. [CrossRef] [PubMed]
2. Stein, C.E.; Birmingham, M.; Kurian, M.; Duclos, P.; Strebel, P. The global burden of measles in the year 2000—A model that uses country-specific indicators. *J. Infect. Dis.* **2003**, *187*, 8–14. [CrossRef] [PubMed]
3. Vynnycky, E.; Adams, E.J.; Cutts, F.T.; Reef, S.E.; Navar, A.M.; Simons, E.; Yoshida, L.M.; Brown, D.W.J.; Jackson, C.; Strebel, P.M.; et al. Using seroprevalence and immunisation coverage data to estimate the global burden of Congenital Rubella Syndrome, 1996–2010: A systematic review. *PLoS ONE* **2016**, *11*, 1996–2010. [CrossRef] [PubMed]
4. World Health Organization Regional Office for the Western Pacific. Expanded Programme on Immunization: Measles and Hepatitis B (WPR/RC54.R3). In Proceedings of the Resolution of Regional Committee for the Western Pacific, Manila, Philippines, 8–12 September 2003. Available online: https://iris.who.int/bitstream/handle/10665/358519/WPR_RC054_Res03_2003_en.pdf (accessed on 1 March 2024).
5. World Health Organization Regional Office for the Western Pacific. Measles Elimination, Hepatitis B Control and Poliomyelitis Eradication (WPR/RC56.R8). In Proceedings of the Resolution of Regional Committee for the Western Pacific, Noumea, New Caledonia, 19–23 September 2005. Available online: https://iris.who.int/bitstream/handle/10665/358495/WPR_RC055_Res08_2005_en.pdf (accessed on 1 March 2024).
6. World Health Organization Regional Office for the Western Pacific. Vaccine Preventable Diseases: Measles Elimination, Hepatitis B Control, and Poliomyelitis Eradication (WPR/RC61.R7). In Proceedings of the Resolution of Regional Committee for the Western Pacific, Putrajaya, Malaysia, 11–15 October 2010. Available online: https://iris.who.int/bitstream/handle/10665/357311/WPR_RC061_Res07_2010_en.pdf (accessed on 1 March 2024).
7. Monthly Measles and Rubella Country Reports to WHO Submitted by 20 March 2024. Available online: https://www.who.int/europe/teams/vaccine-preventable-diseases-immunization/measles-and-rubella--regional-and-country-profiles (accessed on 1 March 2024).

8. World Health Organization Regional Office for the Western Pacific. Elimination of Measles and Acceleration of Rubella Control (WPR/RC63.R5). In Proceedings of the Resolution of Regional Committee for the Western Pacific, Hanoi, Vietnam, 24–28 September 2012. Available online: https://iris.who.int/bitstream/handle/10665/357259/WPR_RC063_Res05_2012_en.pdf (accessed on 1 March 2024).
9. World Health Organization Regional Office for the Western Pacific. Expanded Programme on Immunization (WPR/RC65.R5). In Proceedings of the Resolution of Regional Committee for the Western Pacific, Manila, Philippines, 13–17 October 2014. Available online: https://iris.who.int/bitstream/handle/10665/361132/WPR_RC065_Res05_2014_en.pdf?sequence=3 (accessed on 1 March 2024).
10. Zhang, Y.; Wang, H.; Xu, S.; Mao, N.; Zhu, Z.; Shi, J.; Huang, G.; Liu, C.; Bo, F.; Feng, D.; et al. Monitoring progress toward measles elimination by genetic diversity analysis of measles viruses in China 2009–2010. *Clin. Microbiol. Infect.* **2014**, *20*, 566–577. [CrossRef] [PubMed]
11. Wang, H.; Zhang, Y.; Mao, N.; Zhu, Z.; Cui, A.; Xu, S.; Song, J.; Chen, M.; Fang, X.; Li, C.; et al. Molecular characterization of measles viruses in China: Circulation dynamics of the endemic H1 genotype from 2011 to 2017. *PLoS ONE* **2019**, *14*, 1–13. [CrossRef] [PubMed]
12. Reyes, L. Sustained transmission of measles virus causing outbreaks in the Philippines, 2013–2018. *Int. J. Infect. Dis.* **2019**, *79*, 133. [CrossRef]
13. Centeno, R.; Fuji, N.; Okamoto, M.; Dapat, C.; Saito, M.; Tandoc, A.; Lupisan, S.; Oshitani, H. Genetic characterization of measles virus in the Philippines, 2008–2011 Infectious Diseases. *BMC Res. Notes* **2015**, *8*, 1–9. [CrossRef]
14. Takashima, Y.; Schluter, W.W.; Mariano, K.M.L.; Diorditsa, S.; Castro, M.D.Q.; Ou, A.C. Progress towards measles elimination, Philippines, 1998–2014. *Morb. Mortal. Wkly. Rep.* **2015**, *90*, 149–159.
15. MacIntyre, C.R.; Karki, S.; Sheikh, M.; Zwar, N.; Heywood, A.E. The role of travel in measles outbreaks in Australia—An enhanced surveillance study. *Vaccine* **2016**, *34*, 4386–4391. [CrossRef] [PubMed]
16. Takahashi, T.; Arima, Y.; Kinoshita, H.; Kanou, K.; Saitoh, T.; Sunagawa, T.; Ito, H.; Kanayama, A.; Tabuchi, A.; Nakashima, K.; et al. Ongoing increase in measles cases following importations, Japan, March 2014: Times of challenge and opportunity. *West. Pac. Surveill. Response J. WPSAR* **2014**, *5*, 31–33. [CrossRef] [PubMed]
17. Yang, T.U.; Kim, J.W.; Eom, H.E.; Oh, H.K.; Kim, E.S.; Kang, H.J.; Nam, J.G.; Kim, K.S.; Kim, S.S.; Lee, C.K.; et al. Resurgence of measles in a country of elimination: Interim assessment and current control measures in the Republic of Korea in early 2014. *Int. J. Infect. Dis.* **2015**, *33*, e12–e14. [CrossRef] [PubMed]
18. Kamac, K.; Paterson, B.; Flint, J. Lessons learnt from a measles outbreak in Madang Province, Papua New Guinea, June 2014–March 2015. *West. Pac. Surveill. Response J. WPSAR* **2017**, *8*, 1–5. [CrossRef] [PubMed]
19. World Health Organization. *Health Alert: Suspected Measles Outbreak: Honiara, Solomon Islands, 23 July 2014*; Reliefweb: Geneva, Switzerland, 2014. Available online: http://reliefweb.int/report/solomon-islands/health-alert-suspected-measles-outbreak-honiara-solomon-islands-23-july-2014 (accessed on 1 March 2024).
20. Hagan, J.E.; Takashima, Y.; Sarankhuu, A.; Dashpagma, O.; Jantsansengee, B.; Pastore, R.; Nyamaa, G.; Yadamsuren, B.; Mulders, M.N.; Wannemuehler, K.A.; et al. Risk factors for measles virus infection among adults during a large outbreak in postelimination era in Mongolia, 2015. *J. Infect. Dis.* **2017**, *216*, 1187–1195. [CrossRef] [PubMed]
21. World Health Organization Regional Office for the Western Pacific. *Meeting Report: Sixth Annual Meeting of the Regional Verification Commission for Measles Elimination in the Western Pacific, 12–15 September 2017*; World Health Organization: Manila, Philippines, 2017. Available online: https://iris.who.int/bitstream/handle/10665/259629/RS-2017-GE-49-CHN-eng.pdf?sequence=1 (accessed on 1 March 2024).
22. World Health Organization Regional Office for the Western Pacific. *Meeting Report: 24th Meeting of the Technical Advisory Group on Immunization and Vaccine-Preventable Diseases in the Western Pacific Region, 9–12 June 2015*; World Health Organization: Manila, Philippines, 2015. Available online: https://iris.who.int/bitstream/handle/10665/208792/RS_2015_GE_16_PHL_eng.pdf?sequence=1 (accessed on 1 March 2024).
23. World Health Organization Regional Office for the Western Pacific. Measles and Rubella Elimination (WPR/RC68.R1). In Proceedings of the Resolution of Regional Committee for the Western Pacific, Brisbane, Australia, 9–13 October 2017. Available online: https://iris.who.int/bitstream/handle/10665/361628/WPR-RC068-Res01-2017-en.pdf (accessed on 1 March 2024).
24. World Health Organization Regional Office for the Western Pacific. *Regional Strategy and Plan of Action for Measles and Rubella Elimination in the Western Pacific*; World Health Organization: Manila, Philippines, 2018; ISBN 9789290618515. Available online: https://iris.who.int/bitstream/handle/10665/275089/9789290618515-eng.pdf?sequence=1 (accessed on 1 March 2024).
25. World Health Organization Regional Office for the Western Pacific. *Guidelines on Verification of Measles and Rubella Elimination in the Western Pacific Region*, 2nd ed.; World Health Organization: Manila, Philippines, 2019; ISBN 9789290616290. Available online: https://iris.who.int/bitstream/handle/10665/331139/9789290618607-eng.pdf?sequence=1 (accessed on 1 March 2024).
26. Mahase, E. Measles cases rise 300% globally in first few months of 2019. *BMJ* **2019**, *365*, l1810. [CrossRef] [PubMed]
27. Durrheim, D.N.; Crowcroft, N.S.; Blumberg, L.H. Is the global measles resurgence a public health emergency of international concern? *Int. J. Infect. Dis.* **2019**, *83*, 95–97. [CrossRef] [PubMed]
28. Craig, A.T.; Heywood, A.E.; Worth, H. Measles epidemic in Samoa and other Pacific islands. *Lancet Infect. Dis.* **2020**, *20*, 273–275. [CrossRef] [PubMed]

29. United Nations; Department of Economic and Social Affairs. Population Division. In *World Population Prospects 2022*, Online ed.; United Nations: New York, NY, USA, 2022.
30. Measles-Rubella Bulletin, Western Pacific Region World Health Organization. Available online: https://iris.who.int/handle/10665/375987 (accessed on 1 March 2024).
31. WHO Immunization Data Portal. Available online: https://immunizationdata.who.int (accessed on 1 March 2024).
32. World Health Organization Regional Office for the Western Pacific. *Meeting Report: Fifth Annual Meeting of the Regional Verification Commission for Measles Elimination in the Western Pacific, 20–23 September 2016*; World Health Organization: Manila, Philippines, 2016. Available online: https://iris.who.int/bitstream/handle/10665/252544/RS-2016-GE-25-AUS-eng.pdf?sequence=1&isAllowed=y (accessed on 1 March 2024).
33. World Health Organization Regional Office for the Western Pacific. *Meeting Report: 32nd Meeting of the Technical Advisory Group on Immunization and Vaccine-Preventable Diseases in the Western Pacific Region, 20–23 June 2023*; World Health Organization: Manila, Philippines, 2023. Available online: https://iris.who.int/bitstream/handle/10665/372862/RS-2023-GE-15-PHL-hybrid-eng.pdf?sequence=1 (accessed on 1 March 2024).
34. Ujiie, M. Rubella Resurgence in Japan 2018–2019. *J. Travel Med.* **2019**, *26*, 8129. [CrossRef] [PubMed]
35. World Health Organization Regional Office for the Western Pacific. *Meeting Report: 31st Meeting of the Technical Advisory Group on Immunization and Vaccine-Preventable Diseases in the Western Pacific Region, 21–24 June 2022*; World Health Organization: Manila, Philippines, 2023. Available online: https://iris.who.int/bitstream/handle/10665/365637/RS-2022-GE-09-PHL-eng.pdf?sequence=1 (accessed on 1 March 2024).
36. Durrheim, D.N.; Xu, A.; Baker, M.G.; Hsu, L.Y.; Takashima, Y. China has the momentum to eliminate measles. *Lancet Reg. Health West. Pac.* **2023**, *30*, 1–3. [CrossRef]

vaccines

MDPI

*Article*

# Assessment of Simplified Surveillance for Congenital Rubella Syndrome in Sudan, 2014–2017

**Omayma Abdalla [1], Nada Ahmed [1], Hanan Abdo El-Hag Mukhtar [2], Susan Reef [3], Jose Hagan [3] and Gavin Grant [3,*]**

1 Expanded Program for Immunization, Sudan Ministry of Health, Khartoum P.O. Box 303, Sudan; omeimah6@gmail.com (O.A.); nadajafar@gmail.com (N.A.)
2 Sudan Country Office, World Health Organization, Khartoum P.O. Box 303, Sudan; abdoh@who.int
3 Global Immunization Division, United States Centers for Disease Control and Prevention, Atlanta, GA 30329, USA; susanreef4@gmail.com (S.R.)
* Correspondence: gbgrant@cdc.gov

**Abstract:** Background/Objectives: Congenital rubella syndrome (CRS) is a constellation of serious multi-organ birth defects following rubella virus infection during early pregnancy. Countries in which rubella vaccination has not yet been introduced can have a high burden of this disease. Data on CRS burden and epidemiology are needed to guide the introduction of a rubella vaccine and monitor progress for rubella elimination, but the multi-system nature of CRS manifestations and required specialized testing creates a challenge for conducting CRS surveillance in developing settings such as Sudan. To enhance data quality, we designed and tested a simplified approach for CRS surveillance in Sudan. Methods: Seven CRS surveillance sentinel sites were set up at general pediatric, eye, and cardiology hospitals in Sudan, using standard definitions for reporting and classifying infants with CRS clinical manifestations. Between 2014 and 2017, we evaluated the system using WHO CRS surveillance monitoring indicators, comparing simplified approaches against a comprehensive one. The simplified approaches included (1) an ophthalmic-focused approach; (2) a heart-focused approach; and (3) a cataract-only approach. Results: Surveillance identified 179 infants with suspected CRS via the comprehensive approach, with 25 infants classified as laboratory-confirmed and 6 as clinically compatible. Surveillance sensitivity was highest for the simplified ophthalmic approach, while cataract-based surveillance had the highest proportion of confirmed cases. Conclusions: Simplified CRS surveillance, particularly focusing on detecting cataracts, can significantly contribute to monitoring the impact of rubella vaccine introduction. It could serve as an initial step towards comprehensive CRS surveillance, providing robust evidence to support rubella and CRS elimination efforts.

**Keywords:** surveillance; congenital rubella syndrome (CRS); rubella vaccine introduction; rubella surveillance; congenital birth defects; surveillance trends

## 1. Introduction

Congenital rubella syndrome (CRS) results from a woman acquiring rubella infection during pregnancy, especially when the infection occurs during early pregnancy. As a result of rubella virus infection interrupting fetal development in utero, infants with CRS are born with one or more manifestations that may include congenital cataracts, glaucoma, hearing impairment, cardiac malformations, or developmental delay, each potentially causing life-long disabilities. The disability burden due to CRS is greatest in countries where the rubella vaccine has not yet been introduced. In 2010, the global burden of CRS was estimated at 105,000 CRS cases; in 2019, after 44 additional countries had introduced the rubella-containing vaccine (RCV), this burden decreased to 32,000 [1]. Further reductions in the global CRS burden can be achieved with the introduction of rubella vaccines into the remaining countries, reducing rubella transmission and the incidence of CRS.

By 2023, 175 countries had introduced the RCV. Five of the six World Health Organization (WHO) regions have established rubella and CRS elimination goals. The Eastern Mediterranean Region, of which Sudan is a member-state, is the only region yet to establish a rubella/CRS elimination goal. As of 2023, Sudan had not yet introduced RCV, which would be the first step towards rubella elimination.

Sudan has been collecting case-based rubella data through the measles surveillance system since 2006. The system has demonstrated endemic rubella, including outbreaks of rubella reported in 2014 in the Khartoum, Gezira, and Kasalla states [2]. In addition, previous studies have documented a large rubella immunity gap in Sudanese women of childbearing age in some areas [3,4]. The first study to confirm CRS cases collected clinical specimens in 2005 and 2006 from 31 infants suspected of having CRS from six hospitals in Khartoum. Among these, 11 were laboratory-confirmed with CRS, and rubella viral sequencing identified three genotypes of rubella virus (1E, 2B, and 1G) co-circulating in Sudan [5]. Subsequently, several studies have documented the occurrence of CRS in this country [3,6]. However, no CRS surveillance system has been established in Sudan.

Improving surveillance to better define the epidemiology of CRS in this country can improve the data available to assist decision-makers and program managers on how to prioritize RCV introduction, monitor the impact of its introduction, and, ultimately, assess progress to elimination. CRS surveillance is challenging to implement due to CRS's broad spectrum of clinical manifestations, requiring the involvement of a wide range of clinics at surveillance sites to maximize sensitivity. These include general pediatric clinics and sub-specialty neurological, ophthalmology, otolaryngology, and cardiology clinics. Global standards for CRS surveillance [7] recommend the use of a sentinel site surveillance system to optimize the efficiency of case identification. With the challenges of implementing CRS surveillance, there is a pressing need for alternative approaches in low-resource settings, focusing on the optimal type of sentinel sites and the suspected case definition used to identify cases for notification.

A comprehensive retrospective study in Morocco suggested that congenital cataract surveillance was the most efficient case-finding strategy for CRS [8]. Of the common CRS manifestations, cataracts are among the most visible external manifestations and can be easily detectable by mothers or other community members. Infants with cataracts are, therefore, more likely to be presented for medical care early in life, which presents an opportunity for confirming CRS cases. However, reviews of prospective studies showed only a 16–25% incidence of congenital cataracts in infants with prospectively identified CRS [9,10]. The percentage of all childhood cataracts due to rubella varies depending upon the setting and rates of other infectious and noninfectious etiologies (e.g., genetic causes) [11].

Assessing alternative approaches to CRS surveillance, including simplified suspected case definitions, may improve surveillance quality by focusing on surveillance efforts. In the appropriate setting, a simplified case-based surveillance system where there is the ascertainment of infants with a focused set of clinical CRS manifestations rather than a broad range of manifestations may achieve the goals of CRS surveillance while maximizing sustainability in the country [4]. With cataracts being a possible manifestation that can increase the identification of CRS cases, a suspected case definition focused on congenital cataracts may be a useful approach to simplify the congenital rubella surveillance system. This is further facilitated by potential cataract surgery that often requires pre-operative evaluations that include a detailed cardiac exam. No analysis has been carried out to assess the feasibility and utility of a simplified CRS surveillance system to provide the data needed for decision-makers and program managers.

In Sudan, a CRS surveillance system with seven reporting sites was established, including general pediatrics hospitals, eye hospitals, and a cardiology hospital. We utilized this system to evaluate whether a focused CRS surveillance approach detecting a limited range of manifestations (e.g., ophthalmological or cardiac manifestations) or a focused clinical manifestation of CRS (cataracts) could be beneficial. We assessed this CRS surveillance approach according to the WHO CRS surveillance monitoring criteria and evaluated the performance of the system with three surveillance approaches: (1) simplified site surveillance for eye hospital-based surveillance (simplified-ophthalmic surveillance); (2) simplified site surveillance for heart hospital-based surveillance (simplified-cardiac surveillance); or (3) simplified-cataract-only surveillance for infants diagnosed with cataracts only (simplified-cataract surveillance).

## 2. Materials and Methods

### 2.1. CRS Surveillance System

Sites for the surveillance of CRS were established in seven hospitals in the Khartoum and Gezeira states. At each site, health care providers from relevant clinics were trained to detect and notify surveillance officers of suspected CRS cases for further investigation, with emphasis on the identification of cataracts. Relevant clinics included specialty clinics in cardiology, otolaryngology, ophthalmology, infectious diseases, pediatrics, and neonatology, though not all clinics existed at all sites. Sites themselves had wide, poorly defined catchment areas with cases presented from within two states (that contained 26% of the national population), though one site had referrals from throughout the country.

Infants who met the suspected case definition for CRS were enrolled between 15 February 2014 and 6 June 2017. The suspected case definition for CRS was any infant (less than 1 year of age) with any of the following: (1) ocular manifestations of CRS (e.g., cataract, pigmentary retinopathy or glaucoma), (2) congenital heart disease, (3) suspected hearing impairment, (4) suspected congenital TORCH infection (including toxoplasmosis or other infections (syphilis, varicella, parvovirus B19), rubella, cytomegalovirus, herpes virus), (5) purpura (another visible defect), or (6) clinician suspicion (or confirmation) of rubella infection in the mother during pregnancy.

After a surveillance officer was notified of a suspected CRS case, a case investigation form was completed, and appropriate specimens for rubella testing were collected. Case investigation forms collected data on maternal demographics, child demographics, pregnancy history, infant clinical history, and infant vaccination; clinical history included additional work-up for manifestations associated with CRS. Appropriate specimens included a serum specimen for rubella IgM and IgG testing and a throat swab and urine specimen for reverse-transcription–polymerase chain reaction (RT-PCR) testing. Ophthalmologists were requested to aspirate fluid from lenses removed during cataract surgery for rubella virus testing by RT-PCR whenever possible. Specimens were sent to the national laboratory for testing. Suspected case definition and final case classifications were adapted from the WHO case definitions (Table 1), with the final classification based upon laboratory results and a clinical case definition for cases with inadequate laboratory testing.

### 2.2. Data Analysis

The demographic data of the cases were described by site, sex, year of birth, age at presentation, place of delivery, and clinical presentation. Comparisons of factors between surveillance site and case classification were performed using the chi-square test; surveillance quality indicators for CRS [12] were calculated and compared across these subsets, and continuous variables were assessed by the Kruskal–Wallis test. These subsets evaluated the different approaches to surveillance, comparing comprehensive surveillance (all surveillance sites) with simplified surveillance approaches: simplified-site surveillance (i.e., simplified-ophthalmic surveillance and simplified-cardiac surveillance) and simplified-cataract surveillance by presenting manifestations. As sentinel sites do not have pre-defined catchment areas [13], the denominator used live births calculated based on national estimates for 2018 [14].

**Table 1.** Definitions and criteria used to classify congenital rubella syndrome (CRS) cases.

| Final Case Classification | Definition |
| --- | --- |
| Laboratory-confirmed CRS | A suspected case [1] with one or more Group A symptoms and laboratory confirmation. |
| Clinically compatible CRS | A suspected case [1] with either (1) two or more Group A symptoms, or (2) one Group A and one or more Group B symptoms and inadequate laboratory testing. |
| Discarded case | A suspected case [1] with adequate laboratory testing and no laboratory confirmation, or a case that does not meet the clinically compatible case definition. |
| Congenital rubella infection | A suspected case [1] with no Group A symptoms and laboratory confirmation. |
| Group A symptoms: congenital cataracts, congenital glaucoma, congenital heart disease, hearing impairment, or pigmentary retinopathy. Group B symptoms: purpura, splenomegaly, microcephaly, developmental delay, meningoencephalitis, radiolucent bone disease, and jaundice that begins within 24 h after birth. | |
| Adequate laboratory testing: a single IgM specimen result for <6 months of age, or two sequential IgG test results (at least 2 weeks apart) for children 6 m–<12 m of age. Laboratory confirmation: occurs when an infant has (1) a positive rubella IgM, (2) positive RT-PCR test <12 months of age (no vaccination history), and/or (3) two sequential specimens with stable or increasing IgG levels. | |

[1] The suspected case definition used to ascertain cases was an infant with one or more of the following conditions: cataracts, glaucoma, pigmentary retinopathy, suspected hearing impairment, congenital heart disease, purpura, suspected congenital infection, and suspected or confirmed rubella infection of the mother during pregnancy.

### 2.3. Trend Analysis

To assess the complementarity of surveillance for rubella by undertaking surveillance for CRS, we compared trends in rubella cases to trends of the detected CRS cases. Surveillance for rubella disease in Sudan was conducted through the measles surveillance system, which categorizes acute fever and rash cases as measles, rubella, or non-measles, and non-rubella (discarded) through the testing of sera detected in individuals with a fever, rash, and one or more of three symptoms (cough, coryza, conjunctivitis) using standard protocols (WHO, 2006). Because CRS is a result of rubella infection in a woman during early pregnancy, a well-functioning CRS system should detect trends in CRS that follow trends in rubella corresponding to the remaining gestation time from maternal infection to infant birth. We used cross-correlation to evaluate whether the CRS surveillance detected epidemiological trends that were reflective of the underlying rubella epidemiology in Sudan, specifically assessing the associated lag between rubella and CRS incidence in time series by describing the correlation accounting for the time delay from maternal infection to the onset of CRS (i.e., month of birth). This signal analysis is used to infer a relation between one time series and another; assuming that the specific rubella epidemiology among women of childbearing age is similar to the overall national trends, we would expect a positive cross-correlation between CRS cases and rubella cases, with a time lag corresponding to the remaining gestational time from maternal infection to the birth of the child. All statistical analyses were completed with R 3.2.2 (Vienna, Austria).

## 3. Results

The surveillance sites consisted of three general pediatrics hospitals, three eye hospitals, and one cardiology hospital, with sites including one or more different clinics or wards. Staff at all sites were trained and implemented the standard (comprehensive) protocol for CRS surveillance, with an emphasis on cataract manifestations.

### 3.1. Suspected Cases and Reporting

From 15 February 2014, to 6 June 2017, 179 eligible cases of suspected CRS were detected and notified, and 6 cases were notified beyond one year of age that were previously excluded. Of the total, 31 cases (17%) were reported by cardiology hospitals, 133 (74%)

by eye hospitals, and 15 (8%) by pediatric hospitals (Table 2). A single eye hospital was responsible for 98 (55%) notifications.

**Table 2.** Demographics of suspected cases detected by type of site, including heart, eye, or pediatric hospitals. Associated *p*-values use the Chi-square test of independence for proportions between heart, eye, and pediatric hospitals and the Kruskal–Wallis test for medians.

| | Total/ Comprehensive $n = 179$ | Heart Hospitals $n = 31$ | Eye Hospitals $n = 133$ | Pediatric Hospitals $n = 15$ | Test Statistic |
|---|---|---|---|---|---|
| Age at notification, median days (IQR) | 140 (86, 212) | 155 (87, 236) | 154 (96, 214) | 9 (5, 16.5) | $p < 0.001$ |
| Male Sex, *n* (%) | 94 (53%) | 14 (45%) | 70 (53%) | 10 (67%) | $p = 0.391$ |
| Place of delivery, *n* (%) | | | | | |
| Health facility | 90 (51%) | 20 (67%) | 59 (45%) | 11 (73%) | |
| Home | 81 (46%) | 8 (27%) | 70 (53%) | 3 (20%) | $p = 0.0043$ |
| Not reported | 5 (3%) | 2 (7%) | 2 (2%) | 1 (7%) | |
| Eye findings, *n* (%) | 136 (77%) | 7 (23%) | 127 (97%) | 2 (13%) | $p < 0.0001$ |
| Hearing impairment, *n* (%) | 1 (1%) | 0 (0%) | 0 (0%) | 1 (7%) | $p < 0.085$ |
| Congenital heart disease, *n* (%) | 47 (27%) | 30 (97%) | 11 (8%) | 6 (40%) | $p < 0.001$ |

Overall, infants meeting the suspected case definition were notified at a median age of 140 days (IQR: 86, 212). Age at reporting differed by site as the cardiology hospitals reported a median of 155 days of age (IQR: 87, 236), while pediatric hospitals reported a median of 9 days of age (IQR: 5, 16.5). Place of birth (home or health facility) varied significantly between sites ($p = 0.0043$), including home births being more common among those presenting to eye hospitals, followed by heart hospitals (53% vs. 27%, $p = 0.0043$) (Table 2).

Of the 179 suspected cases, 168 had at least one "Group A" clinical manifestation (Table 3) compatible with CRS, 136 (77%) had at least one eye finding, 47 (27%) had at least one heart finding, and one suspected case (1%) had hearing impairment, while eleven suspected cases did not have any Group A findings. Of the 136 cases with eye findings, 79 (44%) had cataracts, 57 (32%) had glaucoma, and 4 (10%) had pigmentary retinopathy. Among the 47 suspected CRS cases with cardiac manifestations, 30 cases (64%) had patent ductus arteriosus (PDA), 6 had ventricular septal defect (VSD) (13%), and 4 had peripheral pulmonary stenosis (PPS) (9%).

The final classification of the 179 cases was 25 laboratory-confirmed, 6 clinically compatible, and 148 discarded cases (Table 3). Of the seven suspected cases that died, three were lab-confirmed cases, and four were discarded cases. The age of reporting was similar between the final classifications, confirmed, and discarded cases (median 155 vs. 129 days, $p = 0.07$); reporting by sex, 53% were female ($p = 0.13$). None of the 57 suspected cases with glaucoma were laboratory-confirmed as CRS cases (two were clinically compatible), while all four pigmentary retinopathy cases were discarded. A clinical description of a subset of the cases is reported elsewhere [15].

### 3.2. System Performance

We assessed the performance of the different surveillance approaches using the standard surveillance indicators (Table 4), comparing comprehensive surveillance (all cases detected by the entire surveillance system), simplified-site surveillance from simplified-ophthalmic or simplified-cardiac site surveillance, or simplified-cataract surveillance. Comprehensive surveillance from all seven reporting sites had the highest sensitivity (1.32 per 10,000 live births nationwide), with surveillance from eye hospitals (0.98 per $10^4$ live births) and surveillance for cataracts alone (0.58 suspected cases per $10^4$ live births) having the highest sensitivity out of the simplified approaches. The system with the highest rate of case confirmation per suspected case was simplified-cataract surveillance with 24% (19 of 79 cases). Detecting cases early, within the first 3 months of life, was greatest with comprehensive surveillance (23%, 47 of 179 suspected cases). Serologic specimens were collected from 95% or more of cases at all surveillance approaches; simplified-cataract surveillance had the highest collection of virological specimens (61%).

**Table 3.** Demographics of cases by final classification, subdividing the total confirmed cases by those that were confirmed with laboratory results and those that were clinically compatible.

| | Suspected *n* = 179 | All Confirmed *n* = 31 | Lab-Confirmed *n* = 25 | Clinically Compatible *n* = 6 | Discarded *n* = 148 |
|---|---|---|---|---|---|
| Days of age at reporting Median (IQR) | 140 (87–216) | 154 (88–234) | 145 (64–218) | 233 (174–263) | 129 (86–198) |
| Male sex (*n*, %) | 94 (53%) | 12 (39%) | 11 (44%) | 1 (17%) | 82 (55%) |
| Eye findings (*n*, %) | 136 (77%) | 24 (77%) | 19 (76%) | 5 (83%) | 102 (77%) |
| Cataracts | 79 (44%) | 22 (71%) | 19 (76%) | 3 (50%) | 58 (38%) |
| Glaucoma | 57 (32%) | 2 (6%) | 0 (0%) | 2 (33%) | 55 (36%) |
| Pigmentary retinopathy | 4 (2%) | 0 (0%) | 0 (0%) | 0 (0%) | 4 (2%) |
| Hearing Impairment (*n*, %) | 1 (1%) | 0 (0%) | 0 (0%) | 0 (0%) | 1 (1%) |
| Heart findings | 47 (27%) | 19 (61%) | 13 (52%) | 6 (100%) | 28 (19%) |
| Patent ductus arteriosus | 30 (17%) | 14 (45%) | 10 (40%) | 4 (67%) | 16 (11%) |
| Primary pulmonary stenosis | 4 (2%) | 1 (3%) | 1 (4%) | 0 (0%) | 3 (2%) |
| Ventral septal defect | 6 (3%) | 1 (3%) | 1 (4%) | 0 (0%) | 5 (3%) |
| Other defect | 2 (1%) | 0 (0%) | 0 (0%) | 0 (0%) | 2 (1%) |
| Clinical criteria reported | | | | | |
| 2 "A" | 18 (10%) | 13 (43%) | 8(32%) | 5 (83%) | 5 (3%) |
| 1 "A" and ≥1 "B" | 10 (6%) | 3 (10%) | 2 (8%) | 1 (17%) | 7 (5%) |
| 1 "A" and 0 "B" | 137 (78%) | 13 (43%) | 13 (54%) | 0 (0%) | 124 (85%) |
| None of the above | 11 (6%) | 1 (3%) | 1 (4%) | 0 (0%) | 10 (7%) |
| Reporting site | | | | | |
| Cardiology hospital | 31 (17%) | 8 (26%) | 5 (20%) | 3 (50%) | 23 (16%) |
| Eye hospital | 133 (74%) | 19 (61%) | 16 (64%) | 3 (50%) | 114 (77%) |
| Pediatric hospital | 15 (8%) | 4 (13%) | 4 (16%) | 0 (0%) | 11 (7%) |

**Table 4.** Surveillance for congenital rubella syndrome (CRS) indicators comparing the indicators based upon the scope of the surveillance system implemented, from comprehensive assessments to surveillance simplified by site and simplified for cataracts as a major case definition. For each indicator, the box with the most favorable indicator is colored green, and the least favorable is colored gray.

| Type of CRS Surveillance | Comprehensive | Simplified Site | | Simplified Manifestation |
|---|---|---|---|---|
| Indicator | All cases (*n* = 179) | Simplified-cardiac surveillance (*n* = 31) | Simplified-ophthalmic surveillance (*n* = 132) | Simplified-cataract surveillance (*n* = 79) |
| Number of reporting sites/sentinel sites | 7 | 1 | 3 | 5 |
| Sensitivity—national annual rate of suspected CRS cases. Target ≥ 1 per 10,000 live births | 1.32 | 0.23 | 0.98 | 0.58 |
| Case confirmation rate (% efficiency, confirmed cases) | 14% (*n* = 25) | 16% (*n* = 5) | 12% (*n* = 16) | 24% (*n* = 19) |
| Confirmed CRS cases detected within 3 months of birth (%, confirmed cases) | 23% (*n* = 47) | 23% (*n* = 8) | 16% (*n* = 25) | 13% (*n* = 14) |
| Suspected case with adequate blood specimens for serology testing (%, cases) | 95% (*n* = 170) | 87% (*n* = 27) | 96% (*n* = 128) | 95% (*n* = 75) |
| Proportion of serological samples from suspected cases received within 5 days of collection | 95% (*n* = 157) | 96% (*n* = 27) | 95% (*n* = 116) | 96% (*n* = 67) |
| The proportion of suspected cases with an adequate virological specimen | 44% (*n* = 79) | 45% (*n* = 14) | 42% (*n* = 56) | 61% (*n* = 48) |

### 3.3. Trend Analysis

Validating the complementarity of the trend of rubella cases detected through the measles surveillance system, the number of lab-confirmed rubella cases was compared to lab-confirmed CRS cases by month, and the relationship lags in the cross-correlation (Figure 1). Rubella cases are followed by equivalently elevated CRS cases peaking after 8 and 9 months (r = 0.23 and 0.18), which is lower than the 95% confidence band (0.331); observing CRS cases 4 months before rubella peaks, there is also a positive trend (r = 0.31) which could be associated with seasonal differences. This analysis suggests that the peak correlation between rubella and detected CRS cases occurs in CRS cases infected at 1–2 months gestation, though this was not statistically significant.

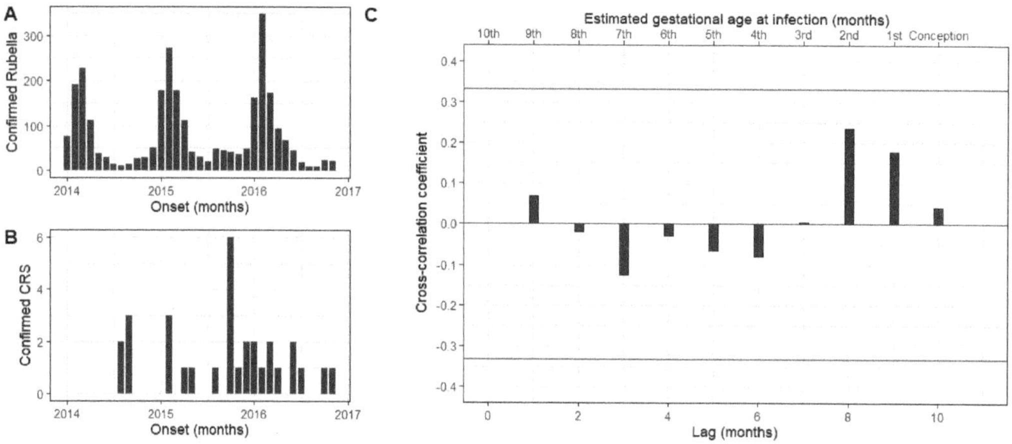


**Figure 1.** Comparison of the time trends of the rubella cases (panel **A**) and laboratory-confirmed congenital rubella syndrome (CRS) cases (panel **B**) in Sudan from January 2014 to December 2017. Panel **C** shows the cross-correlogram of the lag in CRS cases occurring following peaks in rubella cases. This figure indicates a positive (though not statistically significant, within the 95% confidence interval illustrated between the red lines) correlation with a lag of 8–10 months, corresponding to an increase in CRS cases following rubella cases occurring between conception and the third month of gestation.

## 4. Discussion

Decreasing the burden of CRS is the primary purpose of rubella vaccine introduction and monitoring its introduction and impact requires adequate surveillance systems. The progress and achievement of rubella and CRS elimination requires high-quality surveillance to document changes. As expected, the comprehensive surveillance approach has the highest sensitivity, simplified CRS surveillance detection on a more focused and specific set of sites, or specific diagnoses are alternatives when resources are limited. One specific diagnosis that is an especially strong candidate is cataracts, which are one of the few visible CRS manifestations.

The simplified-cataract approach had a higher proportion of suspected cases confirmed as CRS (24%) than the other approaches. Cases identified from eye hospitals included cases with cataracts ($n = 75$), glaucoma ($n = 55$), and pigmentary retinopathy ($n = 1$); however, only cases with cataracts were laboratory-confirmed to be positive ($n = 16$) with two clinically compatible cases. However, two glaucoma cases were also clinically compatible. Notably, glaucoma cases presented at a younger age than cataract cases (median 112 vs. 178 days) and, therefore, are more likely to be positive for IgM testing. Both the simplified-ophthalmic and the simplified-cataract approaches had high rates of serological and virological sample collection but were less likely to detect confirmed CRS cases within the first 3 months of life compared to a simplified-cardiac approach.

While this assessment may reflect the proof of concept of simplified surveillance, these results also reflect the quality of the sites selected. Optimal sentinel site surveillance, including CRS, is driven by careful site selection based on efficiency, patient flow, and other factors. For example, simplified-ophthalmic surveillance performed compared well to a comprehensive surveillance approach involving multiple manifestations of the case definition and various types of surveillance sites. Noting that the simplified-ophthalmic approach was driven by one site with a nationwide referral network, this highlights the value of including surveillance sites with a large catchment area for CRS surveillance. Some selection factors are learned through experience, such as the proportion of cases that are laboratory-confirmed, which varied between similar sites (e.g., between eye hospitals).

Surveillance for CRS may complement rubella surveillance, with temporal trends in CRS being associated with rubella disease. Cross-correlation analysis identified a weak, positive, but not statistically significant correlation between national rubella epidemiology and CRS epidemiology, peaking at around 8 months of lag, which may suggest that the CRS system captures the same epidemiological phenomena as rubella case-based surveillance and, thus, serves as a useful complement to case-based surveillance. Cataracts are most often associated with infection during the second or third month of gestation [16], and the cross-correlation results were consistent with this finding.

CRS surveillance does monitor trends and complements surveillance for rubella, as neither comprehensive nor simplified surveillance approaches capture the total burden of CRS in Sudan, as the true incidence is likely higher. This underestimation of incidence can occur for several reasons, including estimating the catchment area and case ascertainment. The catchment area of all but one of the sites was limited to two of eighteen states (26% of the national population); one eye site had a national catchment. Case ascertainment is not consistent with the expected proportions of CRS-affected infants. For example, hearing impairment is the most common manifestation, seen in approximately 57% of confirmed cases [10] but underreported and identified in only one suspected case. Cataracts are overreported and are expected to be reported in 16–25% of cases [9,10], though they were seen in 64% of confirmed cases from the comprehensive surveillance approach.

The CRS surveillance system in Sudan has similarities and differences to data from other systems prior to the rubella vaccine introduction [17–22]. The CRS incidence for simplified-cataract surveillance (0.58 cases/10,000 live births) and simplified-ophthalmic surveillance (0.98 cases/10,000 live births) in Sudan was similar to 1.0 [18] but lower than two other systems, 3.9, 4.0 [17,22], noting how catchment areas differed to the point that several systems did not attempt to calculate incidence [19,20]. The percentage of suspected cases that were laboratory-confirmed varied between systems, and the system in Sudan (17%) is similar to most systems at 18–22% [17,18,22] but lower than the high of 34% [19]. As expected, the proportion of suspected cases with cataracts from Sudan (44%) was greater than other systems, which ranged from 22% [21] to 37% [19]; concomitantly, a lower percentage of suspected cases with cardiac findings (27%) were reported from Sudan than the other systems which ranged from 46% [17] to 65% [19]. In summary, simplified surveillance (especially cataract and ophthalmic approaches) from Sudan has a greater percentage of cases with cataracts and a lower percentage of positive cases while having similar or lower incidence rates.

This evaluation has several limitations. Clinical case data were limited to a few health facilities in Sudan, which may not reflect the heterogeneity of the disease in Sudan. Surveillance was unable to be continued with high quality beyond 2017 due to funding, staff turnover, and other operational challenges, highlighting the reality of maintaining surveillance systems in low–middle income countries. The analysis focuses on detection but does not account for the human and financial resource burdens of the different surveillance approaches. Most cases were identified through eye hospitals, which had the lowest efficiency rate, highlighting the importance of assessing resources in future evaluations to strike a balance between sensitivity and specificity in system development. The overall background rate of congenital cataracts and their various causes varies globally [23]; this limits between-country incidence, making cataract-based surveillance approaches less comparable between countries. In addition, unique situations in this surveillance system (e.g., an eye hospital with a nationwide catchment area) may limit generalizability. Lastly, the surveillance training had an increased emphasis on the detection of cataracts relative to other symptoms, which may have increased the detection of cataracts compared to other CRS manifestations.

## 5. Conclusions

A comprehensive CRS surveillance system is the standard for monitoring elimination, as defined in the WHO Surveillance Standards [7], complementing surveillance for rubella. A simplified approach may be an alternative where there are limited resources, especially during the rubella vaccine introduction period or when initially establishing a CRS surveillance network. A simplified system can achieve some key goals of CRS surveillance, including documenting the impact of vaccine introduction and identifying infants with CRS to institute control measures and facilitate the early provision of appropriate medical care for the infant. We assessed simplified CRS surveillance within the specific context of Sudan's health care infrastructure and epidemiology. A simplified surveillance system built primarily on eye hospitals or eye findings (either through limiting the scope to eye hospitals and clinics or through a simplified cataract definition for suspected cases) would be effective in detecting CRS cases and may achieve the CRS surveillance goals of this country while reducing the operational burden and improving sustainability. Cases identified by such a system may have different clinical profiles than other CRS surveillance systems. Sudan has a well-developed network of clinical sites for ophthalmological screening and referral for treatment due to a relatively high baseline prevalence of congenital and childhood cataracts [24], making a simplified-ophthalmic approach more feasible than a simplified-cataract approach, which can then be expanded to increase the sensitivity of surveillance for CRS.

While it is rubella vaccines that will decrease the burden of CRS, we conclude that simplified surveillance can play an important role in monitoring the impact of rubella vaccine introduction, while a more sensitive surveillance approach would provide more robust evidence for the elimination of rubella and CRS.

**Author Contributions:** Conceptualization, S.R.; methodology, O.A., N.A., S.R., H.A.E.-H.M., J.H. and G.G.; formal analysis, O.A., J.H. and G.G.; data curation, O.A. and J.H.; writing—original draft preparation, O.A. and J.H.; writing—review and editing, O.A., S.R., J.H. and G.G.; visualization, J.H. and G.G.; supervision, S.R. and N.A.; funding acquisition, H.A.E.-H.M. All authors have read and agreed to the published version of the manuscript.

**Funding:** This research was funded, in part, by the Centers for Disease Control and Prevention to the World Health Organization, grant number 1U66GH000968-3.

**Institutional Review Board Statement:** Ethical and human subject review was conducted and approved by the Community Medicine Council of the Sudan Medical Specialization Board and the research department in the Federal Ministry of Health and the National EPI Research Technical Committee. Written and informed consent of the purpose of this study and the methodology was provided to each person before starting the direct interview and documented on the case report form.

**Data Availability Statement:** The data presented in this study are available on request from the first author due to the data being government data.

**Acknowledgments:** We thank the numerous clinicians, hospital staff, and surveillance officers for their support of the sites and the Sudan Medical Specialization Board. We acknowledge the technical and financial support received for this work from the World Health Organization and the Centers for Disease Control and Prevention. The findings and conclusions in this report are those of the authors and do not necessarily represent the official position of the Centers for Disease Control and Prevention.

**Conflicts of Interest:** The authors declare no conflicts of interest. Staff from the Centers for Disease Control and Prevention supported the design of the study in the collection, analyses, or interpretation of data; in the writing of the manuscript; or in the decision to publish the results.

## References


1. Vynnycky, E.; Knapp, J.K.; Papadopoulos, T.; Cutts, F.T.; Hachiya, M.; Miyano, S.; Reef, S.E. Estimates of the global burden of Congenital Rubella Syndrome, 1996–2019. *Int. J. Infect. Dis.* **2023**, *137*, 149–156. [CrossRef] [PubMed]
2. Ministry of Health Sudan. *Measles and Rubella Surveillance Report*; Ministry of Health Sudan: Khartoum, Sudan, 2014.
3. Adam, O.; Ali, A.K.M.; Hubschen, J.M.; Muller, C.P. Identification of congenital rubella syndrome in Sudan. *BMC Infect. Dis.* **2014**, *14*, 305. [CrossRef] [PubMed]
4. Hamdan, H.Z.; Abdelbagi, I.E.; Nasser, N.M.; Adam, I. Seroprevalence of cytomegalovirus and rubella among pregnant women in western Sudan. *Virol. J.* **2011**, *8*, 217. [CrossRef]
5. Omer, A.; Abdel Rahim, E.H.; Ali, E.E.; Jin, L. Primary investigation of 31 infants with suspected congenital rubella syndrome in Sudan. *Clin. Microbiol. Infect.* **2010**, *16*, 678–682. [CrossRef] [PubMed]
6. Khalfallah, E.A.A. Serodetection of Rubella IgM Antibodies among Newborns delivered at Omdurman Maternity Hospital. Master's Thesis, Sudan University of Science and Technology, Khartoum, Sudan, 2012.
7. World Health Organization. *Congenital Rubella Syndrome: Surveillance Standards for Vaccine-Preventable Diseases*; World Health Organization: Geneva, Switzerland, 2018.
8. Bloom, S.; Rguig, A.; Berraho, A.; Zniber, L.; Bouazzaoui, N.; Zaghloul, Z.; Reef, S.; Zidouh, A.; Papania, M.; Seward, J. Congenital rubella syndrome burden in Morocco: A rapid retrospective assessment. *Lancet* **2005**, *365*, 135–141. [CrossRef] [PubMed]
9. Reef, S.E.; Plotkin, S.A. Chapter 54-Rubella Vaccines. In *Plotkin's Vaccines*, 8th ed.; Orenstein, W., Offit, P., Edwards, K.M., Plotkin, S., Eds.; Elsevier: Philadelphia, PA, USA, 2023; pp. 1025–1056.e1019.
10. Simons, E.A.; Reef, S.E.; Cooper, L.Z.; Zimmerman, L.; Thompson, K.M. Systematic Review of the Manifestations of Congenital Rubella Syndrome in Infants and Characterization of Disability-Adjusted Life Years (DALYs). *Risk Anal.* **2016**, *36*, 1332–1356. [CrossRef] [PubMed]
11. Wu, X.; Long, E.; Lin, H.; Liu, Y. Prevalence and epidemiological characteristics of congenital cataract: A systematic review and meta-analysis. *Sci. Rep.* **2016**, *6*, 28564. [CrossRef]
12. World Health Organization. *WHO-Recommended Surveillance Standards Congenital Rubella Syndrome*; World Health Organization: Geneva, Switzerland, 2018.
13. Murray, J.; Cohen, A.L. Infectious disease surveillance. In *International Encyclopedia of Public Health*; Elsevier: Amsterdam, The Netherlands, 2017; pp. 222–229.
14. Macrotrends. Sudan Population 1950–2024. Available online: https://www.macrotrends.net/global-metrics/countries/SDN/sudan/population (accessed on 17 July 2024).
15. Halees, M.H.; Saleem, M.; Abdalla, A. Rubella Virus in Association with Congenital Cataract at Makkah Eye Complex. *Al-Basar Int. J. Ophthalmol.* **2020**, *7*, 16–20. [CrossRef]
16. Töndury, G.; Smith, D.W. Fetal rubella pathology. *J. Pediatr.* **1966**, *68*, 867–879. [CrossRef]
17. Wondimeneh, Y.; Tiruneh, M.; Ferede, G.; Denekew, K.; Admassu, F.; Tessema, B. Hospital based surveillance of congenital rubella syndrome cases in the pre-vaccine era in Amhara Regional State, Ethiopia: A base line information for the country. *PLoS ONE* **2018**, *13*, e0207095. [CrossRef] [PubMed]
18. Thant, K.Z.; Oo, W.M.; Myint, T.T.; Shwe, T.N.; Han, A.M.; Aye, K.M.; Aye, K.T.; Moe, K.; Thein, S.; Robertson, S.E. Active surveillance for congenital rubella syndrome in Yangon, Myanmar. *Bull. World Health Organ.* **2006**, *84*, 12–20. [CrossRef] [PubMed]
19. Murhekar, M.; Verma, S.; Singh, K.; Bavdekar, A.; Benakappa, N.; Santhanam, S.; Sapkal, G.; Viswanathan, R.; Singh, M.P.; Nag, V.L.; et al. Epidemiology of Congenital Rubella Syndrome (CRS) in India, 2016–2018, based on data from sentinel surveillance. *PLoS Neglected Trop. Dis.* **2020**, *14*, e0007982. [CrossRef] [PubMed]
20. Motaze, N.V.; Manamela, J.; Smit, S.; Rabie, H.; Harper, K.; duPlessis, N.; Reubenson, G.; Coetzee, M.; Ballot, D.; Moore, D.; et al. Congenital Rubella Syndrome Surveillance in South Africa Using a Sentinel Site Approach: A Cross-sectional Study. *Clin. Infect. Dis.* **2019**, *68*, 1658–1664. [CrossRef] [PubMed]
21. Masresha, B.; Shibeshi, M.; Kaiser, R.; Luce, R.; Katsande, R.; Mihigo, R. Congenital Rubella Syndrome in The African Region—Data from Sentinel Surveillance. *J. Immunol. Sci.* **2018**, *2*, 146–150. [CrossRef]
22. Herini, E.S.; Triono, A.; Iskandar, K.; Prasetyo, A.; Nugrahanto, A.P.; Gunadi. Congenital Rubella Syndrome Surveillance After Measles Rubella Vaccination Introduction in Yogyakarta, Indonesia. *Pediatr. Infect. Dis. J.* **2021**, *40*, 1144–1150. [CrossRef] [PubMed]
23. Sheeladevi, S.; Lawrenson, J.; Fielder, A.; Suttle, C. Global prevalence of childhood cataract: A systematic review. *Eye* **2016**, *30*, 1160–1169. [CrossRef] [PubMed]
24. Samy El Gendy, N.M.; Abdel-Kader, A.A. Prevalence of Selected Eye Diseases Using Data Harvested from Ophthalmic Checkup Examination of a Cohort of Two Thousand Middle Eastern and North African Subjects. *J. Ophthalmol.* **2018**, *2018*, 8049475. [CrossRef] [PubMed]

*vaccines*

MDPI

*Article*

# Breakthrough Measles among Vaccinated Adults Born during the Post-Soviet Transition Period in Mongolia

**José E. Hagan [1,*], Stephen N. Crooke [2], Nyamaa Gunregjav [3], Sun B. Sowers [2], Sara Mercader [2], Carole J. Hickman [2], Mick N. Mulders [4], Roberta Pastore [1], Yoshihiro Takashima [1], David N. Durrheim [5], James L. Goodson [6] and Paul A. Rota [2]**

1 Expanded Programme on Immunization, World Health Organization Regional Office for the Western Pacific, 1000 Manila, Philippines
2 Division of Viral Diseases, Centers for Disease Control and Prevention, Atlanta, GA 30329, USA; par1@cdc.gov (P.A.R.)
3 Mongolia National Center for Communicable Diseases, Ulaanbaatar 14210, Mongolia
4 Vaccine Preventable Diseases Laboratory Network, World Health Organization, 1211 Geneva, Switzerland; muldersm@who.int
5 School of Medicine and Public Health, University of Newcastle, Wallsend, NSW 2287, Australia
6 Global Immunization Division, Centers for Disease Control and Prevention, Atlanta, GA 30329, USA
* Correspondence: haganj@who.int; Tel.: +1-4043687294

**Abstract:** Mongolia experienced a nationwide measles outbreak during 1 March 2015–31 December 2016, with 49,077 cases reported to the WHO; many were among vaccinated young adults, suggesting a possible role of vaccine failure. Advanced laboratory methods, coupled with detailed epidemiological investigations, can help classify cases as vaccine failure, failure to vaccinate, or both. In this report, we conducted a study of cases to identify risk factors for breakthrough infection for a subset of laboratory-confirmed measles cases. Of the 193 cases analyzed, only 19 (9.8%) reported measles vaccination history, and 170 (88%) were uncertain. Measles-specific IgG avidity testing classified 120 (62%) cases as low IgG avidity, indicating no prior exposure to measles. Ten of these cases with low IgG avidity had a history of measles vaccination, indicating primary vaccine failure. Overall, sixty cases (31%) had high IgG avidity, indicating breakthrough infection after prior exposure to measles antigen through vaccination or natural infection, but the IgG avidity results were highly age-dependent. This study found that among young children aged 9 months–5 years, breakthrough infection was rare (4/82, 5%); however, among young adults aged 15–25 years, breakthrough infection due to secondary vaccine failure (SVF) occurred on a large scale during this outbreak, accounting for the majority of cases (42/69 cases, 61%). The study found that large-scale secondary vaccine failure occurred in Mongolia, which highlights the potential for sustained outbreaks in post-elimination settings due to "hidden" cohorts of young adults who may have experienced waning immunity. This phenomenon may have implications for the sustainability of measles elimination in countries that remain vulnerable to the importation of the virus from areas where it is still endemic. Until global measles elimination is achieved, enhanced surveillance and preparedness for future outbreaks in post- or peri-elimination countries may be required.

**Keywords:** measles outbreak; vaccine failure; breakthrough infection; IgG Avidity; measles elimination; Mongolia

## 1. Background

Fifty years after the establishment of the Expanded Program on Immunization (EPI) and the widespread use of the measles vaccine globally, worldwide measles mortality has significantly declined from an estimated >2 million deaths per year in 1980 to ~136,000 deaths in 2022; however, the measles virus continues to circulate, causing infections, illness, and over 300 deaths worldwide each day [1]. All six WHO regions have committed to the elimination of endemic measles, but so far, none of them have achieved and sustained this goal [1]. The Region of the Americas achieved measles elimination and was verified in 2016, but subsequent large outbreaks re-established endemic transmission in Venezuela and Brazil. Since 2016, seven other countries across two WHO regions have also seen endemic measles transmission re-established after previously achieving elimination [1].

In Mongolia (population ~3.3 million), a measles-containing vaccine (MCV), administered at 9 months of age, was introduced in the national EPI in 1973, and a second dose of MCV, given at 2 years of age, was introduced in 1989 [2]. A single-antigen measles vaccine was replaced with a measles–mumps–rubella vaccine (MMR) in 2009. Following increasing vaccination coverage and supplemental immunization campaigns, no cases of measles were reported in Mongolia during 2011–2014, and the Regional Verification Commission (RVC) for the WHO Western Pacific Region verified that Mongolia had eliminated endemic measles transmission in July 2014 [3]. However, in March 2015, a nationwide measles outbreak occurred, with 49,077 confirmed or clinically compatible cases reported to the WHO during 1 March 2015–31 December 2016. The outbreak is the largest documented measles outbreak in a post-elimination setting [4]. As the outbreak consisted of an uninterrupted chain of transmission lasting more than 12 months, Mongolia was adjudged by the RVC to have re-established endemic transmission [5].

This outbreak was propagated by transmission among young adults, revealing a large and previously unknown immunity gap in this age group that was belied by the historical routine and supplemental measles immunization coverage reported in these birth cohorts. The initial findings from the outbreak investigation in Mongolia indicated apparent emerging measles susceptibility among vaccinated adults [4], raising questions about whether vaccine failure on a large scale may have contributed to the outbreak.

Outbreaks in several other countries included laboratory-confirmed measles cases among previously vaccinated persons, known as breakthrough infections [6–8]. Breakthrough infections can occur due to primary or secondary vaccine failure. Primary vaccine failure (PVF) is the absence of a measurable antibody response after vaccination (i.e., non-responder), whereas secondary vaccine failure (SVF) is the loss of vaccine-induced immunity over time (i.e., waning immunity), or the inability to achieve a protective titer following vaccination [9–12]. Differentiating PVF and SVF can be achieved by measuring measles IgG antibody avidity, as well as by measuring neutralizing antibody titers [13,14]. As part of the investigation to determine potential root causes of the nationwide measles outbreak in Mongolia, we conducted a cross-sectional study to investigate whether there was laboratory evidence of breakthrough infection and to identify risk factors for breakthrough infection using a subset of laboratory-confirmed measles cases.

## 2. Methods

### 2.1. Study Design and Ethical Clearance

This study used an analytical cross-sectional design to describe the frequency of, and risk factors for, breakthrough measles infection among a sample of laboratory-confirmed cases involving individuals below 30 years of age, as part of the public health response to the nationwide outbreak of measles in Mongolia during 2015–2016. This response activity was reviewed by CDC and Mongolia National Center for Communicable Diseases, deemed not to be human subject research, and was conducted in compliance with applicable federal law and CDC policy.

### 2.2. Case Definition and Sample Selection

The cases studied were a convenience sample of 200 laboratory-confirmed measles virus infections in Mongolia, reported to the Mongolia Ministry of Health and Sports, and investigated by the surveillance team, EPI, Mongolia National Center for Communicable Diseases (NCCD) during 1 March 2015–17 April 2016. These 200 cases were randomly selected from 1665 outbreak cases that met the following eligibility criteria: individuals aged under 30 years, had rash onset during this time period, and an available serological specimen that was collected ≥2 days after rash onset. Cases were investigated and individuals were interviewed by NCCD staff to collect demographic information and self-reported vaccination status.

### 2.3. Laboratory Testing

Cases in this study were selected from outbreak cases that were laboratory-confirmed by the NCCD as being part of an investigation during the national outbreak response, using a commercial enzyme-linked immunosorbent assay ([EIA], Enzygnost™, Siemens, Munich, Germany) for immunoglobulin M (IgM) according to the manufacturer's instructions. To confirm eligibility, serum samples from the 200 cases that were selected for inclusion in this study were tested again at the Centers for Disease Control and Prevention (CDC) using an in-house IgM capture assay [15]. Cases testing negative for IgM by CDC capture assay were excluded from the study.

Measles virus-specific and rubella virus-specific immunoglobulin G (IgG) were detected using commercially available indirect EIAs (Measles IgG Test System, Zeus Scientific, Branchburg, NJ, USA). Cases testing negative for IgG could not be tested for avidity and were excluded from the study. The results of rubella IgG were interpreted together with other results as supporting evidence suggestive of prior vaccination using an MMR vaccine. Measles IgG avidity was measured in serum samples with an end-point dilution assay developed at CDC using a commercial measles IgG EIA (Captia Measles IgG; Trinity BioTech, Jamestown, NJ, USA) modified for use with the denaturing agent diethylamine as previously described [13]. An IgG avidity index of ≤30% was considered low-avidity, 30–70% was considered intermediate-avidity, and >70% was considered high-avidity. An avidity index could not be obtained from specimens that were IgG-positive per the Zeus Measles IgG kit but IgG-negative or indeterminate per the Captia Measles IgG kit; the avidity result for these specimens was reported as undetermined, and they were excluded from analysis [13].

Sera from study cases were also tested at CDC for measles-neutralizing antibody by the plaque reduction neutralization (PRN) assay as previously described [16]. The WHO second international standard anti-measles serum (IS, coded 66/202, National Institute for Biological Standards and Control, South Mimms, UK) was included to calculate the reciprocal of the 50% endpoint titer by the Kärber method. PRN titers were expressed in mIU/mL, with a titer of 1:8 equivalent to a concentration of 8 mIU/mL.

### 2.4. Case Classification and Statistical Analysis

Cases with low, intermediate, and high IgG avidity were compared according to the demographic characteristics and reported vaccination status. Kruskal–Wallis, Fisher's exact, and Chi-square tests were used as appropriate to describe the association between the case characteristics and breakthrough infection status. When calculating $p$-values for differences between low- and high-IgG-avidity cases, intermediate-avidity cases were excluded to avoid a possible misclassification error.

Data were interpreted to classify cases as primary acute infection, primary vaccine failure (PVF), or breakthrough infection due to SVF. Primary acute infection cases were those with low IgG avidity and no history of vaccination. Primary vaccine failure (PVF) cases were those with low IgG avidity and reported history of vaccination. All cases with high IgG avidity were classified as breakthrough infection due to SVF, regardless of the reported history of vaccination. PRN titers were not used for case classification but were used as supportive data to check consistency with primary vs. breakthrough infection classification using IgG avidity [14]. Cases with intermediate avidity were not interpreted with respect to breakthrough infection status.

Vaccine field effectiveness ($VFE_y$) was estimated for 5 age ranges using the following equation derived from the "screening method" described by Chen et al. [17]: $VFE_y = \frac{PCV_y - PPV_y}{(PCV_y - 1) \times PPV_y}$, where $PCV_y$ represents the percent of reinfection cases, and $PPV_y$ represents the estimated historical MCV coverage for a given age cohort $y$. To obtain

$PPV_y$, we determined the highest coverage achieved for MCV1, MCV2, or any SIAs targeting each birth year and calculated the mean of those values among cases aged under 2 years, 2–5 years, 6–14 years, 15–24 years, and 25–29 years.

## 3. Results

Of the 200 cases selected for analysis, 2 suspect cases (1%) had a positive result by Enzygnost IgM EIA but were negative by the CDC IgM capture assay. These were considered to be false-positive IgM results and were excluded from the study. Five additional cases, that were positive by the CDC IgM capture assay, were excluded from the study because sera were negative by IgG EIA and could not be tested for avidity. Of the 193 remaining cases included for analysis, 104 (54%) were male, and the median age was 9 years (interquartile range [IQR], 0.8–20), with a bimodal distribution (Figure 1, Scheme 1) similar to the age and sex distribution of cases observed during the outbreak (Scheme 2). Only 19 (9.8%) of all cases reported a history of measles vaccination, and 170 (88%) cases were uncertain of their vaccination history.

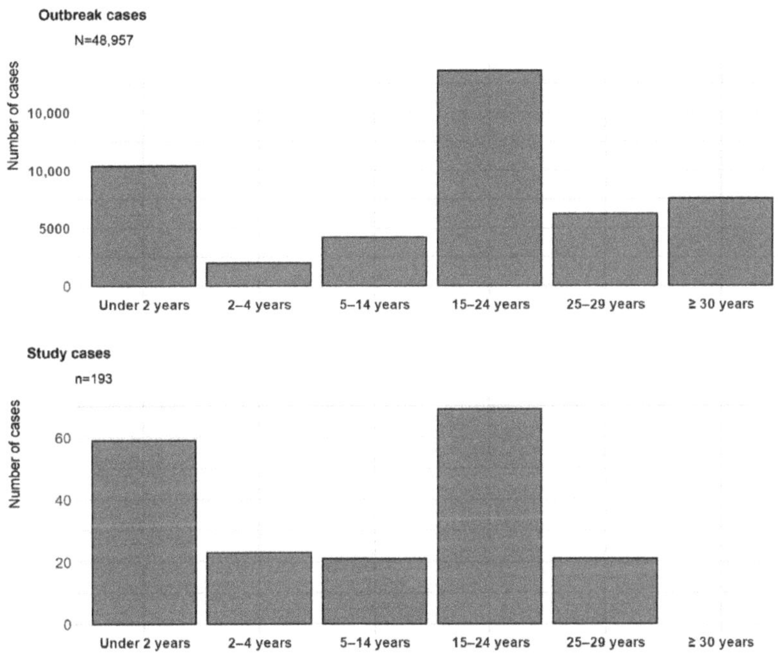


**Figure 1.** Comparison of age distribution of outbreak cases (source: case-based surveillance data officially submitted to WHO) and study cases.

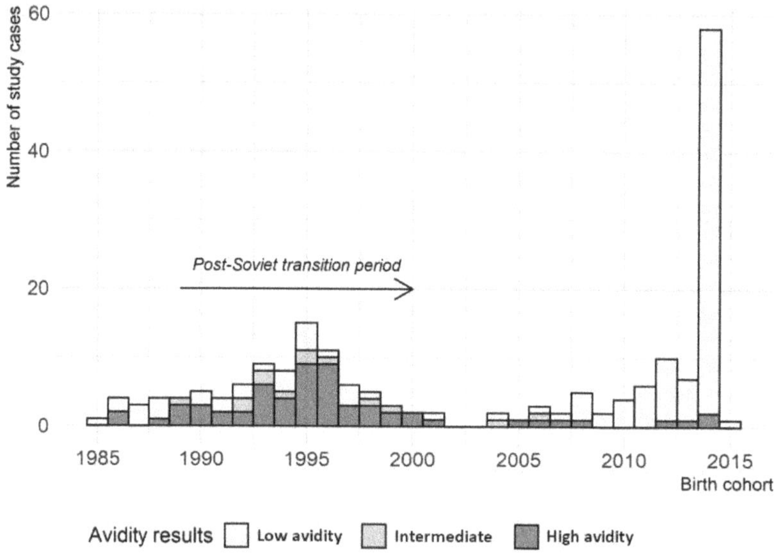


**Scheme 1.** Measles cases, by breakthrough infection classification and by birth year, Mongolia, 1 March 2015–17 April 2016, N = 193.

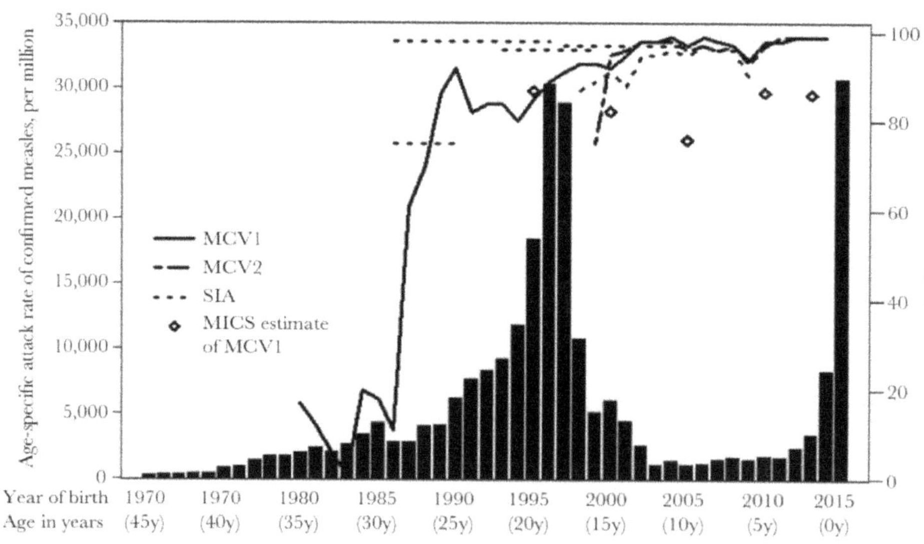


| Year of SIA | Vaccine used | Target age group | Age in 2015 | Number vaccinated | Coverage (%) |
|---|---|---|---|---|---|
| 1994 | Measles | 3–8 years | 24–29 years | 162,751 | 75% |
| 1996 | Measles | 9 mo–10 years | 19–29 years | 541,441 | 98% |
| 2000 | Measles | 9 mo–7 years | 15–22 years | 353,389 | 96% |
| 2007 | Measles | 2–10 years | 10–18 years | 401,575 | 97% |
| 2012 | Measles-Rubella | 3–14 years | 6–17 years | 522,429 | 98% |

**Scheme 2.** Age-specific attack rate during the 2015 outbreak in Mongolia (left y axis) and historical overview of routine and supplemental measles-containing vaccination coverage (right y axis)—Mongolia, 1987–2015. Reproduced with permission from Ref. [4], 2017, Oxford University Press.

Measles-specific IgG avidity testing identified 120 (62%) cases as having low IgG avidity; 110 of these were classified as primary acute infection and 10 of these cases had a history of measles vaccination and were classified as PVF. Sixty cases (31%) had high IgG avidity; nine of these reported a history of vaccination. The other 51 high-IgG-avidity cases did not report a history of vaccination. Thirteen cases (7%) had intermediate avidity. Cases with high-avidity IgG had a significantly higher geometric mean titer (GMT) as measured by PRN compared to primary acute infection, PVF, and intermediate-avidity cases ($p < 0.001$). All high-IgG-avidity cases had a PRN titer of >34,000 mIU/mL. Cases with high-avidity and intermediate-avidity measles-specific IgG were predominantly IgG-positive for rubella (83% and 77%, respectively) compared to the low-avidity cases (31%) ($p < 0.001$).

IgG avidity classification varied significantly by age (Tables 1 and 2, Figure 2). The highest proportion of cases with high IgG avidity (42 cases, 61%) was observed among adults aged 15–24 years (n = 69). In this age group, a further 10 (14%) had intermediate avidity. Among 82 children aged 9 months–5 years, 78 (95%) had low IgG avidity, 4 (5%) had high IgG avidity, and none had intermediate avidity. Reported measles vaccination was nearly twice as common among high-avidity cases (15%) compared to low-avidity cases (8%), although the difference was not statistically significant ($p = 0.172$). Among the four high-avidity cases under 5 years of age, three (75%) were positive for rubella IgG by ELISA, consistent with prior vaccination with MMR vaccine.

**Table 1.** Characteristics of measles cases, by IgG avidity classification, Mongolia, 1 March 2015–17 April 2016.

| Characteristic n (%) or Median (IQR) | Low-Avidity IgG n = 120 | High-Avidity IgG n = 60 | Intermediate-Avidity IgG n = 13 | Total N = 193 | *p*-Value * |
|---|---|---|---|---|---|
| Age in years | 2.0 (0.7–9.5) | 19 (17–22) | 20 (17–22) | 9 (0.8–20) | $p < 0.001$ |
| *Birth cohort (age at infection)* | | | | | |
| 2014–2015 (<2 years) | 57 (47.5) | 2 (3.3) | 0 (0.0) | 59 (30.6) | |
| 2011–2013 (2–4 years) | 21 (17.5) | 2 (3.3) | 0 (0.0) | 23 (11.9) | |
| 2001–2010 (5–14 years) | 14 (11.7) | 5 (8.3) | 2 (15.4) | 21 (10.9) | $p < 0.001$ |
| 1991–2000 (15–24 years) | 17 (14.2) | 42 (70.0) | 10 (76.9) | 69 (35.8) | |
| 1985–1990 (25–29 years) | 11 (9.2) | 9 (15.0) | 1 (7.7) | 21 (10.9) | |
| Male sex | 67 (55.8) | 31 (51.7) | 6 (46.2) | 104 (53.9) | $p = 0.597$ |
| *Symptoms* | | | | | |
| Cough | 48 (40.0) | 17 (28.3) | 7 (53.8) | 72 (37.3) | $p = 0.124$ |
| Coryza | 40 (33.3) | 28 (46.7) | 7 (53.8) | 75 (38.9) | $p = 0.082$ |
| Conjunctivitis | 44 (36.7) | 24 (40.0) | 8 (61.5) | 76 (39.4) | $p = 0.664$ |
| *Recall history of measles vaccine* | | | | | |
| Yes | 10 (8.3) | 9 (15.0) | 0 (0.0) | 19 (9.8) | $p = 0.172$ |
| No or unknown | 110 (91.7) | 51 (85) | 13 (100) | 174 (90.2) | |
| Rubella IgG-positive | 37 (30.8) | 50 (83.3) | 10 (76.9) | 97 (50.3) | $p < 0.001$ |
| PRN Geometric Mean Titer (geometric mean, 95%CI) | 894 (669–1195) | 47,003 (34,970–63,175) | 3695 (957–14,261) | 3371 (2410–4715) | $p < 0.001$ |

* *p*-value comparing cases with high-avidity IgG with low-avidity IgG. *p*-value for PRN titer was calculated by comparing the antilog of the geometric means using Student's *t*-test. Data in the table are presented as n (%) or median (IQR), except in the case of PRN geometric mean titer, which is presented as 95% confidence interval.

**Table 2.** IgG avidity classification and estimated vaccine efficacy by age group, Mongolia, 1 March 2015–17 April 2016.

| Characteristic n (%) | Age in Years (Birth Cohort) | | | | | |
|---|---|---|---|---|---|---|
| | 2014–2015 (<2 Years) n = 59 | 2011–2013 (2–5 Years) n = 23 | 2001–2010 (6–14 years) n = 21 | 1991–2000 (15–24 Years) n = 69 | 1985–1990 (25–29 Years) n = 21 | Total N = 193 |
| Recall measles vaccination | 4 (7%) | 2 (9%) | 1 (5%) | 10 (14%) | 2 (10%) | 19 (10%) |
| Rubella IgG | 7 (12%) | 5 (22%) | 3 (14%) | 61 (88%) | 21 (100%) | 97 (50%) |
| High-avidity | 2 (3%) | 2 (9%) | 5 (24%) | 42 (61%) | 9 (43%) | 60 (31%) |
| Intermediate-avidity | 0 (0%) | 0 (0%) | 2 (10%) | 10 (14%) | 1 (5%) | 13 (7%) |
| Low-avidity | 57 (97%) | 21 (91%) | 14 (67%) | 17 (25%) | 11 (52%) | 120 (62%) |
| PRNT GMT (geometric mean, 95%CI) | 951 (581–1557) | 1970 (917–4341) | 3333 (1142–9726) | 11,139 (6241–19,325) | 4231 (1347–13,294) | 3371 (2410–4715) |
| Historical MCV1 coverage * | 98.1% | 97.8% | 96% | 93.6% | 87.6% | 94.1% |
| Estimated %VE | 94.9% | 94.8% | 93.0% | 75.2% | 82.7% | 91.3% |

* Average administrative immunization coverage with one dose of measles-containing vaccine (data source: World Health Organization. (2023). WHO/UNICEF Immunization Coverage Estimates—2022 revision https://immunizationdata.who.int/global, accessed on 15 January 2024). Data in the table are presented as n (%) or median (IQR), except in the case of PRN geometric mean titer, which is presented as 95% confidence interval.

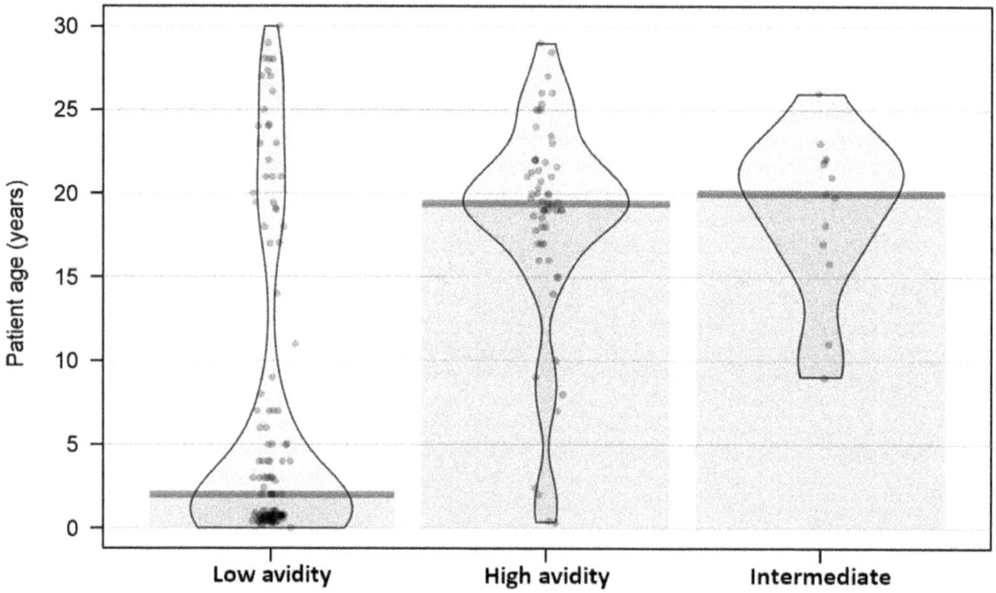


**Figure 2.** Box–violin plot of measles case ages, by IgG avidity classification, Mongolia, 1 March 2015–17 April 2016, N = 193.

The proportion of cases in this study classified as breakthrough infection (i.e., high-IgG-avidity cases), along with historical estimates of routine and supplemental vaccination coverage, were used to estimate vaccine field effectiveness for each age cohort (Table 2). We estimated that vaccine field effectiveness for children aged under 15 years was 93.0–94.9%; however, estimated vaccine effectiveness for adults aged 15–24 years and 25–29 years was 75.2% and 82.8%, respectively.

## 4. Discussion

This study determined that overall, among 193 lab-confirmed measles cases of individuals aged under age 30 years, a substantial proportion (31%) had high-avidity IgG, consistent with breakthrough infection due to SVF. Breakthrough cases occurred overwhelmingly among older age groups, with 61% of cases in the 15–24 years age group and 43% of cases in the 25–29 years age group caused by breakthrough infections. Based on the historical age-specific measles vaccine coverage in Mongolia, we calculated that vaccine field effectiveness for children under age 15 was 93–95%, while for young adults aged 15–29, vaccine effectiveness was 75–83%, insufficient to provide herd immunity against measles outbreaks. These results strongly implicate breakthrough infection due to SVF among young adults as a major contributor to the 2015–2016 outbreak in Mongolia.

Epidemiologically significant SVF breakthrough infection on such a large scale has not previously been described in any other setting. However, our findings should be considered in light of this study's limitations. A great majority (88%) of cases enrolled in this study were uncertain of their measles vaccination status, which is a key piece of information when interpreting avidity results for vaccine failure classifications. The study focused on cases involving individuals under 30, as this age cohort in Mongolia has been highly vaccinated through a combination of routine and supplemental immunization (Scheme 2) and has had very limited risk of measles (or rubella) exposure through natural infection, given the epidemiological history of these diseases in the country. Therefore, in the cases included in this study, serological evidence of previous exposure to measles virus antigen was interpreted as evidence of vaccination. This assumption was further supported by the finding that a very high proportion of cases with both high- and medium-avidity measles IgG were positive for rubella-specific IgG (83% and 77%, respectively) compared to low-avidity cases (31%) ($p < 0.001$). This finding is strongly suggestive of prior vaccination with measles- and rubella-containing vaccine. To eliminate the potential risk of false-positive IgM among previously vaccinated persons, we used PRN titers as complementary evidence of breakthrough infection. All cases classified as breakthrough infection had PRN titers above >34,000 mIU/mL, consistent with previous findings [14]. While all measles cases included in this study were laboratory-confirmed, the sample size was still relatively small and may not be wholly representative of the outbreak population, as it was based on random selection from a convenience sample of cases with available samples collected at least two days after disease onset and with detectable measles-specific IgG. Despite this potential source of bias, the age distribution of this sample was comparable to the age distribution of the overall outbreak (Figure 1). Restricting inclusion criteria to cases that were IgM-positive during initial case investigation may have introduced bias that diluted our findings by potentially excluding some cases of breakthrough infection due to SVF, which may have high-avidity IgG and high titers of neutralizing antibodies without detectable IgM. Finally, as with many large outbreaks, data quality is often limited, particularly relating to clinical presentation and recall vaccination history. For example, we did not observe any significant differences in clinical presentation between breakthrough cases and primary infection cases (Table 1), although the clinical presentation in breakthrough measles cases is generally understood to be mild compared to primary infection [6,18–22]. This may have been due to data quality, the relatively small sample size of the study, or other epidemiological factors of the outbreak.

Receiving two correctly administered, age-appropriate doses of measles vaccine is >95% effective in generating durable protective immunity. Breakthrough measles infections due to PVF and SVF have been reported [23–28] in highly vaccinated populations in countries that have achieved measles elimination [6,18–22,26,29–34] or are approaching measles elimination [35,36]. However, in populations with measles vaccination coverage that meets the 95% target for achieving and sustaining measles elimination, breakthrough measles infection generally accounts for a limited number of cases and has not previously been observed on a mass scale or as a contributing factor to large, prolonged outbreaks. This outbreak in Mongolia is the largest outbreak to date in which breakthrough measles infection was an important factor. The findings of this study point to potential systematic issues occurring during a discrete period in the country's history, specifically impacting young adults aged 15–29 years. Case patients in this age group were born during the decade after the fall of the USSR in 1990 (Scheme 1). During this period, Mongolia experienced significant health system and political transition from central government planning to decentralized health care provision. Suboptimal vaccine storage, handling, or manufacture may have resulted in the widespread administration of a sub-potent measles vaccine that impacted the quality and durability of the immune response for children vaccinated during this period [37,38]. Low vaccine effectiveness due to documented cold-chain inadequacies contributing to a sustained measles outbreak despite high vaccine coverage has been previously described in the Federated States of Micronesia [28]. Unfortunately, in this outbreak, we lacked access to details on the specific vaccines administered, or documented evidence of historical cold-chain failure, which would also have served to definitively pinpoint a systemic cause of vaccine failure. Another potential contributor to the lower vaccine effectiveness observed in this age group may have been age of initial vaccination; although, in Mongolia, the age of first MCV dose has always been at least 9 months, it is unknown whether this schedule was followed strictly in all parts of Mongolia during the history of the immunization program. Brinkman and colleagues reported that 11% of children who received a first dose of measles vaccine before 9 months had neutralizing antibody titers that declined below the minimum protective level by 4 years of age [39]. Infants vaccinated at 6 months, compared to 9 months, develop a less robust immune response to the measles vaccine, even in the absence of maternal antibody [40]. Finally, after years without endemic circulation or large outbreaks in Mongolia to provide periodic exposure to wild measles virus and "boost" immunity among vaccinated people, it is possible that some degree of waning immunity among vaccinated young adults may have occurred. The population aged 15–29 years during the 2015–2016 outbreak appears to have been protected during the large nationwide outbreak that occurred in Mongolia in 2001, when these individuals were aged 1–15 years old [4]. This observation is a compelling suggestion that this immunity gap has emerged over time among a previously immune population.

This study's findings, that breakthrough infection due to SVF may have an epidemiologically important role in large-scale measles infection, have some important implications for the surveillance of measles in the elimination setting. Timely and accurate laboratory confirmation of suspected measles cases is a critical component of surveillance, and the routine method for case confirmation is the detection of measles-specific IgM [41]; however, IgM may not be present in breakthrough cases. Therefore, case confirmation by rRT-PCR has become increasingly useful, particularly in elimination settings [19,20,42]. Targeted use of laboratory techniques such as IgG avidity and PRN testing may be increasingly needed to help to further classify measles cases as primary infection or breakthrough cases to assist our understanding of outbreaks and their root causes.

## 5. Conclusions

In this study, we demonstrated that breakthrough infection due to SVF occurred at a large scale among young adults during the 2015–2016 measles outbreak in Mongolia, a country with a long history of high vaccination coverage that had recently been verified as having eliminated endemic measles. Even when outbreaks occur in highly vaccinated countries where measles is well controlled or eliminated, the vast majority of measles cases still occur in unvaccinated individuals [43], highlighting the continued need for countries to redouble their effort to identify and protect their unreached and underserved populations. However, we are now entering an epoch when a growing number of countries have been free from endemic measles circulation and are thus not experiencing the regular boosting of immunity by wild virus transmission. If the reduced vaccine effectiveness we observed among young adults was due in part to waning immunity from the prolonged absence of exposure to wild virus, the Mongolian experience suggests that there could be expanding cohorts of young adults with waning immunity in other countries as well. As a result, even as countries and regions make progress towards measles elimination, the risk of sustained outbreaks following importation may be steadily increasing. This emerging phenomenon may have important implications for the measles elimination initiative, potentially threatening the sustainability of elimination in countries which remain at risk of importation of the virus from countries where the disease is still endemic. This should serve as a clarion call for urgently accelerated global initiatives to achieve the regional goals of measles elimination in all six WHO regions.

**Author Contributions:** Conceptualization, J.E.H., J.L.G., M.N.M. and P.A.R.; methodology, J.E.H., S.B.S., S.M., C.J.H., M.N.M., J.L.G. and P.A.R.; formal analysis, J.E.H., S.B.S., S.M., C.J.H. and P.A.R.; investigation, J.E.H., N.G., M.N.M., R.P., Y.T. and J.L.G.; resources, Y.T., M.N.M. and P.A.R.; writing—original draft preparation, J.E.H. and S.N.C.; writing—review and editing, S.N.C., S.B.S., S.M., C.J.H., M.M, R.P., D.N.D., J.L.G. and P.A.R.; visualization, J.E.H.; supervision, J.L.G. and P.A.R. All authors have read and agreed to the published version of the manuscript.

**Funding:** This research received no external funding.

**Institutional Review Board Statement:** This outbreak response activity was reviewed by CDC and Mongolia National Center for Communicable Diseases, deemed not to be human subject research, and was conducted in compliance with applicable federal law and CDC policy.

**Informed Consent Statement:** Not applicable. Case data and biological samples were collected as part of a routine outbreak response activity and analyzed to guide public health programming.

**Data Availability Statement:** Restrictions apply to the availability of these data, which were collected during national public health response. Data are available from the authors with permission from the Mongolia Ministry of Health.

**Conflicts of Interest:** The findings and conclusions in this report are those of the authors and do not necessarily represent the official position of the U.S. Centers for Disease Control and Prevention. The authors affiliated with the World Health Organization (WHO) are alone responsible for the views expressed in this publication and they do not necessarily represent the decisions or policies of the WHO. The authors declare no conflicts of interest.

## References

1. Minta, A.; Ferrari, M.; Antoni, S.; Portnoy, A.; Sbarra, A.; Lambert, B.; Hatcher, C.; Hsu, C.; Ho, L.; Steulet, C.; et al. Progress toward Measles Elimination—Worldwide, 2000–2022. *MMWR Morb. Mortal. Wkly. Rep.* **2023**, *98*, 1262–1268. [CrossRef]
2. Rentsen, T.; Enkhtuya, B.; Nymadawa, P.; Kobune, F.; Suzuki, K.; Yoshida, H.; Hachiya, M. Measles outbreak after a post-honeymoon period in Mongolia, 2001. *Jpn J. Infect. Dis.* **2007**, *60*, 198–199. [CrossRef]
3. World Health Organization Regional Office for the Western Pacific. Meeting Report. In *Proceedings of the Third Annual Meeting of the Regional Verification Commission for Measles Elimination in the Western Pacific*; Seoul, Republic of Korea, 18–21 March 2014, World Health Organization: Manila, Philippines, 2016.
4. Hagan, J.; Takashima, Y.; Sarankhuu, A.; Dashpagma, O.; Jantsansengee, B.; Pastore, R.; Nyamaa, G.; Yadamsuren, B.; Mulders, M.; Wannemuehler, K.; et al. Goodson Risk Factors for Measles Virus Infection Among Adults During a Large Outbreak in Postelimination Era in Mongolia, 2015. *J. Infect. Dis.* **2017**, *216*, 1187–1195. [CrossRef]
5. World Health Organization Regional Office for the Western Pacific. Meeting Report. In *Proceedings of the Fifth Annual Meeting of the Regional Verification Commission for Measles Elimination in the Western Pacific*; Sydney, NWS, Australia, 20–23 September 2016, World Health Organization: Manila, Philippines, 2016.
6. Cherry, J.; Zahn, M. Clinical Characteristics of Measles in Previously Vaccinated and Unvaccinated Patients in California. *Clin. Infect. Dis.* **2018**, *67*, 1315–1319. [CrossRef] [PubMed]
7. López-Perea, N.; Fernández-García, A.; Echevarría, J.; de Ory, F.; Pérez-Olmeda, M.; Masa-Calles, J. Measles in Vaccinated People: Epidemiology and Challenges in Surveillance and Diagnosis in the Post-Elimination Phase. Spain, 2014–2020. *Viruses* **2021**, *13*, 1982. [CrossRef] [PubMed]
8. Bianchi, S.; Gori, M.; Fappani, C.; Ciceri, G.; Canuti, M.; Colzani, D.; Dura, M.; Terraneo, M.; Lamberti, A.; Baggieri, M.; et al. Characterization of Vaccine Breakthrough Cases during Measles Outbreaks in Milan and Surrounding Areas, Italy, 2017–2021. *Viruses* **2022**, *14*, 1068. [CrossRef]
9. Wiedermann, U.; Garner-Spitzer, E.; Wagner, A. Primary vaccine failure to routine vaccines: Why and what to do? *Hum. Vaccines Immunother.* **2016**, *12*, 239–243. [CrossRef] [PubMed]
10. Javelle, E.; Colson, P.; Parola, P.; Raoult, D. Measles, the need for a paradigm shift. *Eur. J. Epidemiol.* **2019**, *34*, 897–915. [CrossRef]

11. Sniadack, D.H.; Crowcroft, N.S.; Durrheim, D.N.; Rota, P.A. Roadmap to elimination standard measles and rubella surveillance. *Wkly. Epidemiol. Rec.* **2017**, *9*, 97–105.
12. Pannuti, C.S.; Morello, R.; Moraes, J.; Curti, S.; Afonso, A.; Camargo, M.; Souza, V. Identification of primary and secondary measles vaccine failures by measurement of immunoglobulin G avidity in measles cases during the 1997 São Paulo epidemic. *Clin. Diagn. Lab. Immunol.* **2004**, *11*, 119–122. [CrossRef]
13. Mercader, S.; Garcia, P.; Bellini, W. Measles virus IgG avidity assay for use in classification of measles vaccine failure in measles elimination settings. *Clin. Vaccine Immunol.* **2012**, *19*, 1810–1817. [CrossRef] [PubMed]
14. Sowers, S.; Rota, J.; Hickman, C.; Mercader, S.; Redd, S.; McNall, R.; Williams, N.; McGrew, M.; Walls, M.; Rota, P.; et al. High Concentrations of Measles Neutralizing Antibodies and High-Avidity Measles IgG Accurately Identify Measles Reinfection Cases. *Clin. Vaccine Immunol.* **2016**, *23*, 707–716. [CrossRef] [PubMed]
15. Hummel, K.; Erdman, D.; Heath, J.; Bellini, W. Baculovirus expression of the nucleoprotein gene of measles virus and utility of the recombinant protein in diagnostic enzyme immunoassays. *J. Clin. Microbiol.* **1992**, *30*, 2874–2880. [CrossRef] [PubMed]
16. Cohen, B.J.; Audet, S.; Andrews, N.; Beeler, J. Plaque reduction neutralization test for measles antibodies: Description of a standardised laboratory method for use in immunogenicity studies of aerosol vaccination. *Vaccine* **2007**, *26*, 59–66. [CrossRef] [PubMed]
17. Chen, R.; Orenstein, W. Epidemiologic methods in immunization programs. *Epidemiol. Rev.* **1996**, *18*, 99–117. [CrossRef] [PubMed]
18. Sundell, N.; Dotevall, L.; Sansone, M.; Andersson, M.; Lindh, M.; Wahlberg, T.; Tyrberg, T.; Westin, J.; Liljeqvist, J.; Bergström, T.; et al. Measles outbreak in Gothenburg urban area, Sweden, 2017 to 2018: Low viral load in breakthrough infections. *Eurosurveillance* **2019**, *24*, 1900114. [CrossRef] [PubMed]
19. Gibney, K.; Attwood, L.; Nicholson, S.; Tran, T.; Druce, J.; Healy, J.; Strachan, J.; Franklin, L.; Hall, R.; Cross, G. Emergence of Attenuated Measles Illness Among IgG-positive/IgM-negative Measles Cases: Victoria, Australia, 2008–2017. *Clin. Infect. Dis.* **2020**, *70*, 1060–1067. [CrossRef] [PubMed]
20. Venkat, H.; Briggs, G.; Brady, S.; Komatsu, K.; Hill, C.; Leung, J.; Patel, M.; Livar, E.; Su, C.; Kassem, A.; et al. Measles Outbreak at a Privately Operated Detention Facility: Arizona, 2016. *Clin. Infect. Dis.* **2019**, *68*, 2018–2025. [CrossRef] [PubMed]
21. Seto, J.; Ikeda, T.; Tanaka, S.; Komabayashi, K.; Matoba, Y.; Suzuki, Y.; Takeuchi, S.; Yamauchi, T.; Mizuta, K. Detection of modified measles and super-spreader using a real-time reverse transcription PCR in the largest measles outbreak, Yamagata, Japan, 2017 in its elimination era. *Epidemiol. Infect.* **2018**, *146*, 1707–1713. [CrossRef]
22. Avramovich, E.; Indenbaum, V.; Haber, M.; Amitai, Z.; Tsifanski, E.; Farjun, S.; Sarig, A.; Bracha, A.; Castillo, K.; Markovich, M.; et al. Measles Outbreak in a Highly Vaccinated Population—Israel, July–August 2017. *MMWR Morb. Mortal. Wkly. Rep.* **2018**, *67*, 1186–1188. [CrossRef]
23. Edmonson, M.; Addiss, D.; McPherson, J.; Berg, J.; Circo, S.; Davis, J. Mild measles and secondary vaccine failure during a sustained outbreak in a highly vaccinated population. *JAMA* **1990**, *263*, 2467–2471. [CrossRef] [PubMed]
24. Strebel, P.; Orenstein, W. Measles. *N. Engl. J. Med.* **2019**, *381*, 349–357. [CrossRef] [PubMed]
25. Moss, W. Measles. *Lancet* **2017**, *381*, 2490–2502. [CrossRef]
26. Rosen, J.; Rota, J.; Hickman, C.; Sowers, S.; Mercader, S.; Rota, P.; Bellini, W.; Huang, A.; Doll, M.; Zucker, J.; et al. Outbreak of measles among persons with prior evidence of immunity, New York City, 2011. *Clin. Infect. Dis.* **2014**, *58*, 1205–1210. [CrossRef] [PubMed]
27. Iwamoto, M.; Hickman, C.; Colley, H.; Arciuolo, R.; Mahle, C.; Deocharan, B.; Siemetzki-Kapoor, U.; Zucker, J.; Rosen, J. Measles infection in persons with secondary vaccine failure, New York City, 2018–2019. *Vaccine* **2021**, *39*, 5346–5350. [CrossRef] [PubMed]
28. Hales, C.; Johnson, E.; Helgenberger, L.; Papania, M.; Larzelere, M.; Gopalani, S.; Lebo, E.; Wallace, G.; Moturi, E.; Hickman, C.; et al. Measles Outbreak Associated With Low Vaccine Effectiveness Among Adults in Pohnpei State, Federated States of Micronesia, 2014. In *Open Forum Infectious Diseases*; Oxford University Press: Oxford, UK, 2016; Volume 3.
29. Clemmons, N.; Wallace, G.; Patel, M.; Gastañaduy, P. Incidence of Measles in the United States, 2001–2015. *JAMA* **2017**, *318*, 1279–1281. [CrossRef] [PubMed]
30. Cheng, V.; Wong, S.; Wong, S.; Sridhar, S.; Chen, J.; Yip, C.; Hung, D.; Li, X.; Chuang, V.; Tsang, O.; et al. Measles outbreak from Hong Kong International Airport to the hospital due to secondary vaccine failure in healthcare workers. *Infect. Control Hosp. Epidemiol.* **2019**, *40*, 1407–1415. [CrossRef] [PubMed]
31. Augusto, G.; Silva, A.; Pereira, N.; Fernandes, T.; Leça, A.; Valente, P.; Calé, E.; Aguiar, B.; Martins, A.; Palminha, P.; et al. Report of simultaneous measles outbreaks in two different health regions in Portugal, February to May 2017: Lessons learnt and upcoming challenges. *Eurosurveillance* **2019**, *24*, 1800026. [CrossRef] [PubMed]
32. Komabayashi, K.; Seto, J.; Tanaka, S.; Suzuki, Y.; Ikeda, T.; Onuki, N.; Yamada, K.; Ahiko, T.; Ishikawa, H.; Mizuta, K. The Largest Measles Outbreak, Including 38 Modified Measles and 22 Typical Measles Cases in Its Elimination Era in Yamagata, Japan, 2017. *Jpn J. Infect. Dis.* **2017**, *71*, 413–418. [CrossRef]
33. Eom, H.; Park, Y.; Kim, J.; Yang, J.; Kang, H.; Kim, K.; Chun, B.; Park, O.; Hong, J. Occurrence of measles in a country with elimination status: Amplifying measles infection in hospitalized children due to imported virus. *PLoS ONE* **2018**, *13*, e0188957. [CrossRef]
34. Rota, J.; Hickman, C.; Sowers, S.; Rota, P.; Mercader, S.; Bellini, W. Two case studies of modified measles in vaccinated physicians exposed to primary measles cases: High risk of infection but low risk of transmission. *J. Infect. Dis.* **2011**, *204* (Suppl. S1), S559–S563. [CrossRef] [PubMed]

35. Ma, R.; Lu, L.; Zhangzhu, J.; Chen, M.; Yu, X.; Wang, F.; Peng, X.; Wu, J. A measles outbreak in a middle school with high vaccination coverage and evidence of prior immunity among cases, Beijing, P.A.R. China. *Vaccine* **2016**, *34*, 1853–1860. [CrossRef] [PubMed]
36. Masters, N.; Wagner, A.; Ding, Y.; Zhang, Y.; Boulton, M. Assessing measles vaccine failure in Tianjin, China. *Vaccine* **2019**, *37*, 3251–3254. [CrossRef]
37. Breakwell, L.; Moturi, E.; Helgenberger, L.; Gopalani, S.; Hales, C.; Lam, E.; Sharapov, U.; Larzelere, M.; Johnson, E.; Masao, C.; et al. Measles Outbreak Associated with Vaccine Failure in Adults—Federated States of Micronesia, February–August 2014. *MMWR Morb. Mortal. Wkly. Rep.* **2015**, *64*, 1088–1092. [CrossRef] [PubMed]
38. Fowotade, A.; Okonko, I.; Nwabuisi, C.; Bakare, R.; Fadeyi, A.; Adu, F. Measles vaccine potency and sero-conversion rates among infants receiving measles immunization in Ilorin, Kwara State, Nigeria. *J. Immunoass. Immunochem.* **2015**, *36*, 195–209. [CrossRef] [PubMed]
39. Brinkman, I.; de Wit, J.; Smits, G.; Hulscher, H.T.; Jongerius, M.; Abreu, T.; van der Klis, F.; Hahné, S.; Koopmans, M.; Rots, N.; et al. Early Measles Vaccination During an Outbreak in the Netherlands: Short-Term and Long-Term Decreases in Antibody Responses Among Children Vaccinated Before 12 Months of Age. *J. Infect. Dis.* **2019**, *220*, 594–602. [CrossRef]
40. Gans, H.; Maldonado, Y. Loss of passively acquired maternal antibodies in highly vaccinated populations: An emerging need to define the ontogeny of infant immune responses. *J. Infect. Dis.* **2013**, *208*, 1–3. [CrossRef]
41. WHO Immunization. Vaccines and Biologicals. In *Surveillance Standards for Measles, Rubella and Congenital Rubella Syndrome*; World Health Organization: Geneva, Switzerland, 2018.
42. Kurata, T.; Kanbayashi, D.; Egawa, K.; Kinoshita, M.; Yoshida, H.; Miyazono, M.; Motomura, K. A measles outbreak from an index case with immunologically confirmed secondary vaccine failure. *Vaccine* **2020**, *38*, 1467–1475. [CrossRef]
43. Hübschen, M.; Gouandjika-Vasilache, I.; Dina, J. Measles. *Lancet* **2022**, *399*, 678–690. [CrossRef]

vaccines

MDPI

*Review*

# Measles and Rubella Diagnostic and Classification Challenges in Near- and Post-Elimination Countries

**Thomas D. Filardo *, Stephen N. Crooke, Bettina Bankamp, Kelley Raines, Adria D. Mathis, Tatiana M. Lanzieri , R. Suzanne Beard, Ludmila Perelygina, David E. Sugerman and Paul A. Rota**

Division of Viral Diseases, National Center for Immunization and Respiratory Diseases, Centers for Disease Control and Prevention, Atlanta, GA 30333, USA; qjf9@cdc.gov (S.N.C.); bfb9@cdc.gov (B.B.); pvw2@cdc.gov (K.R.); xda5@cdc.gov (A.D.M.); uyk4@cdc.gov (T.M.L.); zho3@cdc.gov (R.S.B.); ifw0@cdc.gov (L.P.); ggi4@cdc.gov (D.E.S.); par1@cdc.gov (P.A.R.)

* Correspondence: rhx1@cdc.gov

**Abstract:** Measles and rubella are vaccine-preventable viral diseases and can be prevented by safe, highly effective vaccination with measles- and rubella-containing vaccines. Given the myriad causes of febrile exanthems, laboratory surveillance for both measles and rubella is important to document the incidence of these diseases and to track the progress and maintenance of elimination in near- and post-elimination settings. Diagnostic challenges can hinder effective surveillance and classification challenges can hinder efforts to demonstrate achievement or maintenance of elimination. In this report, we review diagnostic and classification challenges for measles and rubella in near- and post-elimination settings.

**Keywords:** measles; rubella; elimination; viral diagnostics

## 1. Introduction

Measles and rubella are vaccine-preventable viral diseases. Both can be prevented by safe, highly effective vaccination with measles- and rubella-containing vaccines, including measles–mumps–rubella (MMR) and measles–rubella (MR) formulations. The elimination of measles and rubella indicates the absence of a continuous endemic transmission of these viruses within a country. In 2012, the World Health Assembly endorsed the Global Vaccine Action Plan (GVAP), with the goal of achieving measles elimination in at least five World Health Organization (WHO) regions by 2020 [1,2]. However, by the end of 2020, none of the six WHO regions had achieved and sustained elimination. The GVAP also included a target to achieve the elimination of rubella in at least five of the six WHO regions by 2020; the Region of the Americas has maintained the elimination of rubella and congenital rubella syndrome (CRS) since 2015 [3]. The WHO remains committed to achieving and sustaining measles and rubella elimination globally, per the Immunization Agenda 2030 [4].

Given the myriad causes of febrile exanthem in both elimination and endemic settings, laboratory surveillance for measles and rubella is important to document the incidence and accurately describe the epidemiology of these diseases so that immunity gaps can be efficiently targeted. Robust laboratory surveillance is key to documenting the course towards elimination in settings where measles and rubella circulate endemically; laboratory surveillance is also critical for documenting the maintenance of elimination. The WHO Global Measles and Rubella Laboratory Network (GMRLN) provides laboratory support for measles and rubella surveillance on a global scale. GMRLN laboratories perform laboratory testing for case confirmation and use molecular epidemiologic methods to monitor viral transmission pathways [5].

Diagnostic challenges can hinder effective surveillance efforts for measles and rubella, particularly accurate and effective contact investigations, which are key components of achieving and maintaining elimination. The classification of cases is also an integral part of achieving and demonstrating the ongoing elimination of measles and rubella at a national and subnational level. Case classification addressed in this discussion includes laboratory confirmation of a measles or rubella case (or the discarding of a suspected case); the differentiation of primary or secondary vaccine failure cases when measles or rubella occurs among those with pre-existing immunity; the determination of vaccine-associated reactions which can mimic measles or rubella; and the classification of measles or rubella cases by source of infection (i.e., imported, import-associated, endemic, or unknown) [6].

In this article, we use a series of fictional, but relatively common, patient-based scenarios to review ongoing diagnostic and classification challenges for measles and rubella which exist in near- and post-elimination countries. These scenarios draw on the experience of measles and rubella national surveillance teams at the United States Centers for Disease Control and Prevention (CDC); these six scenarios are drawn from multiple different suspected and confirmed measles and rubella cases and are fictionalized to maintain privacy.

## 2. Diagnostic Scenarios and Discussion of Management

### 2.1. Scenario 1

A 4-year-old child was seen by her primary care provider with a 2-day history of fever and maculopapular rash. Additional symptoms included coryza and a mild cough that preceded the rash by 3 days. There was no reported exposure to measles, and no reported domestic or international travel in the 21 days prior to symptom onset. The child had received a single dose of MMR vaccination according to the routine U.S. vaccination schedule at 12 months of age [7]. Laboratory testing was limited to the detection of measles-specific IgM in serum, which returned a positive result. Due to delayed reporting, the local public health agency was notified of the positive result 7 days after the case's rash onset, at which time the child had fully recovered.

A public health investigation began. Given that there had been no reported measles cases during the prior 6 months in the state and county of the child's residence, and there were no clear risk factors for measles infection in the child, the possibility of a false–positive measles IgM was considered.

#### 2.1.1. Diagnostic Strategies for Scenario 1

The detection of measles-specific IgM has historically been the primary mode of laboratory confirmation of measles and is recommended by the WHO as the primary test for measles case confirmation. However, the limitations of IgM testing can be seen in settings with low measles incidence. In endemic settings, where the pre-test probability of measles for a patient presenting with a febrile exanthem is high, the positive predictive value (PPV) of IgM tests would be much higher than in elimination settings, where the PPV would be lower due to the low prevalence of the condition within the tested population [8,9]. The concern from the public health agency regarding the possibility of a false–positive IgM result in this scenario is warranted, given the lack of clear measles risk factors and lack of known regional transmission. Measles IgM is known to cross-react with antibodies against other causes of common childhood exanthems, including parvovirus B-19 and human herpesvirus 6 (HHV6), among others [10–12]. False–positive results can also be obtained due to antibody interference (e.g., rheumatoid factor) or other factors [13]. There are also many other potential viral causes of a febrile exanthem that can present clinically as a measles-like illness, including adenovirus, enterovirus, Epstein–Barr virus, and cytomegalovirus, although antibody cross-reactivity has not been routinely demonstrated for these pathogens [14,15].

Options for additional diagnostic testing to discern the likelihood of measles in this case include molecular and serologic testing.

Molecular detection may be challenging in this case since public health notification occurred 7 days after rash onset; however, real-time reverse-transcription polymerase chain reaction (rRT-PCR) can detect measles in respiratory and urine specimens for 10 or more days after rash onset, although the sensitivity of rRT-PCR drops sharply in all specimens after day 7 following rash onset [16–18]. The collection of both a respiratory and urine specimen may improve the sensitivity of testing overall, but negative results for rRT-PCR in this instance would not rule out measles given the declining sensitivity of rRT-PCR testing after day 7. If the original serum specimen from days 0 to 3 after rash onset was available for testing, attempting to detect measles using rRT-PCR in serum may be a viable option for confirming measles, although the sensitivity of serum rRT-PCR may be variable [18–20]. Additionally, serum is not a routinely validated specimen for measles rRT-PCR and testing it may not be possible for diagnostic purposes.

Additional serologic testing may provide supportive information. Serum IgM is generally present for 6–8 weeks after measles infection; therefore, repeating serum IgM may be an option if the patient is able to provide an additional blood specimen [21]. If the initial test was performed with an Enzyme Immunoassay (EIA) using an indirect format, the use of an IgM capture EIA to retest the acute specimen, or the testing of the convalescent specimen, may be beneficial given the generally higher sensitivity and specificity of capture tests compared to indirect tests [22,23]. If acute and convalescent specimens are available for analysis, demonstration of seroconversion or a 4-fold rise in IgG titer using a plaque reduction neutralization test (or another quantitative IgG test validated for this use) can provide additional evidence of acute measles infection. However, it should be noted that the plaque reduction neutralization test is a highly specialized assay that is not available in most laboratories conducting routine public health surveillance.

#### 2.1.2. Scenario 1 Classification Challenges

Additional diagnostic testing, as outlined above, may provide insight into the likelihood of measles infection in this scenario. However, in the absence of additional information, the classification of this case may be challenging in near- or post-elimination settings and may depend upon local guidance. For example, the detection of measles-specific IgM in the absence of recent vaccination is considered laboratory confirmation of measles in the United States, Japan, and England, whereas Canada requires epidemiologic linkage to a PCR positive measles case or known travel to an area of measles activity to consider IgM confirmatory, and Australian guidelines include IgM as "suggestive" but not confirmatory laboratory evidence of infection (Table 1). Guidance available from Mexico suggests that additional testing such as paired samples or IgG avidity can be used to classify IgM positive cases [24]. Therefore, heterogeneity in guidance from elimination settings may alter case classification in a similar scenario depending on the country and on the availability of additional diagnostic testing.

**Table 1.** Use of IgM for measles and rubella case classification by the World Health Organization and select post-elimination countries.

| Country/Jurisdiction | Detection of Measles- or Rubella-Specific IgM | Source |
|---|---|---|
| Australia | Laboratory suggestive evidence; can support probable case definition only. | Measles: https://www.health.gov.au/sites/default/files/documents/2022/06/measles-surveillance-case-definition.pdf Rubella: https://www.health.gov.au/sites/default/files/documents/2022/06/rubella-surveillance-case-definition.pdf |
| Canada | Laboratory confirmation only if case is epidemiologically linked to a PCR confirmed case or has recently travelled to an area of known measles activity. | Measles: https://www.bccdc.ca/health-professionals/clinical-resources/case-definitions/measles# Rubella: http://www.bccdc.ca/health-professionals/clinical-resources/case-definitions/rubella-(german-measles)# |

**Table 1.** *Cont.*

| Country/Jurisdiction | Detection of Measles- or Rubella-Specific IgM | Source |
|---|---|---|
| England | Laboratory confirmation that can support confirmed case definition. | Measles: https://assets.publishing.service.gov.uk/media/65bb924dcc6fd600145dbe4d/20240123_national-measles-guidelines-February-2024.pdf Rubella: https://assets.publishing.service.gov.uk/media/5c35e849ed915d732cade0a5/UK_measles_and_rubella_elimination_strategy.pdf |
| Japan | Laboratory confirmation that can support confirmed case definition. | Measles: https://www.niid.go.jp/niid/images/iasr/35/410/de4101.pdf Rubella: https://www.niid.go.jp/niid/images/iasr/36/425/de4251.pdf |
| Mexico | Can support laboratory confirmation if additional serologic studies (e.g., avidity testing, paired sera) support acute measles infection. | Measles and Rubella: https://www.scielo.org.mx/scielo.php?pid=S0016-38132019000500492&script=sci_arttext&tlng=en |
| United States of America | Laboratory confirmation that can support confirmed case definition. | Measles: https://ndc.services.cdc.gov/case-definitions/measles-2013/ Rubella: https://ndc.services.cdc.gov/case-definitions/rubella-2013/ |
| World Health Organization | Laboratory confirmation that can support confirmed case definition. | Measles: https://www.who.int/publications/m/item/vaccine-preventable-diseases-surveillance-standards-measles Rubella: https://www.who.int/publications/m/item/vaccine-preventable-diseases-surveillance-standards-rubella |

Note: The access date for all listed websites was 15 March 2024.

Additional classification challenges also can occur if serology alone is available for diagnosis. Cases can be classified according to importation status, i.e., whether they were related to importation into a country after exposure during international travel, or if a case was related to transmission occurring within a country. Without genotyping, the determination of the source of infection for the case may remain unknown. If many cases are reported with an unknown import status, this raises concern of missed importations and missed endemic transmission, which can complicate the case of achieving or sustaining elimination for near- and post-elimination countries.

### 2.2. Scenario 2

A 28-year-old woman presents for routine obstetric care at 12 weeks of gestation; as part of routine screening, testing for immunity to rubella is requested. She lives in a country that has verified rubella elimination. The submitting provider orders testing for both IgG and IgM, both of which return positive results. Public health is notified of the positive IgM result. The patient reported prior vaccination against rubella, although she does not have documentation of this vaccination. The public health investigation reveals that the patient traveled internationally 1 month ago for 2 weeks to a region that has not declared rubella elimination; the patient denies any illness prior to, during, or after travel, and does not report any sick contacts during travel. WHO has not reported any recent rubella cases in the WHO region of travel during the preceding 3 months.

#### 2.2.1. Diagnostic Strategies for Scenario 2

The detection of rubella-specific IgM remains the standard for laboratory confirmation of rubella infection. However, like measles, rubella IgM tests can be prone to false positivity. Causes for false–positive rubella IgM include cross-reactivity, test interference, or prolonged

IgM positivity after infection or vaccination [25,26]. The diagnosis of acute rubella during pregnancy is critical in identifying congenital rubella syndrome, which can occur regardless of the clinical severity of maternal infection [26]. The diagnosis of rubella is also complicated by the high proportion of cases that may be asymptomatic [27].

To avoid unnecessary public health investigations, it is important to note that screening for rubella immunity should include only rubella IgG and should not include rubella IgM unless there is concern for recent or acute rubella infection. Testing using IgM for people without the risk of recent or acute rubella infection would be expected to result only in false–positive results.

Additional diagnostic testing for this case would rely on serological methods. Molecular detection of rubella could be attempted in this case, although the detection window for rubella using rRT-PCR is relatively narrow; rubella RNA is reliably detected for at least 4 days after rash onset [27]. However, detection of rubella RNA can occur further out from rash onset in some instances; in one study, up to 50% of oropharyngeal specimens were positive using RT-PCR around day 8–9 after rash onset [28].

The most informative study in this particular situation would be to perform IgG avidity on the original specimen, or a new specimen if the original is unavailable. Given the high efficacy of vaccine protection against rubella illness, high avidity IgG would suggest prior vaccination or remote (three or more months) exposure to rubella and would be inconsistent with a recent infection. The detection of low avidity IgG would confirm recent exposure to wild-type rubella (or rubella vaccination, if applicable). Repeat IgM could also be considered in this case to evaluate the possibility of a false–positive IgM, including a capture IgM if available at a reference laboratory. Given that the patient would be in the convalescent phase of illness, a repeat serum sample for paired IgG titers may not be informative. Of note, in an instance where serologic testing occurs during later stages of pregnancy, high avidity IgG would not be able to differentiate infection earlier in pregnancy (more than three months prior) from prior vaccination or remote exposure to rubella.

#### 2.2.2. Scenario 2 Classification Challenges

Additional diagnostic testing may provide insight into the likelihood of rubella infection in this scenario. However, in the absence of additional laboratory information, the classification of this case may be challenging in near- or post-elimination settings and may depend upon local guidance. As outlined in Table 1, the use of IgM testing as laboratory confirmation varies among different post-elimination settings. As with Scenario 1, additional classification challenges are introduced if serology alone is used for the confirmation of diagnosis, including the concern about missed endemic spread in near- or post-elimination settings.

### 2.3. *Scenario 3*

A 6-year-old male is seen in the emergency department (ED) for a two-day history of fever and cough, followed by an onset of a maculopapular rash just prior to presentation. He arrived in the United States from a measles-endemic country 14 days before being seen in the ED. Ten days ago, he was seen in a refugee clinic for intake examination and, given that he had no available prior vaccine records, was given a dose of MMR vaccine. With concern for measles illness, the emergency clinicians contact local public health authorities, who recommend rRT-PCR testing; rRT-PCR performed on a throat swab returns positive 2 days later, by which time the patient's symptoms have resolved. Local and state public health authorities contact the CDC to help determine if the patient's symptoms were due to wild-type measles infection or a reaction to MMR vaccination.

#### 2.3.1. Diagnostic Strategies for Scenario 3

Patients who receive live attenuated measles-containing vaccine may go on to develop self-limited fever and rash approximately 7–10 days after vaccination, which can be clinically indistinguishable from wild-type measles infection in some cases [21,29]. The presence of respiratory symptoms cannot rule out vaccine reaction, as it may be due to mild respiratory symptoms related to the vaccine reaction itself, or due to concurrent respiratory symptoms related to other infections that commonly occur in children at the age they generally receive MMR vaccination.

Measles can be detected using rRT-PCR during and after wild-type measles infection, as well as through the detection of vaccine-strain measles virus after vaccination with any live attenuated measles-containing vaccine (including MR and MMR). The duration of vaccine-strain detection is unclear; prolonged detection of measles vaccine strain (>100 days after vaccination) has been reported, although such prolonged detection appears to be rare [30]. The differentiation of vaccine strain from wild-type measles is critical when a person has both recent vaccination (i.e., within 21 days of onset of fever and rash) and an epidemiologic risk for measles, as in this case.

Differentiating wild-type from vaccine-strain measles virus can be performed by two methods. First, genotyping can differentiate the two, as the wild-type virus of genotype A (from which all global vaccine strains are derived) no longer circulates in any country globally and would only be detected after vaccination. However, genotyping is time consuming, and results may be required sooner to guide rapid public health response. Delayed recognition of a vaccine reaction by clinicians and public health practitioners may result in an unnecessary public health investigation which can be costly to jurisdictions and burdensome to patients and providers. Another option when rapid results are required is a specialized measles virus genotype A rRT-PCR (MeVA), which can provide rapid differentiation between vaccine strain and wild-type measles virus in approximately 3 h [31]. MeVA is performed in parallel with a standard measles virus rRT-PCR (MeV); a positive result for MeVA in conjunction with a positive MeV result confirms the detection of vaccine-strain measles virus.

In general, in post-elimination settings, MeVA is only required when there is a known epidemiologic risk for wild-type measles. If a patient experiences a febrile rash within 21 days of receipt of MMR (or other measles-containing vaccine), but there is no identified epidemiologic risk, then the syndrome could be clinically diagnosed as a vaccine reaction without additional testing. However, in near-elimination settings, or endemic settings, where epidemiologic risk may be more commonly encountered in domestic settings, further testing may be warranted in a wider set of circumstances.

#### 2.3.2. Scenario 3 Classification Challenges

In near-elimination and endemic settings, classifying vaccine reactions may require advanced molecular diagnostics. In this case, with both recent vaccination and epidemiologic risk for wild-type measles, serology and molecular diagnostics cannot differentiate the immune response to vaccination or the presence or absence of wild-type measles, respectively, without further testing. In post-elimination settings, epidemiologic risk can generally be more carefully defined (when there is no local active transmission), and classification can be performed without advanced diagnostics in most cases [32].

### *2.4. Scenario 4*

A 24-year-old female presented for the evaluation of symptoms. She reported an onset of fever, cough, and coryza 6 days ago, and noticed a faint rash that appeared on her face 4 days ago; the rash subsequently generalized to her trunk and extremities. She was seen in the emergency department and held overnight for observation but released with improving symptoms 3 days ago; measles testing was not performed. On day 4 after rash onset, the patient's primary care provider alerted the health department of the concern for measles. Vaccine records showed receipt of one dose of MMR at age 2 years. A serum and a nasopharyngeal swab were obtained the next day (5 days after rash onset); these specimens' results returned IgG positive, IgM positive, and negative using rRT-PCR. The health department inquires if the case can be ruled out using negative rRT-PCR.

#### 2.4.1. Diagnostic Strategies for Scenario 4

The detection of measles virus using rRT-PCR generally has higher sensitivity and specificity than the detection of IgM, but there are important caveats to the use of rRT-PCR as a broad "rule-out" for measles. While sensitivity of rRT-PCR is high during days 0–3 following rash onset, some reports suggest that sensitivity drops after this timeframe [16,17]. Additionally, patients who develop measles despite pre-existing immunity (i.e., secondary vaccine failure cases) may have lower viral titers overall and may shed measles virus for a shorter time period, as evidenced by a lower risk of secondary transmission from these cases [33]. rRT-PCR sensitivity can also be negatively impacted if specimens are collected, stored, or handled improperly. Therefore, since the timeline for the collection of the specimen after rash onset is critical for the sensitivity and specificity of the rRT-PCR assay, the rRT-PCR results should always be interpreted in the context of epidemiologic risk, clinical presentation, and the results of other laboratory testing.

Additional serologic testing, if available, may provide clarity to the diagnosis of measles. The use of paired acute and convalescent serum specimens may confirm measles infection (as discussed in Scenario 1). Additionally, given that this case was IgG positive, testing for IgG avidity may be useful; the detection of low avidity IgG would confirm recent measles infection in the absence of recent vaccination [34].

#### 2.4.2. Scenario 4 Classification Challenges

As outlined, additional serologic testing may be helpful to provide diagnostic clarity for this case. If additional serologic testing is not available, either because specialized testing such as IgG avidity is unavailable or because a convalescent specimen cannot be obtained, prioritizing one diagnostic result over another may lead to classification challenges (i.e., using rRT-PCR to "rule out" measles cases despite positive serologic testing). Such broad use of rRT-PCR as a "rule out" test may result in missed cases if applied broadly.

### *2.5. Scenario 5*

A 5-year-old male was seen in the emergency room with a 3-day history of subjective fever and coryza, followed by a generalized maculopapular rash that began on his chest and moved to his extremities. He had recently been exposed to a family member who had returned from a measles endemic country with febrile rash illness; however, measles testing had not been pursued for the family member. Due to mild symptoms, the patient's family did not seek care until five days after rash onset. Serologic testing resulted in detectable anti-measles IgM and IgG, and measles virus RNA was detected using rRT-PCR from a nasopharyngeal swab. The patient had written documentation of one MMR dose at 12 months of age.

#### 2.5.1. Diagnostic Strategies for Scenario 5

In this case, the diagnostic challenge lies not in the confirmation of measles, but in classifying the cause of vaccine failure. It is important in elimination settings to attempt to classify measles cases which occur after vaccination as primary vaccine failure (PVF) or secondary vaccine failure (SVF), and to understand the role that vaccine failure cases play in measles outbreaks [35]. PVF to the measles component of MMR occurs in ~2–7% of recipients of MMR at 12 months of age. In PVF, there is a failure to seroconvert after receiving the measles vaccine [36]. In general, almost all people who fail to respond to a first dose would be expected to respond to a second dose with seroconversion, such that the VE for two-dose MMR recipients is higher (97%) than for one-dose recipients (93%) [37]. SVF rarely occurs, generally after prolonged or intense exposures in a household or other congregate setting. Vaccine-derived immunity is more variable and generally shorter lived than immunity acquired after measles infection, such that ~5% of children lose protective antibody levels 10–15 years after vaccination; however, protective immunity may be maintained even in those whose antibody levels decline over time [38]. Additionally, in near- and post-elimination settings, individuals are unlikely to encounter wild-type measles throughout their lifetime, such that there would not be a boosting effect to stimulate maintenance of immunity. Despite these challenges, measles remains largely a condition affecting those unvaccinated against it. During the 15 years after elimination was declared in the US (2001–2015), only 12.9% of measles cases occurred among people documented to have received measles vaccination [39].

2.5.2. Scenario 5 Classification Challenges

The classification of vaccine failure cases relies largely on the measurement of IgG avidity. The presence of IgG at the time of rash onset or prior to rash onset is evidence of pre-existing immunity, and therefore is suggestive of SVF in vaccinated individuals (i.e., it suggests against primary vaccine failure and lack of prior seroconversion) [21]. However, measles is often not recognized until later in the disease course, and the presence of IgG later after rash onset can be characteristic of a primary or secondary immune response. Therefore, when anti-measles IgG is detected, the further characterization of IgG avidity can be used to classify vaccine failure. Low IgG avidity is suggestive of a primary immune response, and therefore suggestive of PVF, if prior vaccination has been documented [40]. High IgG avidity is characteristic of a mature immune response which develops over the course of months; therefore, detection of high avidity IgG is suggestive of SVF. Measles IgG avidity testing is available in specialized laboratories such as the U.S. CDC. Though measurement of IgG avidity is the primary method for discriminating between SVF and PVF, SVF can also be confirmed via detection of high titer (>40,000 mIU/mL) of measles-specific neutralizing antibodies; as previously mentioned, neutralization tests are only available in a few specialized laboratories [40].

*2.6. Scenario 6*

A jurisdiction in a country with sustained measles elimination reported an outbreak of 10 cases of measles because of a community spread of measles from an internationally imported case; transmission was documented in community settings including an elementary school and the waiting room of a healthcare facility. The outbreak was limited to a single county within that jurisdiction. Outbreak-associated cases had rash onsets which spanned from June to July of that year, and the outbreak was declared over after two incubation periods (i.e., 42 days) had passed after the last rash onset associated with the outbreak. Measles genotype D8 was detected in the outbreak.

In September of the same year, two months after the reporting of the outbreak-related cases, the jurisdiction is notified of a patient presenting with measles compatible symptoms who subsequently tested positive for measles RNA using rRT-PCR; genotype D8 was detected. An epidemiologic investigation determined that the patient had no connection to the prior outbreak and had not traveled outside the country during their possible incubation period. Public health authorities sought to determine if the case is related to a separate importation event, or if measles may have resulted from a chain of undetected transmission related to the prior outbreak.

Classification Strategies for Scenario 6

In elimination settings, the identification of the source of infection for measles and rubella cases primarily relies on the epidemiologic investigation, and linkage to known cases or outbreaks can be performed based on epidemiologic investigation. However, such epidemiologic linkages cannot always be identified. Measles and rubella surveillance includes analysis of the molecular epidemiology of these viruses and is used to track importations and transmission patterns globally and within countries. Identical sequences from two cases can provide evidence of a shared chain of transmission, although it is important to note that without accompanying epidemiologic evidence, molecular epidemiology alone cannot prove a direct linkage between cases. Sequences from measles and rubella cases that are distinct can also provide evidence against linkage in the same chain of transmission if there is adequate resolution to identify the distinction between sequences.

Specimens from measles cases can be assigned to 1 of 24 genotypes based on the sequence of the 450 nucleotides coding for the carboxy (COOH) terminal 150 amino acids of the nucleoprotein gene (N-450) [41]. While WHO recognizes 24 genotypes, there has been a substantial reduction in the genetic diversity of circulating measles genotypes, and only genotypes B3 and D8 have been detected since 2021 [42]. Time-based phylogenetic analysis of sequence variations within a genotype can provide evidence for separate chains of transmission. However, the limited sequence information provided by N-450 may not always be sufficient to provide substantial evidence for or against local transmission. Sequencing additional regions of the measles genome by partial or whole-genome sequencing may be able to increase the resolution needed to distinguish between chains of transmission [43,44].

## 3. Discussion and Conclusions

Despite the availability of robust molecular and serologic laboratory tests for the confirmation of measles and rubella infection, diagnostic challenges for measles and rubella persist in near- and post-elimination settings. As highlighted in these scenarios, many diagnostic challenges can be addressed by the combined use of serology and molecular diagnostics, which can provide complementary information. Although rRT-PCR has high sensitivity and specificity during the optimal timeframe for collection (i.e., within 3 days after rash onset), serology maintains utility for cases where there is a delayed recognition of measles or rubella, in cases where presence of measles virus may be short-lived (e.g., in those with pre-existing immunity), and in documentation of prior immunity and classification of vaccine failure where appropriate. However, it is important to note that laboratory testing results alone cannot substitute for thorough epidemiologic investigation of all cases, since case confirmation and classification is based on the evaluation of laboratory and epidemiologic data.

We also highlight the additional diagnostic and classification challenges that can be addressed by advanced laboratory diagnostics, including the differentiation of vaccine strain from wild-type measles infection, and evaluation for undetected chains of transmission. The resolution of sequence analysis will improve as more laboratories move to whole-genome sequencing. For near-elimination countries, establishing a subnational or national network of laboratories capable of performing such advanced diagnostics is important to be able to demonstrate the achievement and maintenance of measles and rubella elimination. The availability of rapid diagnostic tests will also facilitate the development of subnational networks and will improve the time required to confirm measles cases [45]. The use of multiplex testing for a broader array of causes of febrile exanthems may also help detect more common viral etiologies of febrile rash in elimination settings that mimic measles and rubella and may cross-react with serologic testing [46].

The achievement and maintenance of measles and rubella elimination requires intensive case- and laboratory-based surveillance. Diagnostic and classification challenges persist in near- and post-elimination settings. Integrating epidemiologic and laboratory findings, including results from both serologic and molecular modalities, can help alleviate some diagnostic and classification challenges in these settings.

**Author Contributions:** Conceptualization, T.D.F., D.E.S. and P.A.R.; writing—original draft preparation, T.D.F., S.N.C., B.B., T.M.L., R.S.B. and L.P.; writing—review and editing, K.R., A.D.M., D.E.S. and P.A.R.; supervision, D.E.S. and P.A.R. All authors have read and agreed to the published version of the manuscript.

**Funding:** This research received no external funding.

**Conflicts of Interest:** The authors declare no conflicts of interest.

**Note:** The findings and conclusions in this report are those of the authors and do not necessarily represent the official position of the US Centers for Disease Control and Prevention.

## References


1. WHO. Global Vaccine Action Plan 2011–2020. Available online: https://www.who.int/teams/immunization-vaccines-and-biologicals/strategies/global-vaccine-action-plan# (accessed on 7 September 2023).
2. Minta, A.A.; Ferrari, M.; Antoni, S.; Portnoy, A.; Sbarra, A.; Lambert, B.; Hatcher, C.; Hsu, C.H.; Ho, L.L.; Steulet, C.; et al. Progress Toward Measles Elimination—Worldwide, 2000–2022. *MMWR Morb. Mortal. Wkly. Rep.* **2023**, *72*, 1262–1268. [CrossRef] [PubMed]
3. Ou, A.C.; Zimmerman, L.A.; Alexander, J.P., Jr.; Crowcroft, N.S.; O'Connor, P.M.; Knapp, J.K. Progress Toward Rubella and Congenital Rubella Syndrome Elimination—Worldwide, 2012–2022. *MMWR Morb. Mortal. Wkly. Rep.* **2024**, *73*, 162–167. [CrossRef] [PubMed]
4. World Health Organization. Immunization Agenda 2030: A Global Strategy to Leave No One Behind. Available online: https://www.who.int/teams/immunization-vaccines-and-biologicals/strategies/ia2030 (accessed on 7 September 2023).
5. Mulders, M.N.; Rota, P.A.; Icenogle, J.P.; Brown, K.E.; Takeda, M.; Rey, G.J.; Ben Mamou, M.C.; Dosseh, A.R.; Byabamazima, C.R.; Ahmed, H.J.; et al. Global Measles and Rubella Laboratory Network Support for Elimination Goals, 2010–2015. *MMWR Morb. Mortal. Wkly. Rep.* **2016**, *65*, 438–442. [CrossRef] [PubMed]
6. World Health Organization. Measles: Vaccine Preventable Diseases Surveillance Standards. Updated 14 October 2018. Available online: https://www.who.int/publications/m/item/vaccine-preventable-diseases-surveillance-standards-measles (accessed on 15 April 2024).
7. Wodi, A.P.; Murthy, N.; McNally, V.V.; Daley, M.F.; Cineas, S. Advisory Committee on Immunization Practices Recommended Immunization Schedule for Children and Adolescents Aged 18 Years or Younger—United States, 2024. *MMWR Morb. Mortal. Wkly. Rep.* **2024**, *73*, 6–10. [CrossRef] [PubMed]
8. Bolotin, S.; Lim, G.; Dang, V.; Crowcroft, N.; Gubbay, J.; Mazzulli, T.; Schabas, R. The utility of measles and rubella IgM serology in an elimination setting, Ontario, Canada, 2009–2014. *PLoS ONE* **2017**, *12*, e0181172. [CrossRef] [PubMed]
9. Landry, M.L. Immunoglobulin M for Acute Infection: True or False? *Clin. Vaccine Immunol.* **2016**, *23*, 540–545. [CrossRef] [PubMed]
10. Navalpotro, D.; Gimeno, C.; Navarro, D. Concurrent detection of human herpesvirus type 6 and measles-specific IgMs during acute exanthematic human parvovirus B19 infection. *J. Med. Virol.* **2006**, *78*, 1449–1451. [CrossRef] [PubMed]
11. Ciccone, F.H.; Carvalhanas, T.R.; Afonso, A.M.; Flannery, B.; Waldman, E.A. Investigation of measles IgM-seropositive cases of febrile rash illnesses in the absence of documented measles virus transmission, State of São Paulo, Brazil, 2000–2004. *Rev. Soc. Bras. Med. Trop.* **2010**, *43*, 234–239. [CrossRef] [PubMed]
12. Centers for Disease Control and Prevention. Notes from the field: False-positive measles test—Maine, February 2012. *MMWR Morb. Mortal. Wkly. Rep.* **2012**, *61*, 396.
13. Woods, C.R. False-Positive Results for Immunoglobulin M Serologic Results: Explanations and Examples. *J. Pediatr. Infect. Dis. Soc.* **2013**, *2*, 87–90. [CrossRef]
14. Fappani, C.; Gori, M.; Bianchi, S.; Terraneo, M.; Bilardi, E.; Colzani, D.; Tanzi, E.; Canuti, M.; Amendola, A. Differential diagnosis of fever and rash cases negative for measles and rubella to complement surveillance activities. *J. Med. Virol.* **2023**, *95*, e29141. [CrossRef] [PubMed]
15. Davidkin, I.; Valle, M.; Peltola, H.; Hovi, T.; Paunio, M.; Roivainen, M.; Linnavuori, K.; Jokinen, S.; Leinikki, P. Etiology of measles- and rubella-like illnesses in measles, mumps, and rubella-vaccinated children. *J. Infect. Dis.* **1998**, *178*, 1567–1570. [CrossRef] [PubMed]
16. Woo, G.K.S.; Wong, A.H.; Lee, W.Y.; Lau, C.S.; Cheng, P.K.C.; Leung, P.C.K.; Lim, W.W.L. Comparison of laboratory diagnostic methods for measles infection and identification of measles virus genotypes in Hong Kong. *J. Med. Virol.* **2010**, *82*, 1773–1781. [CrossRef] [PubMed]
17. van Binnendijk, R.S.; van den Hof, S.; van den Kerkhof, H.; Kohl, R.H.G.; Woonink, F.; Berbers, G.A.M.; Conyn-van Spaendonck, M.A.E.; Kimman, T.G. Evaluation of serological and virological tests in the diagnosis of clinical and subclinical measles virus infections during an outbreak of measles in The Netherlands. *J. Infect. Dis.* **2003**, *188*, 898–903. [CrossRef]
18. Riddell, M.A.; Chibo, D.; Kelly, H.A.; Catton, M.G.; Birch, C.J. Investigation of optimal specimen type and sampling time for detection of measles virus RNA during a measles epidemic. *J. Clin. Microbiol.* **2001**, *39*, 375–376. [CrossRef] [PubMed]
19. Heywood, A.E.; Gidding, H.F.; Riddell, M.A.; McIntyre, P.B.; MacIntyre, C.R.; Kelly, H.A. Elimination of endemic measles transmission in Australia. *Bull. World Health Organ.* **2009**, *87*, 64–71. [CrossRef] [PubMed]
20. González-Praetorius, A.; Fernández-García, A.; Pérez-Olmeda, M.; García-Rivera, M.V.; Caballero-López, B.; Gilaberte-Reyzabal, S.; Román-Marcos, E.; de Ory-Machón, F.; Echevarría-Mayo, J.E. Measles outbreak in the sanitary area of Guadalajara (Spain): Difficulty in microbiological diagnosis in the era of its elimination. *Enferm. Infecc. Microbiol. Clin. (Engl. Ed.)* **2022**, *40*, 532–538. [CrossRef] [PubMed]
21. Moss, W.J.; Strebel, P.M. Chapter 38—Measles Vaccines. In *Plotkin's Vaccines*, 8th ed.; Orenstein, W., Offit, P., Edwards, K.M., Plotkin, S., Eds.; Elsevier: Philadelphia, PA, USA, 2023; pp. 629–663.e19.
22. Hiebert, J.; Zubach, V.; Charlton, C.L.; Fenton, J.; Tipples, G.A.; Fonseca, K.; Severini, A. Evaluation of Diagnostic Accuracy of Eight Commercial Assays for the Detection of Measles Virus-Specific IgM Antibodies. *J. Clin. Microbiol.* **2021**, *59*, e03161-20. [CrossRef] [PubMed]

23. Helfand, R.F.; Heath, J.L.; Anderson, L.J.; Maes, E.F.; Guris, D.; Bellini, W.J. Diagnosis of measles with an IgM capture EIA: The optimal timing of specimen collection after rash onset. *J. Infect. Dis.* **1997**, *175*, 195–199. [CrossRef]
24. Román-Pedroza, J.F.; Cruz-Ramírez, E.; Landín-Martínez, K.E.; Salas-García, M.; López-Ortiz, E.; Ramírez-González, J.E.; López-Martínez, I.; Díaz-Quiñonez, J.A. Diagnostic algorithm for the confirmation of cases of measles and rubella in Mexico. *Gac. Med. Mex.* **2019**, *155*, 492–495. [CrossRef]
25. Wandinger, K.P.; Saschenbrecker, S.; Steinhagen, K.; Scheper, T.; Meyer, W.; Bartelt, U.; Enders, G. Diagnosis of recent primary rubella virus infections: Significance of glycoprotein-based IgM serology, IgG avidity and immunoblot analysis. *J. Virol. Methods* **2011**, *174*, 85–93. [CrossRef] [PubMed]
26. Best, J.M.; O'Shea, S.; Tipples, G.; Davies, N.; Al-Khusaiby, S.M.; Krause, A.; Hesketh, L.M.; Jin, L.; Enders, G. Interpretation of rubella serology in pregnancy--pitfalls and problems. *BMJ* **2002**, *325*, 147–148. [CrossRef] [PubMed]
27. Reef, S.E.; Plotkin, S.A. Chapter 54—Rubella Vaccines. In *Plotkin's Vaccines*, 8th ed.; Orenstein, W., Offit, P., Edwards, K.M., Plotkin, S., Eds.; Elsevier: Philadelphia, PA, USA, 2023; pp. 1025–1056.e19.
28. Kanbayashi, D.; Kurata, T.; Kaida, A.; Kubo, H.; Yamamoto, S.P.; Egawa, K.; Hirai, Y.; Okada, K.; Kaida, Y.; Ikemori, R.; et al. Shedding of rubella virus in postsymptomatic individuals; viral RNA load is a potential indicator to estimate candidate patients excreting infectious rubella virus. *J. Clin. Virol.* **2023**, *160*, 105377. [CrossRef]
29. Martin, K.G.; Banerjee, E.; McMahon, M.; Kenyon, C.; Strain, A.; Muscoplat, M.H.; Gastanaduy, P.A.; Rota, P.A.; Mody, R.K.; Ehresmann, K. Identifying Vaccine-associated Rash Illness Amidst a Large Measles Outbreak: Minnesota, 2017. *Clin. Infect. Dis.* **2020**, *71*, e517–e519. [CrossRef] [PubMed]
30. McMahon, J.; Mackay, I.M.; Lambert, S.B. Measles Vaccine Virus RNA in Children More Than 100 Days after Vaccination. *Viruses* **2019**, *11*, 636. [CrossRef] [PubMed]
31. Roy, F.; Mendoza, L.; Hiebert, J.; McNall, R.J.; Bankamp, B.; Connolly, S.; Lüdde, A.; Friedrich, N.; Mankertz, A.; Rota, P.A.; et al. Rapid Identification of Measles Virus Vaccine Genotype by Real-Time PCR. *J. Clin. Microbiol.* **2017**, *55*, 735–743. [CrossRef] [PubMed]
32. Association of Public Health Laboratories. Measles Virus Genotype A RT-qPCR (MeVA RT-qPCR). Available online: https://www.aphl.org/Materials/VPD18_MeVA_Assay_CDC_Infosheet_032718.pdf (accessed on 1 February 2024).
33. Fappani, C.; Gori, M.; Canuti, M.; Terraneo, M.; Colzani, D.; Tanzi, E.; Amendola, A.; Bianchi, S. Breakthrough Infections: A Challenge towards Measles Elimination. *Microorganisms* **2022**, *10*, 1567. [CrossRef] [PubMed]
34. Mercader, S.; Garcia, P.; Bellini, W.J. Measles virus IgG avidity assay for use in classification of measles vaccine failure in measles elimination settings. *Clin. Vaccine Immunol.* **2012**, *19*, 1810–1817. [CrossRef] [PubMed]
35. Mercader, S.; Dominguez, A.; Torner, N.; Costa, J.; Sowers, S.B.; Martinez, A.; Bellini, W.J.; Hickman, C.J. Classification of measles breakthrough cases in an elimination setting using a comprehensive algorithm of laboratory results: Why sensitive and specific IgM assays are important. *Int. J. Infect. Dis.* **2021**, *112*, 21–24. [CrossRef]
36. Centers for Disease Control and Prevention. Epidemiology and prevention of vaccine-preventable diseases: Measles [Chapter 13]. In *The Pink Book*, 14th ed.; CDC: Atlanta, GA, USA, 2021. Available online: https://www.cdc.gov/vaccines/pubs/pinkbook/meas.html (accessed on 1 February 2024).
37. McLean, H.Q.; Fiebelkorn, A.P.; Temte, J.L.; Wallace, G.S.; Centers for Disease Control and Prevention. Prevention of measles, rubella, congenital rubella syndrome, and mumps, 2013: Summary recommendations of the Advisory Committee on Immunization Practices (ACIP). *MMWR Recomm. Rep.* **2013**, *62*, 1–34.
38. Moss, W.J.; Griffin, D.E. Global measles elimination. *Nat. Rev. Microbiol.* **2006**, *4*, 900–908. [CrossRef]
39. Clemmons, N.S.; Wallace, G.S.; Patel, M.; Gastañaduy, P.A. Incidence of Measles in the United States, 2001–2015. *JAMA* **2017**, *318*, 1279–1281. [CrossRef]
40. Sowers, S.B.; Rota, J.S.; Hickman, C.J.; Mercader, S.; Redd, S.; McNall, R.J.; Williams, N.; McGrew, M.; Walls, M.L.; Rota, P.A.; et al. High Concentrations of Measles Neutralizing Antibodies and High-Avidity Measles IgG Accurately Identify Measles Reinfection Cases. *Clin. Vaccine Immunol.* **2016**, *23*, 707–716. [CrossRef]
41. Brown, K.E.; Rota, P.A.; Goodson, J.L.; Williams, D.; Abernathy, E.; Takeda, M.; Mulders, M.N. Genetic Characterization of Measles and Rubella Viruses Detected Through Global Measles and Rubella Elimination Surveillance, 2016–2018. *MMWR Morb. Mortal. Wkly. Rep.* **2019**, *68*, 587–591. [CrossRef]
42. World Health Organization. Weekly Epidemiological Record (WER), 30 September 2022, Vol. 97, No. 39. 2022, pp. 481–492. Available online: https://reliefweb.int/report/world/weekly-epidemiological-record-wer-30-september-2022-vol-97-no-39-2022-pp-481-492-enfr (accessed on 1 February 2024).
43. Masters, N.B.; Beck, A.S.; Mathis, A.D.; Leung, J.; Raines, K.; Paul, P.; Stanley, S.E.; Weg, A.L.; Pieracci, E.G.; Gearhart, S.; et al. Measles virus transmission patterns and public health responses during Operation Allies Welcome: A descriptive epidemiological study. *Lancet Public Health* **2023**, *8*, e618–e628. [CrossRef]
44. Gardy, J.L.; Naus, M.; Amlani, A.; Chung, W.; Kim, H.; Tan, M.; Severini, A.; Krajden, M.; Puddicombe, D.; Sahni, V.; et al. Whole-Genome Sequencing of Measles Virus Genotypes H1 and D8 During Outbreaks of Infection Following the 2010 Olympic Winter Games Reveals Viral Transmission Routes. *J. Infect. Dis.* **2015**, *212*, 1574–1578. [CrossRef]

45. Brown, D.W.; Warrener, L.; Scobie, H.M.; Donadel, M.; Waku-Kouomou, D.; Mulders, M.N.; Rota, P.A. Rapid diagnostic tests to address challenges for global measles surveillance. *Curr. Opin. Virol.* **2020**, *41*, 77–84. [CrossRef]
46. Yasuda, M.; Shoji, K.; Tomita, K.; Uchida, Y.; Uematsu, S.; Yoshida, K.; Kono, N.M.; Funatsu, M.M.; Miyairi, I. Clinical and Laboratory Diagnosis of Exanthems Among Japanese Children Younger Than 6 Years Old in the Post-Measles-Rubella Vaccine Era. *Pediatr. Infect. Dis. J.* **2023**, *43*, e44–e48. [CrossRef]

*vaccines*

MDPI

*Review*

# Building Quality Control for Molecular Assays in the Global Measles and Rubella Laboratory Network

**Bettina Bankamp [1,*,†], Raydel Anderson [1,†], Lijuan Hao [1,†], Elena Lopareva [1,†], Min-hsin Chen [1,†], Gimin Kim [1,†], R. Suzanne Beard [1,†], Yoshio Mori [2], Noriyuki Otsuki [2], Akihido Ryo [2] and Paul A. Rota [1,*,†]**

1 Centers for Disease Control and Prevention, 1600 Clifton Road N.E., Atlanta, GA 30329, USA; rdo7@cdc.gov (R.A.); idn1@cdc.gov (L.H.); ecl1@cdc.gov (E.L.); zvp8@cdc.gov (M.-h.C.); ofi6@cdc.gov (G.K.); zho3@cdc.gov (R.S.B.)

2 Department of Virology III, National Institute of Infectious Diseases, Tokyo 208-0011, Japan; yoshiom@niid.go.jp (Y.M.); otsuki@niid.go.jp (N.O.); aryo@niid.go.jp (A.R.)

* Correspondence: bfb9@cdc.gov (B.B.); par1@cdc.gov (P.A.R.)

† CDC disclaimer: The findings and conclusions in this report are those of the authors and do not necessarily represent the official position of the Centers for Disease Control and Prevention.

**Abstract:** More than 100 laboratories in the World Health Organization Global Measles and Rubella Laboratory Network (GMRLN) perform nucleic acid-based methods for case confirmation of measles or rubella infections and/or strain surveillance (genotyping). The quality of laboratory data is critical to ensure that diagnostic results and country reports to regional verification committees are based on accurate data. A molecular External Quality Assurance (mEQA) program was initiated by the US-CDC in 2014 to evaluate the performance of laboratories in the network. The inclusion of testing for measles and rubella viruses, with a focus on detection and genotyping, plus the diversity of assays and platforms employed required a flexible and comprehensive proficiency testing program. A stepwise introduction of new evaluation criteria gradually increased the stringency of the proficiency testing program, while giving laboratories time to implement the required changes. The mEQA program plays an important role in many processes in the GMRLN, including informing plans for the training of laboratory staff, access to reagents, and the submission of sequence data to global databases. The EQA program for Local Public Health Institutes in Japan is described as an example for national mEQA programs. As more laboratories initiate molecular testing, the mEQA will need to continue to expand and to adapt to the changing landscape for molecular testing.

**Keywords:** external quality assessment; genotyping; measles; rubella

## 1. Introduction

The World Health Organization (WHO) Global Measles and Rubella Laboratory Network (GMRLN) comprises more than 700 laboratories that are classified as Sub-National Laboratories (SNLs), National Laboratories (NLs), Regional Reference Laboratories (RRLs), or Global Specialized Laboratories (GSLs) [1]. Almost all of these provide case confirmation for measles and rubella using serological methods, and at least 119 of the laboratories also perform nucleic acid-based molecular methods for case confirmation and/or strain surveillance (genotyping). The most commonly used methods for case confirmation are IgM enzyme immunoassays and real-time RT-PCR (rRT-PCR). The standard method for genotyping is the analysis of the 450 nucleotides at the end of the coding region for the nucleoprotein gene (N450) for the measles virus (MeV) [2] and of the 739 nucleotides in the E1 gene (E1-739) for the rubella virus (RuV) [3]; the sequence data are used to support the classification of cases as either imported or endemic, and are reported to the global sequence databases—MeaNS for MeV and RubeNS for RuV [4,5]. All six WHO regions have set elimination targets for measles and rubella and by 2022, 83 countries had a verified measles elimination status, while 98 countries had verified the elimination of rubella and congenital rubella syndrome [6,7].

The quality of laboratory data is critical to ensure that diagnostic results and genotyping information are based on accurate and reliable laboratory data. Countries are required to include the results of genotyping in the annual report to the Regional Verification Committee, underscoring the need for accurate sequence data. It is important to note that the GMRLN does not prescribe kits or methods for IgM detection, molecular detection, or genotyping; instead, laboratories have the flexibility to choose assays that can generate high-quality data. The GMRLN has implemented multiple steps and procedures to ensure a high quality of laboratory testing including confirmatory testing, distribution of a laboratory manual and protocols [8], an emphasis on quality during training, distribution of quality-controlled reagents through the International Reagent Resource (IRR [9]), accreditation visits, and the use of practice panels and External Quality Assurance (EQA) programs for serology and molecular tests. Many of these approaches are described in a companion publication [1]. This paper focuses on the molecular EQA (mEQA) program.

## 2. Molecular EQA Process

The introduction of a molecular proficiency testing scheme in the GMRLN required a solution to the problem of sample stability during transportation to international laboratories, especially those in countries with high ambient temperature. Flinders Technology Associates (FTA®) cards provide a means to ship samples as non-infectious materials at ambient temperatures [10]. Virus lysates dried onto FTA® elute cards are rendered non-infectious by the chemicals the cards are impregnated with [10,11]. Panels consisting of tubes with 6 mm disks of virus-loaded FTA® cards (Figure 1) provide a cost-effective approach to distributing proficiency samples that can be used for all steps of molecular testing, including RNA extraction.

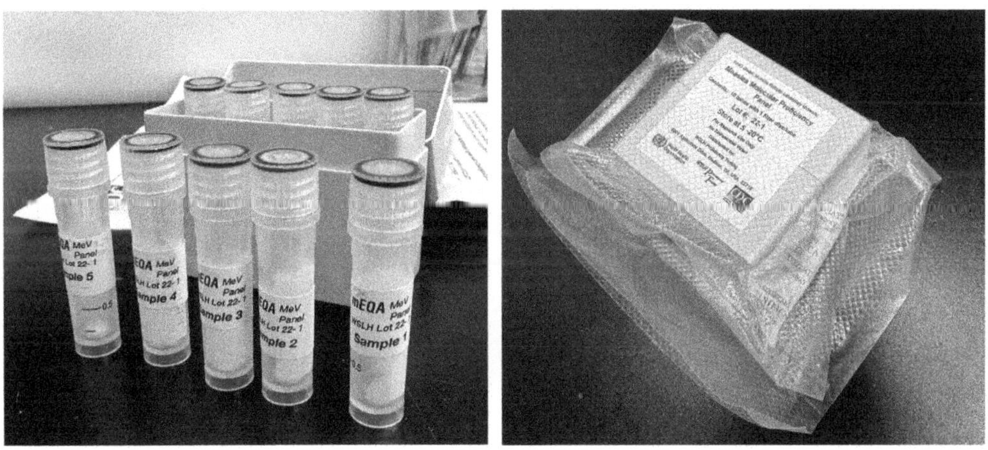

A B

**Figure 1.** Measles and rubella proficiency panels consist of disks of FTA® cards loaded with virus lysates. The figure shows a measles proficiency panel from the 2023 round of the mEQA program. (**A**) Tubes with FTA® card disks. (**B**) Box sealed with desiccant to protect from humidity.

Separate panels are prepared for MeV and RuV testing. Laboratories complete separate report forms for results of the MeV and RuV panels and submit them by email to the US-CDC, together with supplementary raw data such as rRT-PCR results (proprietary files from the platforms, exported data, or pictures of amplification curves), photos of gel electrophoresis, chromatograms, consensus sequences as fasta (text) files, etc. Due to the combination of detection and sequencing and the use of multiple different assays, there is a wide variety of supporting files that can be submitted. The report forms require participants to identify instrumentation, and specify methods, kits and reagents, expiration dates, and controls. This has resulted in a database that has proven useful in cases when laboratories encounter problems; because it allows the US-CDC to connect laboratories that use the same platform or reagents to share experiences. Feedback reports are returned from the US-CDC to the submitter with pass/fail evaluations. Regional laboratory coordinators (RLCs) and the global laboratory coordinator (GLC) are included in all steps of the process, e.g., the identification of laboratories that will participate in upcoming rounds of the mEQA program and the discussion of retest and remedial actions for laboratories with failing scores.

## 3. Changes over the Years

The first lots of the panels were produced at the US-CDC but in 2016, production was moved to a vendor, with most quality control checks of the panels performed at the US-CDC. Initially, this vendor was responsible for shipping the panels but since 2020, shipping has been performed through the IRR [9], which also distributes kits and reagents for the GMRLN. In 2024, the IRR is expected to take over the production of the panels, which will centralize all production of kits and panels at one vendor. After the pilot round in 2014, the US-CDC provided panels for all WHO regions except the European Region, which had a separate mEQA scheme for MeV and RuV, albeit in close collaboration with the US-CDC to harmonize panels and evaluations. Since 2018, the US-CDC has provided panels for all WHO regions. This simplified planning for upcoming rounds of the mEQA program and ensured that laboratories from all WHO regions were evaluated based on the same criteria. Evaluation was divided into detection and genotyping in 2016, and genotyping was further subdivided into evaluation for RT-PCR and sequencing/sequence analysis in 2022. These divisions acknowledge that some laboratories do not perform all three parts of the mEQA program. Division into sections also allows laboratories to separate success in one part of the mEQA program from failure in another (Figure 2).

A

**B. Summary Report**

| | |
|---|---|
| Reviewed by | |
| Feedback report Date | |

**Detection by real-time RT-PCR or endpoint RT-PCR**

| Description | Result | Action Items |
|---|---|---|
| Not evaluated | ☐ | Laboratory did not provide rubella detection results. |
| Passed | ☐ | Laboratory is proficient for detection of rubella RNA |
| Failed | ☐ | Laboratory has failed mEQA for detection of rubella RNA and is not proficient for molecular testing (See comments below). |

**RT-PCR**

| Description | Result | Action Items |
|---|---|---|
| Not evaluated | ☐ | Laboratory did not provide rubella RT-PCR results. |
| Passed | ☐ | Laboratory is proficient for rubella RT-PCR |
| Failed | ☐ | Laboratory has failed mEQA for rubella RT-PCR and is not proficient for rubella RT-PCR (See comments below). |

**Genotyping**

| Description | Result | Action Items |
|---|---|---|
| Not evaluated | ☐ | Laboratory did not provide rubella genotyping results. |
| Passed | ☐ | Laboratory is proficient for rubella genotyping (See comments below) |
| Failed | ☐ | Laboratory has failed mEQA for rubella genotyping and is not proficient for rubella genotyping (See comments below). |

B

**C. Scoring report**

**Detection by real-time RT-qPCR (Points required to pass: 131)**

| Results | Maximum score | Participant score |
|---|---|---|
| Positive control correct result-measles | 10 | |
| Negative control correct result-measles | 10 | |
| Result correct for each sample-measles | 5 x 10 | |
| Positive control correct result-reference gene | 10 | |
| Negative control correct result-reference gene | 10 | |
| Result correct for each sample-reference gene | 5 x 5 | |
| Correct interpretation of all results in report | 5 x 2 | |
| **Assay validation** | | |
| Use of negative extraction control | 5 | |
| Use of positive extraction control or internal control | 5 | |
| All reagents within expiration date | 2 | |
| Submission within two months of receipt of panel | 3 | |
| **Total** | **140** | |

**Figure 2.** Excerpt from the feedback report. Since 2022, evaluation has been divided into three parts: detection, RT-PCR to amplify DNA for sequencing, and genotyping (sequencing and sequence analysis). Laboratories may participate in all or only some parts. Laboratories may pass or fail each part individually; (**A**). Summary report, (**B**). Scoring report.

In 2019, the number of samples in each panel was increased from four to five. In the upcoming round for 2024, a sixth sample will be added to evaluate the ability of participating laboratories to detect samples with low viral load. In 2019, evaluation was changed from a qualitative pass/retest/fail system to a flexible numerical scoring system. This system facilitates the addition of new evaluation criteria and a gradual increase in the number of points awarded for newly added criteria.

## 4. Expansion and a Requirement for Flexibility

The pilot round of the mEQA program was conducted in 2014 with 22 participating laboratories. In the panel for 2022, 119 (MeV) and 108 (RuV) NLs and SNLs from all six WHO regions participated (Figure 3); a similar number is expected to complete the ongoing 2023 mEQA program round.

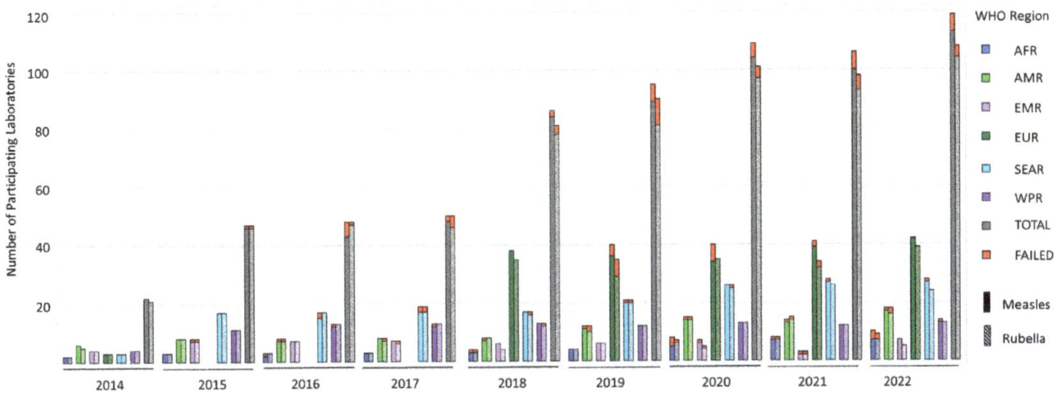


**Figure 3.** Number of participating laboratories per WHO region from 2014 to 2022. "Failed" depicts the number of laboratories that did not pass a retest. Note: The European Region did not participate in 2015–2017.

This expansion was fueled in part by the introduction of molecular methods into many NLs and SNLs during the COVID-19 pandemic. However, the equipment, testing needs, and level of experience vary widely among these laboratories. The African Region has made progress in the past 10 years in increasing the number of laboratories with the capacity to perform molecular assays (and consequently participate in the mEQA program), but is still not on par with other regions. The building of laboratory capacity in the Eastern Mediterranean region has been affected by armed conflicts in the region. The GMRLN is organizing training courses and using a "train the trainers" approach to increase capacity in these regions. In addition, the IRR provides low-income countries with reagents to ensure that measles surveillance is not affected by reagent stock-outs. The inclusion of testing for measles and rubella, a focus on detection and genotyping, plus the diversity of assays and platforms employed required a flexible and comprehensive proficiency testing program. A few laboratories participate only in the MeV or RuV portion of the mEQA program. Some laboratories participate only in the detection part, others in both detection and genotyping and/or sequencing and sequence analysis. Some laboratories perform their own sequencing, others transfer PCR products to sequencing laboratories but analyze the raw sequencing data. This diversity differentiates the MeV and RuV mEQA scheme from other proficiency testing schemes [12–15] and requires corresponding flexibility in the report forms and the evaluation of results; it also requires the evaluators to possess considerable expertise in multiple different assays.

## 5. Improving Quality through Increased Demands in the mEQA Program

The criteria for passing have been significantly strengthened over the years, reflecting the philosophy of the MeV and RuV mEQA program as a constantly evolving process that introduces continuous improvement in quality in participating laboratories. All proposed changes are discussed with RLCs and the GLC before their introduction. New criteria are introduced in a stepwise fashion, usually in the first year as non-scored comments, giving laboratories time to implement the required changes and preventing large numbers of laboratories from failing. In the following year, these new criteria are scored with a low number of points, allowing laboratories to still pass, but highlighting the importance of adapting to the increased demands. For example, a detection assay for a human reference gene is important to assess specimen quality and to distinguish between negative and invalid samples. Increased emphasis on inclusion, correct execution, and interpretation of a reference gene rRT-PCR over several years has reduced the number of laboratories that perform rRT-PCR detection assays without reference genes from 10 in 35 participating laboratories (2017) to 1 in 98 (2022), while keeping the annual number of failures low (Figure 3).

## 6. Remedial Procedures

If a laboratory receives a failing score, the RLC and, in case the failing laboratory is an RRL, the GLC is contacted to discuss options. An immediate retest can be offered in cases where the cause for failure is easily addressed, such as re-analyzing sequence data. In other cases, such as difficulties with interpreting rRT-PCR results, the laboratory will remain in a failed status until either remedial training or a site visit can be conducted. If the problem lies with data management issues (e.g., sending the wrong sequence file), a root cause analysis and corrective action plan will be requested from the laboratory. While a greater number of laboratories may fail initially, this number is reduced after retesting. For example, 14 of 105 laboratories failed the MeV mEQA program in the 2022 round, and 10 of 98 laboratories failed the RuV mEQA program; however, after successful retesting, only 6 and 4 laboratories, respectively, remained in the failed status. Retesting allows laboratories to learn from and correct errors immediately without causing longer-term interruptions.

Over the years, the mEQA program has acquired a central role in many processes in the GMRLN. The results identify training needs in individual laboratories, while trends in inadequate results can inform training activities for entire WHO regions. The successful completion of the mEQA program is required to obtain molecular kits and reagents from the IRR (except for the panels and a small number of kits and reagents to practice the assays). Laboratories that fail the genotyping part of the mEQA program are not allowed to submit sequences to MeaNS or RubeNS, to prevent the submission of potentially incorrect sequences. To prevent interruption in molecular surveillance, these laboratories are required to develop a contingency plan with their RLCs, which may include sending specimens to another laboratory for sequencing and sequence analysis.

## 7. Sub-National mEQA Programs

An increasing number of countries are building sub-national laboratory networks. SNLs decentralize testing, reduce shipping distances, and increase surge capacity to test large numbers of specimens during outbreaks. However, the mEQA program administered by the US-CDC does not have the capacity to provide proficiency panels to SNLs. Instead, countries with large or growing networks of SNLs are encouraged to develop a national mEQA program. One example is the national mEQA program in Japan, where Local Public Health Institutes (LPHIs) have been established by prefectures or government-designated cities as public testing laboratories that contribute to local public health. LPHIs conduct tests for various infectious diseases as defined in the Infectious Diseases Law, and report to the National Institute of Infectious Diseases (NIID) when pathogens are detected.

The Japanese Ministry of Health, Labour and Welfare (MHLW) established guidelines for measles and rubella control in 2007 and 2014, respectively, with the target of eliminating these diseases. Under the guidelines, LPHIs are required to conduct molecular detection for all measles cases starting in 2013 and for RuV cases starting in 2018. Furthermore, if measles or RuV viruses are detected in the tests, LPHLs or the NIID are required to conduct nucleotide sequencing and genotyping.

Since the fiscal year 2016, the MHLW has launched an external quality assessment program for pathogen testing and has commissioned the NIID to conduct the program. Participation is recommended for LPHIs that do not participate in other proficiency testing programs. Two to three pathogen tests are set as assignments each year, from which LPHIs select at least one. For MeV and RuV, molecular detection was tested in the fiscal years 2018 and 2023, and genotyping was evaluated in the fiscal year 2019. Between 68 and 79 LPHIs, which were the majority of laboratories that were conducting measles–rubella testing at that time, participated in these assignments. For assignments in molecular detection, participating laboratories were asked to test multiple blinded samples containing MeV and RuV viruses using the methods that were usually performed. For the genotyping assignment, samples already known to be positive for MeV and RuV were provided for nucleotide sequencing, phylogenetic tree analysis, genotyping, and the naming of viral strains. In these assignments, most LPHIs submitted correct results, but a small number of LPHIs answered incorrectly or had problems (e.g., setting controls). The purpose of this program is not to evaluate or certify the eligibility of laboratories, but to provide an opportunity for each laboratory to check its own testing proficiency. However, when the NIID identifies a false positive or a problem, it points out the problem, provides technical advice and training, and assists the laboratory in solving the problem.

## 8. Considerations for the Development of National EQA Programs

While every country may face unique challenges, there are general considerations that can support the development of a national EQA program, as follows:

1. Identification of laboratories to participate in initial rounds. In some countries participation may be voluntary, while in others, laboratories may be selected by the government.
2. Defining the scope of testing. Countries that are not yet close to the elimination of measles and/or rubella may focus on serological methods for outbreak confirmation and may not need molecular diagnostic assays but should instead focus on strain surveillance by SNLs. On the other hand, some countries may have SNLs that perform molecular diagnostic assays but send positive specimens to the NL for sequencing, obviating the need for an EQA program for strain surveillance. It is also possible to separate the detection and strain surveillance parts into two separate programs.
3. Identification and testing of sample distribution method. Countries with the resources for the fast shipping of frozen samples may choose to generate panels from pooled clinical specimens, which have the advantage of being most like the specimens the laboratories will receive. Countries in which the shipping of frozen samples is logistically challenging may prefer more stable sample types such as FTA® cards. Sample options include cell culture-grown virus stock and extracted RNA. Regardless of sample type, the NL should test the stability of the samples under conditions expected in the field (e.g., elevated ambient temperature).
4. Development of a reporting structure. This includes both the reporting mechanism (email or dedicated website with uploading function) and reporting content. For example, what results should be reported? The mEQA program in the GMLRN created a report form that includes questions about the equipment and reagents used. The report form also explains which additional documents should be submitted (e.g., phylogenetic tree).
5. Execution of a pilot round with a small number of high-performing laboratories. The submitted results should not be scored. Instead, the NL should give feedback to the participants to improve their understanding of expectations and encourage feedback from the participants.
6. Development of a scoring system. The mEQA program in the GMRLN started with a simple pass/fail system but later moved to a numerical scoring system. Stringency should be increased over time to avoid large numbers of participants failing the EQA program.

7. Definition of remedial actions for under-performing laboratories. Will there be an option for a repeat? Will laboratories that do not pass be allowed to continue testing? If yes, what measures will be taken to ensure high-quality results? If no, what steps will be taken to ensure continued molecular surveillance?

## 9. Challenges and Future Developments

Compared to clinical specimens, the RNA copy number in proficiency panels is in the normal-to-high range in the MeV proficiency panels and very high in the RuV panel. Therefore, the panels do not represent the range of viral loads in clinical samples. The copy number was chosen to ensure that the samples give positive signals in detection assays despite inconsistent storage conditions while in transport and can be successfully sequenced. With shipping, the time for testing and possible retesting, and the evaluation of results, a round of the mEQA program takes almost a full year. Over the course of the project, we found that while virus lysates on FTA® cards are more stable than other forms of distribution (e.g., dried RNA), they are not stable at ambient temperature for extended periods of time, especially in tropical countries. However, the high RNA copy number does not allow for an assessment of the sensitivity of detection of the assays used in the participating laboratories. This issue will be addressed in the 2024 round of the mEQA program with the addition of unscored samples with lower RNA copy numbers for MeV and RuV.

Another limitation is that the turnaround time for reporting mEQA program results is currently three months, while laboratories are expected to submit sequence data from current cases to MeaNS/RubeNS within two months of receipt of the specimen. Three months was chosen as the time limit for proficiency testing to give laboratories ample time to complete the genotyping part of the proficiency testing. However, if molecular assays are used to confirm cases, results should be submitted to the national program within four days. RLCs have suggested separate reports for the detection and the sequencing parts of the mEQA program, and this change in reporting will be introduced in the 2025 round of the mEQA program.

A global EQA program faces practical challenges such as stability of the panel during shipping; shipping delays; language issues complicating the use of the report form; staff turnover in participating laboratories affecting access to the IRR for ordering the panels and reagents; laboratories experiencing difficulties in procuring equipment maintenance; and even the possibility of laboratories sharing results. Managers of the mEQA program at the US-CDC Atlanta maintain communications with RLCs to identify and address these challenges, for example, through ongoing stability testing of the panels under elevated temperature conditions for each round of the mEQA program until the testing has been completed in all laboratories; deadlines of three months after receipt of the panel to allow laboratories to address reagent shortages or equipment maintenance problems; communication between evaluators and submitting laboratories if ancillary documents with raw data are missing or questions arise over data entered into the report form; and creation of multiple versions of the panel.

The reduction in circulating MeV genotypes has made routine genotyping data less informative [16] and has created the need to sequence larger regions of the MeV genome, either the non-coding region between the matrix gene and fusion gene coding regions (MF-NCR) or the whole genome [17–20]. Whole genome sequences (WGSs) of RuV are also generated, especially for the analysis of persistent infections [21–23]. Sanger sequencing is used for genotyping in most of the GMRLN laboratories and is also the standard method for the sequencing of the MF-NCR. It is expected that laboratories will transfer the stringent quality control criteria used for routine genotyping to Sanger sequencing of the MF-NCR region. WGSs are usually produced using Illumina® or Oxford Nanopore Technologies® platforms. A separate EQA program for these sequencing methods would ensure that the GMRLN laboratories are proficient in the use of these new sequencing platforms and that

MeV MF-NCR sequences and MeV or RuV WGSs submitted to MeaNS and RubeNS are of high quality.

As stated above, there are no prescribed assays. This flexibility allows laboratories to choose the most appropriate assay, but it complicates the administration of the mEQA program. For example, the introduction of testing for a reference gene was delayed by some laboratories that were reluctant to replace nested end-point RT-PCR assays, which cannot easily accommodate testing for a reference. The different approaches to sequencing (in-house, in a GMRLN RRL, by a commercial vendor) continue to complicate the evaluation of results. The COVID-19 pandemic has initiated a move away from Sanger sequencing towards newer platforms, requiring an adaptation of the evaluation and scoring system.

## 10. Conclusions and Perspective

The success and expansion of the GMRLN is based on the collaboration between colleagues from different regions of the world who all share the goal of improving laboratory testing in support of their countries' measles and rubella elimination goals. The purpose of the MeV and RuV mEQA program is to build capacity for high-quality testing in the network. The mEQA program has proven to be an essential tool for the evaluation of the quality of molecular tests in network laboratories and has acquired a central role in many processes in the GMRLN. The stepwise introduction of increased requirements for passing has improved the quality of molecular testing without putting unnecessary pressure on the laboratories. The mEQA program will need to continue to adapt to the changing landscape in molecular testing, especially considering the rapid evolution of sequencing methods. With the continued expansion of molecular testing, particularly in the African Region, the number of participants in the MeV and RuV mEQA program and the number of countries with independent, sub-national EQA programs are expected to grow.

**Author Contributions:** Writing—original draft preparation, B.B.; writing—review and editing, B.B., R.A., L.H., E.L., M.-h.C., G.K., R.S.B., Y.M., N.O., A.R. and P.A.R.; visualization, B.B. and R.A.; supervision, P.A.R. All authors have read and agreed to the published version of the manuscript.

**Funding:** This research received no external funding.

**Data Availability Statement:** No new data were created.

**Acknowledgments:** The authors are grateful to the Global Coordinator and the Regional Coordinators of the GMRLN for their support of the mEQA program.

**Conflicts of Interest:** The authors declare no conflicts of interest.

## References


1. Rota, P.A.; Evans, R.; Ben Mamou, M.C.; Rey-Benito, G.J.; Sangal, L.; Dosseh, A.R.; Ghoniem, A.; Byabamazima, C.R.; Demanou, M.; Anderson, R.; et al. The Global Measles and Rubella Laboratory Network Supports High Quality Surveillance. *Vaccines* **2024**. *accepted*.
2. World Health Organization. Expanded Programme on Immunization (EPI). Standardization of the nomenclature for describing the genetic characteristics of wild-type measles viruses. *Wkly. Epidemiol. Rec.* **1998**, *73*, 265–269.
3. World Health Organization. Standardization of the nomenclature for genetic characteristics of wild-type rubella viruses. *Wkly. Epidemiol. Rec.* **2005**, *80*, 126–132.
4. Measles Nucleotide Surveillance (MeaNS). MeaNS2. Available online: https://who-gmrln.org/means2 (accessed on 9 May 2024).
5. Rubella Nucleotide Surveillance (MeaNS). RubeNS2. Available online: https://who-gmrln.org/rubens2 (accessed on 9 May 2024).
6. Minta, A.A.; Ferrari, M.; Antoni, S.; Portnoy, A.; Sbarra, A.; Lambert, B.; Hatcher, C.; Hsu, C.H.; Ho, L.L.; Steulet, C.; et al. Progress Toward Measles Elimination—Worldwide, 2000–2022. *MMWR Morb. Mortal. Wkly. Rep.* **2023**, *72*, 1262–1268. [CrossRef]
7. Ou, A.C.; Zimmerman, L.A.; Knapp, J.K.; Antoni, S.; Grant, G.B.; Reef, S.E. Progress Toward Rubella and Congenital Rubella Syndrome Elimination—Worldwide, 2012–2022. *MMWR Morb. Mortal. Wkly. Rep.* **2024**, *73*, 162–167. [CrossRef] [PubMed]
8. *Manual for the Laboratory-Based Surveillance of Measles, Rubella, and Congenital Rubella Syndrome*, 3rd ed.; World Health Organization: Geneva, Switzerland, 2018. Available online: https://www.technet-21.org/en/topics/programme-management/manual-for-the-laboratory-based-surveillance-of-measles-rubella-and-congenital-rubella-syndrome/manual-for-the-laboratory-based-surveillance-of-measles-rubella-and-congenital-rubella-syndrome (accessed on 1 May 2024).
9. IRR International Reagent Resource. Available online: https://www.internationalreagentresource.org/ (accessed on 9 May 2024).

10. Bankamp, B.; Byrd-Leotis, L.A.; Lopareva, E.N.; Woo, G.K.; Liu, C.; Jee, Y.; Ahmed, H.; Lim, W.W.; Ramamurty, N.; Mulders, M.N.; et al. Improving molecular tools for global surveillance of measles virus. *J. Clin. Virol.* **2013**, *58*, 176–182. [CrossRef] [PubMed]
11. Burgoyne, L.A. Solid Medium and Method for DNA Storage. U.S. Patent 5,496,562, 5 March 1996.
12. Buchta, C.; Görzer, I.; Chiba, P.; Camp, J.V.; Holzmann, H.; Puchhammer-Stöckl, E.; Mayerhofer, M.; Müller, M.M.; Aberle, S.W. Variability of cycle threshold values in an external quality assessment scheme for detection of the SARS-CoV-2 virus genome by RT-PCR. *Clin. Chem. Lab. Med.* **2021**, *59*, 987–994. [CrossRef] [PubMed]
13. World Health Organization. Detection of influenza virus subtype A by polymerase chain reaction: WHO external quality assessment programme summary analysis, 2014. *Wkly. Epidemiol. Rec.* **2015**, *90*, 9–16.
14. Pan, P.; Xue, Y.; Gao, J.; Zhu, Q.; Liu, J.; Jiang, Y.; Jin, C. Fifteen years of the proficiency testing program for HIV-1 viral load testing laboratories in China, 2005–2019. *J. Clin. Virol.* **2021**, *142*, 104911. [CrossRef] [PubMed]
15. Potdar, V.; Vijay, N.; Vipat, V.; Jadhav, S.; Gupta, N.; Aggarwal, N. External quality assessment for laboratories in pan-India ILI/SARI surveillance for simultaneous detection of influenza virus and SARS-CoV-2. *Front. Public Health* **2023**, *11*, 1274508. [CrossRef] [PubMed]
16. Bankamp, B.; Kim, G.; Hart, D.; Beck, A.; Ben Mamou, M.; Penedos, A.; Zhang, Y.; Evans, R.; Rota, P.A. Global update on measles molecular epidemiology. *Vaccines* **2024**, *12*, 810.
17. Gardy, J.L.; Naus, M.; Amlani, A.; Chung, W.; Kim, H.; Tan, M.; Severini, A.; Krajden, M.; Puddicombe, D.; Sahni, V.; et al. Whole-Genome Sequencing of Measles Virus Genotypes H1 and D8 During Outbreaks of Infection Following the 2010 Olympic Winter Games Reveals Viral Transmission Routes. *J. Infect. Dis.* **2015**, *212*, 1574–1578. [CrossRef] [PubMed]
18. World Health Organization. The role of extended and whole genome sequencing for tracking transmission of measles and rubella viruses: Report from the Global Measles and Rubella Laboratory Network meeting, 2017. *Wkly. Epidemiol. Rec.* **2018**, *93*, 55–59.
19. Penedos, A.R.; Myers, R.; Hadef, B.; Aladin, F.; Brown, K.E. Assessment of the Utility of Whole Genome Sequencing of Measles Virus in the Characterisation of Outbreaks. *PLoS ONE* **2015**, *10*, e0143081. [CrossRef] [PubMed]
20. Schulz, H.; Hiebert, J.; Frost, J.; McLachlan, E.; Severini, A. Optimisation of methodology for whole genome sequencing of Measles Virus directly from patient specimens. *J. Virol. Methods* **2022**, *299*, 114348. [CrossRef] [PubMed]
21. Abernathy, E.; Chen, M.-H.; Bera, J.; Shrivastava, S.; Kirkness, E.; Zheng, Q.; Bellini, W.; Icenogle, J. Analysis of whole genome sequences of 16 strains of rubella virus from the United States, 1961–2009. *Virol. J.* **2013**, *10*, 32. [CrossRef] [PubMed]
22. Perelygina, L.; Chen, M.-H.; Suppiah, S.; Adebayo, A.; Abernathy, E.; Dorsey, M.; Bercovitch, L.; Paris, K.; White, K.P.; Krol, A.; et al. Infectious vaccine-derived rubella viruses emerge, persist, and evolve in cutaneous granulomas of children with primary immunodeficiencies. *PLoS Pathog.* **2019**, *15*, e1008080. [CrossRef] [PubMed]
23. Zhu, Z.; Chen, M.-H.; Abernathy, E.; Icenogle, J.; Zhou, S.; Wang, C.; Zhao, C.; Wang, Y.; Chen, H.; Si, Y.; et al. Analysis of complete genomes of the rubella virus genotypes 1E and 2B which circulated in China, 2000–2013. *Sci. Rep.* **2016**, *6*, 39025. [CrossRef] [PubMed]

*vaccines*

MDPI

*Article*

# Case Study: Contribution of Extended Sequencing and Phylogeographic Analysis in the Investigation of Measles Outbreaks in Tunisia in 2019

**Anissa Chouikha [1,2,3,*], Marwa Arbi [4], Oussama Souiai [4,5], Henda Touzi [1], Zina Meddeb [1], Essia Ben Farhat [6], Mahrez Yahyaoui [6], Amel Ben Said [6], Chokri Hamouda [6] and Henda Triki [1,2,3]**

1 Laboratory of Clinical Virology, WHO Reference Laboratory for Poliomyelitis and Measles in the Eastern Mediterranean Region, Pasteur Institute of Tunis, University Tunis El Manar (UTM), Tunis 1002, Tunisia; touzihenda@yahoo.fr (H.T.); zinamedeb@gmail.com (Z.M.); henda.triki@pasteur.tn (H.T.)

2 Reasearch Laboratory "Virus, Vectors and Hosts: One Health Approach and Technological Innovation for a Better Health", LR20IPT02, Pasteur Institute, University Tunis El-Manar (UTM), Tunis 1002, Tunisia

3 Clinical Investigation Center (CIC), Institut Pasteur de Tunis, University Tunis El-Manar (UTM), Tunis 1002, Tunisia

4 Laboratory of Bioinformatics, Biomathematics and Biostatistics, Institut Pasteur de Tunis, University of Tunis El-Manar (UTM), Tunis 1002, Tunisia; arbimarwa@gmail.com (M.A.); souiai@gmail.com (O.S.)

5 Higher Institute of Medical Technologies of Tunis, Tunis Al Manar University, Tunis 1068, Tunisia

6 National Program of Immunization Basic Health Care Division, Ministry of Health Tunis, Tunis 1006, Tunisia; essia.hmida@gmail.com (E.B.F.); mahrezyahyaoui@gmail.com (M.Y.); amel3bensaid@gmail.com (A.B.S.); chokri.hamouda@fmt.utm.tn (C.H.)

* Correspondence: chouikhaanissa@gmail.com

**Abstract:** Despite the availability of an effective vaccine for several decades, the measles virus continues to spread worldwide. From 2018 to 2019, several countries experienced large measles outbreaks with genotype B3, including Tunisia. We analyzed 66 samples collected from serologically confirmed measles cases during this outbreak. Fifty-five percent were aged less than 12 months and had not received a measles vaccine. Phylogenetic analysis using the 450 nucleoprotein (N450) window revealed that all strains belonged to genotype B3, with five different variants identified. The N450 sequence of the predominant one, which circulated all through the epidemic period, was identical to the named strain MVs/Kabul.AFG/20.14/3. For better molecular discrimination, the amplification and sequencing of 1018 nucleotides in the non-coding region between the M and F genes (MF-NCRs) revealed higher variability with at least nine clusters. A phylogeographic study using Bayesian methods suggested the Governorate of Kasserine (on the borders of Algeria) as the introduction point with a TMRCA (Time to Most Recent Common Ancestor) for the 2019 sequences estimated around October 2018. These findings emphasize the crucial role of advanced molecular investigations in tracing measles transmission pathways which, together with good vaccine coverage, will help the final success of the global measles elimination program.

**Keywords:** measles; N-450; MF-NCR; Tunisia; epidemic; genotyping; phylogeny; phylogeographic; variability

## 1. Introduction

Measles is a highly contagious, vaccine-preventable disease caused by the measles virus (MeV), a negative-sense RNA virus that belongs to the Morbillivirus genus within the *Paramyxoviridae* family [1]. The standard virus genome size is 15,894 nucleotides (nt) in length and contains six genes encoding different viral proteins: nucleoprotein (N), phosphoprotein (P), matrix protein (M), fusion protein (F), hemagglutinin (H), and polymerase (L). Each coding region is flanked by non-coding regions (NCRs) of variable length. The World Health Organization (WHO) recognizes 24 different MeV genotypes (A, B1-B3, C1-C2, D1-D11, E, F, G1-G3, H1, and H2) based on the nucleotide sequencing of the partial N and the

H genes [2–4]. Since 1963, an effective and safe live-attenuated vaccine has been available and with efficacy against all circulating genotypes. However, measles remains a major cause of infant mortality in the developing world and continues to cause outbreaks in more developed countries [5,6]. In addition to existing gaps in immunization and surveillance programs, the COVID-19 pandemic caused service disruptions and the cancellation of planned supplementary immunization activities, further widening immunity gaps. In response, the WHO collaborated with various stakeholders in 2020 to establish the *Measles and Rubella Global Strategic Framework 2021–2030*, which aims to guide immunization stakeholders at the country, regional, and global levels in planning and implementing more effective measles and rubella elimination efforts, reinforcing the commitment to achieving a world free from these diseases [7].

As laboratory support is crucial for good surveillance, the WHO established the Global Measles and Rubella Laboratory Network (GMRLN) which consists of national, regional, and specialized laboratories that collaborate closely to achieve the global measles elimination goal. These laboratories follow standard procedures to confirm suspected measles cases, either serologically or by the molecular detection of the viral genome, and analyze the genetic characteristics of wild-type MeVs. The laboratories of the network convene annually in a global/regional meeting, are subject to accreditation, undergo yearly external quality control tests, and participate in frequent laboratory training sessions including the serologic and molecular confirmation of suspected cases as well as the genetic characterization of viruses from confirmed cases. MeV genotyping is performed by amplifying and sequencing a 450 nt fragment encoding the COOH terminus of the nucleoprotein according to the WHO manual [8–11]. In 2008, the WHO GMRLN established the Measles Nucleotide Surveillance (MeaNS) database to collect and archive measles virus sequences from all regions. Laboratories within the GMRLN use the MeaNS global database to submit their N450 nucleotide sequences and monitor the global circulation of measles genotypes [3]. Identical N450 sequences are represented by a Distinct Sequence Identification (DSId). Epidemiologically significant sequences that are circulating in several countries are defined as "Named strains" and are used to track transmission patterns for viruses within a single genotype. Circulating strains are linked to named strains which allows a finer mapping of measles transmission than the use of genotyping alone [3].

In recent years, the only reported MeV genotypes are B3 and D8, while the other genotypes have not been detected. This is due to the significant increase in vaccination coverage, which has greatly reduced the diversity of circulating measles viruses [7]. As genetic diversity decreases, the standard N450 sequences may show very low diversity during large outbreaks involving one or multiple countries, with identical sequences. Furthermore, when monitoring measles transmission within a country or region over time, N450 sequences generally do not enable differentiation between ongoing endemic circulation of a MeV variant and multiple new introductions [4,12,13]. To enhance the resolution of molecular epidemiology analysis, especially in this final phase of elimination, sequencing a larger fragment in other hypervariable genomic regions has been proposed. The MF-NCR, located between the fusion and matrix genes, is one of the most variable regions of the measles virus genome and has shown the better resolution of the virus circulation patterns. It is now proposed as a new target for MeV molecular characterization [13–17].

In Tunisia, the measles vaccine was introduced into the national program of immunization in 1983 with two doses of the vaccine given at varying ages: 9 months and 15 months from 1983 to 1998; 15 months and 6 years from 1999 to 2012; and 12 months and 18 months starting from 2013. The vaccination coverage has achieved levels over 90% nationwide over the last decade and, as a results, measles incidence has considerably decreased. The last large outbreak of measles occurred in 1992 with more than 11,000 cases [18]. A measles/rubella national elimination goal was established in 1998 [17]. Since then, few serologically confirmed measles cases have been reported, and are generally less than 20 cases per year except in 2002 (72 confirmed cases) and in 2012 (48 confirmed cases) [18,19].

In 2019, together with many other countries in the world, Tunisia experienced a nationwide measles outbreak [19,20] with a total of 4698 measles cases, among which 1208 were serologically confirmed, 1174 were epi-linked, and 2316 were clinically compatible. The outbreak also resulted in 39 deaths, most of them occurring in infants of less than one year old or in adults suffering from immunodeficiency or other debilitating illnesses [21].

Concurrently, outbreaks occurred in nearby countries, notably Libya and Algeria, as well as in France and Italy, which have substantial population movements with Tunisia. This raised the possibility of virus importation at the origin of the outbreak. The initial cases were detected in two governorates: Kasserine, located in the west near the Algerian border, and Sfax, on the east coast, which frequently receives people from Libya and Algeria for healthcare services. During the 2019 outbreak, Sfax and Kasserine were the most affected areas of the reported cases. However, no epidemiological evidence of importation from Libya to Sfax or from Algeria to Kasserine was found and no clear epidemiological link could be established between the cases in the two Tunisian governorates.

The aim of this study is to assess the genetic variability of MeVs strains from patients infected during the 2019 outbreak in Tunisia and to study the dynamics of virus spread during the outbreak by analyzing the N450 and MF-NCR sequences.

## 2. Materials and Methods

### 2.1. Clinical Specimens

This study was conducted on 88 samples collected from 88 positive cases of serologically confirmed measles (n = 48, throat swab; n = 39, oral fluid; and n = 1, urine). The samples were collected from suspected measles cases in Tunisia between January and December 2019 and were stored at the Laboratory of Clinical Virology in Pasteur Institute of Tunis, which serves as the national laboratory for MeVs detection and genotyping and as a WHO regional reference laboratory in the eastern mediterranean region (EMR).

### 2.2. PCR Amplification and Sequencing

For PCR amplification and sequencing, we used US-CDC RT-PCR methods, as outlined in the WHO lab manual [8]. Viral RNA was extracted using QIAamp viral RNA mini Kit (Qiagen, Hilden, Germany) from 140 µL of clinical specimens, according to the manufacturer's instructions. The extracted RNAs were assessed for virus detection by real time RT-PCR [8] and for genome amplification were reverse transcribed and then amplified by PCR in the nucleoprotein and the MF-NCRs of the genome. In the nucleoprotein region, a 634 nucleotide-long (nt) fragment in the 5′ terminus of the nucleocapsid protein gene was amplified using WHO-recommended primers (MeV216-Forward: 5′-TGG AGC TAT GCC ATG GGA GT-3′; MeV214-Reverse: 5′-TAA CAA TGA TGG AGG GTA GG-3′) provided by CDC-USA. In the MF-NCR, a fragment of 1018 nt was deduced for each samples from two overlapping fragments amplified using the following primers, also provided by US-CDC: fragment 1 (MeV4331-Forward: 5′-CAG ATG CAA GAT AGT AAG AAT CCA G-3′; V4869-Reverse: 5′-CCT GGC CCT CAG TTT TGT TTA G-3′) and fragment 2 (MeVg22-Forward: 5′-CAC AAG CGA CCG AGG TGA C-3′; MeV5145R-Reverse: 5′-GGT TGC CGT GGT CGT GTG TG-3′).

RT-PCR was performed using the One-Step RT-PCR kit (Invitrogen Superscript III One-step RT-PCR with Platinum, Canada) using the CDC-USA standard protocol. In a total volume of 50 µL containing 5 µL extracted RNA, 0.6 µM of each primer, and 0.4 µM of dNTPs were used. The amplification conditions included an initial reverse transcription step of 30 min at 50 °C, followed by a denaturation step of 15 min at 95 °C then by 40 cycles of 95 °C for 30 s, 55 °C (N-gene)/56 °C (MF-NCR) for 30 s, and 72 °C for 30 s, and a final extension step was performed at 72 °C for 10 min.

Amplicons were then purified and sequenced, in both directions, with the ABI Big Dye Terminator Cycle Sequencing Kit (Applied Biosystems, Branchburg, NJ, USA) using the same primers described above and used for PCR amplification.

### 2.3. Sequence Analyses and Phylogeny

The N-450 and MF-NCR sequences of each virus strain were obtained by aligning the forward and reverse sequences using Sequencher® 5.1.4 software. The N450 sequences were submitted to the Measles Nucleotide Sequencing database (MeaNS) and the MF-NCR sequences were submitted to GenBank under accession numbers MT211788-MT211848.

Sequence alignment was performed using MEGA software version 7 and default parameters. The resulting alignment was used to build a maximum likelihood phylogenetic tree using the IQ-TREE web server, supported by 1000 bootstrap replicates (http://iqtree.cibiv.univie.ac.at/) (accessed on 18 May 2024). Midpoint rooting was used for visualization using Figtree software (http://tree.bio.ed.ac.uk/software/figtree/) (accessed on 18 May 2024). The tree was rooted using the midpoint rooting method.

### 2.4. Phylogeography Analysis

Bayesian phylogeography was performed by generating a time-scaled Maximum Clade Credibility (MCC) phylogenetic tree using BEAST v.1.8.4 package. The Bayesian Markov Monte Carlo chain was run for 300 million iterations (sampling every 10,000 states) using the uncorrelated relaxed clock and the skyline tree models. A Bayesian stochastic search variable selection (BSSVS) with a symmetrical discrete trait substitution model and a strict clock assumption were implemented to construct the Bayes factor test and were used to identify the transmission routes between Tunisian regions [22].

The most important parameter estimates (Posterior, Prior, Kappa, clock rate, TMRCA, TreeModel.rootHeight, treeLength, treeLikelihood, and Gamma shape) exhibited a valid effective sampling size (ESS > 200). The MCC tree was generated by Tree Annotator v1.8.4 after removing 10% burn-in and was then visualized in FigTree v.1.4.3 (http://tree.bio.ed.ac.uk/software/figtree/) (accessed on 18 May 2024). The Time To the Most Recent Common Ancestor (TMRCA) and its 95% highest posterior density (95% HPD) was estimated using FigTree v.1.4.3. A posterior probability (pp) of >0.85 means that the MCC tree node has good statistical support [23]. Bayes factors for discrete state transitions were calculated with SpreadD3map of Google Earth Pro (https://www.google.com/earth/versions/) (accessed on 18 May 2024). The Bayes Factor was also calculated with SpreadD3. BF > 3 indicates statistical support for the transitions.

## 3. Results

### 3.1. Epidemiological Data

Of the 88 samples from serologically confirmed cases included in the study, 66 were amplified in the N450 region, among which 61 were also amplified in the MF-NCR. The remaining 22 samples were not amplified in both genomic regions. Their Ct values obtained from the real-time PCR tests were over 34, which indicates a low viral load. The 66 cases comprised 35 females and 31 male, aged 1 month to 62 years. Thirty-six patients were under one year old and were thus unvaccinated, ten were infants aged between 1 and 13 years, and twenty were adults aged between 24 and 62 years.

The studied samples originated from almost all the governorates of Tunisia; only four governorates (Béjà, Jendouba, Medenine, and Siliana) were not represented. These governorates were the less affected by the outbreak, accounting, together, for almost 1% of the nationally recorded measles cases. Figure 1 shows their distribution by date of sample collection together with the total number of suspected cases recorded by the Ministry of Health. The 66 cases were spread across almost the entire outbreak period. Figure S1 shows their distribution by date of sample collection during the outbreak period.

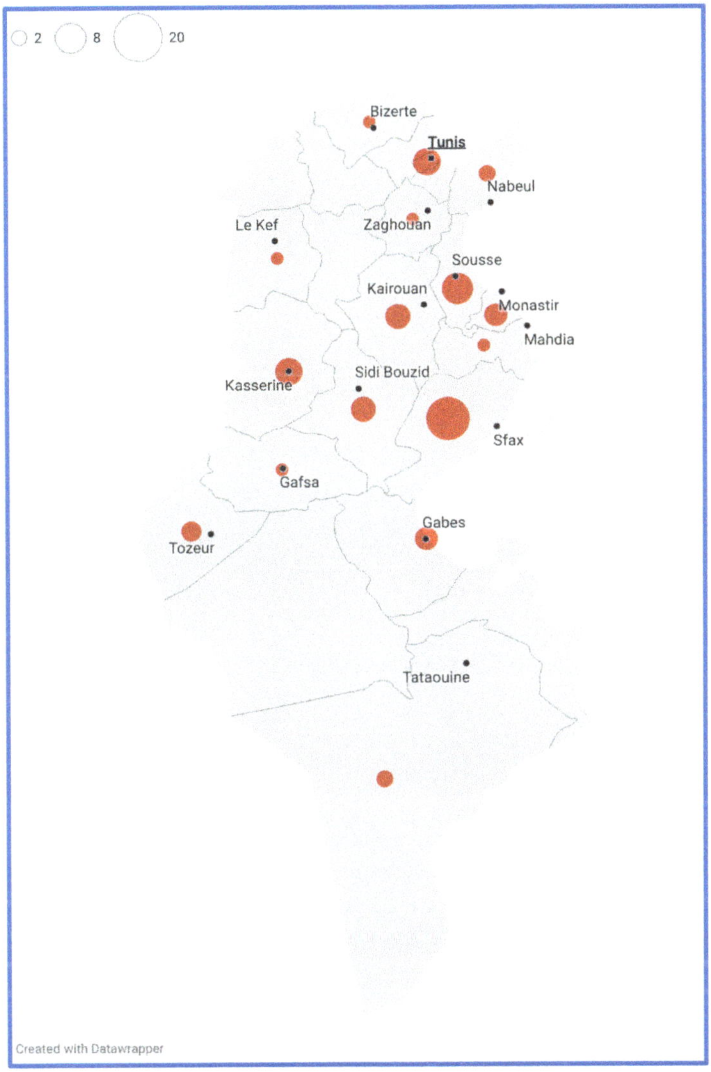


**Figure 1.** Distribution of the 66 genotyped measles cases during the 2019 outbreak in Tunisia by governorate. The map was created with Datawrapper (https://www.datawrapper.de/) (accessed on 18 May 2024). The size of the circles on the map correspond to the number of cases; larger circles indicate a higher number of cases.

### *3.2. Measles Virus Genotyping*

A measles virus genotype was successfully determined by the sequencing of the N450 region of the 66 studied samples obtained from measles-positive cases.

Figure 2 compares the Tunisian sequences with the WHO reference sequences representative of all measles genotypes. The phylogenetic analysis revealed that all Tunisian sequences belonged to genotype B3, according to the topology of the phylogenetic tree shown in Figure 2.

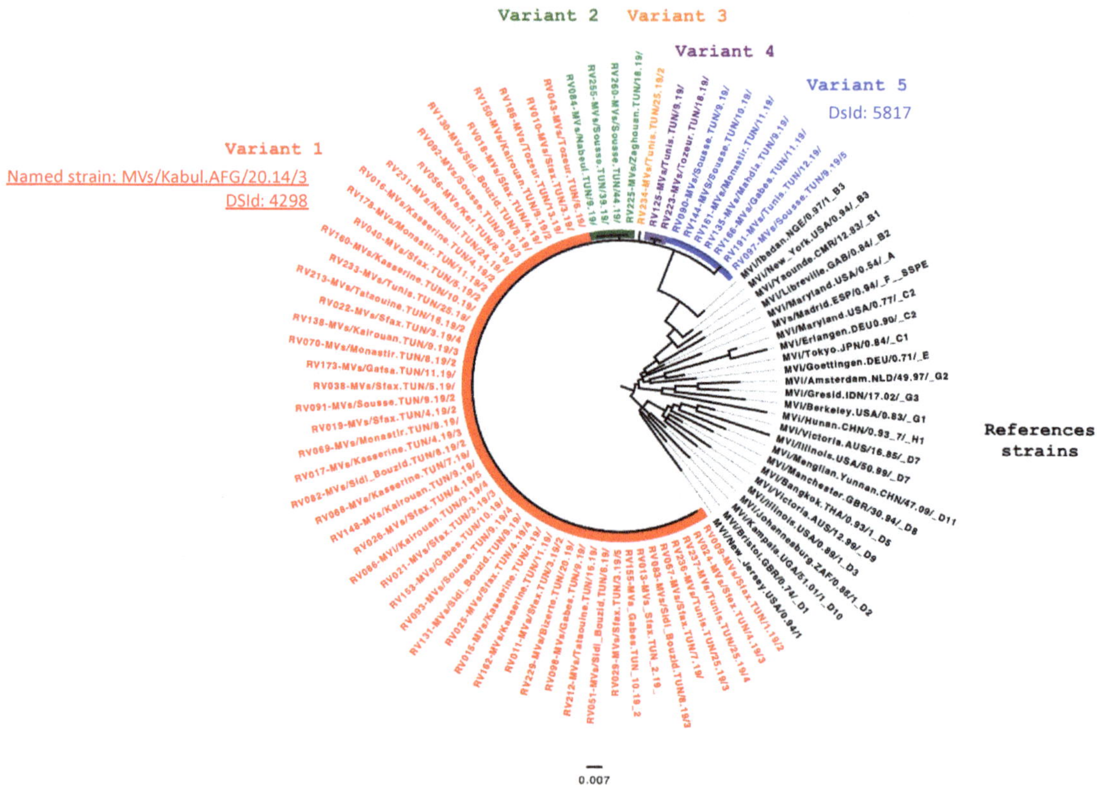


**Figure 2.** Phylogenetic tree of 66 measles virus N450 sequences from Tunisia (2019) compared with the 28 reference sequences. This tree compares 66 N450 sequences of measles viruses collected in Tunisia from week 1 to week 44 in 2019 with 28 reference sequences representing the 24 genotypes (each of the genotypes B3, C2, D5, and D7 are represented by 2 reference sequences). The tree highlights five different variants: Variant 1 (DSId: 4298) (in red) comprises fifty sequences; Variant 2 (DSId: 5847) (in green) comprises four sequences; Variant 3 (DSId: 6067) (in orange) comprises one sequence; Variant 4 (DSId: 5846) (in purple) comprises two sequences; and Variant 5 (DsId: 5817) (in blue) comprises seven sequences. The sequence names are formatted as Lab code–WHO name. The tree was constructed using the maximum likelihood method via the IQ Tree web server and was visualized using FigTree. The topology is supported by 1000 bootstrap replicates.

The most frequently detected variant (Variant 1) represented in red in Figure 3 comprises 50 sequences identical to the named strain MVs/Kabul.AFG/20.14/3 with the Distinct Sequence ID (DSId: 4298). As of 20 May 2024, this strain is widely distributed across 27 countries on 5 continents. The sequences for this variant were obtained from patients from 14 different governorates in Tunisia.

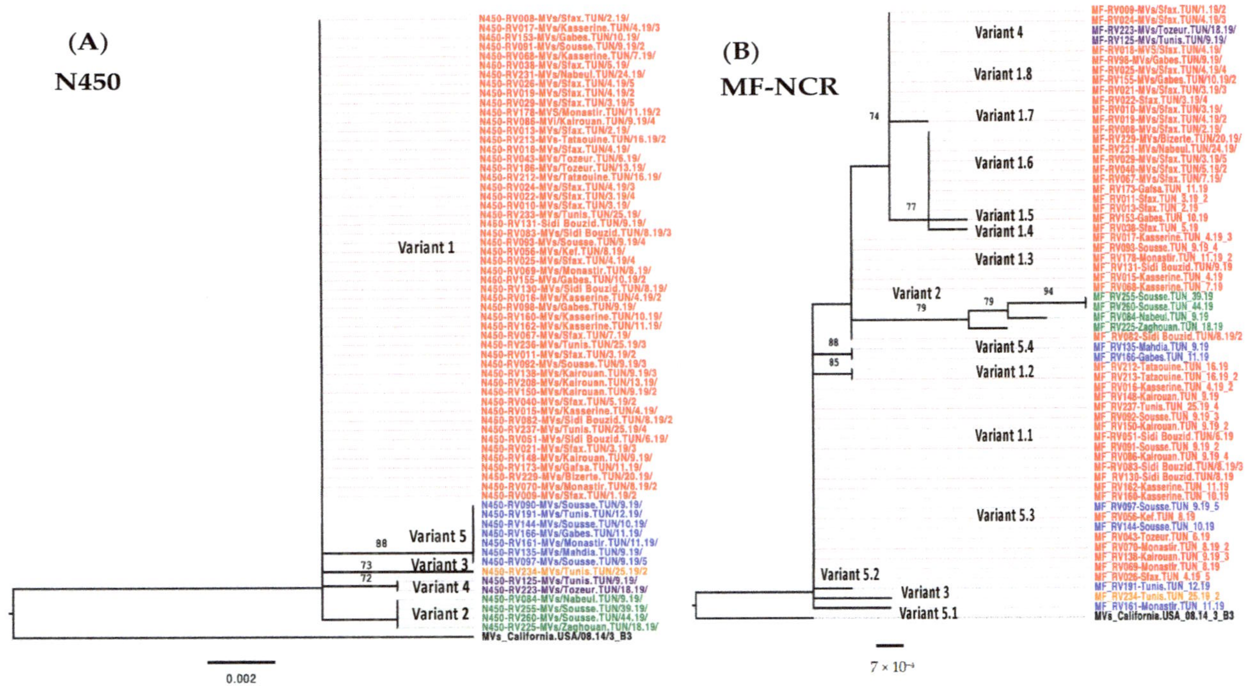


**Figure 3.** Phylogenetic trees comparing the N450 and the MF-NCR sequences of 66 vs. 61 Tunisian sequences, respectively. (**A**) Sequences representing the 450 nt in the C-terminal nucleoprotein gene of the measles genome. (**B**) Sequences representing 1018 nt in the non-coding MF-NCR of the measles genome. The trees were constructed using the maximum likelihood method via the IQ Tree web server and were visualized using FigTree. The topology was supported by 1000 bootstrap replicates.

According to the MeaNS database exact match analysis, no named strain was associated with the sequences of the other four variants. The sequences of Variant 5 (DsId: 5817), shown in blue, originated from four governorates on the eastern coast of Tunisia and were identical to the measles sequences detected in Valence, France, in early 2019.

The sequences from the remaining three Variants 2, 3, and 4 were new and had no identical matches in the MeaNS database with DSIds: 5847, 6067, and 5846, respectively.

Low variability was observed between the different variants in the N450 region as follows: Variants 2 and 4 differed from Variant 1 by one mutation in nucleotides 285 and 312, respectively; Variants 3 and 5 differed from Variant 1 by two mutations in nucleotides 57 and 176 and 13 and 87, respectively.

### 3.3. Phylogenetic Analyses in the MF-NCR

The MF-NCRs of the 61 Tunisian samples were successfully amplified and sequenced. All sequences were 1018 nt in length with no insertions or deletions detected.

The phylogenetic analysis showed a higher genetic variability as compared to the N-450 region, with at least 13 different clusters (Figure 3). The sequences from the major N450 Variant 1 were divided into eight different clusters in the MF-NCR. The sequences obtained from N450 Variant 5 (in blue) were divided into four different clusters in the MF-NCR. The sequences obtained from the N450 Variants 2, 3, and 4 remained together in the MF-NCR (Figure 3).

Figure 4 shows the circulation of the different variants in both N450 (Figure 4A) and MF-NCR (Figure 4B) during the outbreak period. The N450 Variant 1 (red) circulated from week 1 to week 25, suggesting that the same strain would have circulated throughout the outbreak. Concurrently, analysis of the MF-NCR revealed that this variant actually consisted of eight different variants during the same period, all sharing the exact same N450 sequence. For example, Subvariant 1.8 (Figure 4B) circulated from week 1 to week 10, Subvariant 1.6 circulated from week 2 to week 24, and Subvariant 1.1 circulated from week 4 to week 25.

A similar pattern was observed with the N450 Variant 5 (blue), which divided into four distinct variants in the MF-NCR (Figures 3 and 4). This variant was detected from week 9 to week 12. For Variant 3, represented in orange, only one sequence was detected in week 25, while two sequences were identified for Variant 4, represented in purple, detected sporadically in weeks 9 and 18; these sequences clustered alone in both the N450 and the MF-NCR. The N450 Variant 2 (green) included four identical N450 sequences that clustered together in the MF-NCR, despite the few mutations among them. This latter variant would have been circulating at least from week 9 to week 44.

### 3.4. Spatio-Temporal Dynamics of Measles Virus Circulating in Tunisia in 2019

From the dataset composed of the 61 measles MF-NCR sequences (1018 nt), the MCC (Maximum Clade Credibility) tree was built and used to explore the temporal origin of the selected dataset by determining the TMRCA (Time to Most Recent Common Ancestor) (Figure S1). According to the molecular clock analysis, the TMRCA for the measles virus that circulated in Tunisia in 2019 was estimated to be around October 2018 (pp = 0.99) (Figure 5A). For N450, the TMRCA estimation showed that the first introduction of measles virus in Tunisia was in April 2019 (pp = 0.95) (Figure S2.1).

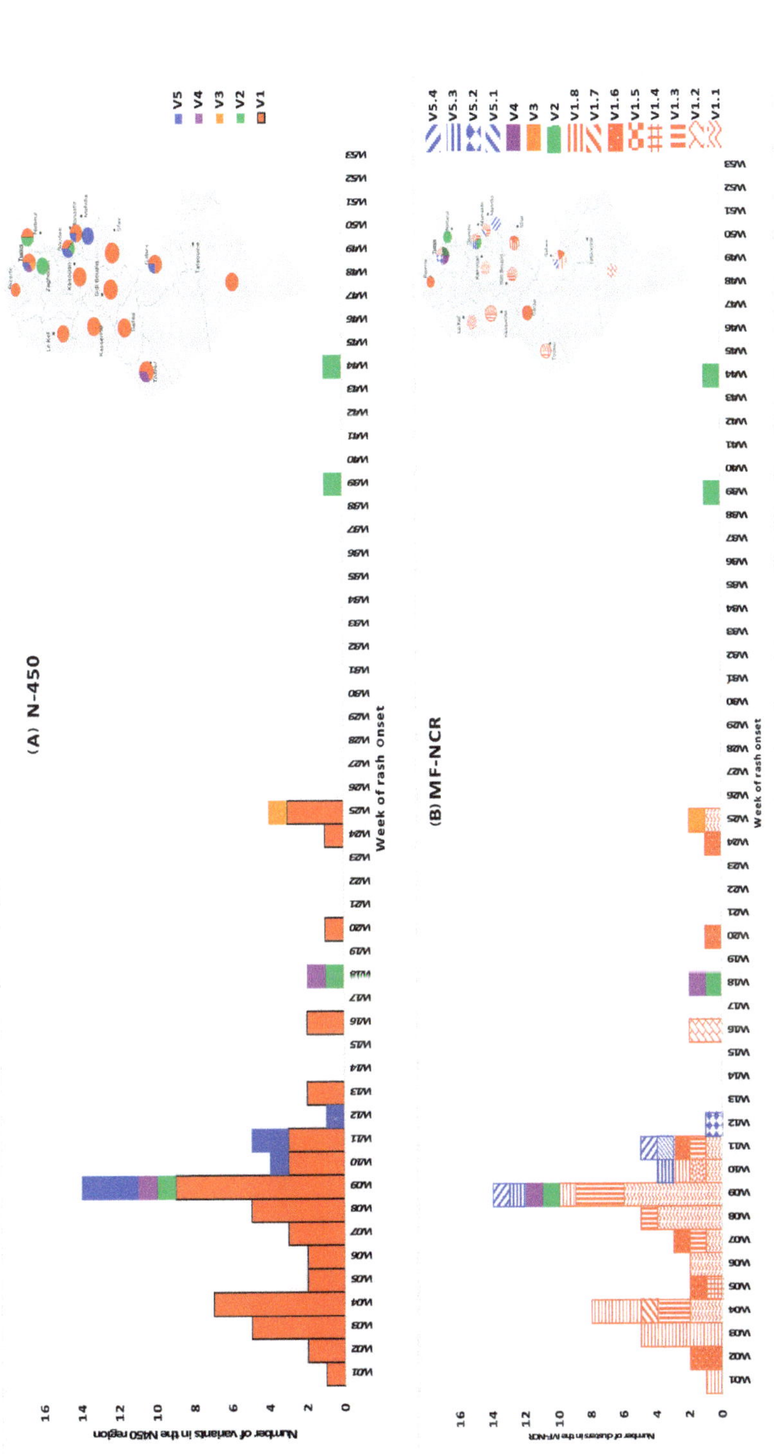


**Figure 4.** Timeline and origin of detection of the different measles virus variants identified in the N450 region (**A**) and in the MF-NCR (**B**), Tunisia 2019.

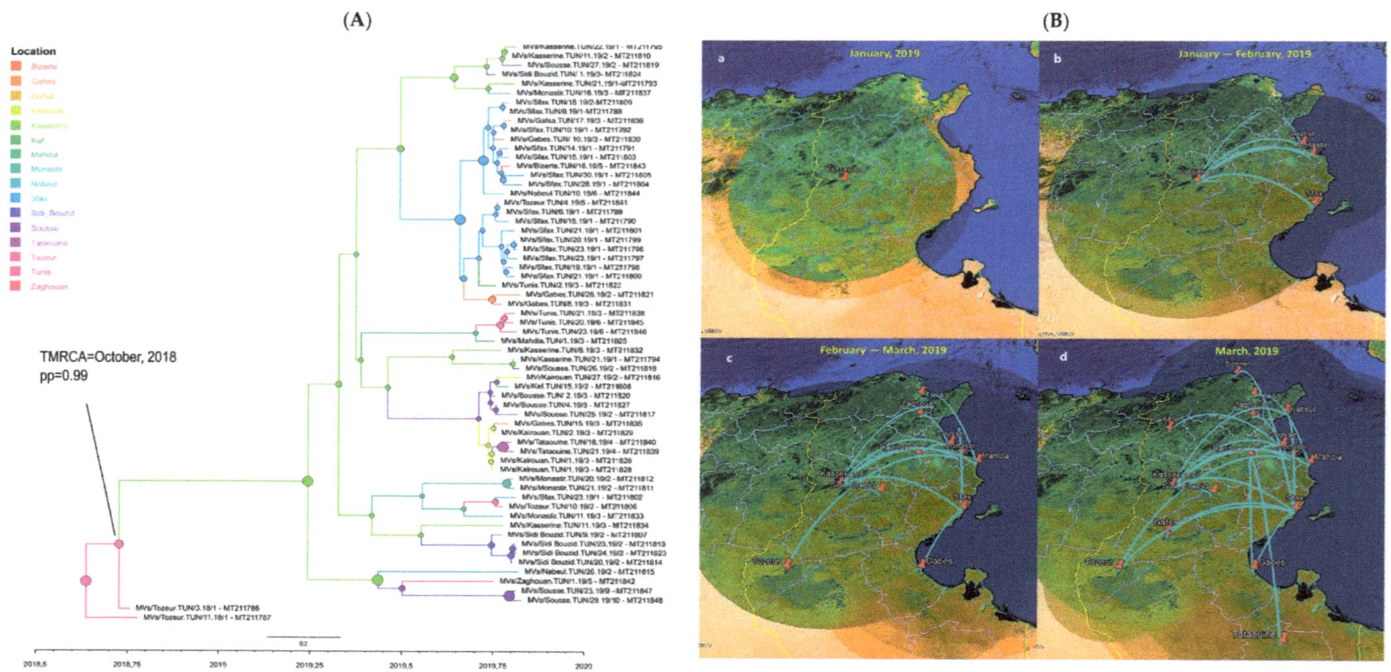


**Figure 5.** The phylodynamics of the measles virus detected in Tunisia in 2019 based on the MF-NCR. (**A**) Bayesian time-scaled MCC tree of the measles virus isolated from Tunisian governorates. The nodes and branches of the MCC tree are colored to illustrate the relevant Tunisian governorates. Node diameters are sized according to posterior probabilities. (**B**) Spatio-temporal dynamics of the B3 measles virus that circulated in Tunisia in 2019 among different Tunisian governorates. The maps (**a–d**) illustrate the various stages of virus spread across the governorates. Transition lines connecting different locations represent the branches in the MCC tree. The diameters of the circles are proportional to the square root of the number of MCC branches that maintain a particular location state at each time point.

To investigate the spatio-temporal dynamics of the B3 measles spread in Tunisia in 2019, a Bayesian phylogeographic framework based on MF-NCR sequences was constructed (Figure 5B). Figure 5(Bb) illustrates the routes of transmission of the epidemic measles viruses from where the outbreak started and how it spread across the country. The generated spatial dynamics confirmed that the initial point of propagation was the governorate of Kasserine (center west of the country), located on the border with Algeria. From Kasserine, the virus spread to other Tunisian governorates (Figure 5(Ba)).

During the January–February period 2019, the virus emerged in the coastal governorates, notably Sousse (BF = 15.59), Monastir (BF = 53), and Sfax (BF = 3.46) (Figure 5(Bb)). By February–March 2019, the epidemic extended further, reaching all governorates, namely in the northern (Zaghouan, Nabeul, Tunis, Kef), in the central (Sidi Bouzid, Kairouan), and in the southern regions (Gafsa, Gabes, Tozeur, Tataouine) of Tunisia (Figure 5(Bc,Bd)). Most of these transitions were statistically supported with BF > 3 (Sfax–Nabeul: BF = 18.05; Kasserine–Sidi Bouzid: BF = 16.07; Sfax–Gafsa: BF = 10.76; Sfax–Gabes: BF = 230.21; Sfax–Tozeur: BF = 12.54).

Based on the N450 analysis, spatio-temporal dynamics revealed that the epidemic of measles virus in Tunisia started from Tunis and spread to Sousse (BF = 5.86) in May 2019 (Figure S2.2A). In July 2019, the virus emerged in the coastal regions (Monastir and Gabes). All these transitions had statistical support (Sousse–Monastir: BF = 4.97; Sousse–Gabes: BF = 7.27) (Figure S2.2B). Then, the transmission zone extended to reach other coastal regions (Mahdia and Sfax) as well as the center of Tunisia (Sidi Bouzid, Kairouan and Kasserine) (Figure S2.2C). Only the transition linking Sousse to Mahdia was supported by a BF equal to 7.94. In October, a total emergence of the virus was observed in many regions in the north (Zaghouan, Nabeul, Bizerte and Kef) and south of Tunisia (Tataouine, Tozeur) (Figure S2.2D). Here, only the Sousse–Zaghouane (BF = 7.45) and Tunis–Tozeur (BF = 30.76) transitions were statistically supported.

## 4. Discussion

In the present work, we found that all the epidemic sequences from Tunisia belong to the B3 genotype. According to the N450 genomic region, most of the sequences (76%, 50 out of 66) belonged to one major variant related to the MVs/Kabul.AFG/20.14/3 named strain (DsId: 4298), which circulated in 17 out of 24 affected governorates of the country and during almost the whole epidemic period, lasting from week 1 to week 25. The N450 phylogenetic analyses identified four other minor variants; one of them was detected in Valence, France, in 2019 and the three others are new and are not yet reported in the MeaNS database. Thus, according to the N-450 genomic region, these minor variants may represent different individual importations while the major variant would be the main virus strain responsible for the outbreak.

We undertook heavy sampling in the early outbreak period and less sampling in the later stages, which may constitute a potential limitation to the accuracy of our findings.

When using the MF-NCR, the findings were clearly different, since more sets of identical sequences were identified. The sequences from the N450 major cluster split into eight subvariants each, with one detected during a shorter period of time.

The use of new sequencing windows, including the MF-NCR as well as whole genome sequencing, has been recommended for improving measles surveillance [15]. A scan of sequence variability across the full MeV genome identified the MF-NCR as the most variable part of the MeV genome [14–16]. The MF-NCR comprises 426 nucleotides of the matrix (M) protein gene its 3′ end, followed by an intergenic region of 3 nucleotides and then 583 nucleotides of the fusion (F) protein gene in its 5′ end. It is the longest non-coding region of the measles virus genome; it is rich in G-C and its functionality is not well understood [17,24]. Previous studies used this genomic region and a found better resolution between measles strains that circulated in concomitant outbreaks or over several years in one country, consistent with epidemiological data [14,15]. However, additional studies in other endemic or epidemic contexts, such as the present work, are needed to better demonstrate the added value of MF-NCR in the molecular investigation of measles transmission. Also, while a large number of sequences are available for the N and the H genes for all genotypes of the measles virus, there are still far fewer sequence data for the MF-NCR. The further identification of MF-NCR sequences from other regions of the world is essential to broaden the number of sequences used in phylogenetic analyses and study transmission patterns at national and international contexts, and our work adds new sequence data from the EMR and north African region.

From the technical side and in the present work, we were able to amplify the MF-NCR of 61 out of 66 samples that showed positive amplification in the N-450 region. Previous authors were also able to obtain MF-NCR sequences from a high proportion of samples that were positive in the N gene region despite the high genetic variability in this region [14]. We did not find deletions or insertions in our B3 MF-NCR sequences, as found in the MF-NCRs of other genotypes [2,11,25,26]. Our results add arguments on the potential easy use of this region as a complementary tool for epidemiological investigation.

The first case of the outbreak was from Kasserine; it was serologically confirmed but no samples for virus detection were collected. Subsequently, several cases were identified in the same governorate and all of these were either serologically confirmed, epi-linked, or clinically confirmed, but no samples for virus detection were collected. The first cases in Kasserine where oral fluid samples were collected had a rash onset on 21st January 2019 and after. On the other hand, the cases identified in Sfax in the same period and starting at the beginning of the outbreak had oral fluid or throat swabs samples collected immediately. The possibility of two routes of transmission was, in fact, raised, but our phylogeographic analyses suggested only one source of transmission, starting from Kasserine. This underscores the value of phylogeographic analyses based on genomic sequences, as the analysis was able to trace the origin of the infection despite the relative delay in obtaining samples from certain regions and the lack of clear epidemiological links between cases as generally provided by the classical epidemiological investigations. The GMRLN does not currently mandate the sequencing of this genomic region; however, many laboratories within the network with sequencing capacities are tracking MeV transmission pathways using MF-NCR sequences. In the present study, we investigated the phylogenetic and phylodynamic analysis of the MF-NCR of the MeV detected in Tunisia during the outbreak of 2019. The phylodynamic study based on the MF-NCR suggests the virus' actual pathways during the outbreak, including the initial point of spread and its subsequent dissemination in the country. Indeed, based on the dates of case notifications to the Ministry of Health, the first cases were from Kasserine with concomitant cases in Sfax starting in week 1, 2019. The notifications started to come from other governorates, and by week 13, the whole country was affected. Our findings align with these epidemiological data as, based on the sequence analysis, the spread of the disease reached all the governorates from which we obtained virus sequences in March. In addition, given the lack of epidemiological link between the cases from different locations, our analyses provide information on the possible routes of transmission from one governorate to another. This outcome aligns with epidemiological information.

Previous phylogenetic and phylodynamic analyses conducted by Jacqueline et al. (2023) and Kim et al. (2021) using MF-NCR sequencing showed that it provided enhanced resolution while tracing the epidemiological routes of measles outbreaks in Spain and South Korea, respectively [27,28]. Our MF-NCR analyses align with epidemiological information based on case notification dates, dates of rash onset, and geographical origin for the measles virus spread. However, we could not perform the analyses for each variant separately as higher numbers of sequences from each variant were needed, and this is one of the limitations of this study. Another limitation is the frequency of sample collection during the outbreak with a lower number of samples collected starting from April and this represents a potential limitation to the accuracy of our phylogenetic analyses.

Our study relies on self-reported data, which may be subject to sampling bias. This could limit the accuracy of the phylogenetic methods, which is due particularly to the unequal distribution of sample sizes over various times and locations.

## 5. Conclusions

In conclusion, this study provides critical baseline data on the wild-type measles viruses that caused the Tunisia outbreak in 2019, which will be very useful for supporting measles elimination in the future. Our study adds evidence that, in addition to sequencing in the N gene, sequencing in the MF-NCR enhances the differentiation of epidemic strains and adds some value towards recommending this supplemental sequencing.

**Supplementary Materials:** The following supporting information can be downloaded at: https://www.mdpi.com/article/10.3390/vaccines12091085/s1, Figure S1: Distribution by week of rash onset of the number of the 66 genotyped measles cases (Histogram in red) and of the number of Measles cases notified to the ministry of health (blue curve) during the MeV outbreak in Tunisia 2019; Figure S2: Phylodynamics of Measles virus detected in Tunisia in 2019 based on N-450 genomic region. 1. Bayesian Time scaled MCC tree of Measles virus isolated from Tunisian governorates. The nodes and branches of MCC tree are colored to express the inferred Tunisian governorates. Node diameters are sized according to posterior prbabilities. 2. Spatio-temporal dynamics of the B3 measles virus that circulated in Tunisia in 2019 among different Tunisian governorates. The snapshots (A–D) illustrate the various stages of virus spread across the governorates. Transition lines connecting different locations represent the branches in the MCC tree. The diameters of the circles are proportional to the square root of the number of MCC branches maintaining a particular location state at each time point.

**Author Contributions:** Conceptualization: A.C. and H.T. (Henda Triki); methodology: H.T. (Henda Touzi), Z.M.; software and bioinformatic analyses: A.C., M.A. and O.S.; validation: A.C. and H.T. (Henda Triki); formal analysis, A.C., M.A. and O.S.; clinical and epidemiological resources: H.T. (Henda Triki), M.Y., A.B.S., C.H. and E.B.F.; data curation: M.Y., E.B.F., A.B.S. and C.H.; original draft preparation: A.C., M.A. and O.S.; review and editing; H.T. (Henda Triki); visualization: A.C., H.T. (Henda Triki), M.A. and O.S.; supervision: H.T. (Henda Triki); project administration: H.T. (Henda Triki), A.B.S., M.Y., C.H. and E.B.F.; funding acquisition: H.T. (Henda Triki). All authors have read and agreed to the published version of the manuscript.

**Funding:** This work was supported by the Tunisia Ministries of Health and of High Education and Research (Reasearch Laboratory "Virus, Vectors and Hosts: One Health Approach and Technological Innovation for a Better Health", LR20IPT02, Institut Pasteur de Tunis, Université Tunis El Manar, Tunis 1002, Tunisia, and the Clinical Investigation Center (CIC), Institut Pasteur de Tunis, Université Tunis El Manar, Tunis 1002, Tunisia). This work was also supported by the WHO Measles and Rubella Elimination Program and the Center of Diseases Control and Prevention, CDC, USA.

**Institutional Review Board Statement:** The samples used in this work were obtained from clinically suspected measles patients for public health and disease control purposes. No personal information on the patients such as name or home address was used in the study.

**Informed Consent Statement:** Not applicable.

**Data Availability Statement:** The original contributions presented in the study are included in the article/Supplementary Materials, further inquiries can be directed to the corresponding author chouikhaanissa@gmail.com.

**Acknowledgments:** Authors express their gratitude to Bettina Bankamp and Raydel Anderson from the CDC, Atlanta, and Amany Ghoniem (WHO EMR Lab Coordinator) and Mick Mulders (WHO Headquarters Lab Coordinator) for their continuous support and guidance. Special appreciation goes to Paul Rota for the useful advice and comments on the manuscript. Additionally, the authors extend their thanks to the measles surveillance teams in the field for their efforts in collecting biological samples and providing clinical and epidemiological data.

**Conflicts of Interest:** The authors declare no conflicts of interest.

## References


1. Griffin, D.E. Measles Virus. In *Fields Virology*, 4th ed.; Knipe, D.M., Howley, P.M., Eds.; Lippincott Williams & Wilkins: Philadelphia, PA, USA, 2001; Volume 1, pp. 1401–1442.
2. Bankamp, B.; Liu, C.; Rivailler, P.; Bera, J.; Shrivastava, S.; Kirkness, E.F.; Bellini, W.J.; Rota, P.A. Wild-type measles viruses with non-standard genome lengths. *PLoS ONE* **2014**, *9*, e95470. [CrossRef]
3. Mulders, M.N.; Paul, R.A.; Brown, K.; Goodson, J. Genetic diversity of wild-type measles viruses and the global measles nucleotide surveillance database (MeaNS). *Wkly. Rep.* **2015**, *90*, 373–380. Available online: https://reliefweb.int/report/world/weekly-epidemiological-record-wer-24-july-2015-vol-90-no-30-pp-373-380-enfr (accessed on 18 May 2024).
4. Brown, K.E.; Rota, P.A.; Goodson, J.L.; Williams, D.; Abernathy, E.; Takeda, M.; Mulders, M.N. Genetic characterization of measles and rubella viruses detected through global measles and rubella elimination surveillance, 2016–2018. *MMWR Morb. Mortal. Wkly. Rep.* **2019**, *68*, 587–591. Available online: https://www.cdc.gov/mmwr/volumes/68/wr/pdfs/mm6826a3-H.pdf (accessed on 18 May 2024). [CrossRef] [PubMed]
5. Rota, P.A.; Moss, W.J.; Takeda, M.; de Swart, R.L.; Thompson, K.M.; Goodson, J.L. Measles. *Nat. Rev. Dis. Primers* **2016**, *2*, 16049. [CrossRef]
6. World Health Organization (WHO). Measles. 2024. Available online: https://www.who.int/news-room/fact-sheets/detail/measles (accessed on 18 May 2024).
7. Minta, A.A.; Ferrari, M.; Antoni, S.; Portnoy, A.; Sbarra, A.; Lambert, B.; Hatcher, C.; Hsu, C.H.; Ho, L.L.; Steulet, C.; et al. Progress Toward Measles Elimination—Worldwide, 2000–2022. *MMWR Morb. Mortal. Wkly. Rep.* **2023**, *72*, 1262–1268. [CrossRef]
8. World Health Organization. Manual for the Laboratory-Based Surveillance of Measles, Rubella, and Congenital Rubella SynDrome; Third Edition, June 2018. Available online: https://www.technet-21.org/fr/manual-introduction (accessed on 18 May 2024).
9. Sniadack, D.H.; Crowcroft, N.S.; Durrheim, D.N.; Rota, P.A. Roadmap to elimination standard measles and rubella surveillance. *Wkly. Epidemiol. Rec.* **2017**, *92*, 97–105. Available online: https://iris.who.int/bitstream/handle/10665/254754/WER9209_10-97-105.pdf?sequence=1 (accessed on 18 May 2024).
10. Rota, P.A.; Brown, K.E.; Hübschen, J.M.; Muller, C.P.; Icenogle, J.; Chen, M.H.; Bankamp, B.; Kessler, J.R.; Brown, D.W.; Bellini, W.J.; et al. Improving global virologic surveillance for measles and rubella. *J. Infect. Dis.* **2011**, *204* (Suppl. 1), S506–S513. [CrossRef] [PubMed]
11. Rota, P.A.; Brown, K.; Mankertz, A.; Santibanez, S.; Shulga, S.; Muller, C.P.; Hübschen, J.M.; Siqueira, M.; Beirnes, J.; Ahmed, H.; et al. Global distribution of measles genotypes and measles molecular epidemiology. *J. Infect. Dis.* **2011**, *204* (Suppl. 1), S514–S523. [CrossRef] [PubMed]
12. Williams, D.; Penedos, A.; Bankamp, B.; Anderson, A.; Hübschen, J.; Ben Mamou, M.; Beck, A.; Brown, D.; Rey-Benito, G.; Evans, R.; et al. Update: Circulation of active genotypes of measles virus and recommendations for use of sequence analysis to monitor viral transmission. *Wkly. Epidemiol. Rec.* **2022**, *39*, 485–492. Available online: https://mectizan.org/wp-content/uploads/2022/11/WER9739-eng-fre.pdf (accessed on 18 May 2024).
13. World Health Organization. The role of extended and whole genome sequencing for tracking transmission of measles and rubella viruses: Report from the Global Measles and Rubella Laboratory Network meeting, 2017. *Wkly. Epidemiol. Rec.* **2018**, *6*, 55–59.
14. Harvala, H.; Wiman, S.; Wallensten, A.; Zakikhany, K.; Englund, H.; Brytting, M. Role of Sequencing the Measles Virus Hemagglutinin Gene and Hypervariable Region in the Measles Outbreak Investigations in Sweden during 2013–2014. *J. Infect. Dis.* **2016**, *213*, 592–599. [CrossRef] [PubMed]
15. Penedos, A.R.; Myers, R.; Hadef, B.; Aladin, F.; Brown, K.E. Assessment of the Utility of Whole Genome Sequencing of Measles Virus in the Characterisation of Outbreaks. *PLoS ONE* **2015**, *10*, e0143081. [CrossRef]
16. Gil, H.; Fernández-García, A.; Mosquera, M.M.; Hübschen, J.M.; Castellanos, A.M.; de Ory, F.; Masa-Calles, J.; Echevarría, J.E. Measles virus genotype D4 strains with non-standard length M-F non-coding region circulated during the major outbreaks of 2011-2012 in Spain. *PLoS ONE* **2018**, *13*, e0199975. [CrossRef] [PubMed] [PubMed Central]
17. Heider, A.; Santibanez, S.; Tischer, A.; Gerike, E.; Tikhonova, N.; Ignatyev, G.; Mrazova, M.; Enders, G.; Schreier, E. Comparative investigation of the long non-coding M-F genome region of wild-type and vaccine measles viruses. *Arch. Virol.* **1997**, *142*, 2521–2528. [CrossRef] [PubMed]
18. Garbouj, M.; Slim, A.; Ghorbal, M.B.; Khamassi, S.; Gaafar, T.; Moshni, E.; Lievano, F. Progress toward interruption of endemic measles transmission in Tunisia. *J. Infect. Dis.* **2003**, *187* (Suppl. 1), S172–S176. [CrossRef] [PubMed]
19. World Health Organization. Disease Outbreak News. Measles—Tunisia. Available online: https://www.who.int/emergencies/disease-outbreak-news/item/2019-DON150#:~:text=To%20date,%20the%20number%20of,48%20cases)%20reported%20in%202012 (accessed on 18 May 2024).
20. World Health Organization. Disease Outbreak News. Measles—Global Situation. 2019. Available online: https://www.who.int/emergencies/disease-outbreak-news/item/2019-DON211 (accessed on 18 May 2024).
21. Mziou, E.; Safer, M.; Hchaichi, A.; Ben Youssef, F.; Letaief, H.; Dhaouadi, S.; Bouabid, L.; Derouiche, S.; Mhadhbi, R.; Bougatef, S.; et al. Measles seroprevalence national survey among a sample of the Tunisian population: Is there an expla-nation for the 2019 measles epidemic in a mostly vaccinated population? *Popul. Med.* **2023**, *5*, A240. [CrossRef]
22. Lemey, P.; Rambaut, A.; Drummond, A.J.; Suchard, M.A. Bayesian phylogeography finds its roots. *PLoS Comput. Biol.* **2009**, *5*, e1000520. [CrossRef] [PubMed]

23. Furuse, Y.; Oshitani, H. Global Transmission Dynamics of Measles in the Measles Elimination Era. *Viruses* **2017**, *9*, 82. [CrossRef] [PubMed]
24. Rima, B.K.; Duprex, W.P. The measles virus replication cycle. *Curr. Top. Microbiol. Immunol.* **2009**, *329*, 77–102. [CrossRef] [PubMed]
25. Al-Tawfiq, J.A.; Memish, Z.A. Measles Outbreaks in the Eastern Mediterranean Region: Urgent Need for Strengthened Vaccination Efforts. *J. Epidemiol. Glob. Health* **2024**, *14*, 252–254. [CrossRef]
26. Ivancic-Jelecki, J.; Slovic, A.; Šantak, M.; Tešović, G.; Forcic, D. Common position of indels that cause deviations from canonical genome organization in different measles virus strains. *Virol. J.* **2016**, *13*, 134. [CrossRef]
27. Jacqueline, C.; Gavilán, A.M.; López-Perea, N.; Penedos, A.R.; Masa-Calles, J.; Echevarría, J.E.; Fernández-García, A.; MMR Study Group. Utility of MF-non coding region for measles molecular surveillance during post-elimination phase, Spain, 2017–2020. *Front. Microbiol.* **2023**, *14*, 1143933. [CrossRef]
28. Kim, J.-M.; Park, S.; Kim, S.; Park, K.R.; Wang, J.S.; Chung, Y.S. Genetic Analysis of the Measles Virus From the Outbreaks in South Korea, 2019. *Front. Microbiol.* **2021**, *12*, 763107. [CrossRef]

vaccines

MDPI

Review

# Global Update on Measles Molecular Epidemiology

Bettina Bankamp [1,*,†], Gimin Kim [1,†], Derek Hart [2,†], Andrew Beck [1,†], Myriam Ben Mamou [3], Ana Penedos [4], Yan Zhang [5], Roger Evans [6] and Paul A. Rota [1,*,†]

1 Centers for Disease Control and Prevention, 1600 Clifton Road NE, Atlanta, GA 30329, USA; ofi6@cdc.gov (G.K.); lpu5@cdc.gov (A.B.)
2 ASRT, Inc., Atlanta, GA 30346, USA; ule1@cdc.gov
3 World Health Organization Regional Office for Europe, 2100 Copenhagen, Denmark; benmamoum@who.int
4 United Kingdom Health Security Agency, London NW9 5EQ, UK; ana.penedos@ukhsa.gov.uk
5 WHO Western Pacific Regional Measles/Rubella Reference Laboratory, National Institute for Viral Disease Control and Prevention, Beijing 100013, China; zhangyan9876543@163.com
6 World Health Organization Western Pacific Regional Office, Manila 1000, Philippines; revans@who.int
* Correspondence: bfb9@cdc.gov (B.B.); par1@cdc.gov (P.A.R.)
† CDC disclaimer: The findings and conclusions in this report are those of the authors and do not necessarily represent the official position of the Centers for Disease Control and Prevention.

**Abstract:** Molecular surveillance of circulating measles variants serves as a line of evidence for the absence of endemic circulation and provides a means to track chains of transmission. Molecular surveillance for measles (genotyping) is based on the sequence of 450 nucleotides at the end of the nucleoprotein coding region (N450) of the measles genome. Genotyping was established in 1998 and, with over 50,000 sequence submissions to the Measles Nucleotide Surveillance database, has proven to be an effective resource for countries attempting to trace pathways of transmission. This review summarizes the tools used for the molecular surveillance of measles and describes the challenge posed by the decreased number of circulating measles genotypes. The Global Measles and Rubella Laboratory Network addressed this challenge through the development of new tools such as named strains and distinct sequence identifiers that analyze the diversity within the currently circulating genotypes. The advantages and limitations of these approaches are discussed, together with the need to generate additional sequence data including whole genome sequences to ensure the continued utility of strain surveillance for measles.

**Keywords:** measles; molecular surveillance; elimination; genotyping

## 1. Introduction

Member states in all six regions of the World Health Organization (WHO) have declared measles elimination goals [1]. Molecular surveillance of circulating measles variants serves as a major line of evidence for the absence of endemic circulation and provides support for the classification of cases as imported, import-related or endemic [2,3]. Based on the sequences of their hemagglutinin and nucleocapsid (N) gene-coding sequences, measles viruses have been divided into 24 genotypes [4–7]. Specimens from new cases are assigned to one of these genotypes by sequencing the 450 nucleotides at the end of the nucleoprotein gene coding region (N450) and comparing these to a set of established reference sequences (Figure 1).

Standard molecular surveillance for measles based on N450 sequencing was established in 1998 [4]; these sequences are submitted to the Measles Nucleotide Surveillance (MeaNS) database which holds >59,000 sequences [8]. Every N450 sequence receives a name ("WHO name") which includes information about the place and time of the case [4]. For example, MVs/Georgia.USA/10.24 would be the sequence name for a case in the state of Georgia, USA in epidemiological week 10 of 2024. The WHO names link the sequence information to epidemiological data. The Global Measles and Rubella Laboratory

Network (GMRLN) in the WHO has standardized naming conventions in a series of publications [4,5,7,9,10]. Countries with endemic measles are encouraged to provide sequences from large outbreaks to generate baseline data that can be used for comparison once these countries get closer to elimination status. Countries in or near elimination status should obtain genotype information from 80% of all chains of transmission, including one case chains [2].

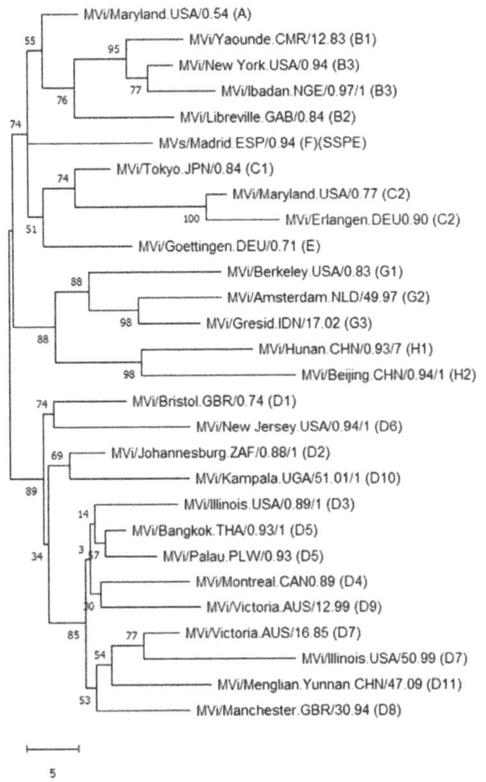


**Figure 1.** Phylogenetic tree with 28 measles N450 reference sequences. Data from MeaNS [8]. The evolutionary history was inferred using the maximum parsimony method. The percentage of replicate trees in which the associated taxa clustered together in the bootstrap test (500 replicates) are shown next to the branches. The tree is drawn to scale, with branch lengths calculated using the average pathway method and are in the units of the number of changes over the whole sequence. Scale bar indicates number of nucleotides.

Through the International Reagent Resource (IRR, [11]) the GMRLN offers kits for Sanger sequencing of N450 and protocols are available from the website of the WHO measles and rubella laboratory manual [12]. Unlike other pathogens, which use sequencing to monitor the development of vaccine or drug escape mutants or to identify candidate strains for updated vaccines [13–19], the major purpose of sequencing measles specimens is to monitor viral transmission and progress toward elimination. Since even a few nucleotide changes may affect the interpretation of sequencing data, the GMRLN has a strong emphasis on sequence quality. Efforts to improve and monitor the quality of molecular testing in laboratories of the GMRLN are described elsewhere [20]. This review describes the reduced diversity of circulating genotypes and the approaches developed by the GMRLN to replace the comparison between genotypes with the interpretation of sequence differences within genotypes. Limitations to the use of the small standard genotyping window, options for extended sequencing and obstacles to the widespread introduction of extended sequencing are discussed.

## 2. Reduced Diversity of Circulating Genotypes

Eighteen co-circulating genotypes were detected in 2003 (Figure 2). The number of genotypes has decreased steadily since then and only two genotypes, B3 and D8, have been detected since 2021 (Figures 2 and 3).

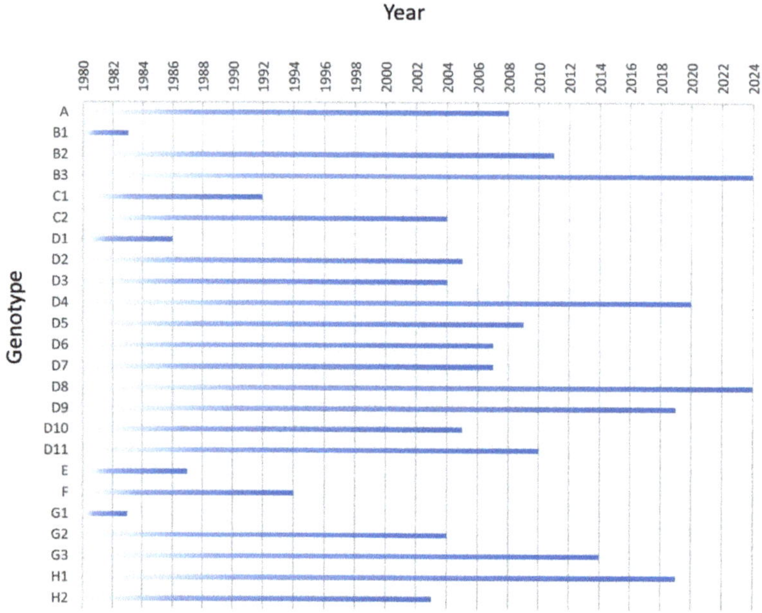


**Figure 2.** Year of last detection of measles genotypes. The last year of documented circulation reported to MeaNS [8] for all 24 genotypes is shown. Viruses with a date of 2024 are currently circulating. All other viruses have had transmission interrupted in the year depicted. Note that the chart does not specify the first year of detection of any genotype.

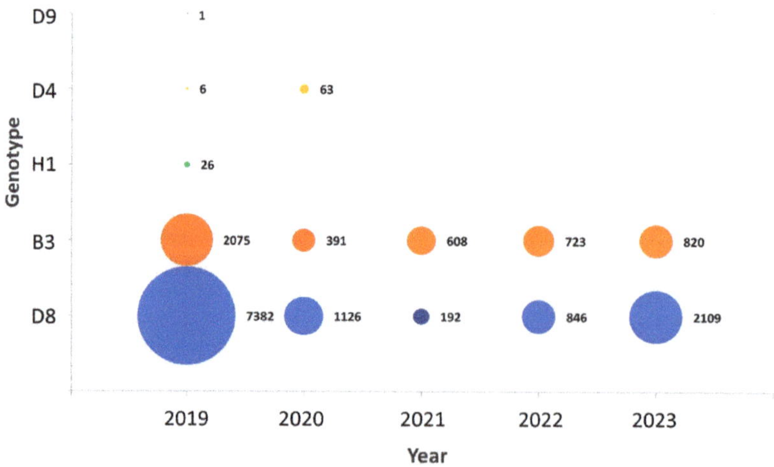


**Figure 3.** Number of submissions per genotype reported to MeaNS [8] 2019–2023.

A caveat to these observations is that the quality of molecular surveillance varies between countries and regions; major surveillance gaps exist in the African, Southeast Asian and Eastern Mediterranean regions. Table 1 shows submissions to MeaNS per WHO region; comparing these to the numbers of estimated cases [21–24] demonstrates the discrepancy between case numbers and genotyping information. Estimated case numbers were not yet available for 2023. The table covers the years of the pandemic and shows that all WHO regions faced difficulties in maintaining molecular surveillance for measles in 2020 and 2021. However, in 2022, the ratio between estimated cases and MeaNS submissions had largely recovered to pre-pandemic levels.

**Table 1.** Estimated cases compared to number of MeaNS submissions, 2019–2023.

| | African Region | | | American Region | | | Eastern Mediterranean Region | | |
|---|---|---|---|---|---|---|---|---|---|
| **Year** | **Cases** * | **MeaNS** # | **Ratio** ^ | **Cases** | **MeaNS** | **Ratio** | **Cases** | **MeaNS** | **Ratio** |
| 2019 | 4,548,000 | 55 | 82,691 | 102,700 | 1397 | 74 | 1,384,500 | 216 | 6410 |
| 2020 | 1,944,700 | 17 | 114,394 | 43,700 | 315 | 139 | 2,043,600 | 121 | 16,889 |
| 2021 | 4,370,190 | 12 | 364,183 | 3410 | 205 | 17 | 2,303,170 | 538 | 4281 |
| 2022 | 5,138,698 | 55 | 93,431 | 825 | 108 | 8 | 1,193,257 | 474 | 2517 |
| | **European Region** | | | **South-East Asian Region** | | | **Western Pacific Region** | | |
| **Year** | **Cases** | **MeaNS** | **Ratio** | **Cases** | **MeaNS** | **Ratio** | **Cases** | **MeaNS** | **Ratio** |
| 2019 | 494,600 | 4356 | 114 | 2,655,000 | 942 | 2818 | 643,700 | 2530 | 254 |
| 2020 | 179,600 | 473 | 380 | 2,552,600 | 556 | 4591 | 784,900 | 128 | 6132 |
| 2021 | 86,190 | 29 | 2972 | 1,702,699 | 13 | 130,977 | 958,395 | 3 | 319,465 |
| 2022 | 63,707 | 133 | 479 | 1,896,917 | 780 | 2432 | 938,883 | 19 | 49,415 |

* Estimated cases [21–24]; # MeaNS submissions [8]; ^ number of estimated cases per MeaNS submission.

While the GMRLN is cautious about declaring genotypes as inactive, it is clear that the number of circulating genotypes has been reduced, suggesting that vaccination efforts have interrupted the transmission of several genotypes. A recent example is the disappearance of genotype H1, which has been endemic in the People's Republic of China (PRC) since the late 1990s [25]. While genotype H1 was frequently exported from the PRC, it never established sustained continued transmission anywhere else. Highly successful vaccination efforts in the PRC appear to have ended circulation of genotype H1 in the country. In 2018, 275 of 316 submissions to MeaNS were genotype H1; in 2019, there were only 21 genotype H1 reports in 427 submissions and the last case with an H1 genotype was reported to MeaNS in September 2019 [8,26]. The last detection of genotype H1 in the PRC corresponds with the failure to detect genotype H1 associated with imported cases globally.

## 3. Utilizing the Diversity within Genotypes

The decrease in the number of circulating genotypes reduced the utility of N450-based genotyping for tracing the pathways of transmission since all sequences are now classified as genotype B3 or D8. However, there is sequence diversity within genotypes and the GMRLN has formalized approaches to characterize this diversity. One tool is the use of a distinct sequence identifier (DSId) [10]. Every novel sequence submitted to MeaNS receives a unique DSId. All submissions of identical sequences receive the same DSId. A MeaNS user with a new sequence can search MeaNS to find identical sequences, i.e., sequences that have the same DSId. The detection of identical sequences in other countries can then be used to support epidemiological data on the import status of a measles case. Different DSIds are prevalent in different parts of the world (Figure 4), indicating the utility of DSIds compared to using genotypes alone.

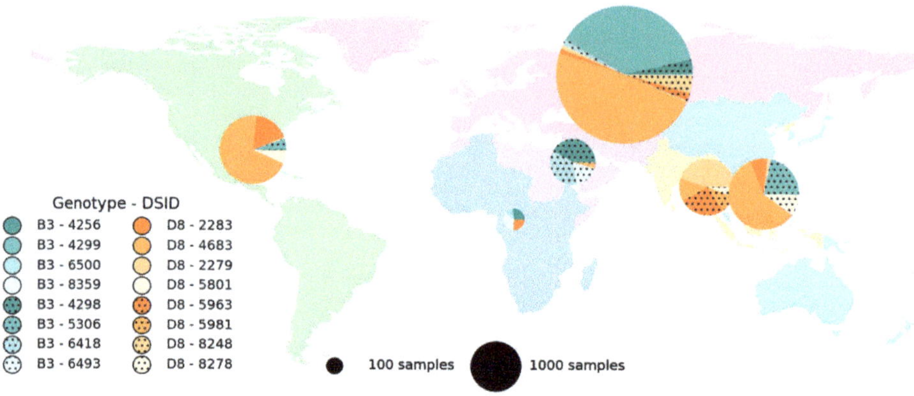


**Figure 4.** Global distribution of major DSIds according to the WHO region, 2019–2023. The genotype is indicated by the color and pattern in each pie chart. The size of the pie chart indicates the number of submissions to MeaNS [8]. Only the eight most frequently detected DSIds are listed.

Information about the detection of DSIds in other countries as well as the global distribution of the DSId should be added to reports to national or regional verification commissions (NVC, RVC) [10], which annually examine the elimination status of countries.

A second tool is the use of named strains (Figure 5). Named strains are identical sequences (i.e., submissions with the same DSId) that have been submitted to MeaNS at least 50 times from multiple countries over the course of the previous two years [9]. Named strains are variants with epidemiological importance as they are widely distributed. The WHO name of the first submission to MeaNS with the relevant N450 sequence is used to identify the named strain. For example, a sequence variant that was found globally in 2018/2019 was MVs/Gir Somnath.IND/42.16, with >6500 submissions to MeaNS. The name of the strain cannot be used as an indication of the source country of an importation, since the very existence of the named strain indicates that this variant is present in multiple countries. Linking a sequence to a named strain in MeaNS implies that the new sequence is part of a lineage with global distribution, which is easier than listing a large number of possible import sources. Figure 6 shows the proportion of the most frequently identified named strains for B3 and D8 from 2019 to 2023, demonstrating the changes in the most commonly found variants over time. Interestingly, the proportion of submitted sequences that are not identical to a named strain (dark green in Figure 6) has continually increased since 2019 and now makes up more than half of all submissions. This may indicate continuing diversification withing the two genotypes or it may be an artifact of surveillance. For example, if a country with highly active surveillance sequences many specimens from a large outbreak of a named strain, those sequences will make up a relatively large proportion of all submitted sequences.

Visualization tools for reports to the NVC or RVC include charts to display DSIds detected by epidemiologic week (Figure 7). The WHO Regional Office for Europe developed an approach that brings together on a single visual all the information about the chains of transmission and sporadic cases in a given country over time with their respective DSIds/named strains, in combination with the epidemiological curve and the information about importations, using data from the NVC's annual report (Annual Status Update) and MeaNS. This approach proved to be a very useful tool to support the decision-making process of the European RVC (Supplementary Figure S1).

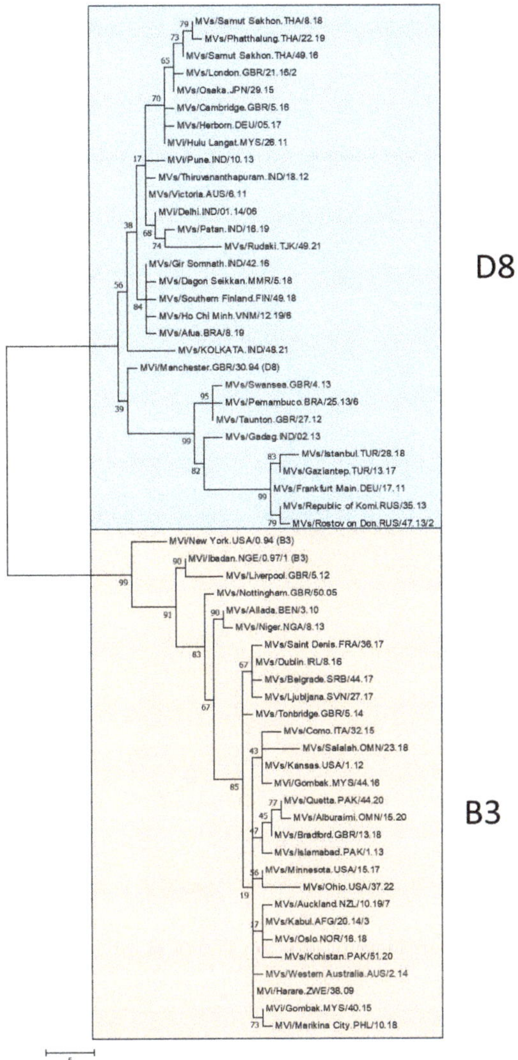


**Figure 5.** Phylogenetic tree of named strains of genotypes B3 and D8. Data from MeaNS [8], accessed 9 April 2024. The percentage of replicate trees in which the associated taxa clustered together in the bootstrap test (500 replicates) are shown next to the branches. The tree is drawn to scale, with branch lengths calculated using the average pathway method and are in the units of the number of changes over the whole sequence. Scale bar indicates number of nucleotides.

Since the initiation of standard protocols for genotyping, adding the genotype information to the WHO name served to describe genetic relatedness between sequences, but the reduction in diversity of circulating viruses now requires a different approach. Efforts are under way to define epidemiologically relevant lineages within genotypes B3 and D8 which will serve as the basis for an updated nomenclature. This nomenclature is expected to maintain the WHO name but add concise information about lineage assignment.

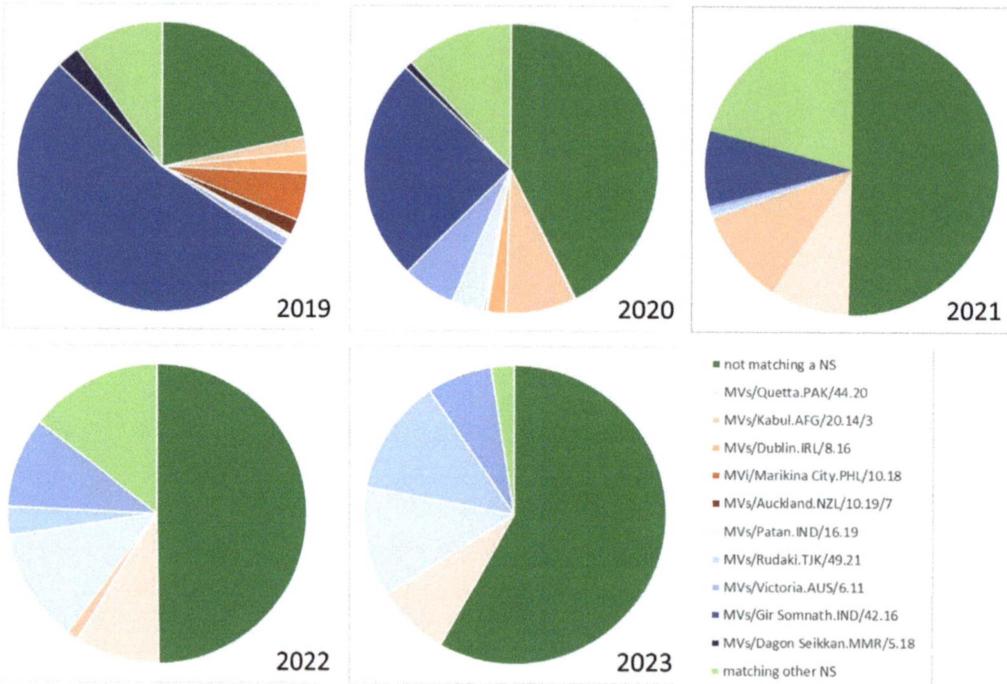


**Figure 6.** Proportion of MeaNS submissions corresponding to the five most frequently reported named strains of genotypes B3 (shades of orange) and D8 (shades of blue), 2019–2023. Data from MeaNS [8], accessed 9 April 2024. NS = named strain.

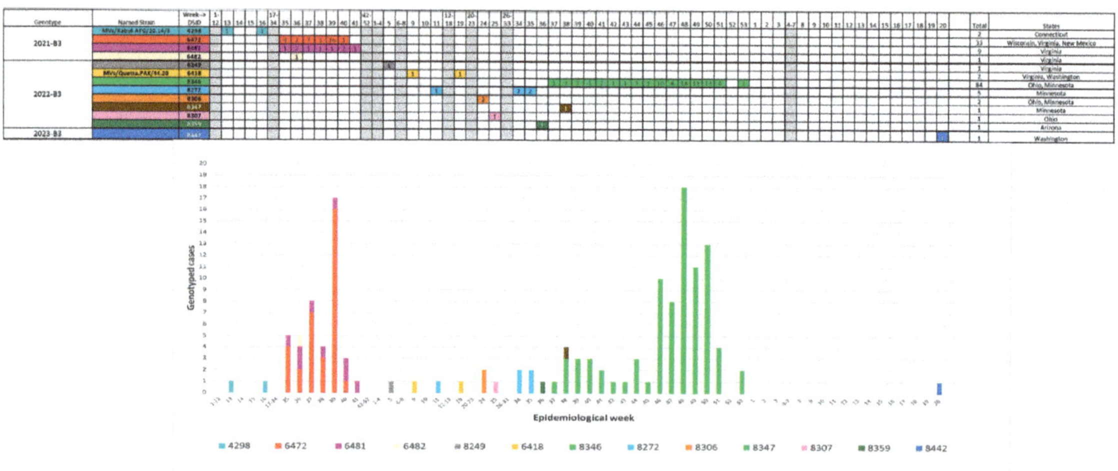


**Figure 7.** Example for reporting to NVC [27]: Genotype B3 cases in the US 2021–2023. (**Top**) Chart format. Columns represent epidemiological weeks. Columns in grey are combined weeks without sequenced cases. The number in each cell indicates the number of identical sequences from cases with onset in that week. (**Bottom**) Curve format. The data and colors are the same as on top. Colors correspond to different DSIds.

## 4. Options for Extended Sequencing

Within a genotype, many sequences are identical to named strains, which are of limited utility for molecular surveillance because of their wide circulation. While N450 sequencing remains the standard in the GMRLN, the resolution offered by a 450-nucleotide window is limited and extended sequencing approaches are required. To provide equitable options to countries needing molecular data for elimination reports, extended sequencing efforts in the GMLRN must consider the varying levels of technical capacity in national laboratories and the funding options for lower-income countries.

Consequently, laboratories have two options for obtaining additional sequence information from measles cases: sequencing the non-coding region between the matrix and fusion protein coding regions (MF-NCR) or whole genome sequencing (WGS). At 1012 nucleotides in length, the MF-NCR is the only long non-coding part and one of the most variable regions of the measles genome. Generally, the acquisition of longer sequence regions or regions of high intratypic diversity provides a better estimate of the substitution patterns along the measles virus (MeV) genome; comparison studies demonstrate that sequencing the MF-NCR offers improved phylogenetic model resolution over N450, especially regarding the statistical support of branching patterns. When molecular clock models are used, the MF-NCR in many cases produces greater certainty (narrower confidence intervals) for posterior estimates of internal node dating (Figure 8). Through the IRR, the GMRLN distributes a kit for Sanger sequencing the MF-NCR to support sequencing in low-income countries and a protocol is available from the WHO Lab Manual website [12].

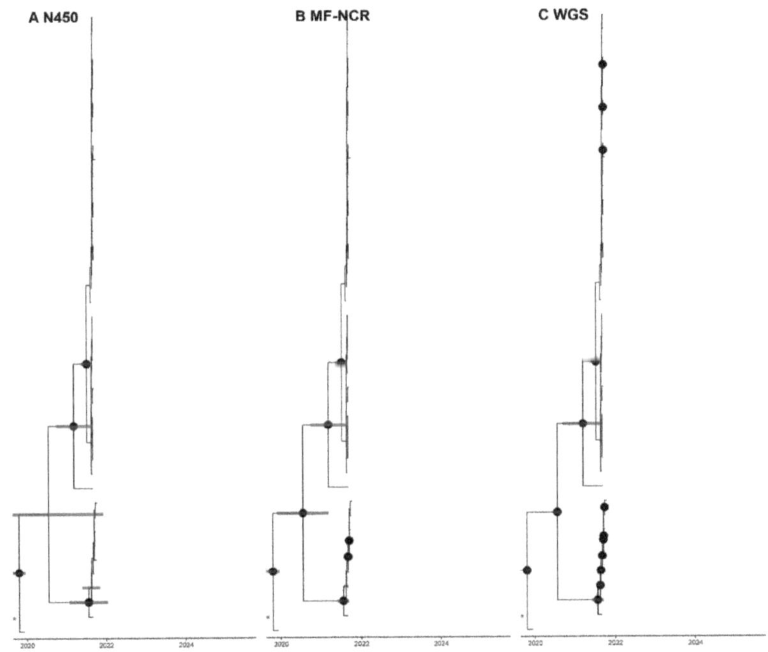


**Figure 8.** Comparison of N450, MF-NCR and WGS. BEAST analysis of (**A**) N450 sequences, (**B**) MF-NCR sequences and (**C**) WGS of the same samples. *X*-axis indicates time scale. Purple bars indicate 95% confidence interval for time points of branching patterns. Black dots indicate high statistical support for branch points. Analysis of longer sequences improves statistical support for branching patterns and narrows confidence intervals. Data are based on published sequences [28], but annotations are simulated to show how the certainty of the tree shape and measurements are likely to change.

WGS provides the most complete reconstructions of MeV evolution; however, it is currently only conducted in a small number of laboratories in the GMRLN. The utility of analysis of WGS has been demonstrated for the analysis of a number of outbreaks. A recent example was the analysis of measles cases observed in Afghan evacuees resettled in the USA following the fall of Kabul, in 2021 (Figure 9 [28]). Methods utilizing well-accepted next-generation sequencing (NGS) platforms (Illumina, Oxford Nanopore Technologies (ONT)) have been developed by several laboratories in the GMRLN. At present, the GMRLN has limited resources to support the widespread implementation of NGS and does not offer protocols or reagents. NGS may be initiated with a regional approach with regional reference laboratories supporting national laboratories.

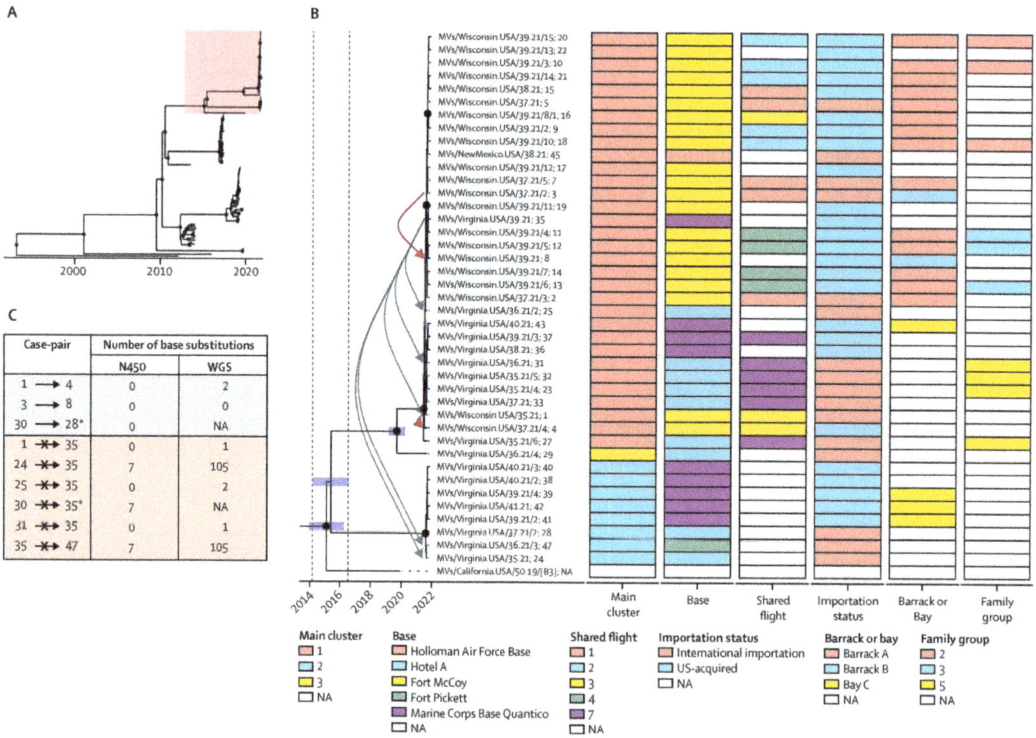


**Figure 9.** From [28], with permission of the authors. Use of WGS in combination with epidemiological data. Measles outbreak among Afghan refugees in the USA in 2021. (**A**) Red square indicates part of tree magnified in B. (**B**) *X*-axis indicates time. Blue bars denote 95% confidence intervals. Red arrows highlight epidemiologically linked cases. Grey arrows highlight cases without epidemiological links. (**C**) High number of nucleotide differences can rule out epidemiological linkage but low numbers do not always serve as proof of linkage. * WGS not available.

Ensuring high-quality sequencing results is more difficult when using NGS methods, due to the complex, multistep nature of the methods and the greater variability in technical approaches. The GMRLN is finalizing a guidance document for quality control of NGS, for both the laboratory and the bioinformatics methods. There are considerable obstacles to the widespread adoption of WGS bioinformatics methods within the GMRLN laboratories. Chiefly, the computational infrastructure required for institutional-grade analyses of NGS data exceeds the capacity of many national laboratories, with respect to both equipment and available bioinformatics expertise. Several laboratories in the GMRLN are in the process of developing sequence analysis pipelines to automate NGS analyses according to the requirements of MeV surveillance. Ideally, these pipelines would be shared or made accessible to contributors from outside the institutions where the pipelines are developed.

The GMRLN has developed guidelines to support decision-making by national laboratories and regional coordinators concerning the need for extended sequencing, whether it is MF-NCR sequencing or WGS [12]. The objective is to recommend extended sequencing to countries in or near elimination where it is expected to bring an added value compared to N450 sequencing. This approach will make a difference for the verification of elimination and provide countries without the capacity for extended sequening access a regional sequencing center.

## 5. Options for Interpreting Sequencing Data

For many years, the standard approach to interpret N450 sequences has been to generate phylogenetic trees that infer relative genetic distances (Figure 1). Capacity building within the GMRLN has led to an increased understanding and use of bootstrap values to evaluate the statistical significance of the results of phylogenetic analysis. However, since the goal of sequencing measles specimens is to determine whether cases are part of the same transmission chain or the result of separate importations, genetic distance alone is ultimately not sufficient to interpret the relevance of a small number of nucleotide changes. One well-accepted software platform for time-based phylogenetic analyses is Bayesian evolutionary analysis by sampling trees (BEAST) [29]. Bayesian tree inference is increasingly popular, accommodating inference of divergence time alongside that of nucleotide substitution patterns. BEAST uses time as the X-axis and inferences can be based on N450 sequences, MF-NCR sequences and WGS (Figures 8 and 9). Bayesian analyses require a large, curated dataset, considerable computational resources, and bioinformatics expertise. An alternative probabilistic approach simplifies the comparison of two sequences [30]. However, it requires reasonable assumptions about the most recent common ancestor of the sequences under comparison and its implementation would require standard nucleotide substitution rates (molecular clocks).

## 6. Molecular Surveillance Supports Development of Diagnostic Assays and Vaccines

While outside the scope of this review, it is worth mentioning that the molecular surveillance of measles viruses generates data for other activities that are essential for measles elimination. First, it provides supporting data to ensure continued functionality of molecular diagnostic assays. Through the IRR, the GMRLN distributes a kit for real-time RT-PCR (rRT-PCR) that is used in many countries for the detection of measles RNA in clinical specimens. The primers and probe for this rRT-PCR assay bind within the standard genotyping window (N450); hence, all genotyping data also monitor the genetic stability of the rRT-PCR primer and probe binding sites. A recent publication [31] identified a lineage of measles virus with nucleotide substitutions in the binding site for the reverse primer of the rRT-PCR assay which led to reduced sensitivity of the diagnostic assay. Consequently, the rRT-PCR reverse primer was modified to restore sensitivity for this measles lineage [32]. While the primers and probe used in the IRR kit are widely used in the GMRLN, many laboratories use other molecular diagnostic assays whose primers and probe bind outside of N450. The increased use of WGS will provide data to monitor the genetic stability of those diagnostic assays.

Secondly, molecular surveillance provides supporting data to monitor the effect of viral evolution on vaccine efficacy. Measles has only one serotype and the vaccine strains developed decades ago still protect against the measles lineages circulating today. However, as an RNA virus, measles is subject to more rapid molecular evolution than DNA viruses [33]. This genetic drift may change epitopes, the protein sequences that are recognized by the immune system, on measles proteins, which could lead to reduced efficacy of the vaccines [34]. WGS provides data for ongoing monitoring of the evolution of immunologically relevant epitopes, and, if necessary, will provide nucleotide sequence data for the development of updated measles vaccines.

## 7. Limitations and Outlook

Any analysis of measles variants is affected by the sequence surveillance gaps present in multiple countries and regions. These gaps widened during the COVID-19 pandemic and surveillance has not yet recovered everywhere. It is expected that this situation will gradually improve as more countries approach elimination; however, surveillance also needs to improve in countries with endemic measles as these are the most frequent sources of imported virus. One reason for the surveillance gaps is a lack of specimens for viral detection and genotyping in many countries. Many national laboratories are proficient in molecular methods, but either do not receive specimens or do not receive the appropriate specimen type. Serology remains the most commonly used method for case confirmation and the collection of throat swabs, nasopharyngeal swabs or urine samples for molecular assays is still not routine in many countries. For example, in the first half of 2023, 33 countries in the European region reported measles cases, but only 18 countries submitted sequences to MeaNS [35]. This is largely due to lack of specimens, as all countries in the European region have access to genotyping, either through their national laboratory or a regional reference laboratory. Improving specimen collection requires training for surveillance staff and program managers as well as the availability of specimen collection kits and adequate specimen shipping and storage.

Adjustments to address the challenge posed by the reduced diversity of circulating viruses have only just begun and will require additional resources, not only for equipment, training, and reagents for extended sequencing but also for staffing to manage the workload. Of course, since extended sequencing has begun only recently, surveillance gaps for MF-NCR sequences and WGS are even larger than the gaps for N450 sequences. Using extended sequencing to trace pathways of transmission is only useful if representative sequences from all countries are available in the database. The COVID-19 pandemic has led to a large increase in NGS sequencing capacity in many laboratories. The challenge for the GMRLN is to leverage this capacity to generate high-quality measles sequences. Establishing regional sequencing centers and developing shared sequencing pipelines will be required to meet the challenge.

Sequencing data cannot substitute for missing epidemiological information. Even WGS cannot distinguish between repeated importations into country A from the same outbreak in country B versus continuous circulation in country A. Epidemiological surveillance and collaboration between laboratory scientists and epidemiologists need to be improved to generate high-quality data for national programs.

## 8. Conclusions

Over more than two decades, the GMRLN has built an effective strain surveillance system that has provided sequence data to monitor pathways of transmission and support for verification of measles elimination. The challenge posed by the decreased number of circulating measles genotypes was addressed by tools that analyze the diversity within the currently circulating genotypes. However, the continued utility of strain surveillance will require the introduction of extended sequencing approaches. While acknowledging the constraints on capacity and funding in national laboratories, the judicious use of existing referral systems and the appropriate introduction of technology to countries, where required, will maintain and develop the strain surveillance system already being provided by the global laboratory network to address the future needs of measles and rubella elimination.

**Supplementary Materials:** The following supporting information can be downloaded at: https://www.mdpi.com/article/10.3390/vaccines12070810/s1, Figure S1: Example for reporting to NVC, Spain 2018–2019. Top: Epidemiological curve. Bars indicate the number of cases per month. Bottom: lineages including non-genotyped sporadic cases. Columns represent weeks from week 1, 2018 to week 52, 2019. Rows are different DSIds or named strains. The genotype is indicated with each DSID. Dashed cells indicate imported case, solid cells represent chains of transmission. The pattern for

D8-Gir Somnath sporadic cases indicates a range of time during which several cases not linked to known chains of transmission occurred.

**Author Contributions:** Writing—original draft preparation, B.B.; writing—review and editing, B.B., A.B., M.B.M., A.P., Y.Z., R.E. and P.A.R.; visualization, B.B., G.K., D.H., A.B. and M.B.M.; supervision, P.A.R. All authors have read and agreed to the published version of the manuscript.

**Funding:** This research received no external funding.

**Acknowledgments:** The authors thank the National Verification Committee, the National Reference Laboratory for measles and rubella at the National Centre for Microbiology (ISCIII), the National Centre for Epidemiology (ISCIII) and the National Epidemiological Surveillance Network from Spain for use of the data that served as the basis for Supplementary Figure S1. The authors thank all laboratories in the GMRLN for contributing sequences to the MeaNS database.

**Conflicts of Interest:** Author Derek Hart was employed by the company ASRT, Inc. The remaining authors declare that the research was conducted in the absence of any commercial or financial relationships that could be construed as a potential conflict of interest.

## References

1. Measles Overview. Available online: https://www.who.int/health-topics/measles (accessed on 9 May 2024).
2. World Health Organization. Monitoring progress towards measles elimination. *Wkly. Epidemiol. Rec.* **2010**, *85*, 490–494.
3. World Health Organization. Guidance for evaluating progress towards elimination of measles and rubella. *Wkly. Epidemiol. Rec.* **2018**, *93*, 544–552.
4. World Health Organization. Standardization of the nomenclature for describing the genetic characteristics of wild-type measles viruses. *Wkly. Epidemiol. Rec.* **1998**, *73*, 265–271.
5. World Health Organization. Update of the nomenclature for describing the genetic characteristics of wild-type measles viruses: New genotypes and reference strains. *Wkly. Epidemiol. Rec.* **2003**, *78*, 229–232.
6. World Health Organization. Global distribution of measles and rubella genotypes-update. *Wkly. Epidemiol. Rec.* **2006**, *81*, 474–479.
7. World Health Organization. Measles virus nomenclature update: 2012. *Wkly. Epidemiol. Rec.* **2012**, *87*, 73–80.
8. Measles Nucleotide Surveillance (MeaNS). Available online: https://who-gmrln.org/means2 (accessed on 9 May 2024).
9. World Health Organization. Genetic diversity of wild-type measles viruses and the global measles nucleotide surveillance database (MeaNS). *Wkly. Epidemiol. Rec.* **2015**, *90*, 373–380.
10. Williams, D.; Penedos, A.; Bankamp, B.; Anderson, R.; Hübschen, J.; Mamou, M.B.; Beck, A.; Brown, D.; Rey-Benito, G.; Evans, R. Update: Circulation of active genotypes of measles virus and recommendations for use of sequence analysis to monitor viral transmission. *Wkly. Epidemiol. Rec.* **2022**, *97*, 485–492.
11. IRR International Reagent Resource. Available online: https://www.internationalreagentresource.org/ (accessed on 9 May 2024).
12. Manual for the Laboratory-Based Surveillance of Measles, Rubella, and Congenital Rubella Syndrome, 3rd ed. 2018. Available online: https://www.technet-21.org/en/topics/programme-management/manual-for-the-laboratory-based-surveillance-of-measles-rubella-and-congenital-rubella-syndrome/manual-for-the-laboratory-based-surveillance-of-measles-rubella-and-congenital-rubella-syndrome (accessed on 9 May 2024).
13. Ávila-Ríos, S.; Parkin, N.; Swanstrom, R.; Paredes, R.; Shafer, R.; Ji, H.; Kantor, R. Next-Generation Sequencing for HIV Drug Resistance Testing: Laboratory, Clinical, and Implementation Considerations. *Viruses* **2020**, *12*, 617. [CrossRef]
14. Bandera, A.; Gori, A.; Clerici, M.; Sironi, M. Phylogenies in ART: HIV reservoirs, HIV latency and drug resistance. *Curr. Opin. Pharmacol.* **2019**, *48*, 24–32. [CrossRef]
15. Deyde, V.M.; Gubareva, L.V. Influenza genome analysis using pyrosequencing method: Current applications for a moving target. *Expert Rev. Mol. Diagn.* **2009**, *9*, 493–509. [CrossRef] [PubMed]
16. McGinnis, J.; Laplante, J.; Shudt, M.; George, K.S. Next generation sequencing for whole genome analysis and surveillance of influenza A viruses. *J. Clin. Virol.* **2016**, *79*, 44–50. [CrossRef]
17. Munyuza, C.; Ji, H.; Lee, E.R. Probe Capture Enrichment Methods for HIV and HCV Genome Sequencing and Drug Resistance Genotyping. *Pathogens* **2022**, *11*, 693. [CrossRef] [PubMed]
18. Van Poelvoorde, L.; Vanneste, K.; De Keersmaecker, S.C.; Thomas, I.; Van Goethem, N.; Van Gucht, S.; Saelens, X.; Roosens, N.H. Whole-Genome Sequence Approach and Phylogenomic Stratification Improve the Association Analysis of Mutations with Patient Data in Influenza Surveillance. *Front. Microbiol.* **2022**, *13*, 809887. [CrossRef]
19. Zhao, X.N.; Zhang, H.-J.; Li, D.; Zhou, J.-N.; Chen, Y.-Y.; Sun, Y.-H.; Adeola, A.C.; Fu, X.-Q.; Shao, Y.; Zhang, M.-L. Whole-genome sequencing reveals origin and evolution of influenza A(H1N1)pdm09 viruses in Lincang, China, from 2014 to 2018. *PLoS ONE* **2020**, *15*, e0234869. [CrossRef] [PubMed]
20. Bankamp, B.; Anderson, R.; Hao, L.; Chen, M.; Kim, G.; Mori, Y.; Rota, P.A. Building quality control for molecular assays in the global measles and rubella laboratory network. *Vaccines* **2024**, accepted.
21. Patel, M.K. Progress toward Regional Measles Elimination—Worldwide, 2000–2019. *MMWR Morb. Mortal. Wkly. Rep.* **2020**, *69*, 1700–1705. [CrossRef] [PubMed]

22. Dixon, M.G. Progress toward Regional Measles Elimination—Worldwide, 2000–2020. *MMWR Morb. Mortal. Wkly. Rep.* **2021**, *70*, 1563–1569. [CrossRef] [PubMed]
23. Minta, A.A. Progress toward Regional Measles Elimination—Worldwide, 2000–2021. *MMWR Morb. Mortal. Wkly. Rep.* **2022**, *71*, 1489–1495. [CrossRef]
24. Minta, A.A. Progress toward Measles Elimination—Worldwide, 2000–2022. *MMWR Morb. Mortal. Wkly. Rep.* **2023**, *72*, 1262–1268. [CrossRef]
25. Xu, W.; Tamin, A.; Rota, J.S.; Zhang, L.; Bellini, W.J.; Rota, P.A. New genetic group of measles virus isolated in the People's Republic of China. *Virus Res.* **1998**, *54*, 147–156. [CrossRef] [PubMed]
26. Wang, H.; Zhu, Z.; Duan, X.; Song, J.; Mao, N.; Cui, A.; Wang, C.; Du, H.; Wang, Y.; Li, F.; et al. Transmission Patterns of Measles Virus Circulating in China During 1993-2021: Genotyping Evidence Supports that China is Approaching Measles Elimination. *Clin. Infect. Dis.* **2023**, *76*, e1140–e1149. [CrossRef] [PubMed]
27. Mathis, D.A. Measles—United States, 1 January 2020–March 28 2024. *MMWR Morb. Mortal. Wkly. Rep.* **2024**, *73*, 295–300. [CrossRef] [PubMed]
28. Masters, N.B.; Beck, A.S.; Mathis, A.D.; Leung, J.; Raines, K.; Paul, P.; E Stanley, S.; Weg, A.L.; Pieracci, E.G.; Gearhart, S.; et al. Measles virus transmission patterns and public health responses during Operation Allies Welcome: A descriptive epidemiological study. *Lancet Public Health* **2023**, *8*, e618–e628. [CrossRef] [PubMed]
29. Bouckaert, R.; Vaughan, T.G.; Barido-Sottani, J.; Duchêne, S.; Fourment, M.; Gavryushkina, A.; Heled, J.; Jones, G.; Kühnert, D.; De Maio, N.; et al. BEAST 2.5: An advanced software platform for Bayesian evolutionary analysis. *PLoS Comput. Biol.* **2019**, *15*, e1006650. [CrossRef]
30. Penedos, A.R.; Fernández-García, A.; Lazar, M.; Ralh, K.; Williams, D.; Brown, K.E. Mind your Ps: A probabilistic model to aid the interpretation of molecular epidemiology data. *EBioMedicine* **2022**, *79*, 103989. [CrossRef] [PubMed]
31. Pérez-Rodríguez, F.J.; Cherpillod, P.; Thomasson, V.; Vetter, P.; Schibler, M. Identification of a measles variant displaying mutations impacting molecular diagnostics, Geneva, Switzerland, 2023. *Eurosurveillance* **2024**, *29*, 2400034. [CrossRef]
32. Beck, A.S.; Lopareva, E.N.; Hwang, H.; Hart, D.; de Almeida, M.; Anderson, R.; Rota, P.A.; Bankamp, B. Evaluation of the Sensitivity of a Measles Diagnostic RT-qPCR Assay Incorporating Recently Observed Priming Mismatch Variants. *Euro Surveill.* **2024**, *29*, 2400410. [CrossRef] [PubMed]
33. Peck, K.M.; Lauring, A.S. Complexities of Viral Mutation Rates. *J. Virol.* **2018**, *92*, e01031-17.
34. Tahara, M.; Ito, Y.; Brindley, M.A.; Ma, X.; He, J.; Xu, S.; Fukuhara, H.; Sakai, K.; Komase, K.; Rota, P.A.; et al. Functional and structural characterization of neutralizing epitopes of measles virus hemagglutinin protein. *J. Virol.* **2013**, *87*, 666–675. [CrossRef]
35. WHO European Region. *WHO EpiBrief: A Report on the Epidemiology of Selected Vaccine-Preventable Diseases in the European Region: No. 2/2023*; WHO Regional Office for Europe: Copenhagen, Denmark, 2023.

*vaccines*

MDPI

*Article*

# The Global Measles and Rubella Laboratory Network Supports High-Quality Surveillance

**Paul A. Rota [1], Roger Evans [2], Myriam Corinne Ben Mamou [3], Gloria Rey-Benito [4], Lucky Sangal [5], Annick Dosseh [6], Amany Ghoniem [7], Charles R. Byabamazima [6], Maurice Demanou [6], Raydel Anderson [1], Gimin Kim [1], Bettina Bankamp [1], R. Suzanne Beard [1], Stephen N. Crooke [1], Sumathi Ramachandran [1], Ana Penedos [8], Vicki Stambos [9], Suellen Nicholson [9], David Featherstone [10] and Mick N. Mulders [11,*]**

1 Centers for Disease Control and Prevention, Atlanta, GA 30329, USA; par1@cdc.gov (P.A.R.); ofi6@cdc.gov (G.K.); bfb9@cdc.gov (B.B.); zho3@cdc.gov (R.S.B.); qjf9@cdc.gov (S.N.C.); dcq6@cdc.gov (S.R.)
2 World Health Organization Western Pacific Regional Office, Manila 1000, Philippines; evansr@who.int
3 World Health Organization European Regional Office, 2100 Copenhagen, Denmark; benmamoum@who.int
4 Pan American Health Organization, Washington, DC 20037, USA; reyglori@paho.org
5 World Health Organization Southeast Asia Regional Office, Delhi 110002, India; sangallu@who.int
6 World Health Organization African Regional Office, Brazzaville P.O. Box 06, Congo; dosseha@who.int (A.D.); byabamazimac@who.int (C.R.B.); demanoum@who.int (M.D.)
7 World Health Organization Eastern Mediterranean Regional Office, Cairo 11371, Egypt; ghoniema@who.int
8 United Kingdom Health Security Agency, London NW9 5EQ, UK; ana.penedos@ukhsa.gov.uk
9 Victorian Infectious Diseases Reference Laboratory, The Royal Melbourne Hospital at the Peter Doherty Institute for Infection and Immunity, Melbourne 3000, Australia; vicki.stambos@mh.org.au (V.S.); suellen.nicholson@mh.org.au (S.N.)
10 Consultant Scientists Ltd., Hastings 4122, New Zealand; featherstoned@gmail.com
11 World Health Organization, 1211 Genève, Switzerland
* Correspondence: muldersm@who.int

**Abstract:** With 762 laboratories, the Global Measles and Rubella Laboratory Network (GMRLN) is the largest laboratory network coordinated by the World Health Organization (WHO). Like the Global Polio Laboratory Network, the GMRLN has multiple tiers, including global specialized laboratories, regional reference laboratories, national laboratories, and, in some countries, subnational laboratories. Regional networks are supervised by regional laboratory coordinators reporting to a global coordinator at WHO headquarters. Laboratories in the GMRLN have strong links to national disease control and vaccination programs. The GMRLN's goal is to support member states in obtaining timely, complete, and reliable laboratory-based surveillance data for measles and rubella as part of the strategy for achieving measles and rubella elimination. Surveillance data are reported to the national program and are included in annual reports on the status of measles and rubella elimination to national verification committees for review by regional verification commissions. Quality within the GMRLN is ensured by monitoring performance through external quality assurance programs, confirmatory and quality control testing, accreditation, and coordination of corrective action and training where needed. The overall performance of the laboratories has remained high over the years despite many challenges, particularly the COVID-19 pandemic. The GMRLN is well-positioned to support high-quality laboratory-based surveillance for measles and rubella and to transition to supporting laboratory testing for other pathogens, including vaccine-preventable diseases.

**Keywords:** measles-rubella laboratory; diagnostics; network; serology; PCR; WHO

## 1. Introduction to GMRLN

The World Health Organization (WHO) Global Measles and Rubella Laboratory Network (GMRLN) was developed using the model of the Global Polio Laboratory Network (GPLN) and the Measles Laboratory Network for the Region of the Americas as its foundation. In 1994, the Region of the Americas was certified as polio-free and, by the latter half of the 1990s, was making progress toward measles elimination. Other WHO regions had also made progress towards achieving polio-free status and were successively implementing a phased approach from control to outbreak prevention to measles elimination phases. By 1998, 115 countries had a measles elimination goal. The laboratory-based surveillance strategies for the first two phases were primarily testing a limited number of cases to confirm outbreaks and suspected spread cases. In the control and outbreak prevention phases, case confirmation was based on the detection of measles- and rubella-specific immunoglobulin M (IgM) in serum samples, though several laboratories were attempting to isolate the virus for genetic characterization. Once countries reached the elimination phase, with an incidence rate of <1 case/100,000 population, laboratories were expected to test all suspected cases and investigate virus transmission patterns to monitor interruption of endemic viral transmission. Specimens testing negative for measles IgM were tested for evidence of rubella IgM.

The GMRLN was built gradually as resources allowed, progress towards disease control was achieved, and elimination goals were set for measles and, later, for rubella. Although the GPLN was used as a model, many more laboratories were needed for the GMRLN, with almost all countries planning to have a measles-rubella laboratory. For the GMRLN, three tiers of laboratories were established. National laboratories (NLs), as nominated by member states, have a close link to national immunization and surveillance programs. Regional reference laboratories (RRLs) were designated from those laboratories demonstrating molecular testing capacity, a strong environment of quality control (QC) and quality assurance (QA), and the capacity to support NLs in their region. Finally, global specialized laboratories (GSLs) with strong technical expertise were established to support the development of protocols, establish QA and QC programs, and provide training and capacity strengthening for network laboratories at all levels. In some large countries, subnational laboratories (SNLs) have been added to the network to share the burden of work. Financial resources were primarily from the US Centers for Disease Control and Prevention (US-CDC), and technical support was provided by WHO, US-CDC, the United Kingdom Health Security Agency (UKHSA), the Victorian Infectious Diseases Reference Laboratory (VIDRL) in Australia, the National Microbiology Laboratory, at the Public Health Agency of Canada, and the National Institute of Infectious Diseases, Japan and RRLs.

Standardization, quality assurance, and timely and accurate reporting were the foundation of the GMRLN. An evaluation of commercially available IgM assays was conducted [1], a laboratory manual was developed and printed in English, French, Chinese, Russian, and Spanish, and annual global serology proficiency and accreditation programs were established in 1999–2000. The standardized WHO nomenclature to describe measles virus genetic characteristics was established at a meeting in 1998 [2]. Since 1997, training workshops covering IgM testing and reporting were held for new laboratories, and essential equipment, test kits, and reagents were provided according to the resource needs of each laboratory. On-site accreditation reviews by laboratory experts enabled the comprehensive, standardized assessment of a laboratory's layout, function, staffing, and interaction with surveillance programs, as well as monitoring performance over the past 12 months. The first GMRLN meeting was held in 2001 to obtain consensus on the development of the laboratory network, strengthen the integration of rubella testing, and develop a plan for improving genetic surveillance and the investigation of new technologies. At the time of the first global meeting, the GMRLN consisted of 3 GSLs, 7 RRLs, and 78 NLs (n = 88). However, the GMRLN expanded rapidly, and by 2012, there were almost 700 laboratories in the network. All countries had access to proficient laboratories or were served by one. In addition, routine testing for measles and rubella IgM exceeded 200,000 tests annually; 10,000 measles and rubella sequences had been submitted to the global databases, and annual proficiency testing, and accreditation programs were in place. The GMRLN continues to expand and support elimination quality surveillance for measles and rubella worldwide.

## 2. Structure and Governance

The GMRLN's goal is to support member states in obtaining timely, complete, and reliable laboratory-based surveillance data for measles and rubella [3]. Surveillance data are reported to the national program and are included in reports to national verification committees (NVC). Quality is ensured by monitoring performance through external quality assurance programs, confirmatory and specialized testing, and accreditation. GSLs and RRLs provide technical assistance to NLs and SNLs for laboratory testing and provide training to expand testing capacity and maintain a stable, competent workforce. GSLs and RRLs also perform specialized and confirmatory testing, develop new assays, and maintain external quality control programs for serologic and molecular testing. It is important to note that some GSLs and RRLs also serve as NLs to support surveillance in their country. The US-CDC supports laboratories in priority countries with laboratory reagents and diagnostic kits through the International Reagent Resource (IRR) program, and the UKHSA maintains the WHO global nucleotide surveillance databases for measles and rubella, Measles Virus Nucleotide Surveillance (MeaNS) and Rubella Virus Nucleotide Surveillance (RubeNS), respectively [4].

The GMRLN is managed by a global laboratory coordinator (GLC) at WHO headquarters in Geneva. Each WHO region has one or more regional laboratory coordinators (RLC) who manage regional activities. The GLC and RLCs, along with staff of the GSLs and RRLs, form the governance structure for GMRLN (Figure 1). In addition, GMRLN has established working groups (WG) to monitor and plan specific activities and develop new approaches. The GMRLN Strategy WG comprises external, non-WHO advisers who are experts in measles and rubella within the context of the global laboratory network. The Strategy WG provides advice and guidance on testing strategies and the introduction of new technologies within the network. The Strategy WG provides input on how to address the demands for laboratory-based surveillance from the global measles and rubella program, and especially regional programs to verify the elimination of measles and rubella. Additional working groups include Next-Generation, Extended Window, and Whole-Genome (NEW) Sequencing, Rapid Diagnostic Tests (RDT), Measles and Rubella Nomenclature, IgM Test Kit Evaluation, Accreditation Checklist, Laboratory Manual, and Seroprevalence. The activities of these WGs will be described in the sections that follow.

A

| WHO Region | GSL | RRL | NL | SNL | Total |
| --- | --- | --- | --- | --- | --- |
| AMR | 1 | 2 | 20 | 116 | 139 |
| EMR | 0 | 3 | 22 | 17 | 42 |
| EUR | 1 | 3 | 49 | 20 | 73 |
| SEAR | 0 | 3 | 18 | 37 | 58 |
| AFR | 0 | 3 | 48 | 4 | 55 |
| WPR w/o PR China | 1 | 2 | 17 | 13 | 33 |
| WPR-China | 0 | 1 | 32* | 339* | 372 |

*For China, the 32 provincial laboratories serve as NLs, while 339 prefecture laboratories are considered SNLs.

B

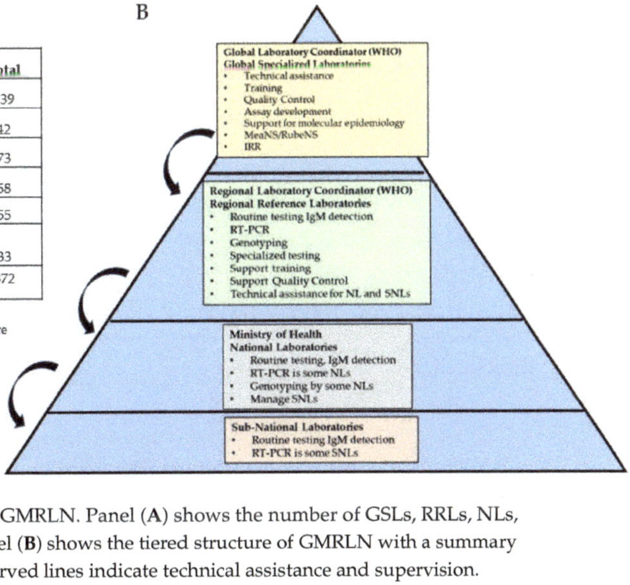


**Figure 1.** Structure and governance of GMRLN. Panel (**A**) shows the number of GSLs, RRLs, NLs, and SNLs by WHO region in 2024. Panel (**B**) shows the tiered structure of GMRLN with a summary of the major functions at each level. Curved lines indicate technical assistance and supervision.

The GMRLN established the MeaNS/RubeNS Steering Committee (SC) as an oversight board to define permissions, access, activities, roles, and responsibilities of database users. The SC also recommends modifications to the website to improve functionality. Every user must agree to the terms of the System Access Agreement and have passed the molecular external quality assurance (mEQA) that is administered by the US-CDC. The website for the databases is administered by the UKHSA and is used exclusively by GMRLN laboratories. Requests for access by non-GMRLN institutions will be considered by the SC.

Two GMRLN meetings take place each year. The winter meeting brings together the GLC, RLCs, GSLs, and other experts to provide a forum to discuss the status of the network and develop an annual work plan. The larger GMRLN meeting occurs later in the year and includes representatives from all GSLs and RRLs, as well as key NLs. At both meetings, the various working groups provide updates on progress.

## 3. Structure of Regional Networks

The GMRLN regional networks align with established WHO regions, the African Region (AFR), the Region of the Americas (AMR), the Eastern Mediterranean Region (EMR), the European Region (EUR), the South-East Asia Region (SEAR), and the Western Pacific Region (WPR). The AFR is divided into three sub-regions: Central Africa, Western Africa, and Eastern and Southern Africa. The number of RRLs in each region varies, and there is at least one NL in most member states (Figures 1 and 2). Many countries have a network of SNLs. All laboratories perform serologic testing, and a growing number of laboratories have molecular testing capacity (Table 1).

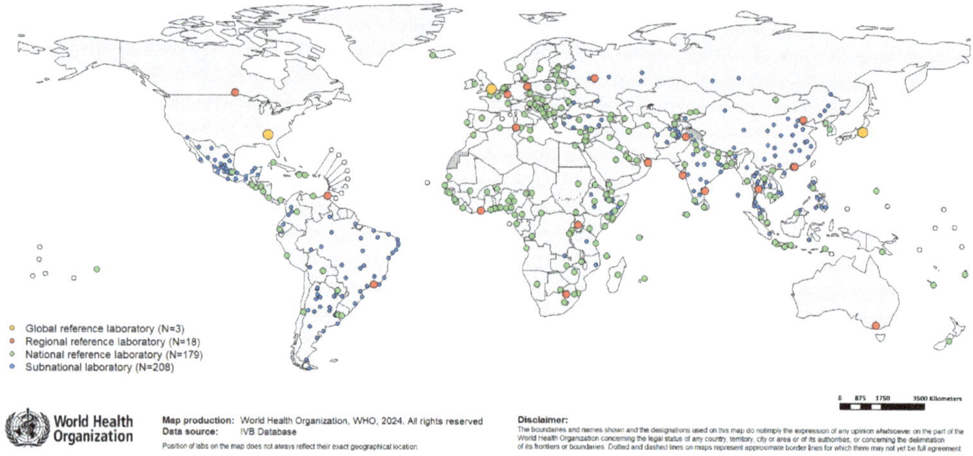


**Figure 2.** Map of GMRLN. Yellow circles indicate the locations of GSLs. Red circles indicate RRLs. Light blue circles indicate NLs. Blue circles indicate SNLs.

**Table 1.** Number of laboratories in the GMRLN performing molecular testing in each WHO region.

| WHO Region | NL Performing Virus Detection | Sequencing Labs |
|---|---|---|
| AMRO | 22 | 9 |
| EMRO | 8 | 7 |
| EURO | 43 | 32 |
| SEARO | 18 | 5 * |
| AFRO | 10 | 6 |
| WPRO | 13 | 45 |

* 5 labs perform sequencing, but 35 perform sequence analysis.

In the AFR, there are three RRLs located in Uganda, South Africa, and Côte d'Ivoire. There are a total of 48 NLs including those in Algeria, Angola, Benin, Botswana, Burkina Faso, Burundi, Cameroon, Central African Republic, Chad, Comoros, Republic of Congo, Democratic Republic of Congo (DRC), Eritrea, Ethiopia, Eswatini, Equatorial Guinea, Gabon, Gambia, Ghana, Guinea, Guinea-Bissau, Kenya, Lesotho, Liberia, Madagascar, Malawi, Mali, Mauritius, Mauritania, Mozambique, Namibia, Niger, Nigeria (7), Rwanda, Seychelles, Senegal, Sierra Leone, South Africa, South Sudan, Tanzania, Togo, Zambia, and Zimbabwe. There are four SNLs in AFR, including one in DRC, two in Ethiopia and one in Mozambique.

In the AMR, there is 1 GSL/RRL, the US-CDC, 2 RRLs located in Brazil and Canada, and 20 NLs including Argentina, Bolivia, Chile, Colombia, Costa Rica, Cuba, Dominican Republic, Ecuador, El Salvador, Guatemala, Haiti, Honduras, Mexico, Nicaragua, Panama, Paraguay, Peru, Uruguay, and Venezuela. The laboratory in Trinidad and Tobago (Caribbean Public Health Agency) functions as a sub-regional reference laboratory for the Caribbean. In addition to WHO-accredited laboratories, some countries independently manage a network of SNLs, including 27 in Argentina, 27 in Brazil, 26 in Canada, 3 in Colombia, 2 in Ecuador, and 31 in Mexico. In the US, the US-CDC supports four vaccine-preventable disease reference centers [5], which provide laboratory testing support to multiple state health laboratories and departments.

In the EMR, there are two RRLs located in Oman and Tunisia, plus a sub-regional reference laboratory located in Pakistan. There are 22 NLs in total in Iran, Iraq, Egypt, Saudi Arabia, Afghanistan, Bahrain, Djibouti, Kuwait, Lebanon, Libya, Morocco, Palestine, Qatar, Somalia, Syria, United Arab Emirates, Tunisia, and 2 in Yemen. There are a few countries with SNL networks, including Afghanistan with 9 and Somalia with 11.

In the EUR, there is one GSL, the UKHSA, and three RRLs located in Luxembourg, Germany, and the Russian Federation. The region includes 49 NLs located in Albania, Armenia, Austria, Azerbaijan, Belarus, Belgium, Bulgaria, Croatia, Cyprus, Czech Republic, Denmark, Estonia, Finland, Georgia, Greece, Hungary, Iceland, Ireland, Israel, Italy, Kazakhstan, Kyrgyzstan, Latvia, Lithuania, Malta, Moldova, Montenegro, North Macedonia, Norway, Poland, Portugal, Romania, Serbia, Slovakia, Slovenia, Spain, Sweden, Switzerland, Tajikistan, Turkey, Turkmenistan, Ukraine, Uzbekistan, 2 in France, 2 in the Netherlands, and 2 in Bosnia and Herzegovina. The EUR region also has countries with SNLs that are part of the GMRLN, including 1 in Kyrgyzstan, 1 in Ukraine, 7 in Turkey, and 10 in the Russian Federation. Three countries (Italy, Kazakhstan, and Ukraine) independently coordinate their own SNL networks, and the NL from four additional countries have collaborating laboratories under their supervision (Finland, Norway, Romania, and Sweden).

In the SEAR, there are three RRLs, one in Thailand and two in India. There is a total of 19 NLs, including 7 in India, 4 in Indonesia, and 1 each in Bangladesh, Bhutan, DPR Korea, Maldives, Myanmar, Nepal, Sri Lanka, and Timor-Leste. The SNL network in SEAR consists of 18 in India, 4 in Indonesia, 1 in Nepal, and 13 in Thailand.

In the WPR, there is 1 GSL, the National Institute for Infectious Disease (NIID), located in Japan, 3 RRLs located in China, Hong Kong, and Australia, and 17 NLs, including 2 in Vietnam and 1 each in Brunei Darussalam, Cambodia, Fiji, French Polynesia, Guam, Lao PDR, Macau, Malaysia, Mongolia, New Caledonia, New Zealand, Papua New Guinea, Philippines, Republic of Korea, and Singapore. There are 13 accredited SNLs in the region: seven in the Philippines, two in Vietnam, and four in Malaysia. China established 32 WHO-accredited provincial and 339 prefectural laboratories accredited by China CDC. The GSL in Japan also independently coordinates its own SNL network.

## 4. Testing and Quality Control in GMRLN

The GMRLN supports measles and rubella surveillance by performing laboratory testing for confirmation of infection and conducting genetic characterization of circulating viruses. All the 762 laboratories perform serologic confirmation for measles and rubella infection. Serologic testing is primarily the detection of measles- and rubella-specific

IgM in serum samples. GMRLN laboratories use commercial kits for IgM detection, and the quality of the kits is monitored by the GMRLN. In 2023, the GMRLN performed over 600,000 serologic tests, a significant increase in testing from 2022 (Table 2). While IgM detection is still considered the standard test for case confirmation, especially in endemic countries, many countries have included the detection of viral RNA by reverse transcription polymerase chain reaction (RT-PCR) in the testing algorithm. As countries move towards the elimination of measles and rubella, molecular testing will play an increasingly important role.

**Table 2.** Workload of the GMRLN in 2022–2023.

| GMRLN Testing by Year | Specimens Received | Specimens Tested |
|---|---|---|
| 2023 | 402,883 | Measles 333,835<br>Rubella 286,780<br>Total tests 620,615 |
| 2022 | 272,990 | Measles 217,179<br>Rubella 209,992<br>Total tests 427,171 |

The GMRLN is responsible for the genetic characterization of wild-type measles and rubella viruses. Laboratories obtain sequence information by amplification of sequencing templates from clinical samples. The current standard protocols call for sequencing either the 450 nucleotides coding for the COOH terminal 150 amino acid region of the measles nucleoprotein gene (N-450) or 739 nucleotides from the rubella E1 gene (E1-739). Sanger sequencing methods are widely used in the GMRLN. Sequence data are submitted to the WHO global nucleotide surveillance databases, MeaNS and RubeNS. It should be noted that sequence analysis is required to distinguish between a measles vaccine reaction and infection with a wild-type virus, though vaccine-specific RT-PCR assays are being introduced in some countries [6]. The GMRLN is developing methods and quality control standards for next-generation sequencing (NGS), which will allow laboratories to obtain whole genome sequences (WGS).

In addition to the standard testing methods, GSLs and RRLs perform referral testing to help with case confirmation and case classification. Testing for immunoglobulin G (IgG) avidity is usually performed in an enzyme-linked immune assay format. High avidity IgG indicates past infection or previous vaccination with measles- or rubella-containing vaccine, while low avidity IgG is consistent with recent vaccination or infection. Avidity testing has been useful for ruling out rubella infections when IgM testing gives false positive results and for distinguishing between primary and secondary vaccine failure in measles breakthrough cases [7].

The GMRLN supports the evaluation of population immunity through serosurveys. Until recently, the most common method was enzyme immunoassay (EIA) to detect measles and rubella IgG. Only a few specialized laboratories can perform virus neutralization assays, which are the most sensitive assays for measuring virus-specific IgG concentrations. More recently, multiplexed bead assays (MBAs) have been employed to measure IgG for measles and rubella [8]. The MBA has a sensitivity equivalent to virus neutralization, is amenable to a high throughput format, and can be performed with a small amount of serum. Simultaneous testing for measles and rubella IgG saves time and resources.

As countries move towards the elimination of measles and rubella, an assessment of the quality of surveillance activities is necessary to demonstrate adequate support for verification of elimination. Five of the eight core surveillance performance indicators assess the quality and timeliness of laboratory testing and should be reported by countries to WHO regional offices. These include a proportion of countries reporting to their WHO regional office on time (target: 100%), reporting discarded non-measles non-rubella cases at the national level (target: $\geq$2 cases per 100,000 population per year), the proportion of suspected cases with adequate specimens for detecting acute measles or rubella infection collected and tested in a proficient laboratory (target: ≥80%), the proportion of laboratory-confirmed chains of transmission with samples adequate for detecting measles or rubella virus collected and tested in an accredited laboratory (target: ≥80%), and proportion of results reported by the laboratory within 4 days of specimen receipt (target: ≥80%). Satisfactory performance by the GMRLN in each country is a prerequisite for verification of elimination.

Quality control is the hallmark of the GMRLN. It is important that all laboratories provide accurate and consistent results to national immunization programs. Quality is improved by sharing protocols for validated methods within the network. The GMRLN has developed a detailed laboratory manual containing chapters on laboratory testing and detailed, regularly updated protocols for standard tests. The latest version of the manual was published in 2018 [9].

The GMRLN laboratories are required to participate in annual proficiency testing (PT) for measles and rubella IgM detection. The serologic PT panels for the NLs are provided by the VIDRL in Melbourne, Australia. As of 2023, there were 144 laboratories participating in the PT program. During the 2023 round of PT, 97% of laboratories submitting measles results and 98% of laboratories submitting rubella results obtained a passing score. As of May 2024, 223 laboratories submitted results for the 2023 PT program; there are additional laboratories still to submit results for this panel. For 2022, 245 laboratories participated in the PT program, and 99% of laboratories submitting measles results and 99% of laboratories submitting rubella results obtained a passing score. For those member states that have large SNL networks, the NLs are responsible for administering country-specific serology PT. The VIDRL provides training workshops for preparing and evaluating PT panels.

To fulfill requirements for WHO accreditation, in addition to passing the PT, NLs need to send 10% of tested specimens or at least 50 specimens annually to the RRL for confirmatory testing. There must be at least 90% concurrence between the results of the NL and the RRL for the NL to obtain full accreditation status. For any laboratory not reaching the minimum concurrence or not submitting samples for QC, its accreditation standing may reflect a provisional status until it returns to compliance.

The purpose of the mEQA program of the GMRLN is to assess the ability of network laboratories to perform molecular testing. Molecular testing includes assays to detect viral RNA, i.e., real-time RT-PCR (rRT-PCR) or endpoint RT-PCR for rubella, as well as assays used for routine genotyping (measles N-450 and rubella E1-739). Additionally, all GMRLN laboratories that report sequences to the global databases, MeaNS and RubeNS, are required to pass the sequencing portion of the mEQA. In 2022, 119 NLs participated in the mEQA for measles, and 108 participated for rubella. Of these, 95% and 96% passed measles and rubella proficiency testing, respectively. Laboratories that fail any portion of the mEQA must pass a repeat test before they can submit sequence data to the global databases. Countries with a large SNL network are responsible for country-specific mEQA. US-CDC provides training workshops to NLs preparing mEQA panels to ensure consistency with proficiency testing.

WHO accredits all GMRLN laboratories based on a standard checklist of requirements. Accreditation is achieved by onsite visits as well as desk reviews. New laboratories will receive an initial onsite accreditation followed by onsite visits every 2–5 years, depending on the region. Most laboratories are required to complete the accreditation checklist for desk review annually. The Accreditation WG completed a revised version of the checklist in 2024.

## 5. Introduction of New Technologies

The GMRLN has designated a working group focusing on developing and deploying rapid diagnostic tests (RDTs) for measles and rubella, including a framework for introducing RDTs to national surveillance programs [10]. RDTs were a game changer during the COVID-19 pandemic, and RDTs are expected to impact the timeliness and sensitivity of measles and rubella surveillance. One challenge considered by the RDT WG is the reporting of negative test results needed to evaluate the performance of national surveillance programs. Along with the WHO, various partners, including the Bill and Melinda Gates Foundation, Gavi the Vaccine Alliance, US-CDC, UKHSA, UNICEF, and FIND, have made great efforts to introduce newly developed measles and rubella testing formats (e.g., RDTs) to the GMRLN. Besides supporting the development and production of RDTs, the WG is developing guidance for the introduction of RDTs.

Three additional WGs with overlapping roles are focusing on improving serologic testing. One WG is involved in the validation of enzyme-linked immune assays. This WG developed a target product profile to define the minimum user requirements of measles and rubella EIA and RDT assays target product profile [11]. The target product profile allows commercial manufacturers of EIA and RDT assays to submit an expression of interest in participating in the evaluation study, which will be advertised in the United Nations Marketplace. One of the RRLs, the Public Health Agency of Canada, has agreed to conduct the laboratory evaluation of the assays and provide a report, which will be evaluated by the GMRLN and made available on the WHO website. Another WG is investigating the reasons for discrepant IgM test results. Recommendations from this WG will be available in the next version of the laboratory manual. A third WG is involved in the development and use of the MBA [8], also called multiplex immunoassay [12], to facilitate seroprevalence studies.

## 6. Molecular Epidemiology

Genetic characterization of wild-type measles and rubella viruses is a critical component of the global surveillance program. Data from virologic surveillance can map viral transmission pathways, allowing linkage of cases and outbreaks and identification of possible sources of importation. Characterization of the genetic properties of circulating wild-type viruses helps monitor progress toward elimination goals. An essential element of verification of measles and rubella elimination is documentation of $\geq$12 months with no continuous circulation of the virus in a country with a well-performing surveillance system; verification of elimination is achieved after $\geq$36 months of uninterrupted endemic viral transmission. Virologic surveillance data provided in each country's annual NVC report to the regional verification commission constitutes a critical line of evidence supporting the verification criteria. The GMRLN plays an essential role in this process by generating high-quality sequence data. At the country level, understanding virus transmission allows the identification of immunization gaps and the tailoring of strategies for the intervention [13].

While WHO recognizes 24 genotypes of measles, the usefulness of standard genotyping for monitoring measles transmission is now limited because only two genotypes, B3 and D8, have been detected since 2021 (Figure 3A). Genetic diversity within a genotype is monitored by using a distinct sequence identifier (DSId) for each unique N-450 sequence. The GMRLN has provided guidance for countries on how to present data from measles N-450 sequences in reports to NVCs [13]. However, with the decrease in genetic diversity, the utility of N-450 sequence analysis to resolve measles transmission pathways is reduced. Increasing the amount of sequence data obtained from each case could improve the resolution of sequence analysis. The GMRLN supports efforts to sequence larger parts of the genome, including using NGS methods for obtaining WGS [14]. The NEW working group evaluated various methods developed by network laboratories for their applicability to virologic surveillance. Guidance for the introduction of new sequencing methods has been published by the NEW working group in the laboratory manual [9]. The NEW working group is involved in defining and developing methods for quality assurance of next-generation sequencing.

Rubella genotypes reported to RubeNS in the last 10 years were genotype 1E (58%) and genotype 2B (42%) (Figure 3B). However, most of the sequences were from outbreaks in only two countries, China, and Japan, highlighting the need to enhance global virologic surveillance for rubella [15]. Analysis of rubella genotypes helped support the verification of the elimination of rubella in the Americas. A nomenclature has been proposed to describe the intergenotypic diversity of rubella viruses [16].

A

| genotype \ year | 2014 | 2015 | 2016 | 2017 | 2018 | 2019 | 2020 | 2021 | 2022 | 2023 | 2024 |
|---|---|---|---|---|---|---|---|---|---|---|---|
| B3 | 1325 | 544 | 640 | 2536 | 2981 | 1943 | 405 | 595 | 740 | 841 | 347 |
| C2 | 0 | 0 | 0 | 0 | 0 | 1 | 0 | 0 | 0 | 0 | 0 |
| D4 | 32 | 59 | 47 | 11 | 19 | 6 | 63 | 0 | 0 | 0 | 0 |
| D5 | 0 | 1 | 0 | 0 | 0 | 0 | 0 | 0 | 0 | 0 | 0 |
| D6 | 1 | 0 | 0 | 0 | 0 | 0 | 0 | 0 | 0 | 0 | 0 |
| D8 | 1043 | 1185 | 1220 | 2303 | 3831 | 7112 | 1091 | 189 | 860 | 2236 | 805 |
| D9 | 82 | 26 | 67 | 45 | 0 | 1 | 0 | 0 | 0 | 0 | 0 |
| G3 | 4 | 0 | 0 | 0 | 0 | 0 | 0 | 0 | 0 | 0 | 0 |
| H1 | 4765 | 3131 | 2546 | 537 | 344 | 26 | 0 | 0 | 0 | 0 | 0 |

B

| genotype \ year | 2014 | 2015 | 2016 | 2017 | 2018 | 2019 | 2020 | 2021 | 2022 | 2023 | 2024 |
|---|---|---|---|---|---|---|---|---|---|---|---|
| 1a | 0 | 1 | 0 | 0 | 0 | 1 | 0 | 0 | 0 | 0 | 0 |
| 1E | 31 | 12 | 10 | 12 | 1091 | 2069 | 47 | 2 | 0 | 0 | 0 |
| 1G | 1 | 2 | 6 | 2 | 0 | 0 | 0 | 0 | 0 | 1 | 0 |
| 1H | 0 | 0 | 1 | 1 | 0 | 0 | 0 | 0 | 0 | 0 | 0 |
| 1J | 1 | 1 | 0 | 0 | 0 | 0 | 0 | 0 | 0 | 0 | 0 |
| 2B | 119 | 387 | 211 | 173 | 145 | 1191 | 44 | 10 | 2 | 1 | 0 |

**Figure 3.** Heatmap showing the number of measles (panel (**A**)) and rubella (panel (**B**)) sequences submitted to MeaNS and RubeNS by genotype for the year 2014 through March 2024.

The Measles and Rubella Nomenclature WG with the GMRLN is analyzing the sequences submitted in MeaNS and RubeNS to define lineages of measles and rubella viruses. This will support a more precise classification of the genetic variants of measles and rubella and improve the ability of sequence data to monitor transmission chains.

## 7. Training

To maintain high-quality work, there is a continual need for training within the GMRLN. Training is provided in multiple formats, hands-on, conducted on-site, or virtually. Most of the recent training activities have focused on methods for molecular biology since serologic testing is well established within the GMRLN; however, training for IgM testing and IgG avidity testing are also offered. Since 2022, twelve regional workshops have been conducted in AFR, AMR, EMR, and EUR, with a focus on molecular and serologic methods (Table 3).

In these workshops, US-CDC provided training to 230 participants from 60 countries through 18 separate workshops (Table 4). Each training workshop serves a unique purpose, with agendas based on regional requirements. On-site workshops involve hands-on training in technical and analytical procedures for rRT-PCR, conventional RT-PCR, and Sanger sequencing associated with the detection and genotyping of measles and rubella viruses. Laboratory exercises are followed by hands-on sequence analysis using RECall® software (version 2.34) and phylogenetic analysis using MEGA® software (version 11). The use of MeaNS and RubeNS databases to track circulating virus lineages and nomenclature for measles and rubella was implemented in the training. Quality control and troubleshooting were also discussed. Follow-up assessments were always conducted to ensure the acceptability of results from the trained laboratories. Participants were provided with practice panels to submit to the CDC for evaluation.

**Table 3.** Regional training activities by the GMRLN in 2022–2023.

| WHO Region | Training | Date | Participants | Lead |
|---|---|---|---|---|
| AFR | Molecular | November 2022 | Eritrea, Kenya, Mauritius, Mozambique, Seychelles, South Africa, Zambia | US-CDC, RRL Uganda Virus Research Institute |
| EUR | Serology webinar | May 2023 | Armenia, Kazakhstan, Kyrgyzstan, Turkmenistan | RRL Moscow |
| EUR | GT/sequencing | May 2023 | Serbia | RRL Luxembourg |
| AFR | Serology | September 2023 | Equatorial Guinea | RRL Pasteur Institute Cote d'Ivoire |
| EUR | Advanced training in serology/molecular | September 2023 | Moscow RRL | RRL Luxembourg |
| EUR | Serology/rRT-PCR/sequence analysis/MeaNS | October 2023 | Entire network (group-specific) | London and US-CDC, RRLs: Luxembourg, Berlin, and Moscow |
| EUR | Measles rRT-PCR hands-on training | November–December 2023 | Kyrgyzstan NL and SNL Uzbekistan Tajikistan | RRL Moscow |
| EMR | ELISA for measles and rubella, measles rRT-PCR | September 2023 | CPHL Kabul | NIH Islamabad |
| EMR | Serological detection of measles and rubella virus | November 2023 | Somalia | RRL Tunisia, Pasteur Institute |
| EMR | MR outbreak simulation exercise | November 2023 | Egypt | Egypt |
| EMR | Workshop on measles and rubella verification of elimination | February 2023 | Kuwait, Qatar, Saudi Arabia, UAE | United Arab Emirates |
| AMR | Measles and rubella rRT-PCR | November 2023 | Nicaragua | AMR |

**Table 4.** Training activities provided by the US CDC and WHO's Regional Offices in 2023.

| Training Location | Training | Date | Participants |
|---|---|---|---|
| Webinar | Webinar on measles and rubella diagnostic real-time RT-PCR | January 2023 | Angola |
| Webinar | Webinar on measles and rubella diagnostic real-time RT-PCR | January 2023 | Armenia, Azerbaijan, Belarus, Kazakhstan, Kyrgyzstan, Moldova, Tajikistan, Turkmenistan, Uzbekistan |
| National Institute of Health, Bangkok, Thailand | Strengthening molecular capacity for the Global Measles and Rubella Laboratory Network in the South-East Asia Region | March 2023 | Bangladesh, Bhutan, Indonesia, Thailand, Maldives, Nepal, Sri Lanka, Timor-Leste |
| Institute of Epidemiological Diagnosis and Reference Laboratory (InDRE), Mexico | Measles and rubella genotyping workshop | September 2023 | Colombia, Mexico, Peru, Trinidad and Tobago, Uruguay |
| Nigeria Centre for Disease Control (NCDC), Nigeria | "Train the Trainers" serology workshop and molecular techniques for the detection of measles and rubella | October 2023 | Lagos Central Public Health Laboratory and the National Reference Laboratory |
| Istanbul, Türkiye | Molecular techniques for the detection of measles and rubella | October 2023 | European countries |
| Webinar | Use of Sequencher® (version 5.4.6) for sequence analysis of measles and rubella | December 2023 | India, Hong Kong, Thailand, Bangladesh |

To build regional training capacity, train the trainers (TTT) workshops have been organized. In addition, the US-CDC has initiated a program to train regional focal points for laboratory training. This TTT is designed to harmonize the approaches to and methods for training and to build regional training capacity. Selected GMRLN scientists spend eight to ten weeks at the US-CDC measles and rubella laboratories in Atlanta, learning techniques, troubleshooting, and analysis, as well as giving presentations. A teach-back session for each method with a hands-on teaching component is part of the TTT workshops to ensure that the knowledge transfer is successful. Ultimately, this TTT program will lead to sustained training capacity in the regions.

## 8. Achievements and Challenges

Overall, the performance of the GMRLN has remained high despite many challenges. While the most significant challenge was the disruption caused by the COVID-19 pandemic, other challenges include limited financial resources for testing and regional coordination, staff turnover in national laboratories, updating molecular epidemiology, integration of new technologies, expansion of the network, lack of serum samples for the serologic proficient testing program, and developing testing strategies for pre- and post-elimination settings. Laboratory surveillance indicators in all regions remain high, although many countries struggle to meet the discard rate of 2/100,000 population.

Now that global travel has returned to pre-pandemic levels, the GMRLN has been able to address staff turnover by providing training opportunities for new staff. These trainings help build a stable and competent workforce, increase capacity, and introduce new or modified testing methods. To address the training needs for this increasing network, regional training capacity will need improvement with the assignment of regional training focal points and continuation of the TTT programs.

The Measles and Rubella Strategic Framework 2021–2030 [17], developed as part of the Immunization Agenda 2030 (IA2030) [18], reinforces measles and rubella elimination as a critical goal. In addition, IA2030 calls for using measles as a tracer to identify weaknesses in immunization programs. Therefore, strong laboratory-based surveillance will be a critical factor in monitoring programmatic achievements. Many countries are now expanding their domestic laboratory capacity by enrolling new laboratories, so the GMRLN keeps expanding. Robust serology and molecular EQA programs monitor the performance of the network laboratories. With that expansion also comes a greater need for EQA programs, creating an increased demand for WHO-coordinated EQA programs. Several countries have established EQA programs for SNLs, and efforts are underway to train national laboratories in larger countries with an SNL network to conduct their own EQA programs. The RLCs have worked with VIRDL to identify sources of serum samples for the serologic proficiency testing program.

The WHO remains committed to continue coordinating the GMRLN through its GLC and RLCs by organizing regular meetings and workshops. Resources are needed to maintain regional coordination for the GMRLN. A game-changer for the network has been the IRR, which took over the provision of proficiency test panels, diagnostic kits, and reagents from the WHO, significantly increasing delivery speed in most countries. RLCs work with the CDC to manage the distribution of materials and monitor inventories to minimize stockouts.

During the pandemic, a major investment was made to introduce molecular testing capacity for SARS-CoV-2 on a wide scale. This created an opportunity to introduce routine molecular testing for other pathogens. Many of the laboratory staff in measles and rubella laboratories have been trained in molecular diagnostics, and with the widespread availability of equipment, many of these laboratories are now adding rRT-PCR for measles and rubella to their portfolio as an added tool to confirm suspect cases. The pandemic also made sequencing accessible to many more laboratories. The GMRLN must make sure network laboratories have the capacity to use rRT-PCR as part of the case confirmation algorithm and generate high-quality sequence data to monitor viral transmission pathways. New, validated protocols and subsequent training will be needed. The GMRLN will continue its reliance on the MeaNS and RubeNS databases, particularly now that many laboratories are transitioning to NGS. Viral genetic diversity has decreased in recent years, creating a need to better describe genetic variability with measles and rubella genotypes. Therefore, there is a critical need to expand capacity for sequencing and to develop an updated nomenclature to describe intragenotype variation.

With an ever-increasing laboratory network, one of the biggest challenges for the GMRLN is its need to diversify its source of funding to maintain and expand its capacity and capability. The US-CDC has been a generous provider of resources to the GMRLN since its inception, not only in funds but also in technical assistance, staff training, and the provision of quality laboratory management programs. This support has been crucial to the GMRLN's development. There has also been a strong reliance on the GPLN since the initiation of the GMRLN. Many investments made into building infrastructure and laboratory capacity in the GPLN have been beneficial to other vaccine-preventable disease laboratory networks such as GMRLN, Yellow Fever, and rotavirus [19]. This synergy has been very beneficial and a cost-effective use of donor support. With polio eradication approaching, a process of transition has been initiated as described in the Strategic Action Plan on Polio Transition [20]. This transition creates a need to integrate activities between polio and other programs, including laboratory networks. A revised action plan is under development to describe the opportunities during transition. The WHO has developed a global strategy for comprehensive vaccine-preventable disease (VPD) surveillance [21,22]. This strategy promotes the development of comprehensive high-functioning surveillance systems that encompass all VPD threats faced by a country in all areas and populations, wherever possible, taking advantage of the shared infrastructure for components of surveillance such as data management and laboratory systems.

One of the five main objectives of the global strategy is to strengthen and expand public health laboratory networks. The GMRLN has an excellent capacity to conduct basic and advanced laboratory testing, as shown by the outcomes of the accreditation and quality control programs. Therefore, the GMRLN is well-positioned to support high-quality laboratory-based surveillance for measles and rubella and to transition to supporting laboratory testing for other pathogens, including vaccine-preventable diseases. Expansion of the GMRLN will be based on the guiding principles of high-quality testing, outstanding quality control, and integration with national and regional disease control plans.

**Author Contributions:** P.A.R., M.N.M., D.F., G.K. and R.A., writing—original draft preparation; R.E., M.C.B.M., G.R.-B., L.S., A.D., A.G., C.R.B., M.D., B.B., R.S.B., S.N.C., S.R., A.P., V.S. and S.N., writing—review and editing; P.A.R. and M.N.M., conceptualization. All authors have read and agreed to the published version of the manuscript.

**Funding:** This research received no external funding.

**Institutional Review Board Statement:** This project was reviewed by the CDC IRB and based on the regulatory definition, this activity was determined not to be human subjects research.

**Informed Consent Statement:** Not applicable.

**Data Availability Statement:** The data presented in this study are available in this article.

**Acknowledgments:** The authors wish to thank Sebastien Antoni for assistance with Figure 2 and Katrina Kretsinger, James Alexander, and Pratima Raghunathan for editorial assistance.

**Conflicts of Interest:** Author David Featherstone was employed by the company Consultant Scientists Ltd. The remaining authors declare that the research was conducted in the absence of any commercial or financial relationships that could be construed as a potential conflict of interest.

**CDC Disclaimer:** The findings and conclusions in this report are those of the authors and do not necessarily represent the official position of the Centers for Disease Control and Prevention.

**WHO Disclaimer:** The findings and conclusions in this report are those of the authors and do not necessarily represent the official position of the World Health Organization.

## References

1. Tipples, G.A.; Hamkar, R.; Mohktari-Azad, T.; Gray, M.; Ball, J.; Head, C.; Ratnam, S. Evaluation of rubella IgM enzyme immunoassays. *J. Clin. Virol.* **2004**, *30*, 233–238. [CrossRef]
2. World Health Organization. Expanded Programme on Immunization (EPI). Standardization of the nomenclature for describing the genetic characteristics of wild-type measles viruses. *Relev. Epidemiol. Hebd.* **1998**, *73*, 265–269.

3. Mulders, M.N.; Rota, P.A.; Icenogle, J.P.; Brown, K.E.; Takeda, M.; Rey, G.J.; Ben Mamou, M.C.; Dosseh, A.R.; Byabamazima, C.R.; Ahmed, H.J.; et al. Global Measles and Rubella Laboratory Network Support for Elimination Goals, 2010–2015. *MMWR. Morb. Mortal. Wkly. Rep.* **2016**, *65*, 438–442. [CrossRef] [PubMed]
4. MeaNS and RubeNS. Available online: https://who-gmrln.org/ (accessed on 11 July 2024).
5. Association of Public Health Laboratories. Vaccine Preventable Diseases. Available online: https://www.aphl.org/programs/infectious_disease/Pages/VPD.aspx (accessed on 12 July 2024).
6. Roy, F.; Mendoza, L.; Hiebert, J.; McNall, R.J.; Bankamp, B.; Connolly, S.; Ludde, A.; Friedrich, N.; Mankertz, A.; Rota, P.A.; et al. Rapid Identification of Measles Virus Vaccine Genotype by Real-Time PCR. *J. Clin. Microbiol.* **2017**, *55*, 735–743. [CrossRef] [PubMed]
7. Sowers, S.B.; Rota, J.S.; Hickman, C.J.; Mercader, S.; Redd, S.; McNall, R.J.; Williams, N.; McGrew, M.; Walls, M.L.; Rota, P.A.; et al. High Concentrations of Measles Neutralizing Antibodies and High-Avidity Measles IgG Accurately Identify Measles Reinfection Cases. *Clin. Vaccine Immunol.* **2016**, *23*, 707–716. [CrossRef]
8. Coughlin, M.M.; Matson, Z.; Sowers, S.B.; Priest, J.W.; Smits, G.P.; van der Klis, F.R.M.; Mitchell, A.; Hickman, C.J.; Scobie, H.M.; Goodson, J.L.; et al. Development of a Measles and Rubella Multiplex Bead Serological Assay for Assessing Population Immunity. *J. Clin. Microbiol.* **2021**, *59*, 6. [CrossRef]
9. World Health Organization. Manual for the Laboratory-based Surveillance of Measles, Rubella, and Congenital Rubella Syndrome. Available online: https://www.technet-21.org/en/manual-introduction (accessed on 22 July 2024).
10. Brown, D.W.; Warrener, L.; Scobie, H.M.; Donadel, M.; Waku-Kouomou, D.; Mulders, M.N.; Rota, P.A. Rapid diagnostic tests to address challenges for global measles surveillance. *Curr. Opin. Virol.* **2020**, *41*, 77–84. [CrossRef] [PubMed]
11. Target Product Profile for Surveillance Tests for Measles and Rubella. Available online: https://www.finddx.org/wp-content/uploads/2024/06/20240613_tpp_measles_rubell_FV_EN.pdf (accessed on 22 July 2024).
12. Smits, G.P.; van Gageldonk, P.G.; Schouls, L.M.; van der Klis, F.R.; Berbers, G.A. Development of a bead-based multiplex immunoassay for simultaneous quantitative detection of IgG serum antibodies against measles, mumps, rubella, and varicella-zoster virus. *Clin. Vaccine Immunol.* **2012**, *19*, 396–400. [CrossRef]
13. Williams, D.; Penedos, A.; Bankamp, B.; Anderson, R.; Hubschen, J.; Ben Mamou, M.; Beck, A.; Brown, D.; Rey, G.; Evans, R.; et al. Update: Circulation of active genotypes of measles virus and recommendations for use of sequence analysis to monitor viral transmission. *Relev. Epidemiol. Hebd.* **2022**, *97*, 485–492.
14. Bankamp, B.; Kim, G.; Hart, D.; Beck, A.; Rota, P.A.; Zhang, Y.; Ben Mamou, M. Global update on measles molecular epidemiology. *Vaccines* **2024**, *12*, 810. [CrossRef] [PubMed]
15. Ou, A.C.; Zimmerman, L.A.; Alexander, J.P., Jr.; Crowcroft, N.S.; O'Connor, P.M.; Knapp, J.K. Progress Toward Rubella and Congenital Rubella Syndrome Elimination—Worldwide, 2012–2022. *MMWR. Morb. Mortal. Wkly. Rep.* **2024**, *73*, 162–167. [CrossRef] [PubMed]
16. Rivailler, P.; Abernathy, E.; Icenogle, J. Genetic diversity of currently circulating rubella viruses: A need to define more precise viral groups. *J. Gen. Virol.* **2017**, *98*, 396–404. [CrossRef] [PubMed]
17. World Health Organization. Measles and Rubella Strategic Framework: 2021–2030. Available online: https://iris.who.int/bitstream/handle/10665/339801/9789240015616-eng.pdf?sequence=1&isAllowed=y (accessed on 22 July 2024).
18. World Health Organization. Immunization Agenda 2030: A Global Strategy to Leave No One Behind. Available online: https://www.who.int/publications/m/item/immunization-agenda-2030-a-global-strategy-to-leave-no-one-behind (accessed on 22 July 2024).
19. Mulders, M.N.; Serhan, F.; Goodson, J.L.; Icenogle, J.; Johnson, B.W.; Rota, P.A. Expansion of Surveillance for Vaccine-preventable Diseases: Building on the Global Polio Laboratory Network and the Global Measles and Rubella Laboratory Network Platforms. *J. Infect. Dis.* **2017**, *216*, S324–S330. [CrossRef]
20. World Health Organization. *Polio Transition and Post-Certification Draft Strategic Action Plan on Polio Transition*; Seventy-first World Health Assembly, A71/9 Provisional Agenda Item; World Health Organization: Geneva, Switzerland, 2018.
21. World Health Organization. Global Strategy for Comprehensive Vaccine-Preventable Disease (VPD) Surveillance. Available online: https://cdn.who.int/media/docs/default-source/immunization/vpd_surveillance/bls20116-ia-global-strategy-english.pdf?sfvrsn=748c3e30_4&download=true (accessed on 22 July 2024).
22. Patel, M.K.; Scobie, H.M.; Serhan, F.; Dahl, B.; Murrill, C.S.; Nakamura, T.; Pallas, S.W.; Cohen, A.L.; Global Comprehensive Vaccine-Preventable Disease Surveillance Working Group. A global comprehensive vaccine-preventable disease surveillance strategy for the immunization Agenda 2030. *Vaccine* **2022**, *42*, S124–S128. [CrossRef] [PubMed]

*vaccines*

MDPI

*Review*

# Use of Measles and Rubella Rapid Diagnostic Tests to Improve Case Detection and Targeting of Vaccinations

**Audrey Rachlin [1,*], Lee M. Hampton [1], Paul A. Rota [2], Mick N. Mulders [3], Mark Papania [1], James L. Goodson [1], L. Kendall Krause [4], Matt Hanson [5], Jennifer Osborn [6], Cassandra Kelly-Cirino [6], Beth Evans [7,8], Antara Sinha [7], Lenesha Warrener [9], David Featherstone [10] and David Brown [9,11]**

1 Global Immunization Division, Centers for Disease Control and Prevention, Atlanta, GA 30329, USA
2 Division of Viral Diseases, Centers for Disease Control and Prevention, Atlanta, GA 30329, USA
3 Department of Immunization, Vaccines and Biologicals, World Health Organization, 1211 Geneva, Switzerland
4 Bill & Melinda Gates Foundation, Seattle, WA 98109, USA
5 Sound Global Health Consulting, LLC, Seattle, WA 98199, USA
6 Foundation for Innovative New Diagnostics (FIND), 1218 Geneva, Switzerland
7 Gavi, the Vaccine Alliance, Global Health Campus, 1218 Geneva, Switzerland
8 Institute of Global Health, Faculty of Medicine, University of Geneva, 1202 Geneva, Switzerland
9 Public Health Microbiology Division, UK Health Security Agency (UKHSA), London NW9 5EQ, UK
10 Consultant Scientists Ltd., Hastings 4122, New Zealand
11 Laboratory of Respiratory Viruses, Exanthematics, Enteroviruses and Viral Emergencies (LVRE), Oswaldo Cruz Institute, FIOCRUZ, Rio de Janeiro 21040-900, Brazil
* Correspondence: rhu0@cdc.gov

**Abstract:** Efforts to control and eliminate measles and rubella are aided by high-quality surveillance data—supported by laboratory confirmation—to guide decision-making on routine immunization strategies and locations for conducting preventive supplementary immunization activities (SIAs) and outbreak response. Important developments in rapid diagnostic tests (RDTs) for measles and rubella present new opportunities for the global measles and rubella surveillance program to greatly improve the ability to rapidly detect and respond to outbreaks. Here, we review the status of RDTs for measles and rubella Immunoglobulin M (IgM) testing, as well as ongoing questions and challenges regarding the operational use and deployment of RDTs as part of global measles and rubella surveillance. Efforts to develop IgM RDTs that can be produced at scale are underway. Once validated RDTs are available, clear information on the benefits, challenges, and costs of their implementation will be critical for shaping deployment guidance and informing country plans for sustainably deploying such tests. The wide availability of RDTs could provide new programmatic options for measles and rubella elimination efforts, potentially enabling improvements and flexibility for testing, surveillance, and vaccination.

**Keywords:** vaccine-preventable disease surveillance; disease elimination; diagnostics; immunization; GMRLN; RDTs

## 1. Introduction

Measles is a highly infectious respiratory disease that requires high population immunity to interrupt transmission. Although measles vaccination is estimated to have prevented 57 million deaths worldwide during 2000–2022, an estimated 136,200 individuals died from measles in 2022 and large or disruptive outbreaks were reported in 37 countries [1]. At the same time, reported rubella cases fell to 17,407 globally in 2022 and 98 countries have been verified as having eliminated rubella [2]. The Immunization Agenda 2021–2030 (IA2030) [3] aims to achieve measles and rubella regional elimination targets as a core indicator of vaccine impact and positions measles as a tracer of a health system's ability to deliver essential childhood vaccines. Efforts to control and eliminate measles and rubella are aided by accurate surveillance data—supported by timely high-quality laboratory testing—to guide decision-making on routine immunization strategies and where to conduct preventive supplementary immunization activities (SIAs) and outbreak response [1,4,5]. Important developments in rapid diagnostic tests (RDTs) for measles and rubella testing, in combination with advances in innovation with molecular detection, present new opportunities for the global measles and rubella surveillance program to greatly improve the ability to rapidly detect and respond to outbreaks. Here, we review the status of RDTs for measles and rubella Immunoglobulin M (IgM) testing, as well as ongoing questions regarding the operational use and deployment of RDTs as part of global measles and rubella surveillance. We also discuss RDT financing challenges in low- and middle-income countries and reflect on the potential ways forward.

## 2. Measles and Rubella Immunization

Vaccines for measles have been in widespread use over the last 50 years, either as a single antigen vaccine or as combination vaccines with rubella, mumps, or varicella antigens [6]. For more than 20 years, the vaccine has been used as part of a global program to control and eliminate measles. The World Health Organization's Strategic Advisory Group of Experts on Immunization (SAGE) recommends the following: two doses of the measles vaccine administered routinely to all children worldwide—in endemic settings, one at nine months and another at 15-18 months of age; and the rubella vaccine should be administered routinely to all children once the member states they live in can achieve levels of population immunity high enough to minimize the risk of rubella infection in unvaccinated females of child-bearing age [6,7]. Complementing routine immunization against measles and rubella, preventive SIAs help close gaps in population immunity and prevent morbidity and mortality against both diseases. Outbreak response vaccination activities are used to control measles and rubella outbreaks and can also further mitigate measles and rubella morbidity and mortality. For both preventive SIAs and outbreak-response activities, timely and reliable surveillance information—including test results and epidemiological data on whom to target for vaccination—can help to reduce the number of unnecessary vaccinations and can make SIAs more effective by identifying at-risk and unreached groups that need to be vaccinated [5,8].

## 3. Laboratory Testing for Measles and Rubella Surveillance to Guide Immunization Programs

Measles virus infection presents as an illness characterized by rash and fever, with a prodromal phase lasting 2 to 4 days that may include symptoms of cough, coryza, and conjunctivitis [9]. The clinical similarities between measles, rubella, and other diseases that can cause fever and maculopapular rash make laboratory confirmation of suspected cases an essential component of surveillance. Lack of laboratory confirmation may lead to misclassification and inaccurate conclusions, for example, that measles or rubella are not circulating in an area where the viruses are responsible for clinical cases, or misclassification leading to mistaken assessments that measles or rubella are responsible for a significant burden of disease, potentially prompting additional response activities unnecessarily [10].

For a number of vaccine-preventable diseases, the lack of timely and accurate laboratory testing capacity has led to challenges in determining when and where to use available vaccines. For example, if a 2015–2016 yellow fever outbreak in Angola—that subsequently spread to the Democratic Republic of Congo—had been more quickly identified and contained through mass vaccination campaigns, it is estimated that not only would there have been significantly fewer yellow fever cases and deaths, but an additional costly mass vaccination campaign could have been unnessary [11]. For cholera, the large number of recorded outbreaks that have occurred since 2021 has led to unprecedented demand for vaccines from impacted countries. In countries where emergency vaccination campaigns have already been implemented, recurring outbreaks have highlighted the need for improved timeliness and accuracy of testing for identifying areas with new or ongoing transmission, enabling more effective and efficient targeting of outbreak responses. In 2023, the Global Task Force on Cholera Control recommended the expanded use of rapid diagnostic tests to strengthen cholera surveillance, to support more timely and accurate confirmation of cholera cases amidst other diarrheal diseases, and enhance the targeting of preventive and response measures such as vaccination [12,13].

Similar to yellow fever and cholera, timely and accurate diagnostic confirmation for measles and rubella may help to identify the geographic areas that need to be prioritized for vaccination, facilitating more efficient and effective use of vaccines. Diagnostic testing can rule out measles or rubella as the cause of an outbreak, avoiding unnecessary outbreak response vaccination campaigns. Similarly, surveillance data with timely and accurate laboratory confirmation for measles and rubella can enable improved understanding of which age groups or populations need to be targeted during any outbreak or vaccination response [5]. Given how quickly measles can spread, rapid detection and response to measles outbreaks is particularly important to minimize the associated morbidity and mortality [14–16].

Accurate and timely surveillance data incorporating laboratory testing results for both measles and rubella can also help monitor the quality of routine immunization services. Increases in cases of measles or rubella can indicate gaps in immunization coverage, including in areas that are otherwise reporting high immunization coverage. For example, an outbreak of measles in Vietnam in 2014 indicated that delays in immunization and lower coverage in specific ethnic groups were creating vulnerabilities masked by high reported overall routine immunization coverage rates [17]. Regular triangulation of vaccine-preventable disease surveillance data with immunization data (e.g., coverage survey data, routine administrative reporting, vaccine stock, etc.) can help identify measles zero-dose or under-immunized children and prompt efforts to vaccinate them [18].

## 4. Measles and Rubella Laboratory Testing

### *4.1. Current Laboratory Testing Methods*

Laboratory-based enzyme immunoassay (EIA) testing of sera for measles and rubella immunoglobulin M (IgM) antibodies is currently the mainstay of testing for both diseases [19]. Measles and rubella EIA testing at national reference laboratories is highly sensitive and specific when performed correctly but has a lower positive predictive value in low-incidence settings [20]. Alternative samples, such as capillary blood and oral fluid that can be tested immediately or collected as dried blood spots, can also be used for IgM antibody detection but they have not been widely adopted for measles and rubella surveillance [10].

Over recent years, quantitative real-time reverse-transcriptase polymerase chain reaction (qRT-PCR) has been used increasingly to complement IgM detection for case confirmation [19]. qRT-PCR has a high sensitivity when specimens are collected soon after the onset of a rash. Other clinical specimens can also be used for quantitative real-time or conventional RT-PCR, including throat or nasal swabs, oral fluid, urine, and capillary blood. Detection of ribonucleic acid (RNA) by RT-PCR also has the added advantage of enabling genotyping, which can be used for molecular epidemiology [21,22].

### *4.2. Role of the Global Measles and Rubella Laboratory Network*

The World Health Organization (WHO) Global Measles and Rubella Laboratory Network (GMRLN), a network of over 700 laboratories operating in 191 countries [23,24], has played a key role in supporting laboratory testing worldwide, including evaluating commercially available measles and rubella EIA test kits. These GMRLN evaluations have resulted in several EIA kits being validated for use in network laboratories. GMRLN laboratories typically receive more than 270,000 samples per year for measles and rubella diagnostic serology from all countries [1,25]. Genotyping and sequencing of measles and rubella viruses also play an increasingly important role in all WHO regions in tracking virus transmission pathways [26]. Virologic surveillance of circulating measles viruses is used to monitor progress toward elimination and GMRLN members update the online Measles Virus Nucleotide Surveillance (MeaNS) and Rubella Virus Nucleotide Surveillance (RubeNS) database once isolates are sequenced [25–27].

### 4.3. *Laboratory Testing Challenges*

Despite these achievements, challenges related to timely and accurate laboratory testing persist, primarily due to limited laboratory and staff capacity and the availability of EIA test kits [28]. In areas with minimal infrastructure or remote locations, these challenges are often intensified by insufficient specimen collection, storage, transport capacity, and laboratory accessibility [29,30]. Blood and other specimens from suspected measles and rubella cases must be carefully transported from the point of collection to the relevant reference laboratory. In hard-to-reach areas, this adds substantially to the time needed to complete testing and may lead to specimens not arriving or being in poor condition if they are not collected, stored, and transported properly [25]. For example, in Nigeria during 2023, only 60.6% of reported measles cases had a blood specimen collected for testing, and among those specimens sent to the lab, only 35.2% arrived within 3 days of collection, falling well below the target for both of these indicators of surveillance system performance of 80% or above [31]. Given these challenges, decentralized testing for measles and rubella, using simplified diagnostic tools, could potentially have significant benefits on the timeliness and utility of measles and rubella diagnostic testing and support timely outbreak-response SIAs.

## 5. Current Status of Measles and Rubella IgM Rapid Diagnostic Tests

### 5.1. *Measles IgM Rapid Diagnostic Tests*

Rapid diagnostic tests (RDTs) based on lateral flow technology are increasingly used for the diagnosis of infections by detection of antibodies or antigens (e.g., malaria, COVID-19, HIV). These tests can be performed at ambient temperature and under field conditions without the use of complex electrical equipment, eliminating the need for reverse cold chain transport of specimens, and with minimal technical training requirements [32,33]. Researchers at the UK Health Security Agency (UKHSA, formerly Public Health England [PHE]) developed an RDT for measles IgM antibodies in 2011 [34]. The test was evaluated using 170 serum specimens collected through measles surveillance or vaccination programs in Ethiopia, Malaysia, and the Russian Federation. An additional 282 oral fluid specimens from the measles, mumps, and rubella (MMR) surveillance program of the United Kingdom of Great Britain and Northern Ireland were also screened, with the Microimmune measles IgM capture EIA (Microimmune Ltd., Hounslow, England) as the gold standard for comparison [34]. With serum specimens, the RDT had a sensitivity of 91% (69/76) and a specificity of 94% (88/94); with oral fluid, the sensitivity was 90% (63/70) and the specificity was 96% (200/208) [34].

The study also demonstrated that the RDT could support measles virologic surveillance, as viral RNA could be extracted from test devices, amplified by standard RT-PCR, and used for sequence analysis to determine the genotype at national or regional laboratories. Here, a panel of 24 oral fluids was used to investigate whether measles virus haemagglutinin (H) and nucleocapsid (N) genes could be amplified by PCR directly from used RDTs. Both H and N genes were reliably detected and the N genes could be sequenced for genotyping. Measles virus genes could be recovered from RDT test strips after storage for five weeks at 20–25 °C [34]. A subsequent evaluation of 103 suspected measles cases during a 2010 nationwide measles outbreak in Zimbabwe confirmed previous findings that it was possible to amplify measles genes from oral fluid using RDT test strips and identify the infecting measles genotype and strain. During the evaluation, there was no loss in the sensitivity of detection of the measles H gene from RDT strips compared to direct detection from oral fluid samples [35].

With support from the Bill & Melinda Gates Foundation (BMGF), this prototype RDT was redesigned into a more robust, cassette-housed device, requiring fewer procedural steps to generate a result, with demonstrated high sensitivity (95%) and specificity (96%) when evaluated on stored sera against the Enzygnost® anti-measles virus IgM EIA reference assay (Siemens Healthcare GmbH, Marburg, Germany) [36,37]. In unpublished field trials from India and Uganda, the sensitivity of measles IgM detection in capillary blood using the RDT was comparable to published performance with RDTs and to current laboratory-based EIA testing; the sensitivity was slightly lower using oral fluid [37].

In a subsequent 2019 field trial in Malaysia, the sensitivity of the measles IgM RDT was lower than reported in earlier evaluations and measles endemic settings. RDT sensitivity using capillary blood was 43% and specificity was 98%; using oral fluid, sensitivity was 26% and specificity was 97% [38]. However, parallel measles and rubella vaccination and mop-up campaigns that occurred within the 8–56 days preceding specimen collection may have led to potential vaccine responses in some cases, contributing to the discordant results. Additionally, measles incidence in Malaysia decreased between the study's design and implementation phases, ultimately resulting in decreased statistical power. These data highlight the need to further evaluate both the performance and potential role of IgM RDTs in low-incidence elimination settings [38].

BMGF and Médecins Sans Frontières have provided further support for a partnership with UK-based Global Access Diagnostics as well as Senegal-based Diatropix, a company associated with the Pasteur Institute in Dakar, to develop a commercially available version of the UKHSA RDT [39,40]. Because of the lower costs and greater ease of use of such lateral flow RDTs—which are similar in operation to home pregnancy tests, COVID-19 at-home tests, and HIV RDTs—their implementation could be scaled up for use in decentralized settings in many countries and used by a wide range of healthcare workers with limited laboratory training.

### 5.2. Rubella IgM Rapid Diagnostic Tests

In contrast to measles IgM RDTs, multiple rubella IgM RDTs are already commercially available, although none have yet been validated by the GMRLN or the WHO. These tests support the diagnosis of recent or active rubella infection, as well as the determination of immune status. Because of the TORCH (toxoplasmosis, others [syphilis, hepatitis B], rubella, cytomegalovirus, and herpes simplex) panel screening among pregnant women and infants in high-income and upper-middle-income countries [41,42], the existing market demand for such tests is substantial. The logistical and operational concerns that make measles IgM RDTs attractive also apply to rubella IgM RDTs. In countries that have not eliminated rubella, pairing measles and rubella IgM RDTs (preferably within a single combined testing platform) would support parallel or sequential measles and rubella testing, which is the standard for EIA testing.

### 5.3. Integration of RDTs into Measles and Rubella Surveillance Programs

Accurate measles and rubella IgM RDTs could eventually create a range of options for more decentralized testing for measles and rubella. For example, an RDT that could test oral fluid and capillary blood specimens would expand who could collect samples and reduce the supplies needed to collect them [37]. Oral fluid and capillary blood specimens are less invasive than whole blood samples and can be collected with less training and equipment than venipuncture. A less-invasive test could potentially result in greater patient testing compliance, therefore improving the representativeness of surveillance [43]. When combined with the simplicity of performing RDTs, a wide range of front-line healthcare workers could utilize such tests. Such characteristics make measles and rubella IgM RDTs particularly attractive for testing in areas in which establishing reference laboratories and transporting specimens are difficult, such as many low- and middle-income countries, Pacific Island countries, areas with civil unrest, and remote, hard-to-reach populations.

The results obtained from measles and rubella IgM RDTs could potentially be integrated into countries' testing systems at different administrative levels, enabling more rapid detection of and timely response to measles cases and outbreaks. For example, RDTs could be used to rapidly expand subnational laboratory networks without the need to equip the laboratory for EIA or qRT-PCR. The GMRLN has a strong training program that could be expanded to include training on the use of RDTs in subnational laboratories. Specimens collected at remote locations and tested by RDTs would be submitted to national laboratories for confirmatory testing by EIA. RDTs with positive results would then be referred to national laboratories or regional laboratories for genotyping or sequencing, as needed. To ensure high-quality standardized testing in subnational laboratories, implementing RDTs in parallel with quality management systems and assurance programs will help to reinforce the validity of the test results, build capacity for the use of RDTs for surveillance, and ensure alignment with global guidance for the post-market surveillance of new diagnostic tools. National labs will likely have a large role to play in the quality management and assurance of RDT use in subnational laboratories if they are to be introduced within a country.

Another option for expanded laboratory diagnostics would be for district surveillance officers to use such RDTs to test suspected measles cases during field investigations. Thorough integration of results from RDT testing into routine health information management systems at both the local and national levels would also help to ensure that testing results are reported and available to guide public health decisions at all administrative levels. This would likely require expansion of the number of variables collected in routine datasets, including RDT usage and results, as well as the strengthening of electronic data reporting in many countries where paper systems are still the current norm.

## 6. Deployment of Measles and Rubella IgM Rapid Diagnostic Tests: Challenges in Low- and Middle-Income Countries

### 6.1. Financing Challenges for Measles and Rubella IgM RDT Deployment

To realize the potential benefits of measles and rubella IgM RDTs to make measles and rubella surveillance in low- and middle-income countries more effective and efficient, such RDTs would need to be deployed at scale in those countries. That deployment would need to balance the timeliness and detail of the data collected with the costs of ongoing distribution and use of the tests so that results can be available to guide decision-making as sustainably as possible. One of the main challenges affecting the development of RDTs for high-priority diseases is the lack of adequate financing. In general, global funding for diagnostics is limited and the lack of incentive from the private sector has been a challenge for the development of diagnostic tests [44–46].

In the long term, RDT use would ideally be funded and supported by government healthcare, public health systems, and private providers. However, in the short term, international groups such as Gavi, the Vaccine Alliance (GAVI) are likely to be major funders for measles and rubella RDT procurement in low- and middle-income countries. Although GAVI is primarily focused on improving the availability of vaccines to low- and middle-income countries and supporting countries in delivering vaccines to their target populations, it has also set up a diagnostic test support program to improve the availability of fit-for-purpose diagnostic tests to make targeted vaccination programs against diseases like measles and rubella more effective, efficient, and equitable [47]. GAVI published a measles IgM RDT market-shaping roadmap describing its expectations on how such a test might be introduced to the market and the potential volume of demand for such a test and is working on a similar rubella RDT roadmap [46]. While GAVI can provide "pull" market incentives (i.e., strategies in which organizations aim to increase the demand for a product and draw ("pull") consumers to the product) to encourage manufacturers to produce diagnostic tests and can fund work to validate test kits and to develop guidelines on how to best use new tests, its procurement funding support is currently limited to the 54 countries eligible for GAVI's support (Figure 1) [48]. As a result, international funding support for the deployment of measles and rubella IgM RDTs outside of those countries will need to come from other sources. Since many countries experiencing large or disruptive measles outbreaks are not eligible for GAVI procurement funding support for diagnostic tests [49], they would likely benefit from funding support from other sources for introducing RDTs.

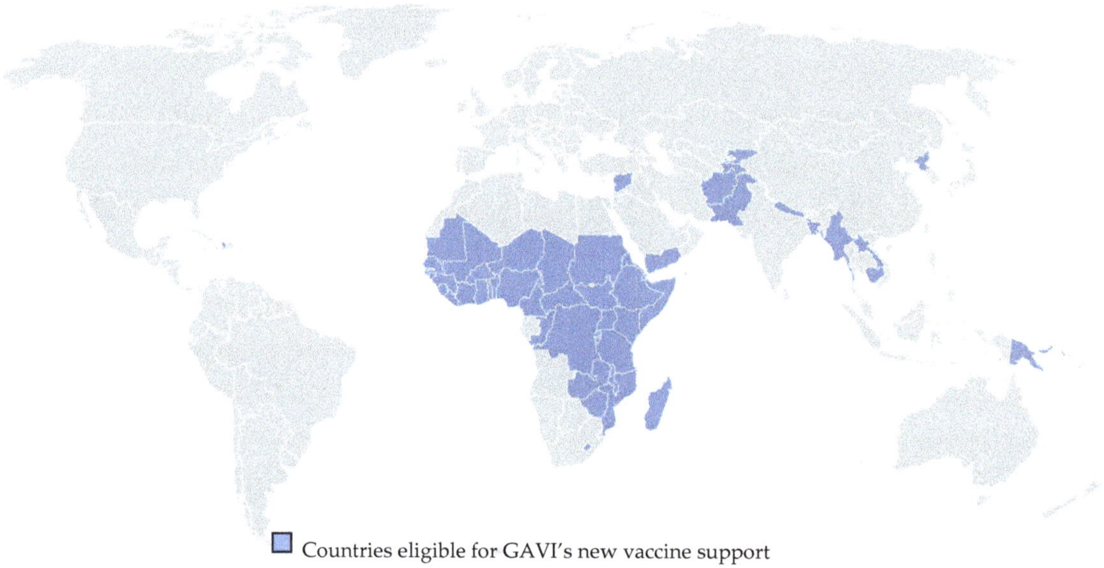


**Figure 1.** Countries eligible for GAVI's new vaccine support in 2024 [48].

A further limitation on widespread deployment is the lack of funding to support rapid development of quality RDTs. GAVI's funding for the purchase of RDTs is applicable as a future incentive but does not directly support the research and development efforts needed to bring RDTs into the market. International funders will be essential to close the funding gaps and ensure timely development of high-performing, tailored, cost-effective tests and their availability for procurement and implementation by GAVI and other partners.

### *6.2. Validation of Commercially Available Measles and Rubella IgM RDTs and Guidance on Deployment*

Validation of diagnostic tests, i.e., evaluation by an independent organization of the accuracy and reliability of a diagnostic test, is essential to indicate to international organizations, national governments, and others involved in diagnostic test procurement which tests are worth procuring and deploying. The GMRLN has for years independently assessed measles and rubella IgM EIA tests and identified those with acceptable performance characteristics for use by national, regional, and global reference laboratories throughout the network. Such assessments have drawn on data from the independent laboratory testing of test kits as well as reviews of test performance and manufacturing quality assurance provided by test producers [23–25]. The GMRLN is positioned to play a similar role for measles and rubella IgM RDTs, helping to guide international organizations, including GAVI, on whether specific RDTs warrant scaling up. The Foundation for Innovative New Diagnostics (FIND), together with the GMRLN and the WHO, have recently published target product profiles (TPPs) for measles and rubella IgM RDTs and EIAs [50]. These TPPs describe the improvements necessary for the development, evaluation, and scale-up of diagnostic tests and will help to indicate to manufacturers the characteristics RDTs will need to have to potentially be procured with funding from international organizations [50].

The development of guidance on RDT deployment can also benefit from a combination of modeling studies and pilot projects. Pilot projects in Uganda, India, and Malaysia with prototype measles IgM RDTs have already demonstrated that such RDTs can be readily used by healthcare workers. For example, during a 2019 field trial in Malaysia, an evaluation team including co-investigators from the Malaysian MOH, U.S. CDC, UKHSA, and WHO implemented a pilot of measles IgM RDT testing in 34 health clinics following standardized one-day regional training. After this one-day training, agreement between readers of the RDTs in health clinics was very high (99% for capillary blood and 97% for oral fluid). A knowledge, attitude, and practices (KAP) survey documented the extensive (92%) previous experience of clinic staff with other RDTs, which was likely an important contributor to the success of using the measles RDT in Malaysian clinics. Furthermore, knowledge was very high (91%) after the formal training and remained high (80%) ≥9 months later among survey respondents. Although not statistically significant, the number of days until public response activities were initiated (e.g., active case detection, mop-up vaccination) decreased by almost five days during the same study, likely related to receiving the RDT results at the point-of-care compared to the time required to perform an EIA in the national laboratory and report results [37,38]. Future pilot studies supported by GAVI in Ethiopia, Zambia, and Nepal will focus on the operational aspects of deploying measles RDTs, and modeling studies are also underway that will assess the tradeoffs between deployment costs and the speed of detection of cases and outbreaks with different strategies for measles and rubella RDTs.

Data on the cost-benefit and effectiveness of measles and rubella RDTs are also needed to make further investment decisions regarding diagnostics development to provide an economic case for future investment in RDTs. There have been estimates of the costs of RDTs for various diseases such as HIV, malaria, and tuberculosis [51–53] that have indicated the decentralization of testing using RDTs is likely to be cost-saving or cost-effective in resource-limited settings [54]. The fast turnaround time of RDTs may also result in a reduction in unnecessary clinical treatment costs, leading to savings for both patients and clinics [55].

While the previous literature has also documented the costs of various aspects of measles and rubella surveillance [56], there is limited information available regarding the costs of implementing measles and rubella RDTs as part of a national surveillance program. Such data would help inform decision-makers and public health planners on the magnitude of resources required for introduction, how these costs may vary across geographies (e.g., rural vs. urban, endemic vs. elimination settings), and how this could impact the public health response during measles and rubella outbreaks. Figure 2 presents the potential benefits and challenges to the introduction and use of RDTs in various settings. The relative benefit of use in these different settings is likely to vary by country and within a country. One benefit is that capillary blood and oral fluid samples could be used at community and health clinic levels, improving patient compliance with testing [37]. However, implementation at these lower levels of the health system would also require reprioritization and optimization of current resources in terms of training, supply logistics, quality control and assurance, and processes for reporting results [32,37,57,58].

| Setting | Device | Community | Health Clinic | Laboratory | Health System |
|---|---|---|---|---|---|
| **Benefits** | • Time to result<br>• Strengthen molecular characterization<br>• Potential cost<br>• Easy to use and interpret<br>• No cold chain required | • Time to result and treatment, less time in clinic<br>• Easy to understand result | • Easy to use and interpret result<br>• Faster time to result<br>• No cold chain required<br>• Realtime reporting<br>• Improved patient compliance<br>• Reduced specimen transport cost | • Simple, cost saving<br>• Timeliness<br>• Easier confirmation of pathogen by extraction of nucleic acid from RDTs | • Time to result and response<br>• Potential cases averted<br>• Cost saving |
| **Challenges** | • Potential interactions with other diseases<br>• Integration with other diagnostic tests<br>• Positive predictive value in endemic vs. elimination settings | • Lack of test understanding/awareness<br>• Distrust<br>• Prefer conventional test | • New reporting processes required<br>• Additional protocols and training required<br>• Additional systems required for logistics | • Potentially additional reporting and logistics<br>• Additional training required<br>• Introduction of new protocols | • Initial introduction costs<br>• Integration with current surveillance systems<br>• Provision of training<br>• Ensuring quality assurance and control |

**Figure 2.** Potential benefits and challenges associated with the introduction of measles and rubella RDTs in various healthcare settings [37,57].

### 6.3. Future Directions and Way Forward

Once the GMRLN has preliminarily identified a measles IgM RDT(s) that meets deployment criteria, the GAVI secretariat is planning to fund pilot projects in multiple countries eligible for GAVI's new vaccine support to assess the costs and effectiveness of different deployment strategies, e.g., placing RDTs in healthcare facilities that would treat suspected measles cases, with district surveillance officers that would investigate such cases. Stocking tests in many sites might speed up the detection of cases and outbreaks while also providing a market incentive to manufacturers to ensure they continue to produce high-quality tests. Without this, given the small commercial market for RDTs, there is a risk that the products will be discontinued or will not be put forward for Stringent Regulatory Authority (SRA) approval. However, this approach may also markedly increase the costs of procuring enough tests to maintain stocks at each site and training staff on their use, so clear information on the benefits and costs of these options will be critical for shaping deployment guidance and informing country plans for sustainably deploying such tests. Once the tests are in use in countries more broadly, careful evaluations of the countries' experiences with deployment can inform further revisions in deployment guidance, country support needed, and how countries implement such tests.

## 7. Conclusions

Measles and rubella IgM RDTs have the potential to markedly improve testing and surveillance for measles and rubella, especially for rapid detection and response to measles and rubella outbreaks. They can potentially contribute to improved effectiveness and efficiency of measles and rubella elimination efforts and vaccination strategies, particularly in low- and middle-income countries. Efforts to develop and validate measles and rubella IgM RDTs that can be produced at scale are underway. International funding will be critical to ensuring the timely development of high-performing, cost-effective tests. Once such validated RDTs are available, funding support will also be needed from international organizations and countries to deploy them. However, since the benefits of use are likely to vary by country and within a country, their implementation will need to carefully balance the costs of ongoing distribution and use so that test results can be available to guide decision-making as sustainably as possible.

**Author Contributions:** Conceptualization: L.M.H., P.A.R., M.N.M., J.L.G. and D.B.; Methodology: L.M.H., P.A.R., M.N.M., J.L.G. and D.B.; Data Curation: P.A.R., M.N.M., M.P., L.K.K., M.H., J.O., C.K.-C., B.E., A.S., L.W., D.F. and D.B.; Formal analysis and investigation: A.R., L.M.H., P.A.R., M.N.M., J.L.G., L.W., D.F. and D.B.; Writing—original draft preparation: A.R. and L.M.H.; Writing—review and editing: A.R., L.M.H., P.A.R., M.N.M., M.P., J.L.G., L.K.K., M.H., J.O., C.K.-C., B.E., A.S., L.W., D.F. and D.B.; Visualization: A.R. and L.M.H.; Supervision: A.R., L.M.H., P.A.R., M.N.M., J.L.G. and D.B.; Project administration: A.R., L.M.H., P.A.R., M.N.M., J.L.G. and D.B. All authors have read and agreed to the published version of the manuscript.

**Funding:** This article was funded by the US Centers for Disease Control and Prevention.

**Institutional Review Board Statement:** This activity was reviewed by the CDC and was conducted consistent with applicable federal law and CDC policy (45 C.F.R. part 46.102(l)(2), 21 C.F.R. part 56; 42 U.S.C. 145 Sect. 241(d); 5 U.S.C. Sect. 552a; 44 U.S.C. Sect. 3501, et seq.).

**Informed Consent Statement:** Not applicable.

**Data Availability Statement:** No new data were created or analyzed as part of this report. Data sharing is not applicable to this article.

**Acknowledgments:** The authors would like to thank the GMRLN as well as the WHO and Ministry of Health collaborators in Malaysia, Uganda, Ghana, Cameroon, India, Brazil, and Zimbabwe. The authors would also like to thank other key collaborators, including Lucky Sangal, Josephine Bwogi, Marilda M. Sequeira, Heather Scobie, Morgane Donadel, and Diane Waku-Kouomou.

**Conflicts of Interest:** L.W. and D.W.B. were supported in part by the Bill & Melinda Gates Foundation grant number OPP1066619 to develop the measles IgM RDT. The rapid diagnostic test has been licensed nonexclusively from the UKHSA to Global Access Diagnostics (GADx) Ltd., England. A modified version of this device is being developed for regulatory approval and commercialization by GADx and Diatropix, a not-for-profit initiative of the Pasteur Institute, Dakar, Senegal, with funding from the Bill & Melinda Gates Foundation, Seattle, WA (grant number INV-003213). L.W. is employed by the UKHSA and has been sub-contracted by the Pasteur Institute, Dakar, to support the technical transfer of measles RDT technology from the UKHSA to GADx and DWB holds a fellowship at Fiocruz in Brazil funded with this grant support. All other authors declared that no competing interests exist.

## References

1. Minta, A.A.; Ferrari, M.; Antoni, S.; Portnoy, A.; Sbarra, A.; Lambert, B.; Hauryski, S.; Hatcher, C.; Nedelec, Y.; Datta, D.; et al. Progress Toward Regional Measles Elimination—Worldwide, 2000–2021. *MMWR Morb. Mortal. Wkly. Rep.* **2022**, *71*, 1489–1495. [CrossRef] [PubMed]
2. Ou, A.C.; Zimmerman, L.A.; Alexander, J.P., Jr.; Crowcroft, N.S.; O'Connor, P.M.; Knapp, J.K. Progress Toward Rubella and Congenital Rubella Syndrome Elimination—Worldwide, 2012–2022. *MMWR Morb. Mortal. Wkly. Rep.* **2024**, *73*, 162–167. [CrossRef] [PubMed]
3. World Health Organisation. Immunization Agenda 2030: A Global Strategy to Leave No One Behind. 2020. Available online: https://www.who.int (accessed on 25 February 2024).
4. Gastanaduy, P.A.; Redd, S.B.; Clemmons, N.S.; Lee, A.D.; Hickman, C.J.; Rota, P.A.; Patel, M. Measles [Chapter 7]. In *Manual for the Surveillance of Vaccine-Preventable Diseases*; US Department of Health and Human Services, CDC: Atlanta, GA, USA, 2023. Available online: https://www.cdc.gov/vaccines/pubs/surv-manual/chpt07-measles.html (accessed on 5 June 2024).
5. Cutts, F.T.; Ferrari, M.J.; Krause, L.K.; Tatem, A.J.; Mosser, J.F. Vaccination strategies for measles control and elimination: Time to strengthen local initiatives. *BMC Med.* **2021**, *19*, 1–8. [CrossRef] [PubMed]
6. World Health Organisation. Measles vaccines: WHO position paper, April 2017–Recommendations. *Vaccine* **2019**, *37*, 219–222. [CrossRef] [PubMed]
7. World Health Organisation. Rubella vaccines: WHO position paper–July 2020–Note de synthèse: Position de l'OMS concernant les vaccins antirubéoleux. *Wkly. Epidemiol. Rec.* **2020**, *95*, 306–324.
8. Gastañaduy, P.A.; Banerjee, E.; DeBolt, C.; Bravo-Alcántara, P.; Samad, S.A.; Pastor, D.; Rota, P.A.; Patel, M.; Crowcroft, N.S.; Durrheim, D.N. Public health responses during measles outbreaks in elimination settings: Strategies and challenges. *Hum. Vaccin Immunother.* **2018**, *14*, 2222–2238. [CrossRef] [PubMed]
9. Moss, W.J. Measles. *Lancet* **2017**, *390*, 2490–2502. [CrossRef]
10. World Health Organisation. *Vaccine Preventable Diseases Surveillance Standards: Measles Chapter*; WHO: Geneva, Switzerland, 2018. Available online: https://www.who.int/publications/m/item/vaccine-preventable-diseases-surveillance-standards-measles (accessed on 28 February 2024).

11. Gavi, the Vaccine Alliance. Improving Yellow Fever Diagnostic Testing for More Efficient, Effective, and Equitable Vaccination. 2021. Available online: https://www.gavi.org/vaccineswork/improving-yellow-fever-diagnostic-testing-more-efficient-effective-and-equitable (accessed on 7 July 2024).
12. World Health Organisation. Global Deployment of Rapid Diagnostic Tests to Boost Fight against Cholera. 2024. Available online: https://www.who.int/news/item/05-04-2024-global-deployment-of-rapid-diagnostic-tests-to-boost-fight-against-cholera (accessed on 9 July 2024).
13. Global Taskforce on Cholera Control. Public Health Surveillance for Cholera: Interim Guidance February 2023. Available online: https://www.gtfcc.org/wp-content/uploads/2023/02/gtfcc-public-health-surveillance-for-cholera-interim-guidance.pdf (accessed on 9 July 2024).
14. Grais, R.F.; Conlan, A.J.; Ferrari, M.J.; Djibo, A.; Le Menach, A.; Bjørnstad, O.N.; Grenfell, B.T. Time is of the essence: Exploring a measles outbreak response vaccination in Niamey, Niger. *J. R. Soc. Interface* **2008**, *5*, 67–74. [CrossRef] [PubMed]
15. Grais, R.F.; Dubray, C.; Fermon, F.; Guerin, P.J. Exploring the time to intervene with a reactive mass vaccination campaign in measles epidemics. *Epidemiol. Infect.* **2006**, *134*, 845–849. [CrossRef]
16. Muscat, M.; Ben Mamou, M.; Reynen-de Kat, C.; Jankovic, D.; Hagan, J.; Singh, S.; Datta, S.S. Progress and Challenges in Measles and Rubella Elimination in the WHO European Region. *Vaccines* **2024**, *12*, 696. [CrossRef]
17. Roberts, L. In Vietnam, an anatomy of a measles outbreak. *Science* **2015**, *348*, 962. [CrossRef] [PubMed]
18. World Health Organization & United States Centers for Disease Control and Prevention. Triangulation for Improved Decision-Making in Immunization Programmes 2020. 2022. Available online: https://www.technet-21.org/media/com_resources/trl/6616/multi_upload/0_Triangulation_CoverOrientation_DRAFT_27Jul2020.pdf (accessed on 25 February 2024).
19. World Health Organisation. *Manual for the Laboratory-Based Surveillance of Measles, Rubella, and Congenital Rubella Syndrome*; World Health Organisation: Geneva, Switzerland, 2018. Available online: https://www.who.int/publications/m/item/chapter-1-manual-for-the-laboratory-based-surveillance-of-measles-rubella-and-congenital-rubella-syndrome (accessed on 21 February 2024).
20. Bolotin, S.; Lim, G.; Dang, V.; Crowcroft, N.; Gubbay, J.; Mazzulli, T.; Schabas, R. The utility of measles and rubella IgM serology in an elimination setting, Ontario, Canada, 2009–2014. *PLoS ONE* **2017**, *12*, e0181172. [CrossRef] [PubMed]
21. Riddell, M.A.; Chibo, D.; Kelly, H.A.; Catton, M.G.; Birch, C.J. Investigation of optimal specimen type and sampling time for detection of measles virus RNA during a measles epidemic. *J. Clin. Microbiol.* **2001**, *39*, 375–376. [CrossRef] [PubMed]
22. van Binnendijk, R.S.; van den Hof, S.; van den Kerkhof, H.; Kohl, R.H.; Woonink, F.; Berbers, G.A.; Conyn-van Spaendonck, M.A.; Kimman, T.G. Evaluation of serological and virological tests in the diagnosis of clinical and subclinical measles virus infections during an outbreak of measles in The Netherlands. *J. Infect. Dis.* **2003**, *188*, 898–903. [CrossRef] [PubMed]
23. Mulders, M.N. Global measles and rubella laboratory network support for elimination goals, 2010–2015. *MMWR Morb. Mortal. Wkly. Rep.* **2016**, *65*, 438–442. [CrossRef] [PubMed]
24. Strebel, P.; Grabowsky, M.; Hoekstra, E.; Gay, A.; Cochi, S. Evolution and Contribution of a Global Partnership against Measles and Rubella, 2001–2023. *Vaccines* **2024**, *12*, 693. [CrossRef]
25. Mulders, M.N.; Serhan, F.; Goodson, J.L.; Icenogle, J.; Johnson, B.W.; Rota, P.A. Expansion of Surveillance for Vaccine-preventable Diseases: Building on the Global Polio Laboratory Network and the Global Measles and Rubella Laboratory Network Platforms. *J. Infect. Dis.* **2017**, *216*, S324–S330. [CrossRef] [PubMed]
26. Brown, K.E.; Rota, P.A.; Goodson, J.L.; Williams, D.; Abernathy, E.; Takeda, M.; Mulders, M.N. Genetic characterization of measles and rubella viruses detected through global measles and rubella elimination surveillance, 2016–2018. *MMWR Morb. Mortal. Wkly. Rep.* **2019**, *68*, 587–591. [CrossRef]
27. Williams, D.; Penedos, A.; Bankamp, B.; Anderson, R.; Hübschen, J.; Mamou, M.B.; Beck, A.; Brown, D.; Rey-Benito, G.; Evans, R.; et al. *Update: Circulation of Active Genotypes of Measles Virus and Recommendations for Use of Sequence Analysis to Monitor Viral Transmission*; World Health Organization: Geneva, Switzerland, 2022.
28. Patel, M.K.; Gibson, R.; Cohen, A.; Dumolard, L.; Gacic-Dobo, M. Global landscape of measles and rubella surveillance. *Vaccine* **2018**, *36*, 7385–7392. [CrossRef] [PubMed]
29. Scobie, H.M.; Ilunga, B.K.; Mulumba, A.; Shidi, C.; Coulibaly, T.; Obama, R.; Tamfum, J.J.M.; Simbu, E.P.; Smit, S.B.; Masresha, B.; et al. Antecedent causes of a measles resurgence in the Democratic Republic of the Congo. *Pan Afr. Med. J.* **2015**, *21*, 30. [CrossRef]
30. Orenstein, W.A.; Hinman, A.; Nkowane, B.; Olive, J.M.; Reingold, A. Measles and Rubella Global Strategic Plan 2012-2020 midterm review. *Vaccine* **2018**, *36* (Suppl. 1), A1–A34. [CrossRef]
31. Nigeria Centers for Disease Control. An Update of Measles Outbreak in Nigeria Measles Situation Report. Abuja, Nigeria. 2023. Available online: https://ncdc.gov.ng/diseases/sitreps/?cat=11&name=An%20Update%20of%20Measles%20Outbreak%20in%20Nigeria (accessed on 2 March 2024).
32. Pai, N.P.; Vadnais, C.; Denkinger, C.; Engel, N.; Pai, M. Point-of-care testing for infectious diseases: Diversity, complexity, and barriers in low-and middle-income countries. *PLoS Med.* **2012**, *9*, e1001306. [CrossRef]
33. Osorio, L.; Garcia, J.A.; Parra, L.G.; Garcia, V.; Torres, L.; Degroote, S.; Ridde, V. A scoping review on the field validation and implementation of rapid diagnostic tests for vector-borne and other infectious diseases of poverty in urban areas. *Infect. Dis. Poverty* **2018**, *7*, 1–18. [CrossRef]

34. Warrener, L.; Slibinskas, R.; Chua, K.B.; Nigatu, W.; Brown, K.E.; Sasnauskas, K.; Samuel, D.; Brown, D. A point-of-care test for measles diagnosis: Detection of measles-specific IgM antibodies and viral nucleic acid. *Bull. World Health Organ.* **2011**, *89*, 675–682. [CrossRef]
35. Shonhai, A.; Warrener, L.; Mangwanya, D.; Slibinskas, R.; Brown, K.; Brown, D.; Featherstone, D.; Samuel, D. Investigation of a measles outbreak in Zimbabwe, 2010: Potential of a point of care test to replace laboratory confirmation of suspected cases. *Epidemiol. Infect.* **2015**, *143*, 3442–3450. [CrossRef] [PubMed]
36. Warrener, L.; Andrews, N.; Koroma, H.; Alessandrini, I.; Haque, M.; Garcia, C.C.; Matos, A.R.; Caetano, B.; Lemos, X.R.; Siqueira, M.M.; et al. Evaluation of a rapid diagnostic test for measles IgM detection; accuracy and the reliability of visual reading using sera from the measles surveillance programme in Brazil, 2015. *Epidemiol. Infect.* **2023**, *151*, e151. [CrossRef]
37. Brown, D.W.; Warrener, L.; Scobie, H.M.; Donadel, M.; Waku-Kouomou, D.; Mulders, M.N.; Rota, P.A. Rapid diagnostic tests to address challenges for global measles surveillance. *Curr. Opin. Virol.* **2020**, *41*, 77–84. [CrossRef]
38. Senin, A.A.; Noordin, N.M.; Sani, J.A.M.; Mahat, D.; Donadel, M.; Scobie, H.M.; Omar, A.; Chem, Y.K.; Zahari, M.I.; Ismail, F.; et al. A measles IgM rapid diagnostic test to address challenges with national measles surveillance and response in Malaysia. *PLoS ONE* **2024**, *19*, e0298730. [CrossRef]
39. Institut Pasteur Dakar. Launch of the Rapid Diagnostic Test Production Platform at the Institut Pasteur in Dakar. 2020. Available online: https://www.fondation-merieux.org/en/news/inauguration-of-the-diatropix-production-platform-at-the-institut-pasteur-of-dakar/ (accessed on 5 March 2024).
40. Médecins Sans Frontières. RDTs: Measles and Meningitis. Geneva, Switzerland. Available online: https://fondation.msf.fr/en/projects/rdts-measles-and-meningitis#in-detail (accessed on 16 March 2024).
41. United States Centers for Disease Control and Prevention. Serology Testing for Rubella and Congenital Rubella Syndrome (CRS). 2023. Available online: https://www.cdc.gov/rubella/lab/serology.html (accessed on 6 March 2024).
42. Cullen, A.; Brown, S.; Cafferkey, M.; O'Brien, N.; Griffin, E. Current use of the TORCH screen in the diagnosis of congenital infection. *J. Infect.* **1998**, *36*, 185–188. Available online: https://www.sciencedirect.com/science/article/pii/S016344539880011X (accessed on 6 March 2024). [CrossRef] [PubMed]
43. Jin, L.; Vyse, A.; Brown, D.W. The role of RT-PCR assay of oral fluid for diagnosis and surveillance of measles, mumps and rubella. *Bull. World Health Organ.* **2002**, *80*, 76–77.
44. The Academy of Medical Sciences. Improving the Development and Deployment of Rapid Diagnostic Tests in Lmics, Workshop Report, 21 November 2016. London, United Kingdom. 2016. Available online: https://acmedsci.ac.uk/file-download/18597310 (accessed on 8 June 2024).
45. PATH. Market Failures and Opportunities for Increasing Access to Diagnostics in Low- and Middle-Income Countries. PATH: Seattle. 2022. Available online: https://www.path.org/resources/market-failures-andopportunities-for-increasing-access-to-diagnosticsin-low-and-middle-income-countries/ (accessed on 10 June 2024).
46. Yimer, S.A.; Booij, B.B.; Tobert, G.; Hebbeler, A.; Oloo, P.; Brangel, P.; Jackson, M.L.A.; Jarman, R.; Craig, D.; Avumegah, M.S.; et al. Rapid diagnostic test: A critical need for outbreak preparedness and response for high priority pathogens. *BMJ Glob. Health* **2024**, *9*, e014386. [CrossRef]
47. Gavi, the Vaccine Alliance. Measles Rapid Diagnostics Capacity Roadmap: Public Summary. *Geneva, Switzerland.* 2023. Available online: https://www.gavi.org/sites/default/files/about/market-shaping/roadmaps/Public-Summary_Measles-Diagnostics-Roadmap-2023.pdf (accessed on 10 March 2024).
48. Gavi, the Vaccine Alliance. Eligibility. Geneva, Switzerland. 2024. Available online: https://www.gavi.org/types-support/sustainability/eligibility (accessed on 10 March 2024).
49. World Health Organisation. Global Measles and Rubella Monthly Update 2024. Geneva, Switzerland. 2024. Available online: https://cdn.who.int/media/docs/default-source/immunization/immunization-coverage/global_mr_update.pptx?sfvrsn=c83eebae_147 (accessed on 10 March 2024).
50. Foundation for Innovative New Diagnostics (FIND). Target Product Profile for Surveillance Tests for Measles and Rubella. Geneva, Switzerland. 2024. Available online: https://www.finddx.org/wp-content/uploads/2024/06/20240613_tpp_measles_rubell_FV_EN.pdf (accessed on 17 June 2024).
51. Abimbola, T.O.; Marston, B.J.; Date, A.A.; Blandford, J.M.; Sangrujee, N.; Wiktor, S.Z. Cost-effectiveness of tuberculosis diagnostic strategies to reduce early mortality among persons with advanced HIV infection initiating antiretroviral therapy. *JAIDS J. Acquir. Immune Defic. Syndr.* **2012**, *60*, e1–e7. [CrossRef] [PubMed]
52. de Oliveira, M.R.F.; Giozza, S.P.; Peixoto, H.M.; Romero, G.A. Cost-effectiveness of diagnostic for malaria in Extra-Amazon Region, Brazil. *Malar. J.* **2012**, *11*, 1–10. [CrossRef] [PubMed]
53. Doyle, N.M.; Levison, J.E.; Gardner, M.O. Rapid HIV versus enzyme-linked immunosorbent assay screening in a low-risk Mexican American population presenting in labor: A cost-effectiveness analysis. *Am. J. Obstet. Gynecol.* **2005**, *193*, 1280–1285. [CrossRef] [PubMed]
54. Sohn, H.; Kasaie, P.; Kendall, E.; Gomez, G.B.; Vassall, A.; Pai, M.; Dowdy, D. Informing decision-making for universal access to quality tuberculosis diagnosis in India: An economic-epidemiological model. *BMC Med.* **2019**, *17*, 155. [CrossRef] [PubMed]
55. Odaga, J.; Sinclair, D.; Lokong Adaktar, J.; Donegan, S.; Hopkins, H.; Garner, P. Rapid diagnostic tests versus clinical diagnosis for managing people with fever in malaria endemic settings. *Cochrane Database Syst. Rev.* **2014**, *4*, CD008998. [CrossRef] [PubMed]

56. Thompson, K.M.; Odahowski, C.L. Systematic Review of Health Economic Analyses of Measles and Rubella Immunization Interventions. *Risk Anal.* **2016**, *36*, 1297–1314. [CrossRef] [PubMed]
57. Pai, N.P.; Wilkinson, S.; Deli-Houssein, R.; Vijh, R.; Vadnais, C.; Behlim, T.; Steben, M.; Engel, N.; Wong, T. Barriers to Implementation of Rapid and Point-of-Care Tests for Human Immunodeficiency Virus Infection: Findings From a Systematic Review (1996–2014). *Point Care* **2015**, *14*, 81–87. [CrossRef]
58. Asiimwe, C.; Kyabayinze, D.J.; Kyalisiima, Z.; Nabakooza, J.; Bajabaite, M.; Counihan, H.; Tibenderana, J.K. Early experiences on the feasibility, acceptability, and use of malaria rapid diagnostic tests at peripheral health centres in Uganda-insights into some barriers and facilitators. *Implement Sci.* **2012**, *7*, 1–12. [CrossRef]

vaccines

MDPI

Article

# "Anees Has Measles": Storytelling and Singing to Enhance MMR Vaccination in Child Care Centers Amid Religious Hesitancy

Therdpong Thongseiratch [1,*], Puttichart Khantee [2], Naphat Jaroenmark [1], Napatsaree Nuttapasit [1] and Nithida Thonglua [1]

[1] Child Development Unit, Department of Pediatrics, Faculty of Medicine, Prince of Songkla University, Songkhla 90110, Thailand; natpat.nay@hotmail.com (N.J.); napatsaree.nut@gmail.com (N.N.); thonglua31@gmail.com (N.T.)

[2] Infectious Disease Unit, Department of Pediatrics, Faculty of Medicine, Prince of Songkla University, Songkhla 90110, Thailand

* Correspondence: ttherd@gmail.com; Tel.: +66-843099325

**Abstract:** This study explores the enhancement of MMR vaccination rates in the deep south of Thailand through a culturally tailored intervention that incorporates storytelling and singing, aligning with local cultural and religious values. The "Anees has Measles" intervention, developed with input from community stakeholders including health workers, religious leaders, and parents, featured traditional melodies in its singing activities. The intervention comprised two main components: storytelling sessions and singing activities, both utilizing culturally resonant content and formats to effectively engage the community. Conducted from December 2019 to March 2020 across eight districts in five provinces, the study targeted children aged 18 months to 5 years in government child care centers. Results indicated a substantial increase in MMR vaccination coverage from 44.3% to 72.0% twelve months post-intervention, and further to 77.0% at 48 months post-intervention, representing a significant and sustained improvement ($p < 0.001$). This marked and continuous increase demonstrates the effectiveness of culturally adapted health education in areas with significant vaccine hesitancy. The findings highlight the importance of integrating culturally and religiously sensitive methods into public health strategies, significantly enhancing vaccine acceptance and coverage in diverse and conservative settings. This approach suggests a broader applicability for similar interventions in comparable contexts globally.

**Keywords:** MMR vaccination; cultural adaptation; storytelling; singing; health education; vaccine hesitancy

## 1. Introduction

Measles is a highly contagious viral disease that is spread through the air by respiratory droplets when infected individuals cough or sneeze [1]. If left untreated, measles can lead to serious complications such as encephalitis, pneumonia, and even death [2]. The measles vaccine, often administered as part of the combined measles, mumps, and rubella (MMR) vaccine, is a highly effective measure to prevent the spread of the disease [3]. The World Health Organization (WHO) recommends that children receive two doses of the vaccine for maximum protection [4,5]. The vaccine has been instrumental in reducing measles cases globally, and high vaccination coverage is essential for achieving herd immunity and preventing outbreaks [6].

In recent years, measles outbreaks have increasingly occurred in communities with low vaccination rates [7–9]. Unvaccinated children are at a higher risk of contracting measles and contributing to the spread of the virus [10]. These outbreaks are particularly concerning in regions where healthcare access is limited, and the capacity to manage large-scale measles cases is inadequate. The resurgence of measles in certain areas highlights the importance of maintaining high vaccination coverage to prevent the disease's spread [11–13].

Religious and cultural beliefs contribute to vaccine hesitancy [14]. For instance, in parts of Southern Thailand, there are misconceptions about the MMR vaccine not being halal, leading to lower vaccination rates among Muslim populations [15–17]. The perception that vaccines contain ingredients forbidden in Islam has fueled skepticism and fear, resulting in decreased uptake of essential immunizations like the measles vaccine [18,19].

To address the challenges posed by MMR vaccine hesitancy, various interventions have been implemented [20]. These include educational campaigns to dispel myths about vaccines, engagement with religious and community leaders to endorse vaccination, and culturally sensitive health communication strategies [21–24]. Many factors influence parental decisions to vaccinate, and parents who actively decline immunization often believe that vaccines are unsafe and ineffective, that the diseases they are meant to prevent are mild and uncommon, and may mistrust their health professionals [25]. Nevertheless, such attitudes could shift during an outbreak [26,27]. To date, there has been limited research assessing the uptake of the MMR vaccine following measles outbreaks in communities with historically low vaccination rates. This information is crucial for managing future outbreaks in similar contexts.

Since 2000, measles cases in Thailand have generally trended downwards, but the deep southern provinces have experienced recurring epidemics every 3–5 years, leading to disability and mortality. These provinces, where Muslims are the majority, reported the highest incidence rates in the country, with 126 cases per 100,000 population, and notably low MMR vaccine coverage of around 70% from 2014 to 2018 [28–30]. The region's overall childhood vaccine coverage is among the lowest in Thailand, compounded by them having the highest frequency of measles outbreaks. In November 2018, more than 20 cases of measles-related deaths were reported for that year's outbreak, highlighting the severe impact of these epidemics [28–32]. In this area, vaccine acceptance is significantly influenced by Islamic practices and religious leaders, contrasting with other Thai communities, predominantly Buddhist, who generally perceive vaccines as protective against disease [33]. This pattern is similar to that observed in Malaysian Muslim communities, where vaccine hesitancy is also prevalent [34].

In this study, we explored the impact of a measles outbreak and a targeted two-pronged immunization campaign on MMR vaccine uptake at local child care centers in a region with notable religious hesitancy. In Southern Thailand, initiatives employing design thinking methods have been used to empathize with community concerns and develop new strategies to boost MMR vaccination. These efforts focus on creating culturally resonant narratives and imagery to enhance health literacy and promote vaccine acceptance among child care center staff and parents. The objectives of the study were to (a) describe and compare the uptake of MMR at the local child care centers with that of the wider regional and national levels, (b) assess trends in immunization coverage and evaluate any increases in relation to the timing of the outbreak and the immunization campaign, and (c) gather quantitative and qualitative feedback from child care center staff regarding the impact of the immunization campaign.

## 2. Materials and Methods

### *2.1. Study Population*

The study population included parents, child care center staff, and religious counselors associated with children aged 18 months to 5 years in subdistrict local government child care centers across 8 districts with recorded measles mortality, located in 5 provinces in the deep south of Thailand. The data collection period spanned from 1 December 2019 to March 2020. During this time, an immunization campaign was implemented, which included distributing a culturally adapted storybook and organizing measles prevention activities such as storytelling and singing at the child care centers. These districts were selected based on their historically low uptake of the MMR vaccine and recent reports of measles outbreaks, targeting areas where the intervention could have the most significant impact.

### 2.2. *Storytelling and Singing Intervention*

The intervention included two main components designed to increase MMR vaccination rates among the target population: the distribution of a specially designed storybook and the conducting of related singing activities.

Storybook Development

The storybook titled "Anees has Measles" (Figure 1) was crafted using a design thinking approach to deeply understand and empathize with the community's concerns about MMR vaccination. This creative process involved various stakeholders from the community, including parents, health workers, and religious leaders, who shared their insights on cultural nuances and common hesitancies surrounding vaccines. Their contributions ensured the content was culturally relevant and sensitive to the audience's beliefs and practices.

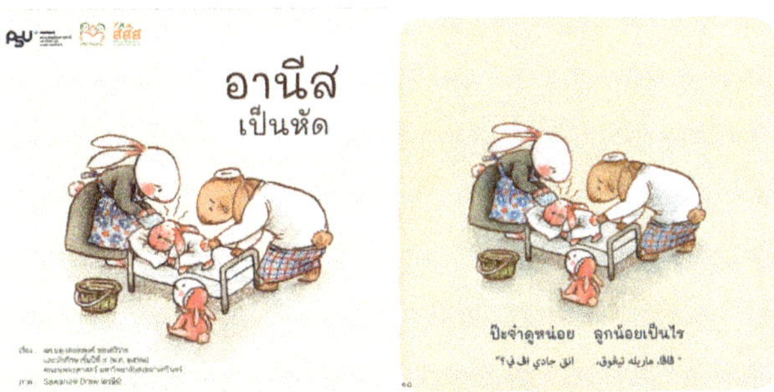


**Figure 1.** The storybook, titled "Anees has Measles".

The storybook aims to engage both children and their parents with its culturally resonant narratives and appealing imagery, making the topic of vaccination approachable and understandable. It consists of the following components:

(1) The Story of Anees: A narrative about a girl named Anees who contracts measles, illustrating the severity of the disease. It underscores the message that vaccines can be deemed halal when necessary to save lives, aligning with religious considerations.
(2) Insights from the Muslim Organization of Thailand: This section highlights the importance of vaccinations and reassures that they can be considered halal, addressing a significant cultural concern within the community.
(3) Educational Q&A on MMR Vaccine: Eight carefully crafted questions and answers designed to educate the community about the MMR vaccine, addressing common doubts and misinformation.
(4) Vaccine EPI Schedule Table of Thailand: An informative table presenting the official vaccination schedule, helping parents understand when their children should receive their shots.
(5) Vaccine Song Lyrics: Lyrics of a song related to the MMR vaccine, designed to be catchy and memorable, which helps reinforce the information about vaccination in a fun and engaging way.

Singing Activity: Alongside the storybook, a singing activity was integrated into the intervention. This activity utilized traditional Muslim melodies to reinforce the messages in the storybook, emphasizing the benefits of vaccination and the risks of measles. The singing sessions were designed to be interactive, involving both children and their parents, and thereby fostering a community-based learning environment that supports behavioral change towards the utilization of health practices. The complete videos of the songs performed in the intervention can be accessed via https://photos.app.goo.gl/GYm4Ft5

pBEY2Fbjw5 (accessed on 1 July 2024). All teachers, medical students, and children featured in these videos have provided their consent.

### 2.3. Targeted Vaccination Categories

This study focused exclusively on a catch-up vaccination approach:

C1 (Catch-up Vaccination): Targeted children aged 18 months to 5 years who had not previously received any MMR doses. These children were offered their first dose of MMR, with the recommendation to receive a second dose at least one month later.

C2 (Catch-up Vaccination): Consisted of children who had already received one dose of MMR. These children were provided a second dose to complete their immunization against measles.

### 2.4. Data Sources and Collection

Privacy, confidentiality, and the rights of patients were rigorously protected throughout the study in accordance with local health information policies. Data were primarily collected from two main sources:

Local Health Data, including details extracted from the local health information system, such as gender, birth date, and dates of MMR immunizations for children.

Immunization Records, meticulously checked by child care center staff before and after the intervention; these records, combined with secondary data from the local health data system, were used to verify the immunization status of each child.

### 2.5. Data Analysis

Vaccination Uptake Analysis: MMR vaccination coverage at 12 and 48 months was assessed based on records from the local health clinics and compared with broader regional and national data. The differences in vaccination rates before and after the intervention were analyzed using the Wilcoxon signed-rank test due to the non-normal distribution of the data (as indicated by the Shapiro–Wilk test). Statistical significance was determined at a level of $p < 0.05$. Confidence intervals (CI) for the changes in vaccination rates were calculated to provide a measure of the precision of the estimated effects.

Trend Analysis in Immunization Coverage: The monthly administration of MMR doses during 2020 was tracked alongside significant outbreak events and compared with historical data from 2018 to 2019 to identify any significant changes in vaccination trends. The analysis involved comparing the pre-intervention and post-intervention periods, with statistical significance determined using appropriate non-parametric tests.

Quantitative and Qualitative Feedback: Gathered feedback from child care staff regarding the intervention's impact, analyzed quantitatively and thematically to identify key themes affecting the program's success.

All statistical analyses were performed using STATA/IC version 16.0, focusing on the differences in vaccination uptake before and after the intervention, and evaluating the effectiveness of the culturally tailored educational strategies implemented during the measles outbreak.

## 3. Results

The study population consisted of 983 children aged 18 months to 5 years old in a government child care center as of 1 December 2019; 49% were male.

### 3.1. Vaccination Uptake at Local Health Center, Provincial, and National Levels

Vaccination coverage was closely monitored at the local health center and compared with regional and national levels. Initially, the local health center reported an MMR2 coverage rate of 44.3% (435/983) before the intervention. This rate increased significantly to 72.0% (708/983) twelve months after the intervention and further to 77.0% (734/953) by the 48-month mark post-intervention (Table 1).

Compared to broader geographical vaccination trends, the local health center's pre-intervention coverage was considerably lower than the regional and national averages. The deep-south region's coverage was 50.8% initially, rising to 66.7% at 12 months but slightly declining to 65.7% at 48 months. Nationally, Thailand started at 89.7% and saw a slight increase to 90.5% at 12 months, reaching 92.5% at 48 months.

**Table 1.** Vaccination coverage at the local health center, in the deep-south region, and at the national level (Thailand).

| Geographical Area | MMR2 Coverage at Pre-Intervention (%) | MMR2 Coverage at 12 Months (%) | MMR2 Coverage at 48 Months (%) |
|---|---|---|---|
| Local health center | 435/983 (44.3) | 708/983 (72.0) | 734/953 (77.0) |
| Deep south region | 50.8 | 66.7 | 65.7 |
| Thailand | 89.7 | 90.5 | 92.5 |

### 3.2. *Statistical Analysis of Vaccination Rate Changes*

The effectiveness of the "Anees has Measles" storybook intervention on MMR vaccination rates was statistically analyzed. The Shapiro–Wilk test indicated non-normal distribution of vaccination rate changes ($W = 0.775$, $p < 0.001$). Consequently, the Wilcoxon signed-rank test was applied, confirming a significant increase in vaccination rates from an initial 44.3% to 72.0% post-intervention, an increase of 27.77 percentage points ($Z = 31{,}180.5$, $p < 0.001$). This substantial increase underscores the intervention's success in boosting MMR vaccination uptake in the target child care centers. These findings demonstrate notable improvements in MMR vaccination rates at the local health center, highlighting the significant impact of the targeted educational intervention. Despite remarkable progress, local rates still lag behind national averages, emphasizing the need for continued efforts to enhance vaccination coverage.

### 3.3. *Quantitative Child Care Staff Feedback*

Following the evaluation of vaccination coverage, an additional aspect of the study involved assessing the satisfaction levels of staff from the Subdistrict Administrative Organization and child care centers regarding the "Anees has Measles" storybook intervention. A survey was conducted to gather these insights, with the results highlighting a positive reception towards the project's execution and outcomes.

#### 3.3.1. Satisfaction Survey Results

Program Appropriateness: A large majority of respondents felt the program's format was highly suitable, with 28.39% rating it as mostly appropriate and 54.20% as appropriate, summing to an overall satisfaction rate of 80.21%.

Program Duration: Similarly, the duration of the program was deemed appropriate by 26.27% and very appropriate by 65.68%, yielding a combined approval of 79.86%.

Knowledge/Benefit Gained: The educational benefit of the project "Anees has Measles" was acknowledged, with 83.57% of participants reporting they gained knowledge or benefits from the program.

Increased Vaccine Awareness: The importance of measles vaccination was more widely recognized post-intervention, as indicated by an 88.39% agreement rate among the respondents.

Data Collection and Transfer: The project's data management was praised, with 80.77% satisfaction regarding the ability to collect and transfer complete and accurate data.

The overall satisfaction with the project was noted at 83.22%, indicating strong approval of the initiative's impact and execution.

#### 3.3.2. Book Feedback and Impact

Increased Disease Understanding: 80.51% of respondents felt their understanding of measles improved significantly.

Perceived Vaccine Importance: 81.65% recognized the increased importance of vaccination.

Confidence in Vaccination: An increased confidence in vaccinating was reported by 81.14% of participants.

Religious Context Understanding: The project facilitated a better understanding of religious stipulations regarding vaccination, with 79.62% acknowledging this aspect.

### 3.4. Qualitative Child Care Staff Feedback

In addition to the quantitative satisfaction survey, qualitative feedback was collected from participants to gain deeper insights into the experiences and perceptions surrounding the "Anees has Measles" storybook intervention. Through thematic analysis of the qualitative data, several key themes emerged that provided a nuanced understanding of the intervention's impact and areas for improvement.

Themes from Qualitative Feedback:

1. Continuity and Frequency of Programs

Participants emphasized the need for regular and ongoing interventions to maintain high levels of awareness and prevention.

> *"We need this measles prevention project every year. It helps in keeping the community alert and prepared against the disease."*

2. Community and Multi-sectoral Engagement

The importance of collaborative efforts among healthcare providers, parents, and community leaders was highlighted as crucial for the success of the program.

> *"It's crucial that everyone gets involved, not just the healthcare workers. Parents, teachers, and local leaders need to understand and support the initiative for it to be successful."*

3. Project Duration and Reach

Respondents suggested that a longer project duration and broader reach would enhance the effectiveness of the intervention.

> *"The program was great, but it felt rushed. Extending the duration and covering more areas could help reach more families and have a stronger impact."*

4. Field Activities

Theme: The need for more interactive and on-site activities was identified to strengthen the program's impact and community engagement.

> *"Having more activities in our community would make the message stronger. People need to see and experience the benefits of vaccination firsthand."*

5. Sustainability of Educational Efforts

Ongoing educational initiatives were deemed necessary to improve vaccine uptake and health literacy continuously.

> *"Continuous education on not just measles but all vaccine-preventable diseases is needed to keep our community healthy. This should be an ongoing effort."*

6. Barriers to Engagement

Participants noted several barriers to engagement, including logistical issues and the accessibility of educational materials.

> *"The storybook was a good idea, but my work schedule didn't allow me to participate much. Also, some parents mentioned that the text and pictures were too small for the kids to see clearly."*

7. Enhanced Educational Materials

Feedback indicated a need for more appealing and accessible educational materials to effectively convey the message.

*"The storybook should have larger print and more colorful pictures to attract the children's attention. Making the material more engaging will help in delivering the message effectively."*

These themes and quotations encapsulate the multifaceted perspectives on the "Anees has Measles" storybook intervention, highlighting the program's successes and areas for improvement. The feedback underscores the necessity for adaptable, engaging, and sustained efforts to combat vaccine hesitancy and promote public health in the community.

## 4. Discussion

The effectiveness of the "Anees has Measles" storybook intervention, complemented by singing activities, in increasing MMR vaccination rates among young children in the deep south of Thailand is a testament to the power of culturally and religiously sensitive health communication strategies. By integrating stakeholders from the community in the development process—including parents, health workers, and religious leaders—the intervention was tailored to resonate with the local cultural and religious ethos, which played a crucial role in its acceptance and success. This approach is consistent with previous studies that emphasize the importance of community involvement in health interventions to ensure cultural compatibility and increase the likelihood of positive outcomes [35–37].

Utilizing storytelling and singing, which are culturally familiar methods of communication, the intervention presented the vaccination message in an engaging and non-confrontational manner. This strategy proved effective in not only increasing the understanding of and trust in vaccinations but also in making the educational process enjoyable for children and their parents [38–41]. Similar approaches have been documented in other settings, where integrating health education into local cultural practices significantly improved public health initiatives' receptiveness and effectiveness [42].

The substantial increase in vaccination rates post-intervention highlights the potential of targeted educational strategies to modify health behaviors, particularly in areas with initial vaccine hesitancy and low vaccine coverage. This aligns with findings from other regions where tailored communication strategies have successfully addressed vaccine hesitancy. Moreover, the use of specific educational tools within the storybook, such as the Q&A section and vaccination schedule, helped demystify the MMR vaccine and addressed prevalent misconceptions, a method supported by literature on health education [43–45]. Despite the intervention's success, challenges such as logistical issues and limited reach were noted, suggesting the need for ongoing support and resources to ensure wider accessibility and consistency in vaccine delivery.

The study, while insightful, presents several limitations that should be considered when interpreting the results. Firstly, the absence of a control group limits the ability to conclusively attribute the observed improvements in vaccination rates solely to the intervention, despite comparisons with regional and national data. This limitation makes it challenging to definitively isolate the effect of the intervention from other external factors that may have influenced the outcomes. Secondly, the findings are based on a relatively small sample size and are confined to specific child care centers in Southern Thailand, which may not fully represent broader populations or different cultural contexts. Thirdly, the reliance on voluntary participation could introduce selection bias, as those who chose to participate might inherently have different attitudes towards vaccination compared to the general population. Additionally, we did not collect detailed information on the sociodemographic features of parents, which could provide further insights into factors affecting vaccination uptake. While the 48-month follow-up period provided valuable longitudinal data, the study could benefit from exploring other aspects such as the continuity of vaccination behavior beyond the immediate aftermath of the intervention and the long-term acceptance of vaccines in the community. These limitations underscore the need for further research with a more robust experimental design, including a control group and broader demographic sampling, to validate and expand upon these initial findings.

The findings from this study have important implications for both clinical practice and future research. Clinically, the integration of culturally appropriate educational materials and methods into routine vaccination campaigns could enhance vaccine uptake in other regions with similar cultural and religious considerations. For future research, this study highlights the need for larger-scale interventions and longer follow-up periods to verify the findings and assess the long-term sustainability of the intervention effects. It also underscores the importance of exploring different types of educational interventions that could cater to diverse cultural groups, thereby enhancing the overall effectiveness of public health campaigns aimed at increasing vaccine coverage. Further studies could also investigate the impact of combining multiple communication strategies on vaccine hesitancy to identify the most effective approaches for various populations.

## 5. Conclusions

Overall, the "Anees has Measles" intervention illustrates that culturally tailored educational strategies that employ engaging and familiar communication formats can effectively enhance vaccination uptake in communities with significant vaccine hesitancy due to religious beliefs. The positive outcomes of this study provide valuable insights for designing future public health programs that aim to bridge the gap between cultural beliefs and health behaviors, emphasizing the importance of a sustained and adaptive approach to health education and community involvement.

**Supplementary Materials:** The following supporting information can be downloaded at: https://www.mdpi.com/article/10.3390/vaccines12070819/s1. PDF S1: "Anees has Measles" storybook.

**Author Contributions:** Conceptualization, T.T. and N.J.; methodology, T.T. and N.J.; software, T.T.; validation, T.T., N.J. and N.N.; formal analysis, T.T., P.K. and N.N.; investigation, T.T., P.K. and N.J.; resources, T.T. and N.J.; data curation, T.T. and N.J.; writing—original draft preparation, T.T.; writing—review and editing, T.T., P.K., N.J., N.N. and N.T.; visualization, T.T. and N.T.; supervision, T.T. and N.T.; project administration, T.T.; funding acquisition, T.T. All authors have read and agreed to the published version of the manuscript.

**Funding:** This research was funded by the Faculty of Medicine, Prince of Songkla University. The APC was funded by the Faculty of Medicine, Prince of Songkla University.

**Institutional Review Board Statement:** The study was conducted in accordance with the Declaration of Helsinki, and approved by the Institutional Review Board of the Faculty of Medicine, Prince of Songkla University. The ethics approval code for our study is REC.67-231-1-1.

**Informed Consent Statement:** Informed consent was obtained from all subjects involved in the study.

**Data Availability Statement:** Data supporting the reported results can be reached by contacting the corresponding author. Where no new data were created, or where data are unavailable due to privacy or ethical restrictions, please see the supplemental files associated with this publication.

**Acknowledgments:** The authors would like to express their gratitude for the administrative and technical support provided by the Faculty of Medicine, Prince of Songkla University. Additionally, heartfelt thanks are extended to the Thai Creative for Reading Culture Promotion Foundation and the Thai Health Promotion Foundation for their comprehensive support throughout all phases of publishing this storybook. We also wish to acknowledge the contributions of the group of 4th year Medical students for the Health Promotion block, who utilized design thinking methods to develop the first prototype of the storybook and song, Rapeepat Thewamit, co-advisor of the project, Rapeephan Pattanavech, the editor, Sawanee Draw, the illustrator, Sudjai Bhromkoed, chairman of The Creative for Reading Culture Promotion Foundation (CRF), and the Southernmost Reading Power Network for the development and distribution of the storybook. Your collective efforts have made this project possible, and we are deeply grateful for your dedication and hard work.

**Conflicts of Interest:** The authors declare no conflicts of interest. The funders had no role in the design of the study; in the collection, analyses, or interpretation of data; in the writing of the manuscript; or in the decision to publish the results.

## References


1. Naim, H.Y. Measles virus: A pathogen, vaccine, and a vector. *Hum. Vaccin. Immunother.* **2015**, *11*, 21–26. [CrossRef]
2. Centers for Disease Control and Prevention (CDC). Increased transmission and outbreaks of measles—European Region, 2011. *Morb. Mortal. Wkly Rep.* **2011**, *60*, 1605–1610.
3. Di Pietrantonj, C.; Rivetti, A.; Marchione, P.; Debalini, M.G.; Demicheli, V. Vaccines for measles, mumps, rubella, and varicella in children. *Cochrane Database Syst. Rev.* **2021**, *11*, CD004407.
4. Moss, W.J.; Griffin, D.E. Measles. *Lancet* **2012**, *379*, 153–164. [CrossRef]
5. Bester, J.C. Measles and Measles Vaccination: A Review. *JAMA Pediatr.* **2016**, *170*, 1209–1215. [CrossRef] [PubMed]
6. Hughes, S.L.; Bolotin, S.; Khan, S.; Li, Y.; Johnson, C.; Friedman, L.; Tricco, A.C.; Hahné, S.J.; Heffernan, J.M.; Dabbagh, A.; et al. The effect of time since measles vaccination and age at first dose on measles vaccine effectiveness—A systematic review. *Vaccine* **2020**, *38*, 460–469. [CrossRef] [PubMed]
7. Clemmons, N.; Wallace, G.S.; Patel, M.; Gastañaduy, P.A. Incidence of Measles in the United States, 2001–2015. *JAMA* **2017**, *318*, 1279. [CrossRef] [PubMed]
8. Dabbagh, A.; Laws, R.L.; Steulet, C.; Dumolard, L.; Mulders, M.N.; Kretsinger, K.; Alexander, J.P.; Rota, P.A.; Goodson, J.L. Progress Toward Regional Measles Elimination—Worldwide, 2000–2017. *Morb. Mortal. Wkly Rep.* **2018**, *67*, 1323–1329. [CrossRef]
9. Patel, M.; Lee, A.D.; Clemmons, N.S.; Redd, S.B.; Poser, S.; Blog, D.; Zucker, J.R.; Leung, J.; Link-Gelles, R.; Pham, H.; et al. National Update on Measles Cases and Outbreaks—United States, January 1–October 1, 2019. *Morb. Mortal. Wkly. Rep.* **2019**, *68*, 893–896. [CrossRef]
10. Guerra, F.; Bolotin, S.; Lim, G.; Heffernan, J.; Deeks, S.L.; Li, Y.; Crowcroft, N.S. The basic reproduction number (R0) of measles: A systematic review. *Lancet Infect. Dis.* **2017**, *17*, e420–e428. [CrossRef]
11. Zucker, J.R.; Rosen, J.B.; Iwamoto, M.; Arciuolo, R.J.; Langdon-Embry, M.; Vora, N.M.; Rakeman, J.L.; Isaac, B.M.; Jean, A.; Asfaw, M.; et al. Consequences of Undervaccination—Measles Outbreak, New York City, 2018–2019. *N. Engl. J. Med.* **2020**, *382*, 1009–1017. [CrossRef]
12. Phadke, V.K.; Bednarczyk, R.A.; Omer, S.B. Vaccine Refusal and Measles Outbreaks in the US. *JAMA* **2020**, *324*, 1344–1345. [CrossRef] [PubMed]
13. Dimala, C.A.; Kadia, B.M.; Nji, M.; Ndemazie, N.B. Factors associated with measles resurgence in the United States in the post-elimination era. *Sci. Rep.* **2021**, *11*, 51. [CrossRef]
14. Nuwarda, R.F.; Ramzan, I.; Weekes, L.; Kayser, V. Vaccine Hesitancy: Contemporary Issues and Historical Background. *Vaccines* **2022**, *10*, 1595. [CrossRef]
15. Alsuwaidi, A.R.; Hammad, H.A.A.; Elbarazi, I.; Sheek-Hussein, M. Vaccine hesitancy within the Muslim community: Islamic faith and public health perspectives. *Hum. Vaccin. Immunother.* **2023**, *19*, 2190716. [CrossRef]
16. Jinarong, T.; Chootong, R.; Vichitkunakorn, P.; Songwathana, P. Muslim parents' beliefs and factors influencing complete immunization of children aged 0–5 years in a Thai rural community: A qualitative study. *BMC Public. Health* **2023**, *23*, 1348. [CrossRef]
17. Trangerud, H.A. "What is the problem with vaccines?" A typology of religious vaccine skepticism. *Vaccine X* **2023**, *14*, 100349. [CrossRef]
18. Ahmed, A.; Lee, K.S.; Bukhsh, A.; Al-Worafi, Y.M.; Sarker, M.M.R.; Ming, L.C.; Khan, T.M. Outbreak of vaccine-preventable diseases in Muslim majority countries. *J. Infect. Public. Health* **2018**, *11*, 153–155. [CrossRef] [PubMed]
19. Ansari, M.T.; Jamaluddin, N.N.; Ramlan, T.A.; Zamri, N.; Majeed, S.; Badgujar, V.; Sami, F.; Hasnain, M.S.; Singh, H.K.B. Knowledge, attitude, perception of Muslim parents towards vaccination in Malaysia. *Hum. Vaccin. Immunother.* **2021**, *17*, 785–790. [CrossRef] [PubMed]
20. Nayar, R.K.; Nair, A.T.; Shaffi, M.; Swarnam, K.; Kumar, A.; Abraham, M.; Lordson, J.; Grace, C. Methods to overcome vaccine hesitancy. *Lancet* **2019**, *393*, 1203–1204. [CrossRef]
21. Le Menach, A.; Boxall, N.; Amirthalingam, G.; Maddock, L.; Balasegaram, S.; Mindlin, M. Increased measles-mumps-rubella (MMR) vaccine uptake in the context of a targeted immunisation campaign during a measles outbreak in a vaccine-reluctant community in England. *Vaccine* **2014**, *32*, 1147–1152. [CrossRef] [PubMed]
22. Jarrett, C.; Wilson, R.; O'Leary, M.; Eckersberger, E.; Larson, H.J. Strategies for addressing vaccine hesitancy—A systematic review. *Vaccine* **2015**, *33*, 4180–4190. [CrossRef] [PubMed]
23. Kompithra, R.Z.; Magdalenal, R.; Mathew, L.G.; Verghese, V.P. A High Volume, User-Friendly Immunization Clinic in Vellore, India: A Model for Urban Hospitals. *J. Immun.* **2016**, *1*, 1–8. [CrossRef]
24. Krishnendhu, V.K.; George, L.S. Drivers and barriers for measles rubella vaccination campaign: A qualitative study. *J. Fam. Med. Prim. Care* **2019**, *8*, 881–885. [CrossRef]
25. Olson, O.; Berry, C.; Kumar, N. Addressing Parental Vaccine Hesitancy towards Childhood Vaccines in the United States: A Systematic Literature Review of Communication Interventions and Strategies. *Vaccines* **2020**, *8*, 590. [CrossRef] [PubMed]
26. Phadke, V.K.; Bednarczyk, R.A.; Salmon, D.A.; Omer, S.B. Association Between Vaccine Refusal and Vaccine-Preventable Diseases in the United States. *JAMA* **2016**, *315*, 1149. [CrossRef] [PubMed]
27. Chung, Y.; Schamel, J.; Fisher, A.; Frew, P.M. Influences on Immunization Decision-Making among US Parents of Young Children. *Matern. Child. Health J.* **2017**, *21*, 2178–2187. [CrossRef]

28. Ministry of Public Health. Department of Disease Control. Thailand Measles Situation Report 2018 to 2019. 2019. Available online: https://ddc.moph.go.th/uploads/files/1112120200121090145.pdf (accessed on 10 April 2022).
29. Ministry of Public Health. Department of Disease Control. Thailand Measles Database 2018. 2018. Available online: https://apps-doe.moph.go.th/measles/ (accessed on 15 April 2022).
30. Ministry of Public Health. Department of Disease Control. Annual Epidemiological Surveillance Report 2019. 2021. Available online: https://ddc.moph.go.th/uploads/publish/1129820210620030431.pdf (accessed on 10 April 2022).
31. Daya, S.; Lillahkul, N.; Noin, J. Experience of parents of Thai Muslim Childhood aged 0–5 years in Yala Province who rejected the service of expanded program immunization with vaccine. *J. Dept. Med. Serv.* **2018**, *43*, 137–141. Available online: https://he02.tci-thaijo.org/index.php/JDMS/article/view/247857 (accessed on 12 April 2023).
32. Puti, S.; Pilate, A.; Puti, S.; Talalama, I.; Muputi, N. *Health Status, Beliefs, and Health Behaviors of People in the Southern Border Provinces*; Thai Muslim's Health Promotion Program: Bangkok, Thailand, 2018.
33. Yotawut, M. Maternal perceptions of Childhood Vaccinations: A case study of Banphaeo General Hospital Samutsakorn Province. *J. Nurs. Health Care.* **2019**, *37*, 32–41. Available online: https://he01.tci-thaijo.org/index.php/jnat-ned/article/view/232339 (accessed on 12 April 2023).
34. Lim, W.Y.; Amar-Singh, H.S.S.; Jeganathan, N.; Rahmat, H.; Mustafa, N.A.; Yusof, M.; Rahman, F.-S.; Itam, R.; Chan, S.C.H.; N-Julia, M.S. Exploring immunisation refusal by parents in the Malaysian context. *Cogent Med.* **2016**, *3*, 1142410. [CrossRef]
35. Nixon, L.S.; Hudson, N.; Culley, L.; Lakhanpaul, M.; Robertson, N.; Johnson, M.R.D.; McFeeters, M.; Johal, N.; Hamlyn-Williams, C.; Boo, Y.Y.; et al. Key considerations when involving children in health intervention design: Reflections on working in partnership with South Asian children in the UK on a tailored Management and Intervention for Asthma (MIA) study. *Res. Involv. Engag.* **2022**, *8*, 9. [CrossRef] [PubMed]
36. Radhamony, R.; Cross, W.M.; Townsin, L.; Banik, B. Perspectives of culturally and linguistically diverse (CALD) community members regarding mental health services: A qualitative analysis. *J. Psychiatr. Ment. Health Nurs.* **2023**, *30*, 850–864. [CrossRef] [PubMed]
37. Ferdinand, A.; Lambert, M.; Trad, L.; Pedrana, L.; Paradies, Y.; Kelaher, M. Indigenous engagement in health: Lessons from Brazil, Chile, Australia and New Zealand. *Int. J. Equity Health* **2020**, *19*, 47. [CrossRef] [PubMed]
38. Daykin, N.; Mansfield, L.; Meads, C.; Julier, G.; Tomlinson, A.; Payne, A.; Duffy, L.G.; Lane, J.; D'innocenzo, G.; Burnett, A.; et al. What works for wellbeing? A systematic review of wellbeing outcomes for music and singing in adults. *Perspect. Public Health* **2018**, *138*, 39–46. [CrossRef] [PubMed]
39. Feng, L.; Romero-Garcia, R.; Suckling, J.; Tan, J.; Larbi, A.; Cheah, I.; Wong, G.; Tsakok, M.; Lanskey, B.; Lim, D.; et al. Effects of choral singing versus health education on cognitive decline and aging: A randomized controlled trial. *Aging* **2020**, *12*, 24798–24816. [CrossRef] [PubMed]
40. Black, L.W.; Wolfe, A.W.; Han, S.-H. Storytelling and Deliberative Play in the Oregon Citizens' Assembly Online Pilot on COVID-19 Recovery. *Am. Behav. Sci.* **2023**, *67*, 963–981. [CrossRef] [PubMed]
41. Lober, A.; Komnenich, P. Storytelling as a Teaching Approach for Breastfeeding Education. *Nurs. Women's Health* **2020**, *24*, 440–445. [CrossRef] [PubMed]
42. Shruti, T.; Govindraju, H.A.; Sriranga, J. Incorporation of Storytelling as a Method of Oral Health Education among 3–6-year-old Preschool Children. *Int. J. Clin. Pediatr. Dent.* **2021**, *14*, 349–352. [CrossRef]
43. Meyer, B.A.; Viskupič, F.; Wiltse, D.L. Pharmacists to partner with religious leaders to overcome vaccine hesitancy among Christians. *J. Am. Pharm. Assoc.* **2022**, *62*, 302–304. [CrossRef]
44. Hicken, A.; Jones, P.; Menon, A.; Rozek, L.S. Can endorsement by religious leaders move the needle on vaccine hesitancy? *Vaccine* **2024**, *42*, 918–923. [CrossRef]
45. Thomas, B.; Flood, C.M. Eliminating Religious and Philosophical Exemptions: The Next Step in Ontario's Campaign against Vaccine Hesitancy. *Healthc. Policy* **2020**, *16*, 14–20. [CrossRef] [PubMed]

vaccines

MDPI

*Article*

# A Cross-Sectional Study of Measles-Specific Antibody Levels in Australian Blood Donors—Implications for Measles Post-Elimination Countries

**Kirsten M. Williamson [1,2,*], Helen Faddy [3,4], Suellen Nicholson [5,6], Vicki Stambos [5], Veronica Hoad [3], Michelle Butler [1], Tambri Housen [2,7], Tony Merritt [1] and David N. Durrheim [1,7]**

1 Hunter New England Population Health, Hunter New England Local Health District, Locked Bag 10, Wallsend, NSW 2287, Australia; michelle.butler@health.nsw.gov.au (M.B.); tony.merritt@health.nsw.gov.au (T.M.); david.durrheim@health.nsw.gov.au (D.N.D.)
2 National Centre for Epidemiology and Population Health, Australian National University, 62 Mills Road, Acton, ACT 2601, Australia; tambri.housen@newcastle.edu.au
3 Australian Red Cross Lifeblood, P.O. Box 354, South Melbourne, VIC 3205, Australia; hfaddy@usc.edu.au (H.F.); vhoad@redcrossblood.org.au (V.H.)
4 School of Health, University of the Sunshine Coast, P.O. Box 200, Petrie, QLD 4502, Australia
5 Victorian Infectious Diseases Reference Laboratory, Royal Melbourne Hospital, The Peter Doherty Institute for Infection and Immunity, 792 Elizabeth Street, Melbourne, VIC 3000, Australia; suellen.nicholson@vidrl.org.au (S.N.); vicki.stambos@mh.org.au (V.S.)
6 Department of Infectious Diseases, University of Melbourne, Grattan Street, Parkville, VIC 3010, Australia
7 School of Medicine and Public Health, University of Newcastle, University Drive, Callaghan, NSW 2308, Australia
* Correspondence: kirsten.williamson@health.nsw.gov.au

**Abstract:** Passive immunisation with normal human immunoglobulin (NHIG) is recommended as post-exposure prophylaxis (PEP) for higher-risk measles contacts where vaccination is contraindicated. However, the concentration of measles-specific antibodies in NHIG depends on antibody levels within pooled donor plasma. There are concerns that measles immunity in the Australian population may be declining over time and that blood donors' levels will progressively decrease, impacting levels required to produce effective NHIG for measles PEP. A cross-sectional study of Australian plasmapheresis donors was performed using an age-stratified, random sample of recovered serum specimens, collected between October and November 2019 ($n$ = 1199). Measles-specific IgG antibodies were quantified by ELISA (Enzygnost anti-measles virus IgG, Siemens), and negative and equivocal specimens ($n$ = 149) also underwent plaque reduction neutralisation testing (PRNT). Mean antibody levels (optical density values) progressively decreased from older to younger birth cohorts, from 2.09 [±0.09, 95% CI] to 0.58 [±0.04, 95% CI] in donors born in 1940–1959 and 1990–2001, respectively ($p < 0.0001$). This study shows that mean measles-specific IgG levels are significantly lower in younger Australian donors. While current NHIG selection policies target older donors, as younger birth cohorts become an increasingly larger proportion of contributing donors, measles-specific antibody concentrations of NHIG will progressively reduce. We therefore recommend monitoring measles-specific antibody levels in future donors and NHIG products in Australia and other countries that eliminated measles before the birth of their youngest blood donors.

**Keywords:** measles; antibody; immunity; immunoglobulin; IgG; donor; NHIG

## 1. Introduction

Australia's comprehensive national immunisation program and control initiatives have achieved the elimination of endemic measles in Australia [1]. However, measles-specific antibody levels tend to be lower in individuals where immunity is vaccine-derived rather than derived from wild measles virus infection [2]. Declining measles antibody levels have been found in populations where widespread immunisation has led to the interruption of wild-type measles transmission [3,4]. There are concerns that the Australian population may also be experiencing a waning of measles immunity over time.

Normal human immunoglobulin (NHIG) is recommended as post-exposure prophylaxis (PEP) for measles in higher-risk contacts where vaccination is contraindicated [5]. Australian guidelines currently recommend 0.2 mL/kg for infants and pregnant women and 0.5 mL/kg, to a maximum of 15 mL, for immunocompromised people via intramuscular injection [6].

NHIG is a sterile solution containing antibodies against various pathogens [7]. Virus-specific antibodies within the preparation bind to the corresponding target, thus preventing or attenuating disease [8]. In Australia, NHIG is produced by CSL Behring through fractionation of human plasma donated to the Australian Red Cross Lifeblood (hereafter "Lifeblood") [7,9]. Donors must be aged 18 to 75 years or over 75 years if they have donated previously and are medically fit [10].

The effectiveness of NHIG in preventing measles is dependent on the concentration of measles-specific antibodies within the preparation [11]. The concentration of measles-specific antibodies within NHIG depends on the antibody levels within the pooled donor plasma from which it is produced [12]. While the minimum effective dose of measles-specific antibodies required (based on contemporary IG products) is unclear, a dose–response effect has been clearly observed [13].

Studies in the US, Germany, New Zealand, Canada, and the UK have found that those born after widespread measles vaccination was introduced, and subsequently living without circulating measles virus, had lower measles-specific antibody levels [14,15]. Corresponding decreases in the measles-specific antibody levels of immunoglobulin products have also been observed [16,17]. Consequently, some countries have increased the dosage and/or changed the route of administration of NHIG, or required that NHIG products achieve a specific measles antibody level [17–22]; however, Australian recommendations remain unchanged [6]. Contrastingly, in Australia, NHIG must have a minimum level of hepatitis A virus (HAV) antibodies to be released by CSL Behring. Since 2017, Lifeblood has preferentially directed whole blood-derived plasma from donors aged 60 years and over to CSL Behring for NHIG production, as older donors have been demonstrated to have higher HAV antibody levels [internal data, Lifeblood]. Preferencing donations from older cohorts may affect other specific antibody levels within NHIG.

The objective of this study was to establish if mean measles-specific IgG antibody levels differ between birth cohorts of Australian plasma donors to provide guidance to policymakers.

## 2. Materials and Methods

### 2.1. Study Population and Design

A cross-sectional study of measles-specific antibody levels in Australian plasmapheresis donors was performed. Subjects had donated at Lifeblood collection centres across Australia between 29 October and 14 November 2019. Recovered serum specimens (residual sera remaining after routine testing) were stratified and randomly selected from the following five age groups, which represented the corresponding birth-year cohorts: (A) 18–29 years old (1990–2001); (B) 30–39 years old (1980–1989); (C) 40–49 years old (1970–1979); (D) 50–59 years old (1960–1969); and (E) 60+ years old (1940–1959).

Demographic data (date of birth, gender, residential postcode, and donation type) were obtained prior to de-identification with a unique study number. Serum (≥1 mL) was aliquoted, and specimens were frozen (−30 °C) and stored before transfer to the Victorian Infectious Diseases Reference Laboratory (VIDRL), Melbourne.

### 2.2. Sample Size Calculation

For estimating the mean antibody level with effect size 0.3 and 90% power, the calculated target sample size per age group was 233 (total target sample size of 1165) [23]. This equated to approximately 10% of plasmapheresis donor specimens received by the Sydney processing centre for specialised testing over one month and approximately 0.25% of the total Australian donor population [24].

### 2.3. Laboratory Testing

All individual specimens were tested using the Enzygnost anti-measles virus IgG diagnostic kit (Siemens Healthcare Diagnostics, Marburg, Germany) on the BEP®® 2000 ELISA processor (Siemens Healthcare Diagnostics) as per manufacturer's instructions. Measles-specific antibody levels were recorded as optical density (OD) values. The results were classified as positive (OD > 0.2, with OD 0.2–0.4 being 'low positive'); equivocal (OD 0.1–0.2); or negative (OD < 0.1). Equivocal and negative specimens were retested twice, and the result used was based on concordance with the result interpretation. Previous studies have shown that samples reactive by this ELISA in the range of corrected OD 0.1–0.2 generally have measles-virus neutralising antibody levels of >120 mIU/mL on plaque reduction neutralisation testing (PRNT) [25–29]. Levels ≥120 mIU/mL are considered protective [30,31].

Because PRNT is more sensitive at lower antibody concentrations, all specimens that tested equivocal and negative on ELISA also underwent PRNT [29]. PRNT was performed according to the protocol established for the WHO measles immunogenicity studies of aerosol vaccination project by Cohen et al. [31], based on the original method developed by Albrecht et al. [32]. The 50% neutralising antibody end-point titres ($ND_{50}$) were calculated using the Karber formula, and the results were standardised against the WHO 3rd International Standard (IS) (NIBSC code 97/648) for measles antibodies containing 3000 mIU/mL. The WHO 3rd IS was diluted and tested over a series of ten valid assay runs to determine the geometric mean titre (GMT) and +/− two standard deviations as per recommendation by Cohen et al. [31]. All subsequent assay runs included the diluted WHO 3rd IS for validation purposes and to calculate the sample titres in mIU/mL.

### 2.4. Data Analysis

Statistical analysis was performed with Stata version 14.0. Mean OD values were compared using Student's *t*-test for variables with two levels (gender, donation type, and donation frequency) and one-way ANOVA with post hoc analysis using Tukey HSD for birth year cohorts. Regarding Student's *t*-test, the assumption of normality was met by the central limit theorem (i.e., large sample size), and equal variance was observed between groups using a variance ratio test. Although age-group/birth-cohort data appeared skewed, one-way ANOVA was deemed appropriate. Because the ANOVA test is robust, especially as sample size increases and sample sizes for all levels are equal, violations of rules of normality and equal variance that are not extreme can be considered not serious [33]. As per Sullivan (2011), if the largest standard deviation of the groups is less than two times the smallest standard deviation, then the assumption can be considered not violated [34].

Kruskal–Wallis test was used to compare median OD values between states/territories due to large differences in sample sizes across the levels. The correlation between OD values and year of birth was determined using the Pearson correlation coefficient.

Multivariate analysis was performed using a backward, stepwise, linear regression. Variables were initially included, where $p < 0.25$ on parametric tests, and then removed one by one until only significant variables remained. Year of birth was included as a numerical variable, and gender and donation frequency were considered categorical variables. Post-estimation P-P plot, Q-Q plot, and RVF plot were visualised (Appendix A).

## 3. Results

Measles-specific IgG antibody levels were measured in a total of 1200 plasmapheresis donors, with 232 to 245 subjects in each of the five birth year cohorts. One subject was excluded due to discordant results between initial ELISA testing with PRNT and further testing with a second ELISA assay. Therefore, the final study population was $n = 1199$.

The mean OD value was 1.28 (±0.05 95% CI; range 0.00–3.52), well above the assay's positive cut-off (OD > 0.2). However, there was a consistent, downward trend in the mean measles-specific IgG antibody levels from older to younger donor cohorts. The mean antibody levels were higher in females when adjusted for age. There was no difference in levels based on state/territory of residence or donation type (Table 1).

**Table 1.** Measles-specific IgG antibody levels measured by ELISA (optical density (OD) values) in Australian plasmapheresis donors, 29 October to 14 November 2019, by demography.

| | *n* (%) | Mean OD [95% CI] | Standard Deviation | Range | *p*-Value |
|---|---|---|---|---|---|
| Total | 1199 | 1.28 [1.23–1.33] | | 0.00–3.52 | |
| Birth Year Cohort (Age) | | | | | |
| 1940–1959 (60+ years) | 232 (19.4) | 2.09 [2.00–2.18] | 0.71 | 0.36–3.52 | |
| 1960–1969 (50–59 years) | 239 (19.9) | 1.87 [1.76–1.97] | 0.82 | 0.05–3.17 | |
| 1970–1979 (40–49 years) | 241 (20.1) | 1.18 [1.06–1.29] | 0.90 | 0.00–3.22 | **<0.0001** |
| 1980–1989 (30–39 years) | 242 (20.2) | 0.74 [0.65–0.83] # | 0.72 | 0.00–3.00 | |
| 1990–2001 (18–29 years) | 245 (20.4) | 0.58 [0.52–0.64] # | 0.47 | 0.00–2.79 | |
| Gender | | | | | |
| Female | 565 (47.1) | 1.32 [1.24–1.40] | 0.95 | 0.00–3.52 | 0.179 |
| Male | 634 (52.9) | 1.25 [1.17–1.32] | 0.95 | 0.00–3.33 | |
| Donation Type | | | | | |
| Source plasma | 1142 (95.3) | 1.28 [1.23–1.34] | 0.95 | 0.00–3.52 | 0.840 |
| Clinical apheresis | 57 (4.7) | 1.26 [1.01–1.51] | 0.96 | 0.04–3.17 | |
| Donation Frequency | | | | | |
| First-time apheresis donor | 440 (36.7) | 1.09 [1.01–1.18] | 0.90 | 0.00–3.52 | **<0.0001** |
| Repeat apheresis donor | 759 (63.3) | 1.39 [1.32–1.46] | 0.96 | 0.00–3.40 | |
| | ***n*(%)** | **Median OD** | **Interquartile Range** | **Range** | ***p*-Value** |
| State/Territory | | | | | |
| Australian Capital Territory | 46 (3.8) | 1.24 | 0.54–2.13 | 0.07–3.00 | |
| New South Wales | 275 (22.9) | 1.03 | 0.39–1.98 | 0.00–3.52 | |
| Northern Territory | 3 (0.3) | 2.55 | 1.03–3.00 | 1.03–3.00 | |
| Queensland | 261 (21.8) | 1.01 | 0.45–2.10 | 0.00–3.33 | |
| South Australia | 104 (8.7) | 1.44 | 0.58–2.31 | 0.09–3.12 | 0.112 |
| Tasmania | 41 (3.4) | 1.34 | 0.61–2.34 | 0.03–3.00 | |
| Victoria | 315 (26.3) | 0.98 | 0.42–1.88 | 0.00–3.40 | |
| Western Australia | 154 (12.8) | 1.18 | 0.37–2.14 | 0.00–3.15 | |

# $p < 0.05$ for all birth year cohorts except 1980–1989 and 1990–2001.

### 3.1. Measles-Specific IgG Antibody Levels by Subgroup

Although antibody levels were widely dispersed within each age group, there was a clear downward trend in OD values from older to younger cohorts (Figure 1). All 232 donors born before 1960 and 98.7% (236/239) born from 1960 to 1969 had OD values > 0.2, suggesting measles immunity. By comparison, 88.4% (213/241), 81.8% (198/242), and 78.4% (192/245) of donors born in the years 1970–1979, 1980–1989, and 1990–2001, respectively, had OD values > 0.2 ($p < 0.001$).

The mean measles-specific antibody levels decreased significantly from older to younger cohorts (1940–1959: OD 2.09 ± 0.09, vs. 1990–2001: OD 0.58 ± 0.04, 95% CI). Differences between groups were statistically significant in all birth year cohorts ($p < 0.05$) except for the 1980–1989 and 1990–2001 cohorts (Figure 2). There was no significant change to the results when the 1940–1959 cohort ($n = 232$) was separated into two groups (1940–1949 and 1950–1959) nor when subjects in the 1940–1949 group ($n = 43$) were excluded. There was a moderate, negative correlation between measles-specific antibody ELISA OD values and year of birth (Pearson's r = −0.629, $p < 0.0001$) (Appendix A).

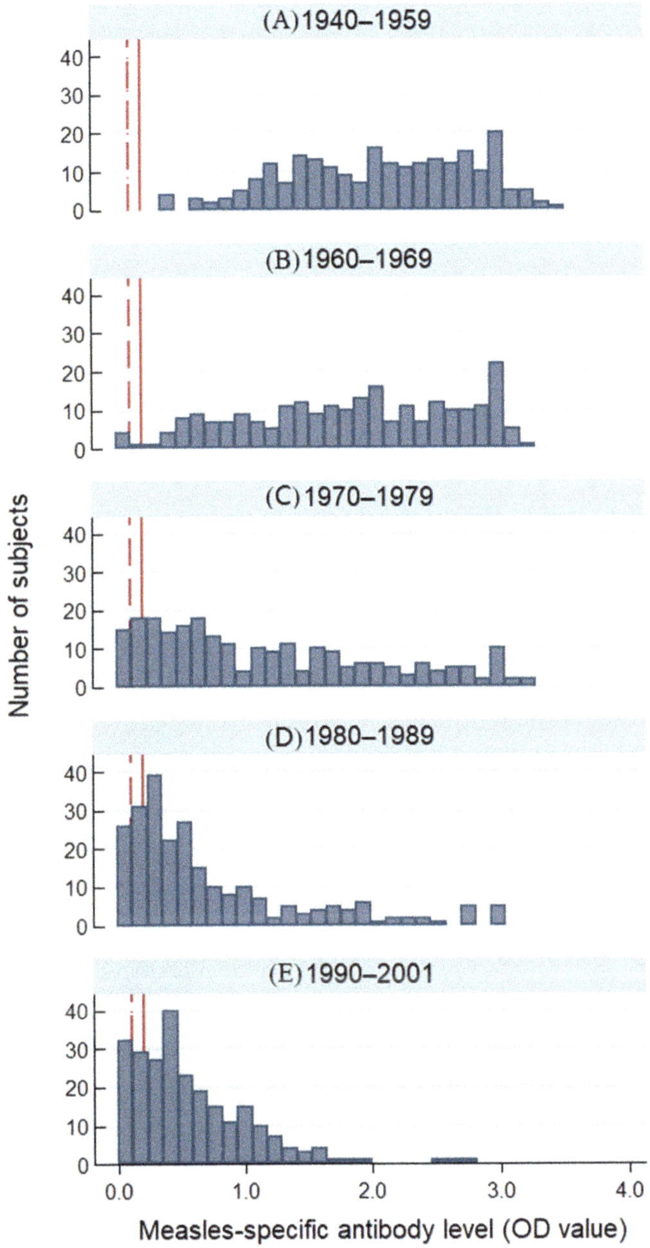


**Figure 1.** Distribution of measles-specific IgG antibody levels measured by ELISA (optical density values) in Australian plasmapheresis donors that donated from 29 October to 14 November 2019, by birth year cohorts: (**A**) 1940–1959, (**B**) 1960–1969, (**C**) 1970–1979, (**D**) 1980–1989, and (**E**) 1990–2001. The dark red line shows a positive cut-off for assay (OD = 0.2). OD values >0.2 suggest immunity. The dark red dotted line shows an equivocal cut-off (OD = 0.1). OD values 0.1–0.2 are considered equivocal; OD values < 0.1 are negative and therefore considered non-immune.

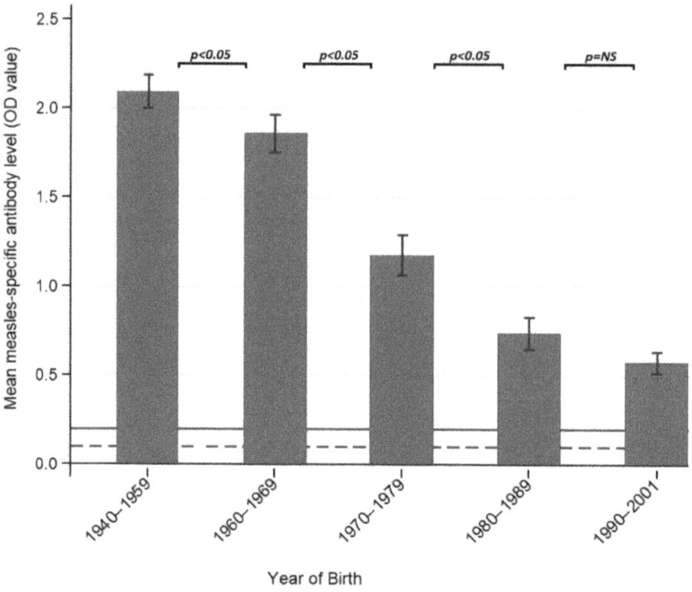


**Figure 2.** Mean measles-specific IgG antibody optical density (OD) values as measured by ELISA in Australian plasmapheresis donors who donated from 29 October to 14 November 2019, by birth year cohorts. Error bars (vertical) show 95% confidence intervals. Difference bars (horizontal) depict the significance of difference in means between cohorts using one-way ANOVA and Tukey HSD analysis. The dark red line shows a positive cut-off for assay (OD = 0.2). OD values > 0.2 suggest immunity. The dark red dotted line shows an equivocal cut-off (OD = 0.1). OD values 0.1–0.2 are considered equivocal; OD values < 0.1 are negative and therefore considered non-immune.

Univariate analysis did not detect a significant difference in the mean OD values between females (OD 1.32 ± 0.08, 95% CI) and males (1.25 ± 0.07, 95% CI) ($p = 0.179$); however, there was a significant difference when adjusted for age/year of birth ($p = 0.016$) (Appendix A).

There was a significant difference in the mean measles-specific antibody levels between first-time apheresis donors (OD = 1.09 ± 0.08, 95% CI) and repeat donors (OD = 1.39 ± 0.07, 95% CI) ($p < 0.0001$); however, when adjusted for age and gender, the effect of donor status was no longer significant ($p = 0.524$). First-time apheresis donors were generally younger than repeat donors [median age (IQR) 38 years (28–51) vs. 48 years (35–59), respectively]; thus, the relationship between donation frequency and antibody levels was likely confounded by age/year of birth.

Study population proportions by gender and residential state/territory (Table 1) were similar to the broader Australian plasmapheresis donor population (Appendix A). There was no significant difference in the median antibody levels between states and territories ($p = 0.112$).

### 3.2. Multivariate Analysis

Multiple linear regression was performed to predict measles-specific antibody OD value from the year of birth, gender, and first-time vs. repeat donor status. Year of birth and gender added statistically significantly to the prediction ($p < 0.001$ and $p < 0.01$), whilst donor status did not ($p = 0.981$); therefore, donor status was removed from the model. The final model was significant; however, it only explained 40% of the variance in OD values [$F(2, 1196) = 397.76$, $p < 0.0001$, $R^2 = 0.399$]. It was predicted that as donor age decreased by one year, the OD value decreased by 0.04. Males were predicted to have an OD value of 0.12

less than females of the same age. Post-regression visualisations appeared acceptable for the normality of residuals (P-P and Q-Q plot); the RVF plot was slightly curved, suggesting some heteroscedasticity (Appendix A).

### 3.3. Plaque Reduction Neutralisation Testing (PRNT)

A total of 150 specimens underwent PRNT to determine what proportion of subjects with negative or equivocal ELISA results were still above the assumed correlate of protection. One subject was excluded due to discordant results (see above). This gave a final sample size of $n$ = 149, which included all ELISA negative ($n$ = 66) and equivocal ($n$ = 63) specimens, plus a small random selection of low-positive ($n$ = 10) and positive specimens ($n$ = 10).

Younger birth cohorts were over-represented amongst the ELISA negative and equivocal specimens: Overall, 75.8% (50/66) and 76.2% (48/63) of negative and equivocal specimens, respectively, came from subjects born after 1979. By contrast, none (0/7) of the negative, equivocal, or low-positive specimens were from subjects born prior to 1960 (Appendix A). Of the 66 specimens that were ELISA-negative, 56.1% (37/66) were above the assumed correlate of protection on PRNT. Of the 63 specimens that were equivocal on ELISA, 96.8% (61/63) were above the assumed correlate of protection. All low-positive (10/10) and positive (10/10) ELISA specimens tested were above the correlate of protection (Table 2).

**Table 2.** Measles-specific IgG antibody categories measured by ELISA and corresponding measles-neutralising antibody categories by plaque reduction neutralisation testing (PRNT) in a subset of Australian plasmapheresis donors ($n$ = 149), 29 October to 14 November 2019.

| ELISA Result | PRNT Result | | |
|---|---|---|---|
| | **Above Correlate of Protection ≥120 mIU/mL $n$ (%)** | **Below Correlate of Protection <120 mIU/mL $n$ (%)** | **Total** |
| Negative | 37 (56.1) | 29 (43.9) | 66 |
| Equivocal | 61 (96.8) | 2 (3.2) | 63 |
| Low-positive | 10 (100.0) | 0 (0.0%) | 10 |
| Positive | 10 (100.0) | 0 (0.0%) | 10 |
| Total | 118 (79.2) | 31 (20.8) | 149 |

## 4. Discussion

The effectiveness of NHIG as measles post-exposure prophylaxis is dependent on measles-specific antibody levels in the blood donor population from whom plasma is fractionated to make IG products. This study demonstrated a significant decrease in the mean measles-specific IgG antibody levels from older to younger Australian donor cohorts. The present Lifeblood policy of preferentially using plasma from whole blood donors aged over 60 provides higher antibody levels in current products; however, older birth cohort donors will progressively be replaced by younger ones over decades. In the future, this may result in a decline in measles antibody levels in Australian NHIG and a corresponding reduction in the protection provided to high-risk measles contacts by NHIG, unless measures are taken.

A similar decrease in measles-specific antibody levels was observed across US plasma donor birth cohorts. A sharp decline was noted in donors born after 1963, which coincided with the introduction of measles vaccination in the USA. Levels appeared to plateau in cohorts born in the 1970s and 1980s, followed by another decline after the introduction of a second dose of vaccine in 1989. Another plateau was described in those born after 1990 [14,15].

In our study of Australian plasmapheresis donors, the decline in antibody levels was particularly evident in donors born from the late 1960s onwards (Figure 3). This corresponds with the introduction and subsequent funding of the measles vaccine in Australia in 1968 and 1970, respectively [35]. A steady decrease was observed until the 1990–2001 birth year cohort. A prospective study is required to determine if antibody levels will continue to decline in subsequent birth year cohorts or reach a "steady state" as suggested by the US study.

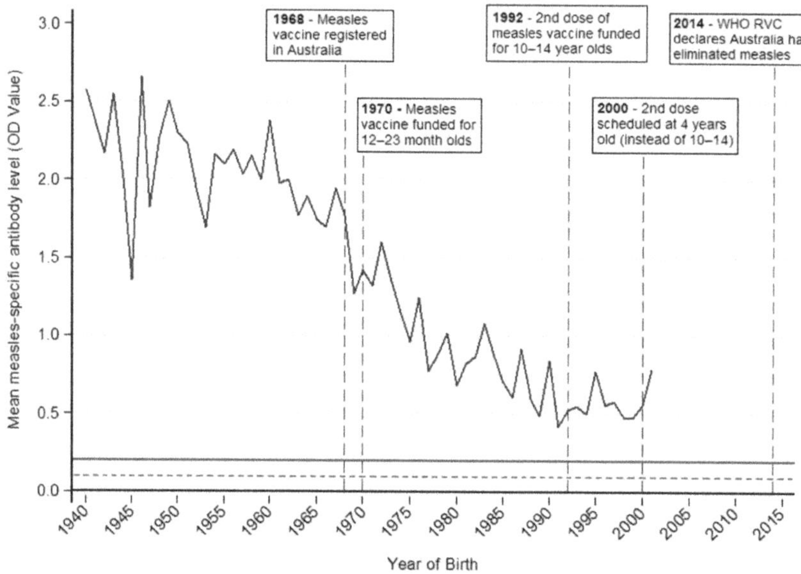


**Figure 3.** Mean measles-specific IgG antibody levels optical density (OD) values measured by ELISA in Australian plasmapheresis donors who donated from 29 October to 14 November 2019 by year of birth, and milestones for vaccination and control of measles in Australia [35,36]. The dark red line shows a positive cut-off for assay (OD = 0.2). OD values > 0.2 suggest immunity. The dark red dotted line shows an equivocal cut-off (OD = 0.1). OD values 0.1–0.2 are considered equivocal; OD values < 0.1 are negative and therefore considered non-immune.

Australia was verified to have eliminated endemic measles by the World Health Organization in 2014 [36]. However, the absence of endemic transmission in Australia can be demonstrated as early as 2009 and likely occurred even earlier than this [37]. There is an increasing cohort of Australians, born after 2009, who have lived solely in a post-elimination environment and have thus not been exposed to wild-type measles. This cohort is currently too young to be captured by this study; therefore, it would be wise to monitor the measles-specific antibody levels of Australian plasma donor cohorts on a regular basis in the future.

Given the decreasing trend across birth cohorts found by our study, it is anticipated that the mean measles-specific antibody levels of the overall Australian donor population, and thus overall donations, will decrease in the future. The mean antibody level (OD value) for our overall study population was 1.28. It is assumed that donors born after 1970 will form a larger proportion of the total Australian donations in the future. By extrapolating from age-specific levels in our study, the mean antibody level of 2.09 for those 60 years and over in 2019 was estimated to decrease to 1.87 in 2029 and 1.18 in 2039. When adjusted for age, the estimated mean level for total Australian blood donations (plasma and whole blood) received from all age groups in 2019 was 1.30. This was estimated to decrease to 1.01 in 2029 and 0.74 in 2039 (Appendix A). Our estimates suggest that in 10 years' time, the mean measles-specific antibody levels for donations from those 60 years and over and the annual total Australian donations will be approximately 90% and 80%, respectively, of what they are now. In 20 years, the mean measles-specific antibody levels for donations from individuals 60 years and over, and the total Australian donations, will be approximately 60% of their current level. This is assuming that a "steady state" is maintained in donors born after 1990 and that there is no decay in an individual's antibody levels over time.

The mean measles-specific antibody levels were slightly higher in females than males in our study. Nonetheless, both genders showed the same trend towards lower levels in younger birth cohorts. An Australian national rubella serosurvey in 2012–2013 found a lower proportion of rubella seropositive males in the 30–44-year age group, which was thought to reflect the initial vaccination program targeting females only. However, at this time, separate monovalent vaccines were used for rubella and measles, with measles vaccination recommended and funded for both males and females; therefore, it is unlikely to account for the difference in measles immunity between genders [35,38]. However, there is an increasing body of evidence that females typically develop higher antibody responses to a range of vaccines, including the measles–mumps–rubella vaccine [39–41]. This has been attributed to hormonal and potentially epigenetic and environmental differences between males and females [40]. However, most vaccine studies do not stratify their data by gender; thus, this area remains under-researched.

Measles vaccines are part of Australia's National Immunisation Program and vaccine schedule changes are synchronised across states and territories [35]; thus, similar median antibody levels were expected, although our study was not specifically powered for this. While first-time donors tended to be younger, there was no significant difference in the mean antibody levels between first-time and repeat donors when adjusted for age and gender. The multivariate analysis supported that birth year and gender significantly predicted measles antibody levels, while donation frequency did not. However, the model only explained 40% of the variability in OD values. In future studies, additional variables such as previous measles infection or immunisation would likely improve the model.

Young et al. measured the measles-specific antibody titres in Australian NHIG manufactured between 2010 and 2014 [42], acknowledging that their study was conducted prior to 2017 when Lifeblood began prioritising older donors for NHIG production and therefore titres are expected to have increased. Titres in intramuscular products ranged from 51 to 76 IU/mL when measured by PRNT, which equated to 1.5 to 2.3 times the US Centre for Biologics Evaluation and Research (CBER) standard. Titres did not appear to decrease between products from earlier and later years; however, the study's time span and sample size were limited.

If NHIG with a measles antibody concentration of 51 IU/mL was administered using the current Australian guidelines, this would equate to delivery of measles-specific antibodies of at least 10.2 IU/kg for immunocompetent contacts and 25.5 IU/kg for immunocompromised contacts. A study by Endo et al. found that an intramuscular NHIG dose of 10.9 IU/kg given within 5 days prevented clinically evident disease in five out of six (83.3%) paediatric close contacts. Doses of ≥13.2 IU/kg prevented disease in 13 out of 13 (100%) paediatric close contacts [11]. Subsequent modelling by Young et al. estimated that to achieve protection in measles-naïve contacts, an intramuscular dose of 17.5 IU/kg measles-specific antibodies was required [43]. Thus, assuming a measles-specific antibody concentration of NHIG of 51 IU/mL, the current Australian dose of 0.2 mL/kg would under-dose measles-naïve contacts. The decreasing mean antibody levels of Australian blood donor populations forecast by our study and the observed decrease in potency of overseas NHIG products suggest that the measles antibody concentration of Australian NHIG will also fall in the future [16].

Multiple international bodies and national studies have recommended an increase in the dose of NHIG as measles PEP [19,20,43,44]. Unlike other countries, routine monitoring of measles-specific antibody concentrations in IG products is not required in Australia [1,22]. The downward trend in antibody levels demonstrated by our study supports the need for monitoring antibody levels in Australian donors and NHIG in the future.

Measures to increase the effectiveness of NHIG include the prioritisation of plasma from older donors, and potential prioritisation from female donors and/or those with a history of measles infection for fractionation. Existing Lifeblood policies mean that, in Australia, male plasma is used solely for direct transfusion, and therefore more female plasma is already directed to plasma for fractionation. Fortunately, because this strategy also works for other diseases for which NHIG-VF is indicated, such as hepatitis A and rubella, this is likely to have enabled Australian products to maintain their efficacy where other countries may not. If antibody levels fall in the future, measles-specific IG products or monoclonal antibodies could be explored, although the manufacture of disease-specific IG precludes the production of other IG from the same source plasma [45]. Revaccination of plasma donors by Modrof et al. showed an increase in measles-specific antibody levels at one month; however, after one year, the levels returned close to baseline [15].

This study has limitations. Firstly, due to the sampling approach, first-time apheresis donors were over-represented, and whole blood donors, who are preferentially recruited to provide NHIG, were excluded from the study. As plasma collection volumes increase, the yield of IgG may decrease. As whole blood donors donate less plasma, there may be more IgG per 100 mL. Whilst very frequent plasma donations may cause a decrease in IgG levels [46], the mean apheresis donation frequency in Australia is under four per annum. Additionally, study samples were collected pre-donation. Therefore, it is unlikely this would have significantly altered the findings. Secondly, younger birth cohorts from a post-measles elimination period were too young to be sampled by our study; therefore, we recommend repeating the study regularly in the future. Thirdly, we did not measure antibody levels in NHIG products from the time period.

PRNT is more sensitive for detecting measles-specific antibodies at lower antibody concentrations; therefore, it was possible that antibody levels below the positive cut-off (OD < 0.2) were underestimated by ELISA. PRNT is the gold standard for estimating measles immunity. However, when compared with ELISA, PRNT is technically demanding, expensive, and difficult to standardise between different laboratories [25,41,47,48]. PRNT detects only functional neutralising antibodies against specific proteins, while ELISA detects antibodies against all viral proteins; additionally, the neutralising antibodies measured by PRNT could belong to all classes of antibodies, while ELISA measures specific classes (IgG and/or IgM and/or IgA) [47].

Previous studies have used ELISA with duplicate testing of a subset of samples using PRNT and observed high agreement of IgG titres between ELISA and PRNT results [25,49], although ELISA values tend to be higher than those of PRNT [47,48]. Somewhat reassuringly in our study, 97% of specimens with "equivocal" ELISA were still above the correlate of protection (120 mIU/mL) on PRNT. This suggests that Australia may have more time before the mean population measles immunity falls below protective levels; however, the overall findings of our study support the need to monitor younger birth cohorts' immunity in the future. This finding is likely to be shared across countries that achieved interruption of endemic measles transmission before the births of their youngest donors, an effect of delaying concerted efforts to achieve global eradication of measles. Achieving measles eradication would remove the concern about decreasing measles-specific antibody levels.

## 5. Conclusions

Measles-specific antibody levels decreased significantly from older to younger Australian plasmapheresis donors. In the future, when blood donor cohorts targeted for NHIG production progressively include the youngest cohorts, this may impact the measles-specific antibody content of NHIG and jeopardise its effectiveness for passive immunisation against measles. Monitoring measles-specific antibody levels in future blood donor cohorts and NHIG products is recommended in Australia and other countries that eliminated measles before the birth of their youngest donors.

**Author Contributions:** Conceptualisation, D.N.D., H.F., S.N. and K.M.W.; methodology, H.F., S.N., D.N.D., K.M.W., T.M. and T.H.; specimen collection, H.F.; laboratory processing, analysis, and technical support, S.N. and V.S.; statistical analysis, K.M.W. and M.B.; data curation, H.F., S.N., V.H. and K.M.W.; writing—original draft preparation, K.M.W.; writing—review and editing, H.F., S.N., V.S., V.H., M.B., T.H., T.M. and D.N.D.; supervision, D.N.D., T.M. and T.H.; funding acquisition, D.N.D., H.F. and S.N. All authors have read and agreed to the published version of the manuscript.

**Funding:** This research was funded by the University of Newcastle post-graduate health protection research grant and in-kind support provided by the Australian Red Cross Lifeblood Service, Victorian Infectious Disease Reference Laboratory. The Australian Government funds the Australian Red Cross Lifeblood to provide blood, blood products, and services to the Australian community. K.M. Williamson undertook this study as part of the Australian National University Master of Philosophy in Applied Epidemiology (MAE) Program. The MAE Program is funded by Australian federal, state, and territory health departments.

**Institutional Review Board Statement:** This study was conducted in accordance with the National Statement on Ethical Conduct in Human Research (2007) under the *National Health and Medical Research Council Act* 1992. Ethics approval was obtained from the Australian Red Cross Lifeblood Ethics Committee (Ref No. 02102019, 14 October 2019) and the Australian National University Human Research Ethics Committee (Ref No. 2019/859, 31 October 2019). Samples provided by Australian blood donors can be used for ethically approved research studies with consent provided during the routine blood donation process.

**Informed Consent Statement:** Not applicable.

**Data Availability Statement:** Data may be made available through the corresponding authors to qualified and interested investigators upon reasonable request.

**Acknowledgments:** Australian governments fund Australian Red Cross Lifeblood to provide blood, blood products, and services to the Australian community. The authors gratefully acknowledge staff at the Australian Red Cross Lifeblood Service and Victorian Infectious Disease Reference Laboratory; particular thanks are due to Lina Rustanti and Chiara Carnevali for assisting with sample identification and stratification; Glen Shuttleworth for providing donor demographic data; Rianne Brizuela and Daniel Simons for performing the ELISA testing; and Macy Chirambo, Alma Redzic, and Kate Sharma for assisting with the PRNT. We also gratefully thank Paul Rota, Michael Catton, and Alice Richardson for their technical advice.

**Conflicts of Interest:** The authors declare no conflicts of interest.

## Appendix A

**Table A1.** Number and proportion of recovered serum specimens from plasmapheresis donors received by the Australian Red Cross Lifeblood Sydney processing centre in the month of November 2019 [Internal data, Lifeblood].

| (A) Age and Gender | | | | (B) State/Territory | |
|---|---|---|---|---|---|
| **Age Group** | **Gender** | **No. by Age & Gender** | **No. by Age (%)** | **State/Territory** | **No. (%)** |
| 18–29 years | Female<br>Male | 1954<br>1611 | 3565 (28.5%) | ACT | 636 (5.1%) |
| 30–39 years | Female<br>Male | 1351<br>1529 | 2880 (23.0%) | NSW<br>NT | 3237 (25.9%)<br>168 (1.3%) |
| 40–49 years | Female<br>Male | 1059<br>1158 | 2217 (17.7%) | QLD<br>SA | 2595 (20.8%)<br>1014 (8.1%) |
| 50–59 years | Female<br>Male | 900<br>1122 | 2022 (16.2%) | TAS<br>VIC | 451 (3.6%)<br>3079 (24.6%) |
| 60+ years | Female<br>Male | 749<br>1071 | 1820 (14.6%) | WA | 1324 (10.6%) |
| All Ages | Female<br>Male | 6013 (48.1%)<br>6491 (51.9%) | 12,504 (100%) | All States/Territories | 12,504 (100%) |

**Table A2.** Demographics of a subset of study population ($n$ = 149) that underwent measles-specific IgG antibody testing by ELISA and measles neutralising antibody testing by PRNT.

| | All Study Subjects | Subset of Subjects Who Underwent PRNT | | | | |
|---|---|---|---|---|---|---|
| | $n$ (%) | Total $n$ (%) | ELISA Negative $n$ (%) | ELISA Equivocal $n$ (%) | ELISA Low Positive $n$ (%) | ELISA Positive $n$ (%) |
| Total | 1199 | 149 (100) | 66 (100) | 63 (100) | 10 (100) | 10 (100) |
| Birth Year Cohort (Age) | | | | | | |
| 1940–1959 (60+ years) | 232 (19.4) | 7 (4.7) | 0 (0.0) | 0 (0.0) | 0 (0.0) | 7 (70.0) |
| 1960–1969 (50–59 years) | 239 (19.9) | 6 (4.0) | 2 (3.0) | 1 (1.6) | 0 (0.0) | 3 (30.0) |
| 1970–1979 (40–49 years) | 241 (20.1) | 30 (20.1) | 14 (21.2) | 14 (22.2) | 2 (20.0) | 0 (0.0) |
| 1980–1989 (30–39 years) | 242 (20.2) | 49 (32.9) | 20 (30.3) | 24 (38.1) | 5 (50.0) | 0 (0.0) |
| 1990–2001 (18–29 years) | 245 (20.4) | 57 (38.3) | 30 (45.5) | 24 (38.1) | 3 (30.0) | 0 (0.0) |
| Gender | | | | | | |
| Female | 565 (47.1) | 55 (36.9) | 17 (25.8) | 30 (47.6) | 3 (30.0) | 5 (50.0) |
| Male | 634 (52.9) | 94 (63.1) | 49 (74.2) | 33 (52.4) | 7 (70.0) | 5 (50.0) |

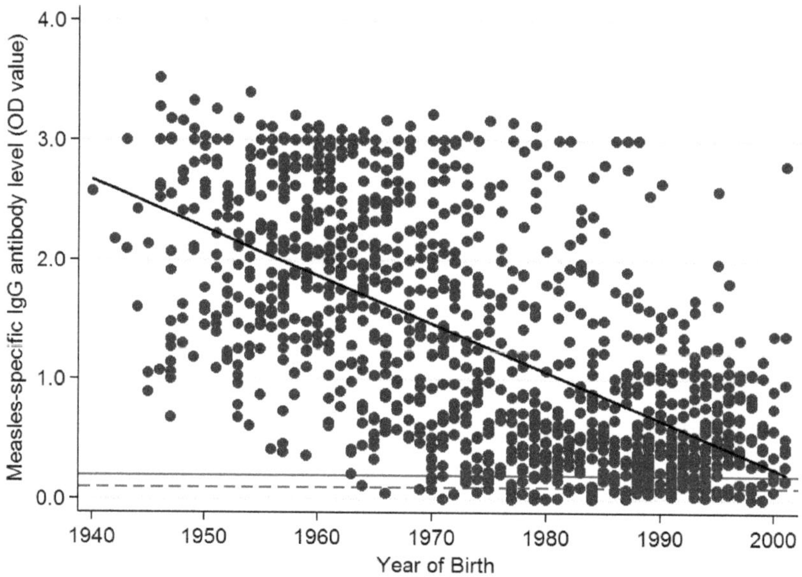


**Figure A1.** Measles-specific IgG antibody levels (optical density values) measured by ELISA, by year of birth in Australian plasmapheresis donors who donated from 29 October to 14 November 2019. The black line shows the line of best fit. The dark red line shows a positive cut-off for assay (OD = 0.2). OD values > 0.2 suggest immunity. The dark red dotted line shows an equivocal cut-off (OD = 0.1). OD values 0.1–0.2 are considered equivocal; OD values < 0.1 are negative and therefore considered non-immune.

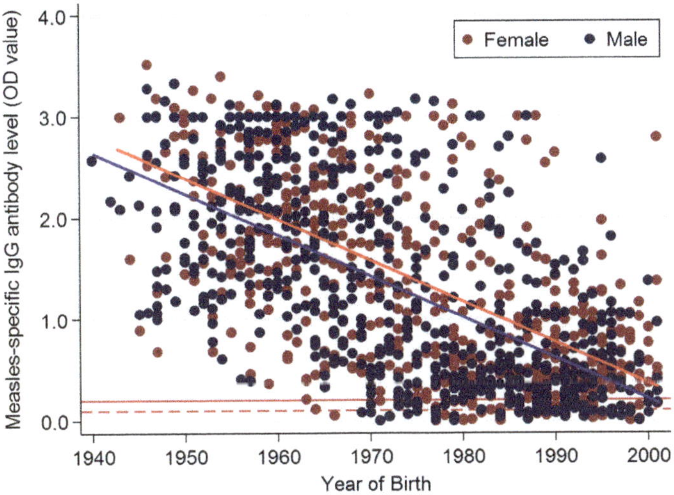


**Figure A2.** Measles-specific IgG antibody level (optical density values) measured by ELISA by year of birth in Australian plasmapheresis donors who donated from 29 October to 14 November 2019, by gender. Red dots represent female donors and the light red line indicates the line of best fit. Blue dots represent male donors and the blue line indicates the line of best fit. The dark red line shows a positive cut-off for assay (OD = 0.2). OD values > 0.2 suggest immunity. The dark red dotted line shows an equivocal cut-off (OD = 0.1). OD values 0.1–0.2 are considered equivocal; OD values < 0.1 are negative and therefore considered non-immune.

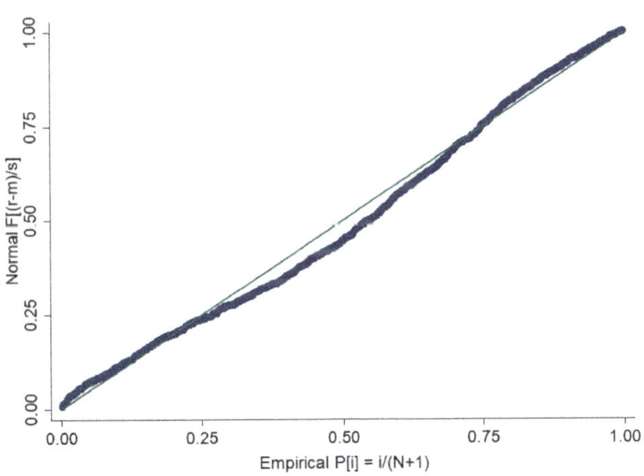


**(A)**

**Figure A3.** *Cont.*

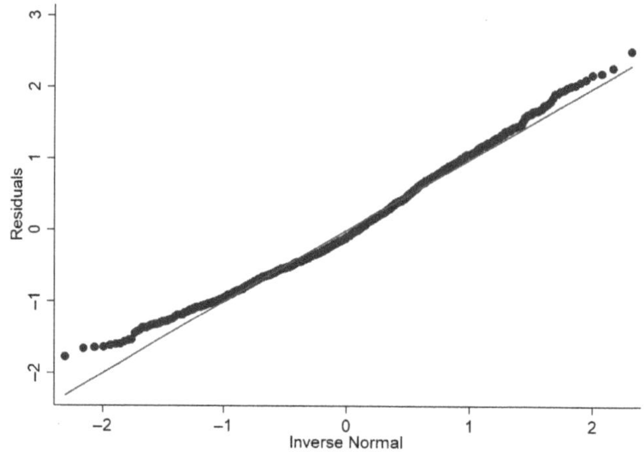


(B)

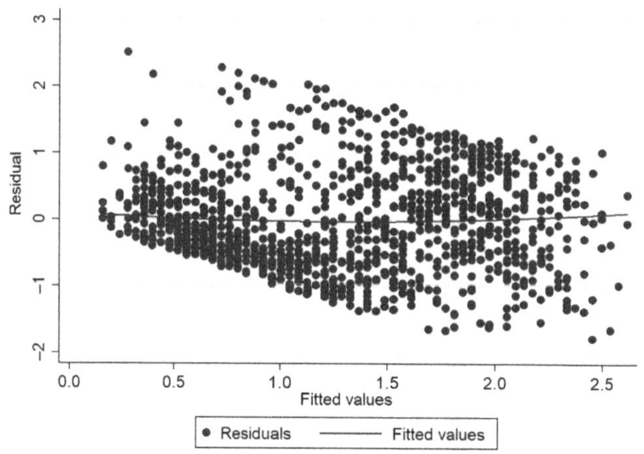


(C)

**Figure A3.** (**A**) P-P plot, (**B**) Q-Q plot, and (**C**) RVF plot of residuals following multiple linear regression analysis of OD value by birth year and gender.

**Appendix B. Estimation of Levels in Current and Future Australian Donor Populations**

Age-group-specific mean OD values obtained from this study were applied to the total Australian blood donation (whole blood and plasma) demographics for the year 2019 [internal data, Lifeblood], to estimate an age-adjusted mean antibody level for the total Australian blood donations in 2019 (see Appendix B Table A3). Estimation of the mean measles-specific antibody levels for future total Australian blood donations (whole blood plus plasma) in the years 2029 and 2039 were made using the following assumptions:

1. The distribution of whole blood and plasma donations across age groups in the future will be similar to that of the Australian donations in 2019.
2. The current age groups in this study and their corresponding age-specific mean antibody level will become the next consecutive age group and antibody level in ten years' time; that is, the current 30–39-year age group in 2019 with mean antibody level = X

will become the 40–49-year age group in 2029 whose mean antibody level = X, and the 50–59-year age group in 2039 whose mean antibody level = X.

3. There is no decay of antibody levels within donors as they age; that is, the mean antibody level = X for 30–39-year-olds in 2019 will become the mean antibody level = X for 40–49-year-olds in 2029 without any waning.
4. As the antibody levels of youngest donors (18–29-year-olds) in future cohorts cannot be predicted, the mean antibody level for 18–29-year-olds in 2019 is used for 18–29-year-olds in 2029 and 2039, acknowledging that this may be an overestimate.

**Table A3.** Total Australian blood donations (whole blood and plasma) by age group in 2019 [internal data, Lifeblood]. Age-specific mean measles IgG antibody levels in Australian blood donors in 2019 based on study results; estimated age-adjusted mean antibody levels for the total Australian blood donations in 2019; predicted age-adjusted mean antibody levels for total Australian blood donations in 2029 and 2039.

| Age Group (Years) | Number of Total Blood Donations (Plasma + Whole Blood) in 2019 | % | Mean Measles-Specific IgG Antibody Levels in 2019 [95% CI] | Estimated Mean Antibody Levels in 2029 * | Estimated Mean Antibody Levels in 2039 * |
|---|---|---|---|---|---|
| 18–29 | 327,130 | 22.14% | 0.58 [0.52–0.64] | 0.58 | 0.58 |
| 30–39 | 278,054 | 18.81% | 0.74 [0.65–0.83] | 0.58 | 0.58 |
| 40–49 | 258,875 | 17.52% | 1.18 [1.06–1.29] | 0.74 | 0.58 |
| 50–59 | 291,846 | 19.75% | 1.87 [1.76–1.97] | 1.18 | 0.74 |
| 60+ | 321,959 | 21.79% | 2.09 [2.00–2.18] | 1.87 | 1.18 |
| Total | 1,477,864 | 100.00% | | | |
| Age-adjusted mean antibody level for annual total Australian blood donations | | | 1.30 | 1.01 | 0.74 |

* Assumed that the current age groups in the study and their mean antibody level will become the next consecutive age group in 10 years (e.g., current 18–29-year-olds with a mean OD value of 0.58 will become the 30–39-year age group in 2029). Assumed antibody levels plateau in donors born after 1990 (which is unconfirmed); therefore, projected age-adjusted levels for 2029 and 2039 may be overestimated.

## References


1. Chiew, M.; Dey, A.; Martin, N.; Wang, H.; Davis, S.; McIntyre, P.B. Australian vaccine preventable disease epidemiological review series: Measles 2000–2011. *Commun. Dis. Intell.* **2015**, *39*, E1–E9.
2. Viana, P.O.; Ono, E.; Miyamoto, M.; Salomao, R.; Costa-Carvalho, B.T.; Weckx, L.Y.; de Moraes-Pinto, M.I. Humoral and cellular immune responses to measles and tetanus: The importance of elapsed time since last exposure and the nature of the antigen. *J. Clin. Immunol.* **2010**, *30*, 574–582. [CrossRef] [PubMed]
3. Davidkin, I.; Jokinen, S.; Broman, M.; Leinikki, P.; Peltola, H. Persistence of measles, mumps, and rubella antibodies in an MMR-vaccinated cohort: A 20-year follow-up. *J. Infect. Dis.* **2008**, *197*, 950–956. [CrossRef]
4. Waaijenborg, S.; Hahné, S.J.M.; Mollema, L.; Smits, G.P.; Berbers, G.A.M.; van der Klis, F.R.M.; de Melker, H.E.; Wallinga, J. Waning of maternal antibodies against measles, mumps, rubella, and varicella in communities with contrasting vaccination coverage. *J. Infect. Dis.* **2013**, *208*, 10–16. [CrossRef] [PubMed]
5. Australian Technical Advisory Group on Immunisation. *Australian Immunisation Handbook*; Australian Government Department of Health: Canberra, ACT, Australia, 2018.
6. Communicable Diseases Network Australia. *National Guidelines for Public Health Units: Measles*; Communicable Diseases Network Australia: Canberra, ACT, Australia, 2019. Available online: https://www1.health.gov.au/internet/main/publishing.nsf/Content/cdna-song-measles.htm (accessed on 17 December 2019).
7. CSL Behring. *Australian Product Information—Normal Immunoglobulin-VF (Human Normal Immunoglobulin)*; CSL Behring: Broadmeadows, VIC, Australia, 2020.
8. Keller, M.A.; Stiehm, E.R. Passive immunity in prevention and treatment of infectious diseases. *Clin. Microbiol. Rev.* **2000**, *13*, 602–614. [CrossRef]
9. National Blood Authority Australia. *Annual Report 2017–2018*; National Blood Authority Australia: Lyneham, ACT, Australia, 2018.
10. Australian Red Cross Lifeblood. How Does Age Affect My Ability to Donate? 2020. Available online: https://www.donateblood.com.au/faq/age (accessed on 16 September 2020).
11. Endo, A.; Izumi, H.; Miyashita, M.; Taniguchi, K.; Okubo, O.; Harada, K. Current efficacy of post exposure prophylaxis against measles with immunoglobulin. *J. Pediatr.* **2001**, *138*, 926–928. [CrossRef] [PubMed]

12. Young, M.K.; Cripps, A.W.; Nimmo, G.R. The use of normal human immunoglobulin (NHIG) for public health purposes in Queensland 2004–2014 and Australia 2014–2016. *Commun. Dis. Intell.* **2019**, *43*. [CrossRef]
13. Young, M.K.; Nimmo, G.R.; Cripps, A.W.; Jones, M.A. Post-exposure passive immunisation for preventing measles. In *Cochrane Database of Systematic Reviews*; John Wiley & Sons, Inc.: Hoboken, NJ, USA, 2014.
14. Simon, T.L.; FitzGerald, P.; Kühne, M.; Farrar, C.; Knowles, J.; Bycholski, K.; Zenker, O. Longitudinal changes in measles antibody titers in plasma donors and minimum antibody levels of immunoglobulin products for treatment of primary immunodeficiency. *Transfusion* **2018**, *58* (Suppl. S3), 3065–3071. [CrossRef]
15. Modrof, J.; Tille, B.; Farcet, M.R.; McVey, J.; Schreiner, J.A.; Borders, C.M.; Gudino, M.; Fitzgerald, P.; Simon, T.L.; Kreil, T.R. Measles virus neutralizing antibodies in intravenous immunoglobulins: Is an increase by revaccination of plasma donors possible? *J. Infect. Dis.* **2017**, *216*, 977–980. [CrossRef]
16. Audet, S.; Virata-Theimer, M.L.; Beeler, J.A.; Scott, D.E.; Frazier, D.J.; Mikolajczyk, M.G.; Eller, N.; Chen, F.; Yu, M.Y.W. Measles-Virus–Neutralizing Antibodies in Intravenous Immunoglobulins. *J. Infect. Dis.* **2006**, *194*, 781–789. [CrossRef]
17. Sinden, J. *Post Exposure Prophylaxis for Measles*; New Zealand Blood Service: Auckland, New Zealand, 2012.
18. Matysiak-Klose, D.; Santibanez, S.; Schwerdtfeger, C.; Koch, J.; von Bernuth, H.; Hengel, H.; Littmann, M.; Terhardt, M.; Wicker, S.; Mankertz, A.; et al. Post-exposure prophylaxis for measles with immunoglobulins revised recommendations of the standing committee on vaccination in Germany. *Vaccine* **2018**, *36*, 7916–7922. [CrossRef] [PubMed]
19. Ramsay, M.; Manikkavasagan, G.; Brown, K.; Craig, L. *Post Exposure Prophylaxis for Measles: Revised Guidance*; Health Protection Agency: London, UK, 2009.
20. Tunis, M.C.; Salvadori, M.I.; Dubey, V.; Baclic, O.; National Advisory Committee on Immunization. Updated NACI recommendations for measles post-exposure prophylaxis. *Can. Commun. Dis. Rep.* **2018**, *44*, 226–230. [CrossRef] [PubMed]
21. McLean, H.Q.; Fiebelkorn, A.P.; Temte, J.L.; Wallace, G.S.; Centers for Disease Control & Prevention. Prevention of measles, rubella, congenital rubella syndrome, and mumps, 2013: Summary recommendations of the Advisory Committee on Immunization Practices (ACIP). In *Morbidity and Mortality Weekly Report (MMWR)*; Centers for Disease Control and Prevention: Atlanta, GA, USA, 2013; Volume 62, pp. 1–34.
22. US Food and Drug Administration. *Code of Federal Regulations Title 21, Volume 7, Part 640, Subpart J, Section 640.104: Additional Standards for Human Blood and Blood Products, Immune Globulin (Human), Potency*; US Food and Drug Administration: Silver Spring, MD, USA, 2019.
23. Hajian-Tilaki, K. Sample size estimation in epidemiologic studies. *Caspian J. Intern. Med.* **2011**, *2*, 289–298. [PubMed]
24. Kirby Institute; UNSW Sydney; Australian Red Cross Lifeblood. *Transfusion-Transmissible Infections in Australia: 2019 Surveillance Report*; Kirby Institute: Kensington, NSW, Australia, 2019.
25. Cohen, B.J.; Doblas, D.; Andrews, N. Comparison of plaque reduction neutralisation test (PRNT) and measles virus-specific IgG ELISA for assessing immunogenicity of measles vaccination. *Vaccine* **2008**, *26*, 6392–6397. [CrossRef] [PubMed]
26. Cohen, B.; Parry, R.; Doblas, D.; Samuel, D.; Warrener, L.; Andrews, N.; Brown, D. Measles immunity testing: Comparison of two measles IgG ELISAs with plaque reduction neutralisation assay. *J. Virol. Methods* **2006**, *131*, 209–212. [CrossRef] [PubMed]
27. Ratnam, S.; Gadag, V.; West, R.; Burris, J.; Oates, E.; Stead, F.; Bouilianne, N. Comparison of commercial enzyme immunoassay kits with plaque reduction neutralization test for detection of measles virus antibody. *J. Clin. Microbiol.* **1995**, *33*, 811–815. [CrossRef]
28. Tischer, A.; Andrews, N.; Kafatos, G.; Nardone, A.; Berbers, G.; Davidkin, I.; Aboudy, Y.; Backhouse, J.; Barbara, C.; Miller, E.; et al. Standardization of measles, mumps and rubella assays to enable comparisons of seroprevalence data across 21 European countries and Australia. *Epidemiol. Infect.* **2007**, *135*, 787–797. [CrossRef] [PubMed]
29. Tischer, A.; Gassner, M.; Richard, J.L.; Suter-Riniker, F.; Mankertz, A.; Heininger, U. Vaccinated students with negative enzyme immunoassay results show positive measles virus-specific antibody levels by immunofluorescence and plaque neutralisation tests. *J. Clin. Virol.* **2007**, *38*, 204–209. [CrossRef] [PubMed]
30. Chen, R.T.; Markowitz, L.E.; Albrecht, P.; Stewart, J.A.; Mofenson, L.M.; Preblud, S.R.; Orenstein, W.A. Measles antibody: Reevaluation of protective titers. *J. Infect. Dis.* **1990**, *162*, 1036–1042. [CrossRef]
31. Cohen, B.J.; Audet, S.; Andrews, N.; Beeler, J.; WHO Working Group on Measles Plaque Reduction Neutralization Test. Plaque reduction neutralization test for measles antibodies: Description of a standardised laboratory method for use in immunogenicity studies of aerosol vaccination. *Vaccine* **2007**, *26*, 59–66. [CrossRef]
32. Albrecht, P.; Herrmann, K.; Burns, G.R. Role of virus strain in conventional and enhanced measles plaque neutralization test. *J. Virol. Methods* **1981**, *3*, 251–260. [CrossRef] [PubMed]
33. Pennsylvania State University. STAT 500 Applied Statistics: 10.2.1.—ANOVA Assumptions. 2022. Available online: https://online.stat.psu.edu/stat500/lesson/10/10.2/10.2.1 (accessed on 23 February 2022).
34. Sullivan, M. *Fundamentals of Statistics*; Pearson Prentice Hall: London, UK, 2011.
35. National Centre for Immunisation Research and Surveillance. Significant Events in Measles, Mumps and Rubella Vaccination Practice in Australia. *December 2019*. Available online: http://ncirs.org.au/sites/default/files/2019-12/Measles-mumps-rubella-history-Dec%202019.pdf (accessed on 28 April 2020).
36. Australian Government Department of Health. Measles—Elimination Achieved in Australia. 20 March 2014. Available online: https://www1.health.gov.au/internet/main/publishing.nsf/Content/ohp-measles-elim-announce-2014.htm (accessed on 2 August 2020).

37. Gidding, H.F.; Martin, N.V.; Stambos, V.; Tran, T.; Dey, A.; Dowse, G.K.; Kelly, H.A.; Durrheim, D.N.; Lambert, S.B. Verification of measles elimination in Australia: Application of World Health Organization regional guidelines. *J. Epidemiol. Glob. Health* **2016**, *6*, 197–209. [CrossRef] [PubMed]
38. Edirisuriya, C.; Beard, F.H.; Hendry, A.J.; Dey, A.; Gidding, H.F.; Hueston, L.; Dwyer, D.E.; Wood, J.G.; Macartney, K.K.; McIntyre, P.B. Australian rubella serosurvey 2012–2013: On track for elimination? *Vaccine* **2018**, *36*, 2794–2798. [CrossRef] [PubMed]
39. Klein, S.L.; Marriott, I.; Fish, E.N. Sex-based differences in immune function and responses to vaccination. *Trans. R. Soc. Trop. Med. Hyg.* **2015**, *109*, 9–15. [CrossRef]
40. Fischinger, S.; Boudreau, C.M.; Butler, A.L.; Streeck, H.; Alter, G. Sex differences in vaccine-induced humoral immunity. *Semin. Immunopathol.* **2019**, *41*, 239–249. [CrossRef] [PubMed]
41. Mossong, J.; O'Callaghan, C.J.; Ratnam, S. Modelling antibody response to measles vaccine and subsequent waning of immunity in a low exposure population. *Vaccine* **2000**, *19*, 523–529. [CrossRef] [PubMed]
42. Young, M.K.; Bertolini, J.; Kotharu, P.; Maher, D.; Cripps, A.W. Do Australian immunoglobulin products meet international measles antibody titre standards? *Hum. Vaccines Immunother.* **2017**, *13*, 607–612. [CrossRef] [PubMed]
43. Young, M.K.; Ng, S.K.; Nimmo, G.R.; Cripps, A.W. The optimal dose of disease-specific antibodies for post-exposure prophylaxis of measles and rubella in Australia: New guidelines recommended. *Expert Opin. Drug Metab. Toxicol.* **2018**, *14*, 663–669. [CrossRef]
44. Public Health England. *Guidelines on Post-Exposure Prophylaxis for Measles June 2019*; Wellington House: London, UK, 2019.
45. Galardi, D.A.; Herson, N. Pricing of blood products. *Am. J. Health-Syst. Pharm.* **2000**, *57*, 2061. [CrossRef]
46. Hoad, V.C.; Castrén, J.; Norda, R.; Pink, J. A donor safety evidence literature review of the short- and long-term effects of plasmapheresis. *Vox Sang.* **2024**, *119*, 94–101. [CrossRef] [PubMed]
47. Siennicka, J.; Czescik, A.; Trzcinska, A. The significance for epidemiological studies anti-measles antibody detection examined by enzyme immunoassay (EIA) and plaque reduction neutralization test (PRNT). *Prz. Epidemiol.* **2014**, *68*, 417–420, 527–529.
48. Terletskaia-Ladwig, E.; Enders, G.; Meier, S.; Dietz, K.; Enders, M. Development and evaluation of an automatable focus reduction neutralisation test for the detection of measles virus antibodies using imaging analysis. *J. Virol. Methods* **2011**, *178*, 124–128. [CrossRef] [PubMed]
49. Kang, H.J.; Han, Y.W.; Kim, S.J.; Kim, Y.-J.; Kim, A.-R.; Kim, J.A.; Jung, H.-D.; Eom, H.E.; Park, O.; Kim, S.S. An increasing, potentially measles-susceptible population over time after vaccination in Korea. *Vaccine* **2017**, *35*, 4126–4132. [CrossRef] [PubMed]

*vaccines*

MDPI

*Review*

# A World without Measles and Rubella: Addressing the Challenge of Vaccine Hesitancy

**David M. Higgins and Sean T. O'Leary ***

Adult and Child Center for Outcomes Research and Delivery Science (ACCORDS), Children's Hospital Colorado, University of Colorado School of Medicine, Aurora, CO 80045, USA; david.higgins@cuanschutz.edu
* Correspondence: sean.oleary@cuanschutz.edu; Tel.:+1-303-724-1582

**Abstract:** The worldwide elimination of measles and rubella is feasible, but not without overcoming the substantial challenge of vaccine hesitancy. This challenge is complicated by the spread of misinformation and disinformation fueled by rapidly progressing technologies and evolving forms of online communication. The recent COVID-19 pandemic has only added further complexity to this challenge. However, considerable progress has been made in understanding the scope of the problem and the complex factors that influence vaccine hesitancy. Our understanding of evidence-based strategies for addressing vaccine hesitancy has grown significantly, including evidence for effective communication and behavioral interventions. In this article, we review measles and rubella vaccines and vaccine hesitancy. We then provide an overview of evidence-based strategies for addressing vaccine hesitancy, including communication strategies and behavioral interventions. This article is relevant to healthcare professionals, health system leaders, public health professionals, policymakers, community leaders, and any individuals who have a role in addressing vaccine hesitancy in their communities. Finally, we review future directions and major areas of research need.

**Keywords:** vaccination; vaccine hesitancy; vaccine delay; vaccine refusal; measles; rubella

## 1. Introduction

The measles and rubella viruses continue to cause over 9 million cases of disease and 136,000 deaths worldwide every year despite the availability of effective, safe, and inexpensive vaccines for over half a century [1]. As obligate human pathogens, eradicating measles and rubella worldwide is technically feasible. However, despite all six World Health Organization regions committing to elimination, no region has achieved and maintained elimination. Disruptions to vaccination programs during the coronavirus-19 (COVID-19) pandemic resulted in significant setbacks to measles and rubella elimination efforts, which have yet to be reversed [1].

Efforts to eradicate measles and rubella from the world must address the substantial challenge of vaccine hesitancy to be successful. Vaccine hesitancy, defined by the WHO as a "delay in acceptance or refusal of vaccines despite availability of vaccination services", can lead to measles and rubella vaccine delay or refusal, which undermines elimination efforts [2,3]. Factors influencing vaccine hesitancy are complex and involve historical, socio-cultural, environmental, institutional, economic, political, and individual/group factors [2]. These factors are further influenced by rapidly changing technologies that allow for the rapid and ubiquitous spread of information, misinformation, and disinformation. Fortunately, since vaccine hesitancy has been around since the development of vaccines, there is a long history of experience and evidence to inform efforts to address vaccine hesitancy.

In this article, we review the history and current state of measles and rubella vaccine hesitancy. We then provide an overview of evidence-based strategies for addressing vaccine hesitancy, including communication strategies and behavioral interventions that can be implemented within systems and organizations. These strategies are relevant to healthcare providers, health system leaders, public health professionals, policymakers, community leaders, and any individuals who have a role in addressing vaccine hesitancy in their communities. Finally, we review future directions and major areas of need for research.

With effective, safe, and inexpensive vaccines, every illness, complication, or death from measles and rubella is unacceptable. Using evidence-based strategies to address vaccine hesitancy and a re-commitment worldwide to improve vaccine uptake, measles and rubella can be eradicated.

## 2. History of Measles and Rubella Disease and Vaccination

Before the development and widespread availability of vaccines in the late 20th century, measles and rubella plagued humanity for thousands of years, with no effective tools to prevent their consequences [4,5]. Measles disease was first described in the 7th century, although the infectious pathogen would not be identified until the early 20th century [5]. Measles is a highly contagious viral disease that classically begins with a prodrome of fever, cough, coryza, conjunctivitis, and spots on the buccal mucosa (Koplik spots), followed by a maculopapular rash which starts on the head and neck and spreads to the rest of the body [6]. While some individuals have a resolution of these symptoms, many will develop complications, including diarrhea, otitis media, pneumonia, encephalitis, subacute sclerosing panencephalitis, or death. Rubella was initially thought to be a variant of measles but was first identified as a separate disease in 1814 [4]. Rubella is a viral disease that begins with a prodrome of mild fever, malaise, lymphadenopathy, and upper respiratory symptoms before the appearance of a maculopapular rash [6]. While complications of rubella are rare in many individuals, for pregnant persons, rubella infection can lead to congenital rubella syndrome (CRS), which can result in miscarriages, stillbirths, and severe birth defects in infants [6].

For centuries, measles and rubella have caused significant public health burdens worldwide. Measles is estimated to have caused greater than 2–3 million deaths worldwide every year before the availability of vaccines [5]. While precise historical estimates of the public health burden of rubella are lacking, during the last major rubella epidemic in the United States in 1964–1965, there were an estimated 12.5 million rubella cases with 30,000 affected pregnancies leading to 6250 spontaneous abortions and 2100 newborns who died at or shortly after birth [4]. Another 20,000 children were born with CRS, resulting in approximately 11,600 infants who were deaf, 3580 who were blind, and 1800 who were mentally disabled.

Scientific advancements in the 18th, 19th, and 20th centuries culminated in the successful development of safe and effective vaccines against both measles and rubella [4,5]. Two measles vaccines (an inactivated and live attenuated vaccine) were developed and licensed in the United States in 1963 [5]. The inactivated vaccine was later withdrawn due to poor effectiveness. Over the next five years, further attenuated live measles vaccines were developed and licensed, showing improved side-effect profiles over the originally licensed live attenuated vaccine [5]. Four rubella vaccines were developed and licensed in the United States and Europe during the 1960s–1970s [4]. Eventually, one rubella vaccine became the predominant vaccine licensed and available worldwide due to superior effectiveness and a preferable side-effect profile. In 1971, the measles and rubella vaccines were licensed as a combined measles, mumps, and rubella (MMR) vaccine [5]. Later, in 2005, the combined measles, mumps, rubella, and varicella (MMRV) vaccine was licensed [5].

Aside from clean water, vaccines arguably reduced more diseases and deaths worldwide than any other public health achievement in human history, and measles and rubella vaccines are important contributors to this accomplishment [7]. With the widespread availability of measles and rubella vaccines and improvements in worldwide vaccination rates in the early 21st century, significant progress has been made toward eliminating measles and rubella [1]. From 2000 to 2022, the measles vaccine alone is estimated to have prevented 57 million deaths worldwide [1]. By 2022, 51% of the world's countries had eliminated rubella disease [8].

Despite the incredible success of measles and rubella vaccination programs worldwide, these diseases remain a significant public health threat. It is estimated that measles caused 136,200 deaths worldwide in 2022, and rubella caused an estimated 32,000 cases of CRS in 2019 [1,9]. Gains in worldwide measles and rubella vaccination experienced significant setbacks during the COVID-19 pandemic, which have yet to recover [1,8]. The setbacks experienced during the COVID-19 pandemic are due to various factors, including major disruptions in measles and rubella vaccination programs and changes in attitudinal barriers to vaccination, including vaccine hesitancy. With widely available, effective, low-cost vaccines, the eradication of measles and rubella is technically feasible, but first, the challenge of vaccine hesitancy must be considered and addressed.

## 3. History and Current State of Measles and Rubella Vaccine Hesitancy

### *3.1. Brief History of Measles and Rubella Vaccine Misinformation and Antivaccine Activism*

Vaccine hesitancy is primarily fueled by antivaccine activism, which has a history as long as vaccines themselves (Figure 1). Shortly after the introduction and use of the smallpox vaccine in the late 18th and early 19th centuries, opposition to vaccination was first led, in part, by medical professionals on the fringes of the medical and health professions [2]. This opposition to smallpox vaccination led to dropping vaccination rates, the resurgence of smallpox outbreaks, and the establishment of compulsory vaccination laws in the 19th century [2]. These laws differed from modern mandatory vaccination laws, which impose penalties for not vaccinating, as compulsory vaccination meant individuals had no choice in whether they received a vaccine. In response to enacting these compulsory vaccine laws, the antivaccine movement capitalized on perceived violations of personal freedoms, a tactic still used today, and successfully repealed some compulsory smallpox vaccination laws [2].

The middle of the 20th century saw a relative lull in the antivaccine movement, with improvements in the manufacture and delivery of vaccines and public health infrastructure [2]. However, in the 1970s and 1980s, the antivaccine movement again gained traction with the spread of both misinformation and disinformation about whole-cell pertussis vaccines and the establishment of several antivaccine organizations by antivaccine activists in the U.S., Australia, and Europe [2]. Misinformation is defined as false information that is shared by people who do not realize it is false and do not mean any harm, whereas disinformation is false information that is spread with malicious intent [10].

Within the context of this revitalized antivaccine movement came arguably the most damaging modern-day antivaccine misinformation incident. In 1998, Andrew Wakefield, a since-discredited British physician, published an article in the Lancet suggesting a link between the MMR vaccine and autism in 12 children [11]. This article was later found to be false and fraudulent [12]. The journal eventually retracted this now-infamous article. Andrew Wakefield was stripped of his license to practice medicine, and many large studies have confirmed there is no causal link between MMR and autism; the damage from this fraudulent article was already done [12]. The article received widespread media attention, and antivaccine activists jumped at the opportunity to add this misinformation to their reasons for vaccine opposition [13]. The fallout from this incident resulted in significant declines in MMR vaccination and inestimable preventable harm around the world.

Complicating the MMR and autism myth during the 1990s were concerns about the safety of thimerosal, a mercury-based preservative used in some vaccines [13]. Although there was no evidence that the dose of thimerosal in vaccines causes significant harm, in 1999, the U.S. Public Health Service agencies, the American Academy of Pediatrics, and vaccine manufacturers agreed to reduce or eliminate the use of thimerosal in vaccines [14,15]. While this action in the U.S. was taken as a precautionary measure, it sent mixed messages to the public about the safety of vaccines and added to antivaccine controversies. In the U.S., thimerosal was removed from all vaccines by 2001, except multi-dose influenza vaccine vials [14]. It is still used throughout the world with no evidence of harm.

Throughout the start of the 21st century, the spread of vaccine misinformation, disinformation, and antivaccine activism has been fueled by rapidly progressing technologies and evolving forms of online communication. In 2002, researchers studied online antivaccination information and concluded, "There is a high probability that parents will encounter elaborate antivaccination material on the world wide web. Factual refutational strategies alone are unlikely to counter the highly rhetorical appeals that shape these sites" [16]. Since then, with advancements in online technology and the explosion of social media use, vaccine misinformation and disinformation have spread rapidly. As Larson et al. noted in an editorial in 2022, "The role of social media in fueling the spread of vaccine hesitancy and its increasingly documented health consequences cannot be overstated" [17].

Although antivaccine sentiments and vaccine hesitancy have been studied and reported on most frequently in the US, similar patterns have taken shape worldwide, including in low- and middle-income countries (LMICs) [2,18]. Using data from 290 surveys conducted between 2015 and 2019 across 149 countries, researchers found varying determinants of vaccine hesitancy between countries, including perceptions of the importance, safety, and effectiveness of vaccines and changes in vaccine confidence over time [18]. Ultimately, the rising global threat of antivaccine sentiments and vaccine misinformation contributed to the WHO classifying vaccine hesitancy as a top ten global health threat in 2019 [19].

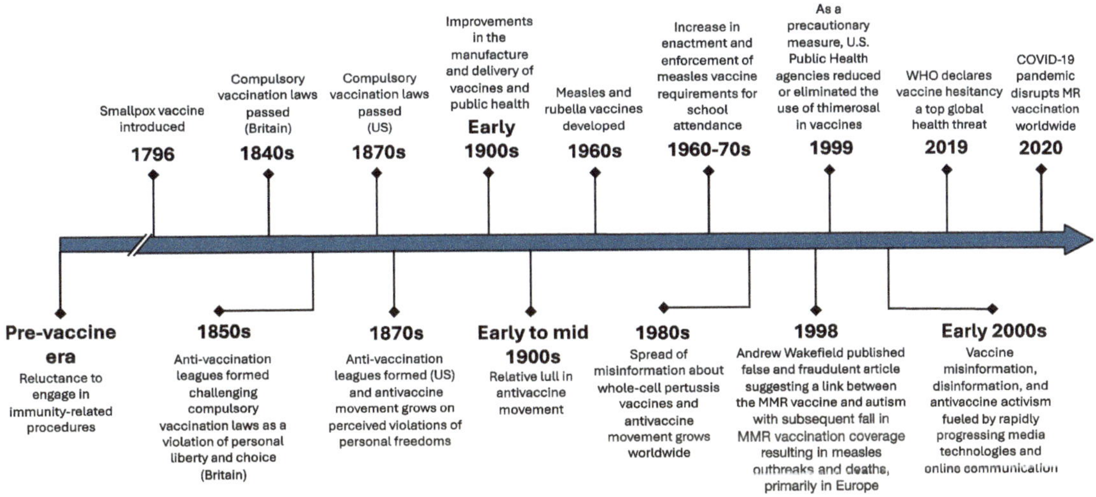


**Figure 1.** Timeline of significant events in vaccine hesitancy [2,20].

### 3.2. *Definitions of Vaccine Hesitancy, Confidence, Acceptance, and Refusal*

The clarity of terms when considering vaccine hesitancy is critical. Mixing terms or unclear definitions may add to confusion about vaccine attitudes and intentions and undermine attempts to communicate productively on these topics, especially when terms are used in public discourse [21,22]. There must also be an appreciation that terms such as vaccine hesitancy occur on a spectrum of attitudes and intentions, which is challenging to define. Attempts to have productive discussions about vaccine hesitancy should clarify terminology before use and recognize the common and practical uses and public perception of terms.

While many definitions for vaccine hesitancy have been proposed or reported in the literature, the WHO Strategic Advisory Group of Experts (SAGE) working group on vaccine hesitancy defined vaccine hesitancy as "... delay in acceptance or refusal of vaccination despite the availability of vaccination services. Vaccine hesitancy is complex and context-specific, varying across time, place, and vaccines. It is influenced by factors such as complacency, convenience, and confidence [3]". As Bedford et al. point out, due to its wide use in public discourse, the term vaccine hesitancy may incorrectly be assumed to be a behavior when it is a psychological state that influences behavior or inaccurately used to explain all undervaccination in a population when other causes may be responsible, such as access barriers [22].

According to the WHO SAGE working group on vaccine hesitancy, vaccine confidence refers to vaccine safety and efficacy, the healthcare workers delivering vaccines, and those making decisions regarding vaccine approval in a population [2,3]. Other definitions of vaccine confidence include confidence in the processes and policies that lead to vaccine development, licensure, manufacturing, and use recommendations [23]. Vaccine acceptance has been described as "the degree to which individuals accept, question or refuse vaccination [24]", and vaccine refusal as an "unwillingness to allow oneself or family member to be immunized against a preventable contagious disease [2]". Other descriptions of vaccine acceptance and refusal have been proposed [2].

### 3.3. *Common Determinants of Vaccine Hesitancy*

The WHO categorized the determinants of vaccine hesitancy into a framework that includes three major categories: (1) contextual influences, (2) individual and group influences, and (3) issues related directly to a vaccine or vaccination [3]. The contextual influences include the media environment, leaders and anti- or pro-vaccine figures, historical perspectives, and religious, cultural, socio-economic, political, or geographic influences. Individual and group factors include personal, family, or community experiences with vaccination, general beliefs and attitudes about health and prevention, knowledge and awareness about vaccination, trust in health systems and professionals, perceived risks/benefits of vaccines, and social norms. Issues related directly to a vaccine or vaccination include the scientific evidence, introduction of new vaccines, the mode of administration, type of vaccination program, vaccine schedule, costs, and the knowledge, attitudes, and strength of recommendation of healthcare professionals.

These determinants of vaccine hesitancy can negatively or positively influence vaccine attitudes. Also, for each individual or community, multiple determinants work in complex ways to influence attitudes and intentions around vaccines. For example, media may be a source of widespread vaccine misinformation, but it also can be used to communicate important information regarding vaccination. Synergistically, either anti- or pro-vaccine leaders may use media or other contextual factors to enhance the influence of these determinants. Furthermore, the clustering of religious, cultural, and individual or group factors can create communities with unique vaccine hesitancy determinants influencing their attitudes and intentions. Therefore, any evaluation of the determinants of vaccine hesitancy in a population or individual should consider the broad range of factors that contribute to attitudes and intentions. Assuming a community is influenced by only one of these determinants alone may prevent the optimal use of strategies to address vaccine hesitancy.

### 3.4. *Measurement of Vaccine Hesitancy*

Vaccine hesitancy falls on a spectrum of vaccine attitudes and intentions. Several typologies of parental vaccine hesitancy have been described [2,25–27]. These vaccine hesitancy typologies generally span from those who recognize the importance of vaccines and accept all vaccines on one end of the spectrum to those who refuse all vaccines, often have mistrust in the medical system, or have other strong religious or personal beliefs, and their beliefs about vaccines are fixed [27]. These typologies help to describe general observations about the spectrum of vaccine hesitancy and can be used as a tool for tailoring vaccine communication; however, they do not entirely describe the heterogeneity found within the spectrum of vaccine hesitancy. Also, these typologies may evolve and must be adapted for different population contexts. Additionally, these typologies are not unique to measles and rubella vaccines. Furthermore, if these typologies are inappropriately used to mislabel individuals, this may inhibit honest and respectful communication.

Multiple vaccine hesitancy and confidence measures have been developed, and some of them validated, to describe where individuals are on the spectrum of vaccine hesitancy attitudes and intentions [2]. Some of the most commonly used and validated measures include the Parent Attitudes about Childhood Vaccines (PACV) [28], Vaccine Confidence Scale (VCS) [29], Vaccine Hesitancy Scale (VHS) [30], 5C Antecedents of Vaccine Acceptance (5C) [31], and Caregiver Vaccination Attitudes Scale (CVAS) [32]. It is important to note that these scales have limited validation studies except for the PACV and VCS [2]. Also, most of these measures were developed in high-income countries (HIC), and their utility in other populations has yet to be validated. Additionally, it is worth noting that these tools are not specific to measles or rubella vaccines. While an adaptation of the VHS survey tool for measuring measles vaccine confidence was used (aMVHS), it was limited in predicting a child's measles vaccination status [33].

In general, these vaccine hesitancy measurement tools use at least several questions to measure some combination of constructs, including belief in the importance of vaccines, trust in vaccines and the professionals and processes that approve and recommend vaccines, perceived safety of vaccines, perceived risks of infectious diseases, and responsibility to the greater community [2]. Most of these measures' conceptual basis is grounded in the Health Belief Model, where individuals' vaccination behaviors are influenced by their perceptions of the vaccine and vaccine-preventable disease [34]. Unfortunately, most vaccine hesitancy measurement tools have limited psychometric validation and replication to ensure they measure what they are designed to measure [2]. Further studies validating these tools in different populations and correlating measurements with actual vaccination behavior are warranted, and caution should be used in interpreting these measurements.

Finally, the measurement of vaccine hesitancy at the population level is often reported by polling with methodologies that may or may not have been validated and are not always transparent [35–37]. These polls still have value in informing trends in vaccine hesitancy but are often misinterpreted by the media or the general public to reflect something they may not have measured. For instance, a poll asking a single question about support for vaccine requirements to attend school may be misinterpreted as reflecting the full spectrum of vaccine hesitancy attitudes in a population. Unfortunately, until validated vaccine hesitancy measures are more consistently applied and used, policymakers and health professionals are left with these data types to monitor vaccine hesitancy, guide policy, appropriately target populations with vaccine hesitancy interventions, and inform policy.

### *3.5. Epidemiology of Measles and Rubella Vaccine Hesitancy*

A precise understanding of the epidemiology of measles and rubella vaccine hesitancy is inhibited by using different and sometimes unvalidated measurement tools, as described above, which are implemented inconsistently across populations and time. Additionally, vaccine hesitancy may vary by type of vaccination, and validated measures specific to measles and rubella vaccines are lacking and have not been widely used. Furthermore, since vaccine hesitancy is on a spectrum, classifying individuals as having vaccine hesitancy for epidemiologic assessment is challenging and varies between methodologies and measures. For these reasons, many countries or jurisdictions rely on vaccine uptake alone to estimate vaccine hesitancy in populations. However, these data cannot differentiate between attitudinal, behavioral, and access causes for undervaccination [2]. In response to these shortcomings, experts have called for standardized, timely, and actionable surveillance systems for vaccine hesitancy [38–40].

Despite these limitations, some epidemiologic data about the prevalence of vaccine hesitancy are critical to understand. U.S. studies have consistently shown that the proportion of parents with vaccine hesitancy leading to the outright refusal of all vaccines for their children is small (1–3%) [26,27,41,42]. These data suggest that the proportion of individuals with absolute fixed beliefs is small, and a majority fall somewhere on the vaccine hesitancy spectrum where they have potentially movable vaccine attitudes and intentions.

Based on a recent meta-analysis with studies from over 30 different countries, the worldwide cumulative prevalence of vaccine hesitancy among parents of children aged 0–6 years old has been estimated to be ~20% [43]. However, this prevalence varies greatly by country. Additionally, in this meta-analysis, there were variations in the definitions of vaccine hesitancy, a range of different measures used, differences in country income levels, and dissimilarities in the approved and recommended vaccines, leading to a high degree of heterogeneity among the studies. These global data mirror studies in the U.S., which estimate that the prevalence of overall vaccine hesitancy is around 20% [40,44].

There are ongoing global efforts to describe measles and rubella vaccine hesitancy and confidence at national levels [39,45]. However, for a disease as contagious as measles, even local pockets of vaccine hesitancy leading to undervaccination can result in disease outbreaks, and the evidence-based approaches to addressing vaccine hesitancy discussed below are difficult to implement at a national level. Therefore, more granular geospatial surveillance of vaccine hesitancy is necessary to have actionable data on vaccine hesitancy.

As stated previously, worldwide vaccination with measles and rubella vaccines decreased in the years following the start of the COVID-19 pandemic; however, it is unclear if this decrease is due primarily to disruptions in vaccination programs or significant changes in hesitancy toward measles and rubella vaccines. Several studies and polls in the U.S. and Canada have not shown significant changes in childhood vaccine hesitancy since the start of the COVID-19 pandemic [36,40,46,47]. On the other hand, global survey data demonstrated a decrease in the perception of the importance of vaccines for children in many countries before and after the start of the pandemic [48,49]. Further data are needed to fully understand the relationship between post-pandemic decreases in measles and rubella vaccination and changes in vaccine hesitancy. It is also critical to determine whether pandemic-related changes to vaccine hesitancy to measles and rubella vaccines, if present, are transient or long-lasting.

## 4. Communication Strategies to Improve Measles and Rubella Vaccine Acceptance

In light of the challenge of vaccine hesitancy described above, what can be done to overcome vaccine hesitancy and, ultimately, improve measles and rubella vaccine uptake? Over the past several decades, many approaches for individual and public communication and healthcare system, organizational, and public health strategies to address vaccine hesitancy have been recommended or implemented. However, rigorous evidence supporting these strategies was largely lacking until recently. There are multiple ongoing trials and studies to evaluate strategies to improve vaccine uptake, and our understanding is continually evolving and improving.

Despite the rising threat of vaccine hesitancy in LMICs, most of the research on communication strategies to address vaccine hesitancy has been conducted in HICs. Behavioral research on improving vaccine uptake in LMICs has primarily focused on promoting the demand for vaccinations through social mobilization which includes the involvement of a wide range of national and local partners to raise the demand for vaccines [50,51]. Studies from LMICs are included, where appropriate, to the strategies discussed below; however, there is a significant evidence gap for high-quality research on communication and behavioral strategies to address vaccine hesitancy in LMICs. Multiple studies in LMICs are ongoing that will improve the evidence for strategies in LMICs [51].

While more work to gather evidence for communication strategies is ongoing and needs to be completed, several strategies have more evidence than others in improving vaccine acceptance [2]. The following is not a comprehensive review of every strategy used but an overview of strategies with the most robust evidence that are most commonly used. Although all the strategies discussed here have not been studied for effectiveness in improving measles or rubella vaccine uptake specifically, the principles are likely generalizable to all childhood vaccines. Also, many of these strategies have been used in multi-component interventions, making it difficult to determine the isolated effectiveness of individual strategies.

### 4.1. Healthcare Professional Communication Strategies

As trusted sources about vaccines, healthcare professionals have the potential to influence vaccination attitudes and behaviors [52]. A recommendation from a healthcare professional is one of the most important predictors of vaccine acceptance [27].

Healthcare professionals should be prepared to answer vaccine-related questions or concerns and be knowledgeable about the facts related to vaccines and vaccine-preventable diseases. In populations where a lack of awareness or understanding of vaccination is a barrier, providing education and information about vaccines can improve uptake [53]. For instance, in some LMICs, studies have shown education and information about vaccines can improve vaccine uptake [51,54–57]. However, a growing body of evidence has shown that unless there is a significant knowledge gap, simply educating parents on the facts about vaccines may improve parents' knowledge about vaccines but results in little to no difference in parental attitudes toward vaccines or intention to vaccinate [53,58].

Training healthcare professionals on vaccine communication strategies is critical, and many of these professionals report a need for further education [27]. However, training healthcare professionals on information about vaccines alone has not been found to improve vaccine uptake [59].

Establishing an honest dialogue, actively listening, and welcoming questions are all critical to the vaccination discussion [27]. Although many strategies have been proposed for healthcare professionals to communicate with vaccine-hesitant parents or patients, only in recent years have some strategies been rigorously tested in large, randomized controlled trials (RCTs) [27]. These strategies can be used concurrently or as needed based on the flow of the vaccine discussion. Additionally, although most frequently studied in clinicians in ambulatory healthcare settings, these strategies should translate to other health professionals who play a role in vaccination delivery processes in various settings. The following strategies have evidence supporting their effectiveness in improving vaccine uptake (Table 1) [27]:

- Providing a strong and high-quality recommendation;
- Using the presumptive format for initiating vaccine communication ("Johnny's due for three shots today");
- Pursuing adherence despite initial parental reluctance;
- Using motivational interviewing for parents or patients who express hesitancy.

**Table 1.** Healthcare professional communication strategies to address vaccine hesitancy [1].

| Strategy | Examples/Recommendations |
|---|---|
| Provide a strong recommendation for vaccination | • A strong recommendation from a healthcare professional is one of the best ways to improve vaccine acceptance<br>• The strength and quality of the recommendation are important<br>• Missed opportunities to recommend vaccination are frequent and correlate with decreased vaccine uptake |
| Use the presumptive format for initiating vaccine communication | • Example: "Today we're going to do 3 shots"<br>• Example: "John's due for 2 vaccines today"<br>• Example: "I know you have had concerns before, but Sara is due for 3 shots today"<br>• Tone and body language matter<br>• A presumptive format can be used even if resistance has been voiced previously |
| Pursue adherence despite initial reluctance | • Example: "The MMR vaccine is very important for Jack to receive"<br>• Pursuing adherence is in contrast to immediately acquiescing when parents express initial reluctance |

**Table 1.** *Cont.*

| Strategy | Examples/Recommendations |
| --- | --- |
| Use motivational interviewing for individuals who express reluctance | • Open ended questions: try to understand the individual's stance on vaccination.<br>• Example: "Can you tell me more about what you've heard?"<br>• Affirmations: help the individual to feel supported, appreciated, and understood.<br>• Example: "It is clear that you care about your child's health."<br>• Reflections: reflect the individual's words to encourage partnership and build rapport.<br>• Example: "It sounds like you are worried about side effects of the MMR vaccine."<br>• Ask Permission to Share: ask before sharing information to increase individual's receptiveness.<br>• Example: "Can I share what I know about the MMR vaccine with you?"<br>• Autonomy Support: enhance the individual's sense of control.<br>• Example: "Ultimately, this is a decision only you can make." |

[1] Adapted from: O'Leary ST, Opel DJ, Cataldi JR, et al. Strategies for Improving Vaccine Communication and Uptake. Pediatrics; 2024 [27].

There is good evidence that a strong recommendation for vaccination from a healthcare professional increases vaccine acceptance [60]. When a parent or patient hears a recommendation for vaccination, they are more likely to receive a vaccine than if no recommendation is made [61]. While this strategy may seem self-evident, studies have found that missed opportunities to recommend vaccination are frequent and correlate with decreased vaccine uptake [62–64]. The strength of the vaccine recommendation is also important and correlates with improved vaccine uptake [27].

Another communication strategy that can be used with a strong recommendation for vaccination is the presumptive approach when initiating vaccine communication, where vaccine communication is initiated with a closed-ended statement such as "Jack is due for several vaccines today" [65–69]. The presumptive approach contrasts with a participatory approach, where an open-ended question is used. Presenting vaccination as the default option presents vaccination as an opt-out decision, making it more likely for the parent or patient to stick to the status quo and accept vaccination [70,71]. Multiple studies have shown that the presumptive approach for initiating vaccination communication is associated with increased vaccine uptake, even among parents who have negative attitudes toward vaccines. Furthermore, clinicians report high satisfaction with using the presumptive approach and improvements in the efficiency of vaccine discussions [72]. Strongly recommending a course of action or using opt-out default language when communicating about any health intervention must only be performed when there is a clear low risk and high benefit to an intervention, such as with measles and rubella vaccination [73].

Another complementary strategy with some evidence supporting its effectiveness is pursuing adherence despite initial parental reluctance [27]. An example of this strategy would be to reemphasize the importance of a vaccine despite the parent expressing some reluctance to vaccinate. Additionally, despite non-acceptance at an initial visit, pursuing adherence with follow-up communication or repeating recommendations at future visits is associated with improved vaccine acceptance [74,75]

When individuals still express reluctance to vaccinate following a strong presumptive recommendation, motivational interviewing (MI) is another strategy that can be used [27]. Motivational interviewing is a patient-centered approach to enhancing behavior change by leveraging a patient's inherent motivations [76,77]. The evidence for using MI when addressing vaccine-hesitant patients or parents is growing, and additional studies are ongoing [78–83]. Multiple RCTs have found that training providers on MI strategies improved HPV vaccine uptake [78,80,84].

Other proposed strategies exist with limited evidence to date including (1) health professionals using their own experiences with vaccine-preventable diseases or vaccines, (2) mentioning strategies available to minimize the pain associated with vaccination, and (3) bundling all vaccines that a child is eligible for at a visit with a single recommendation [27]. Additionally, including non-clinician personnel such as front desk staff, medical assistants, nurses, and other health professionals in all the vaccine communication processes discussed here may enhance their effectiveness and create a culture of vaccination in the healthcare setting. In LMICs, several studies have demonstrated that trained community members can use vaccine communication strategies to improve vaccine acceptance [54,56,85].

Finally, healthcare professionals should be prepared to answer vaccine-related misinformation or myths. There is emerging evidence to guide providers in carefully debunking a myth or misinformation that follows the fact, warning, fallacy, fact approach [27,86]. In this approach, debunking should start with the fact, followed by a warning about the myth, then briefly explaining the fallacy of the myth, followed by repeating the fact. It is also helpful to highlight the potential hidden motives of people who spread disinformation.

### 4.2. Individual Communication Strategies

With improvements in technology, there has been significant interest in individual or tailored communication strategies such as apps and web-based interventions to improve vaccine uptake with mixed success [2,87,88]. An RCT of delivering web-based vaccine messages tailored to parents' vaccine attitudes did not improve infant vaccine uptake [89]. Multiple similar apps or websites have been developed; however, most of these did not evaluate or demonstrate improvements in vaccine uptake [90–96]. However, many of these apps or web-based tools have been shown to improve vaccine knowledge, attitudes, or beliefs. For example, a parent-centered, gamified mobile intervention about the MMR vaccine increased parents' knowledge, intention to vaccinate, and confidence in the vaccination decision [94].

Further work is warranted on individual-level strategies using apps and web-based tools. Concerns about these tools' usability, scalability, and availability for different populations and settings still need to be addressed. In addition to demonstrating positive effects on vaccine uptake, these dissemination, equity, and sustainability issues must be addressed.

### 4.3. Mass Communication Strategies

While there is broad interest in using mass communication (social media, website, TV, etc.) to improve vaccine attitudes and uptake, evidence for the effectiveness of messages and mass communication strategies is lacking [2]. Few large-scale and robust studies exist to inform whether these platforms actually improve vaccine uptake [88,97]. Unfortunately, some well-meaning strategies have even been shown to backfire among the most hesitant parents. For instance, a web-based intervention aimed to improve MMR vaccination by sharing one of four different types of information with parents (information explaining the lack of evidence that MMR causes autism; information about the dangers of measles, mumps, and rubella; images of children who have measles, mumps, and rubella; or a dramatic narrative about an infant who almost died of measles) increased misperceptions about the MMR vaccine or reduced vaccination intention [98].

Despite a lack of robust evidence, different mass communication strategies have been recommended, including the promotion of vaccines from healthcare professionals or other trusted messengers, the use of influencers or celebrities, using narratives, specifically targeting parents, and framing messages in a way that optimizes vaccination behavior change [99]. Unfortunately, due to anti-physician and anti-establishment sentiments and the algorithms that curate media echo chambers online, many of these strategies may not effectively reach the most vaccine-hesitant individuals or influence their attitudes or behaviors [99].

Unfortunately, the use of mass communication for spreading vaccine misinformation and disinformation, which contributes to vaccine hesitancy, is well documented [2,100]. The need for evidence-based strategies to address the spread of mis/disinformation through mass communication has been identified as a public health priority by the Surgeon General of the United States and WHO and is a critical area of future research [100–102].

## 5. Healthcare System, Organization, and Public Health Strategies to Improve Measles and Rubella Vaccine Acceptance

Beyond communication strategies to improve vaccine acceptance, multiple healthcare system, organizational, and public health strategies improve vaccine uptake [2]. These strategies may not be intended to address vaccine hesitancy directly; however, they may effectively overcome low to moderate levels of vaccine hesitancy by lowering or incentivizing the activation energy required for vaccination.

### *5.1. Healthcare System/Organizational Strategies to Improve Vaccine Uptake Reminder*

There are a variety of healthcare systems or organizational strategies to improve vaccine uptake, and they are often used concurrently with communication interventions. For instance, these strategies decrease missed opportunities to make a strong presumptive recommendation for vaccination or increase the repeated use of those communication strategies. The following healthcare system/organizational strategies have evidence supporting their effectiveness in improving vaccine uptake [87]:

- Reminder/recall;
- Standing orders;
- Provider assessment/feedback;
- Provider reminders.

Reminder and recall systems encompass various methods to identify and remind or notify individuals or parents when vaccines are due. Reminder and recall can be conducted using mail, phone, text, apps, other media, and electronic health records. These notifications are sometimes tailored to individuals and can be accompanied by educational messages [92]. Both observational studies and RCTs in HICs and LMICs have shown evidence that these methods increase vaccine uptake and they are often combined with other strategies [51,103–105].

Standing orders allow healthcare professionals to administer vaccines according to a protocol approved by a supervising authorized practitioner. While no RCTs exist for this strategy, observational studies have demonstrated improved vaccine uptake [88]. Standing orders can reduce missed opportunities for vaccination and empower non-clinician healthcare personnel to have a significant role in vaccine delivery [88]. Most of the evidence for standing orders comes from the U.S.; contextual differences in healthcare infrastructure and authority for different healthcare professionals to administer vaccinations may limit its generalizability to other countries.

Provider assessment and feedback include strategies whereby healthcare professionals receive their vaccination rates and feedback on improvement [87,106]. Although several studies failed to demonstrate improved vaccine uptake with audit and feedback alone, other studies showed improvements in vaccine uptake, especially when used concurrently with other strategies [87,88].

Provider reminders include a variety of methods to remind providers about when patients are due for vaccinations [87,88]. Provider reminders can be performed in various ways, including written notes, chart flags, or electronic health record alerts. Multiple studies have shown the effectiveness of provider reminders for vaccine uptake, and this strategy is often combined with others [107–109].

Finally, immunization information systems (IISs), which serve as a confidential central source of vaccination information for a geographic area, can enhance the availability and use of multiple strategies, including provider reminders, audit and feedback, and reminder and recall strategies [88].

### *5.2. Strategies to Improve Access to Vaccination Services*

While a comprehensive review of strategies to improve access to vaccination services is beyond the scope of this article, it is important to recognize that the use of the evidence-based strategies discussed above depends on access to high-quality vaccination services such as health professionals with adequate training on vaccine communication and healthcare systems or organizations that can use evidence-based methods to promote vaccination. Individuals are unlikely to be exposed to these strategies to address vaccine hesitancy without improving access to vaccination services.

Reducing or eliminating costs for vaccines such as the MMR vaccine is one of the most effective ways to improve access and increase vaccine uptake [87]. In the U.S., most children can receive vaccines at no cost through health insurance or the Vaccines for Children (VFC) program, which provides vaccines for individuals who are uninsured, underinsured, have public insurance (Medicaid), or are American Indian/Alaska Native. Since the VFC program was implemented in 1994, MMR vaccination rates in the U.S. have risen significantly to over 90% [1,110]. Globally, the Measles and Rubella Partnership works with countries and populations to ensure sustainable financing for measles and rubella vaccination services [111]. Preventing measles and rubella through vaccination has a very high return on investment. Vaccination scenarios to reach worldwide measles and rubella elimination have been shown to be more cost-effective than current trends for both measles and rubella [112].

Vaccination programs in communities, including schools, childcare centers, community gathering places, and homes, successfully improve vaccine uptake [87]. School- or childcare-based vaccination programs are particularly helpful for children less likely to access healthcare, and this approach has been used in many countries.

### *5.3. Incentives and Requirements to Improve Vaccine Uptake*

Incentives and requirements for vaccination are often considered strategies to improve vaccine uptake in those who are willing to be vaccinated. These evidence-based strategies, though, are grounded in behavioral science and often can overcome low to moderate levels of vaccine hesitancy and improve vaccination uptake.

Using incentives has been shown to improve vaccination uptake [87]. For instance, in one RCT, the chance of winning a monetary prize was associated with increased vaccine uptake [113]. Other studies have shown that different incentives, such as tying vaccination to insurance-related incentives or public benefits, can improve vaccine uptake [87]. However, incentive programs may be cost-prohibitive outside of large organizations or insurers. In LMICs, several studies of offering small monetary or non-monetary incentives demonstrated improved vaccine uptake [114–116].

Requiring vaccines for schools or childcare attendance can improve vaccine uptake [87]. Many countries have some vaccine requirements for school or childcare attendance with differing degrees of requirements and enforcement [117]. Although there is significant heterogeneity in requirements between countries, several common patterns have been identified. First, the public reaction to vaccine requirements influences the persistence of these requirements within a country. Second, when vaccine-preventable outbreaks occur, this often leads to the introduction of requirements. Third, issues with vaccine access, exemptions, and the enforcement of laws mean the effects of these requirements are variable and context-specific [117].

## 6. Future Directions and Major Research Needs

Although considerable progress has been made in understanding measles and rubella vaccine hesitancy and the evidence for interventions that improve uptake, substantial work remains. Major measles and rubella vaccine hesitancy research needs fall into one of three significant categories of research priorities: (1) further describing the epidemiology and the social and behavioral determinants of vaccine hesitancy, (2) building the evidence for interventions to improve vaccine uptake, and (3) expanding research into LMICs countries and marginalized communities.

Significant work remains to describe the epidemiology of vaccine hesitancy further. We agree with the calls from others to create standardized, timely, and actionable surveillance systems for vaccine hesitancy. These systems need to be grounded in understanding the behavioral and social determinants of vaccine hesitancy, utilize measures validated and used by other countries and jurisdictions, be geospatially granular enough to represent local communities, and be timely and actionable by local vaccination programs [38]. These systems must also be refined in response to evolving evidence, culturally tailored, appropriately representing marginalized communities, and available in multiple languages. Additionally, efforts to address measles and rubella would benefit from a deeper understanding of vaccine hesitancy's social and behavioral determinants, which inform tailored and culturally relevant interventions.

Communication interventions from healthcare professionals and the implementation of these tools need to be studied further to be improved and optimized. Additionally, evidence for interventions to address the increasing spread of vaccine misinformation, disinformation, and antivaccine activism in online communication is in its infancy, and more research with rigorous methods is needed. Using online communication to improve vaccine confidence also needs to be studied more in-depth to better harness the power of these tools.

Finally, many of the resources described here were studied in well-resourced countries. Research in LMICs is necessary to determine which interventions are the most effective and can be implemented and disseminated sustainably and equitably within these countries.

## 7. Discussion

This article reviewed evidence-based strategies for addressing measles and rubella vaccine hesitancy to improve vaccine uptake and, ultimately, eliminate measles and rubella. The strategies reviewed here should not be viewed as stand-alone nor as immutable. These strategies are best applied in combination and must be tailored to the unique contexts of the communities in which they are being used. Additionally, the evidence for these strategies continues to evolve, as do the recipients of these strategies and the context in which they are delivered. With rapid changes in how information is shared and disseminated, changes in human behaviors and social dynamics, and the lingering effects of the COVID-19 pandemic, ongoing research on the best strategies to address vaccine hesitancy and optimal implementation of these strategies is desperately needed. Vaccine hesitancy is a complex issue that requires cross-discipline collaboration. Funding must be increased for all research investigating attitudinal barriers to vaccination because vaccines alone do not save lives; vaccinations save lives.

Finally, while this article aims to provide background on measles and rubella vaccine hesitancy and an overview of evidence-based strategies for addressing measles and rubella vaccine hesitancy, the problem of access cannot be ignored. The strategies discussed in this article are significantly influenced by the social determinants of health, including equitable access to affordable and quality healthcare services [118]. The availability of health professionals skilled at culturally relevant vaccine communication, health systems with the infrastructure to implement vaccine uptake strategies, health insurance coverage, and reduced or no-cost preventive care services influence the success of vaccine-hesitancy interventions. Tackling these barriers must involve deeper collaboration between healthcare providers, health system leaders, public health professionals, policymakers, and community leaders. Efforts must be made to improve the implementation and availability of evidence-based strategies for addressing vaccine hesitancy to improve vaccine uptake and, ultimately, eradicate measles and rubella worldwide.

**Author Contributions:** Writing—original draft preparation, D.M.H. and S.T.O.; writing—review and editing, D.M.H. and S.T.O.; visualization, D.M.H. and S.T.O. All authors have read and agreed to the published version of the manuscript.

**Funding:** This research received no external funding.

**Acknowledgments:** D.H. is supported by the Health Resources and Services Administration (HRSA) of the U.S. Department of Health and Human Services (HHS) under grant number T32HP42016 for Research in Primary Care for USD 2,225,097 over 5 years, 0% financed with nongovernmental sources. This information or content and conclusions are those of the author and should not be construed as the official position or policy of, nor should any endorsements be inferred by HRSA, HHS, or the U.S. government.

**Conflicts of Interest:** The authors declare no conflicts of interest.

## References

1. Minta, A.A.; Ferrari, M.; Antoni, S.; Portnoy, A.; Sbarra, A.; Lambert, B.; Hatcher, C.; Hsu, C.H.; Ho, L.L.; Steulet, C.; et al. Progress Toward Measles Elimination—Worldwide, 2000–2022. *MMWR Morb. Mortal. Wkly. Rep.* **2023**, *72*, 1262–1268. [CrossRef] [PubMed]
2. Omer, S.B.; O'Leary, S.; Danchin, M. Chapter 84—Vaccine Hesitancy and Behavioral Factors Associated With Vaccine Uptake. In *Plotkin's Vaccines*, 8th ed.; Orenstein, W., Offit, P., Edwards, K.M., Plotkin, S., Eds.; Elsevier: Philadelphia, PA, USA, 2023; pp. 1696–1703.e1694. [CrossRef]
3. MacDonald, N.E. Vaccine hesitancy: Definition, scope and determinants. *Vaccine* **2015**, *33*, 4161–4164. [CrossRef] [PubMed]
4. Reef, S.E.; Plotkin, S.A. Chapter 54—Rubella Vaccines. In *Plotkin's Vaccines*, 8th ed.; Orenstein, W., Offit, P., Edwards, K.M., Plotkin, S., Eds.; Elsevier: Philadelphia, PA, USA, 2023; pp. 1025–1056.e1019. [CrossRef]
5. Moss, W.J.; Strebel, P.M. Chapter 38—Measles Vaccines. In *Plotkin's Vaccines*, 8th ed.; Orenstein, W., Offit, P., Edwards, K.M., Plotkin, S., Eds.; Elsevier: Philadelphia, PA, USA, 2023; pp. 629–663.e619. [CrossRef]
6. Committee on Infectious Diseases, American Academy of Pediatrics; Kimberlin, D.W.; Barnett, E.D.; Lynfield, R.; Sawyer, M.H.R. *Red Book: 2021–2024 Report of the Committee on Infectious Diseases*; American Academy of Pediatrics: Elk Grove Village, IL, USA, 2021.
7. Orenstein, W.A.; Offit, P.A.; Edwards, K.M.; Plotkin, S.A. *Plotkin's Vaccines, E-Book*; Elsevier Health Sciences: Amsterdam, The Netherlands, 2022.
8. Ou, A.C.; Zimmerman, L.A.; Alexander, J.P., Jr.; Crowcroft, N.S.; O'Connor, P.M.; Knapp, J.K. Progress Toward Rubella and Congenital Rubella Syndrome Elimination—Worldwide, 2012–2022. *MMWR Morb. Mortal. Wkly. Rep.* **2024**, *73*, 162–167. [CrossRef] [PubMed]
9. Vynnycky, E.; Knapp, J.K.; Papadopoulos, T.; Cutts, F.T.; Hachiya, M.; Miyano, S.; Reef, S.E. Estimates of the global burden of Congenital Rubella Syndrome, 1996–2019. *Int. J. Infect. Dis.* **2023**, *137*, 149–156. [CrossRef] [PubMed]
10. United Nations Children's Fund. *Vaccine Misinformation Management Field Guide*; United Nations Children's Fund: New York, NY, USA, 2020.
11. Wakefield, A.J. MMR vaccination and autism. *Lancet* **1999**, *354*, 949–950. [CrossRef] [PubMed]
12. Omer, S. The discredited doctor hailed by the anti-vaccine movement. *Nature* **2020**, *586*, 668–669. [CrossRef]
13. Nuwarda, R.F.; Ramzan, I.; Weekes, L.; Kayser, V. Vaccine Hesitancy: Contemporary Issues and Historical Background. *Vaccines* **2022**, *10*, 1595. [CrossRef] [PubMed]
14. Center for Disease Control and Prevention. Thimerosal and Vaccines. Available online: https://www.cdc.gov/vaccinesafety/concerns/thimerosal/index.html (accessed on 30 March 2024).
15. Centers for Disease Control and Prevention (CDC). Thimerosal in vaccines: A joint statement of the American Academy of Pediatrics and the Public Health Service. *MMWR Morb. Mortal. Wkly. Rep.* **1999**, *48*, 563–565.
16. Davies, P.; Chapman, S.; Leask, J. Antivaccination activists on the world wide web. *Arch. Dis. Child.* **2002**, *87*, 22–25. [CrossRef]
17. Larson, H.J.; Gakidou, E.; Murray, C.J.L. The Vaccine-Hesitant Moment. *N. Engl. J. Med.* **2022**, *387*, 58–65. [CrossRef]
18. de Figueiredo, A.; Simas, C.; Karafillakis, E.; Paterson, P.; Larson, H.J. Mapping global trends in vaccine confidence and investigating barriers to vaccine uptake: A large-scale retrospective temporal modelling study. *Lancet* **2020**, *396*, 898–908. [CrossRef] [PubMed]
19. World Health Organization. Ten Threats to Global Health in 2019. Available online: https://www.who.int/news-room/spotlight/ten-threats-to-global-health-in-2019 (accessed on 12 May 2024).
20. Wolfe, R.M.; Sharp, L.K. Anti-vaccinationists past and present. *BMJ* **2002**, *325*, 430–432. [CrossRef] [PubMed]
21. Dudley, M.Z.; Privor-Dumm, L.; Dubé, È.; MacDonald, N.E. Words matter: Vaccine hesitancy, vaccine demand, vaccine confidence, herd immunity and mandatory vaccination. *Vaccine* **2020**, *38*, 709–711. [CrossRef] [PubMed]
22. Bedford, H.; Attwell, K.; Danchin, M.; Marshall, H.; Corben, P.; Leask, J. Vaccine hesitancy, refusal and access barriers: The need for clarity in terminology. *Vaccine* **2018**, *36*, 6556–6558. [CrossRef] [PubMed]
23. U.S. Department of Health and Human Services. Featured Priority: Vaccine Confidence. Available online: https://www.hhs.gov/vaccines/featured-priorities/vaccine-confidence/index.html (accessed on 1 April 2024).
24. Dubé, È.; Ward, J.K.; Verger, P.; MacDonald, N.E. Vaccine Hesitancy, Acceptance, and Anti-Vaccination: Trends and Future Prospects for Public Health. *Annu. Rev. Public Health* **2021**, *42*, 175–191. [CrossRef] [PubMed]

25. Leask, J.; Kinnersley, P.; Jackson, C.; Cheater, F.; Bedford, H.; Rowles, G. Communicating with parents about vaccination: A framework for health professionals. *BMC Pediatr.* **2012**, *12*, 154. [CrossRef] [PubMed]
26. Gust, D.; Brown, C.; Sheedy, K.; Hibbs, B.; Weaver, D.; Nowak, G. Immunization attitudes and beliefs among parents: Beyond a dichotomous perspective. *Am. J. Health Behav.* **2005**, *29*, 81–92. [CrossRef] [PubMed]
27. O'Leary, S.T.; Opel, D.J.; Cataldi, J.R.; Hackell, J.M.; Committee on Infectious Diseases; Committee on Practice and Ambulatory Medicine; Committee on Bioethics. Strategies for Improving Vaccine Communication and Uptake. *Pediatrics* **2024**, *153*, e2023065483. [CrossRef] [PubMed]
28. Opel, D.J.; Mangione-Smith, R.; Taylor, J.A.; Korfiatis, C.; Wiese, C.; Catz, S.; Martin, D.P. Development of a survey to identify vaccine-hesitant parents: The parent attitudes about childhood vaccines survey. *Hum. Vaccin.* **2011**, *7*, 419–425. [CrossRef]
29. Gilkey, M.B.; Magnus, B.E.; Reiter, P.L.; McRee, A.L.; Dempsey, A.F.; Brewer, N.T. The Vaccination Confidence Scale: A brief measure of parents' vaccination beliefs. *Vaccine* **2014**, *32*, 6259–6265. [CrossRef]
30. Larson, H.J.; Jarrett, C.; Schulz, W.S.; Chaudhuri, M.; Zhou, Y.; Dube, E.; Schuster, M.; MacDonald, N.E.; Wilson, R. Measuring vaccine hesitancy: The development of a survey tool. *Vaccine* **2015**, *33*, 4165–4175. [CrossRef]
31. Betsch, C.; Schmid, P.; Heinemeier, D.; Korn, L.; Holtmann, C.; Böhm, R. Beyond confidence: Development of a measure assessing the 5C psychological antecedents of vaccination. *PLoS ONE* **2018**, *13*, e0208601. [CrossRef] [PubMed]
32. Wallace, A.S.; Wannemuehler, K.; Bonsu, G.; Wardle, M.; Nyaku, M.; Amponsah-Achiano, K.; Dadzie, J.F.; Sarpong, F.O.; Orenstein, W.A.; Rosenberg, E.S.; et al. Development of a valid and reliable scale to assess parents' beliefs and attitudes about childhood vaccines and their association with vaccination uptake and delay in Ghana. *Vaccine* **2019**, *37*, 848–856. [CrossRef]
33. Sabahelzain, M.M.; Dubé, E.; Moukhyer, M.; Larson, H.J.; van den Borne, B.; Bosma, H. Psychometric properties of the adapted measles vaccine hesitancy scale in Sudan. *PLoS ONE* **2020**, *15*, e0237171. [CrossRef]
34. Rosenstock, I.M.; Strecher, V.J.; Becker, M.H. Social learning theory and the Health Belief Model. *Health Educ. Q.* **1988**, *15*, 175–183. [CrossRef]
35. Lopes, L.; Schumacher, S.; Sparks, G.; Presiado, M.; Hamel, L.; Brodie, M. KFF COVID-19 Vaccine Monitor: December 2022. Available online: https://www.kff.org/coronavirus-covid-19/poll-finding/kff-covid-19-vaccine-monitor-december-2022/ (accessed on 12 May 2024).
36. Pew Research Center. Americans' Largely Positive Views of Childhood Vaccines Hold Steady. Available online: https://www.pewresearch.org/science/2023/05/16/americans-largely-positive-views-of-childhood-vaccines-hold-steady/ (accessed on 16 May 2024).
37. Angus Reid Institute. Parental Opposition to Childhood Vaccination Grows as Canadians Worry about Harms of Anti-Vax Movement. Available online: https://angusreid.org/wp-content/uploads/2024/02/2024.02.28_vaccine.pdf (accessed on 10 April 2024).
38. Gilkey, M.B.; Brewer, N.T. It's Time for a National Surveillance System for Vaccine Confidence and Hesitancy. *Pediatrics* **2023**, *152*, e2023063169. [CrossRef]
39. Kumar, D.; Mathur, M.; Tanu, T.; Singh, M.; Kumari, N.; Mathur, M.; Lahariya, C.; Kapoor, N.; Mohapatra, A.; Rana, R.K.; et al. Setting up an epidemiological surveillance system for vaccine hesitancy outbreaks and illustration of its steps of investigation. *Fam. Med. Community Health* **2021**, *9*, e001080. [CrossRef]
40. Higgins, D.M.; Moss, A.; Blackwell, S.; O'Leary, S.T. The COVID-19 Pandemic and Parental Attitudes Toward Routine Childhood Vaccines. *Pediatrics* **2023**, *152*, e2023062927. [CrossRef] [PubMed]
41. Gust, D.A.; Darling, N.; Kennedy, A.; Schwartz, B. Parents with doubts about vaccines: Which vaccines and reasons why. *Pediatrics* **2008**, *122*, 718–725. [CrossRef]
42. Daley, M.F.; Reifler, L.M.; Shoup, J.A.; Narwaney, K.J.; Kharbanda, E.O.; Groom, H.C.; Jackson, M.L.; Jacobsen, S.J.; McLean, H.Q.; Klein, N.P.; et al. Temporal Trends in Undervaccination: A Population-Based Cohort Study. *Am. J. Prev. Med.* **2021**, *61*, 64–72. [CrossRef]
43. Abenova, M.; Shaltynov, A.; Jamedinova, U.; Semenova, Y. Worldwide Child Routine Vaccination Hesitancy Rate among Parents of Children Aged 0–6 Years: A Systematic Review and Meta-Analysis of Cross-Sectional Studies. *Vaccines* **2024**, *12*, 31. [CrossRef] [PubMed]
44. Santibanez, T.A.; Nguyen, K.H.; Greby, S.M.; Fisher, A.; Scanlon, P.; Bhatt, A.; Srivastav, A.; Singleton, J.A. Parental Vaccine Hesitancy and Childhood Influenza Vaccination. *Pediatrics* **2020**, *146*, e2020007609. [CrossRef] [PubMed]
45. Vaccine Confidence Project. Available online: https://www.vaccineconfidence.org (accessed on 30 March 2024).
46. Opel, D.J.; Furniss, A.; Zhou, C.; Rice, J.D.; Spielvogle, H.; Spina, C.; Perreira, C.; Giang, J.; Dundas, N.; Dempsey, A.; et al. Parent Attitudes Towards Childhood Vaccines After the Onset of SARS-CoV-2 in the United States. *Acad. Pediatr.* **2022**, *22*, 1407–1413. [CrossRef] [PubMed]
47. Humble, R.M.; Scott, S.D.; Dubé, E.; Olson, J.; MacDonald, S.E. The impact of the COVID-19 pandemic on parents' perceptions and acceptance of routine childhood vaccination in Canada: A national longitudinal study. *Vaccine* **2023**, *41*, 407–415. [CrossRef] [PubMed]
48. Eagan, R.L.; Larson, H.J.; de Figueiredo, A. Recent trends in vaccine coverage and confidence: A cause for concern. *Hum. Vaccin. Immunother.* **2023**, *19*, 2237374. [CrossRef] [PubMed]
49. United Nations Children's Fund. *The State of the World's Children 2023: For Every Child, Vaccination*; UNICEF Innocenti—Global Office of Research and Foresight: Florence, Italy, 2023.

50. Jalloh, M.F.; Wilhelm, E.; Abad, N.; Prybylski, D. Mobilize to vaccinate: Lessons learned from social mobilization for immunization in low and middle-income countries. *Hum. Vaccin. Immunother.* **2020**, *16*, 1208–1214. [CrossRef] [PubMed]
51. Merriam, S.; Behnrendt, H. *Increasing Vaccine Uptake in Low- and Middle-Income Countries*; The Behavioural Insights Team: London, UK, 2020.
52. Freed, G.L.; Clark, S.J.; Butchart, A.T.; Singer, D.C.; Davis, M.M. Sources and perceived credibility of vaccine-safety information for parents. *Pediatrics* **2011**, *127* (Suppl. S1), S107–S112. [CrossRef] [PubMed]
53. Kaufman, J.; Ryan, R.; Walsh, L.; Horey, D.; Leask, J.; Robinson, P.; Hill, S. Face-to-face interventions for informing or educating parents about early childhood vaccination. *Cochrane Database Syst. Rev.* **2018**, *5*, Cd010038. [CrossRef] [PubMed]
54. Powell-Jackson, T.; Fabbri, C.; Dutt, V.; Tougher, S.; Singh, K. Effect and cost-effectiveness of educating mothers about childhood DPT vaccination on immunisation uptake, knowledge, and perceptions in Uttar Pradesh, India: A randomised controlled trial. *PLoS Med.* **2018**, *15*, e1002519. [CrossRef]
55. Usman, H.R.; Rahbar, M.H.; Kristensen, S.; Vermund, S.H.; Kirby, R.S.; Habib, F.; Chamot, E. Randomized controlled trial to improve childhood immunization adherence in rural Pakistan: Redesigned immunization card and maternal education. *Trop. Med. Int. Health* **2011**, *16*, 334–342. [CrossRef]
56. Owais, A.; Hanif, B.; Siddiqui, A.R.; Agha, A.; Zaidi, A.K. Does improving maternal knowledge of vaccines impact infant immunization rates? A community-based randomized-controlled trial in Karachi, Pakistan. *BMC Public. Health* **2011**, *11*, 239. [CrossRef] [PubMed]
57. Usman, H.R.; Akhtar, S.; Habib, F.; Jehan, I. Redesigned immunization card and center-based education to reduce childhood immunization dropouts in urban Pakistan: A randomized controlled trial. *Vaccine* **2009**, *27*, 467–472. [CrossRef] [PubMed]
58. Danchin, M. Does informing or educating parents about early childhood vaccination improve uptake? *J. Paediatr. Child Health* **2019**, *55*, 1142–1144. [CrossRef] [PubMed]
59. Guide to Community Preventive Services. Vaccination Programs: Provider Education When Used Alone. Available online: https://www.thecommunityguide.org/findings/vaccination-programs-provider-education-when-used-alone.html (accessed on 10 April 2024).
60. Smith, L.E.; Amlôt, R.; Weinman, J.; Yiend, J.; Rubin, G.J. A systematic review of factors affecting vaccine uptake in young children. *Vaccine* **2017**, *35*, 6059–6069. [CrossRef] [PubMed]
61. Dempsey, A.F.; Pyrzanowski, J.; Lockhart, S.; Campagna, E.; Barnard, J.; O'Leary, S.T. Parents' perceptions of provider communication regarding adolescent vaccines. *Hum. Vaccin. Immunother.* **2016**, *12*, 1469–1475. [CrossRef] [PubMed]
62. Sabnis, S.S.; Pomeranz, A.J.; Amateau, M.M. The effect of education, feedback, and provider prompts on the rate of missed vaccine opportunities in a community health center. *Clin. Pediatr.* **2003**, *42*, 147–151. [CrossRef] [PubMed]
63. Szilagyi, P.G.; Rodewald, L.E. Missed opportunities for immunizations: A review of the evidence. *J. Public Health Manag. Pract.* **1996**, *2*, 18–25. [CrossRef] [PubMed]
64. Sridhar, S.; Maleq, N.; Guillermet, E.; Colombini, A.; Gessner, B.D. A systematic literature review of missed opportunities for immunization in low- and middle-income countries. *Vaccine* **2014**, *32*, 6870–6879. [CrossRef] [PubMed]
65. Hofstetter, A.M.; Robinson, J.D.; Lepere, K.; Cunningham, M.; Etsekson, N.; Opel, D.J. Clinician-parent discussions about influenza vaccination of children and their association with vaccine acceptance. *Vaccine* **2017**, *35*, 2709–2715. [CrossRef]
66. Opel, D.J.; Mangione-Smith, R.; Robinson, J.D.; Heritage, J.; DeVere, V.; Salas, H.S.; Zhou, C.; Taylor, J.A. The Influence of Provider Communication Behaviors on Parental Vaccine Acceptance and Visit Experience. *Am. J. Public Health* **2015**, *105*, 1998–2004. [CrossRef]
67. Opel, D.J.; Heritage, J.; Taylor, J.A.; Mangione-Smith, R.; Salas, H.S.; Devere, V.; Zhou, C.; Robinson, J.D. The architecture of provider-parent vaccine discussions at health supervision visits. *Pediatrics* **2013**, *132*, 1037–1046. [CrossRef] [PubMed]
68. Opel, D.J.; Robinson, J.D.; Heritage, J.; Korfiatis, C.; Taylor, J.A.; Mangione-Smith, R. Characterizing providers' immunization communication practices during health supervision visits with vaccine-hesitant parents: A pilot study. *Vaccine* **2012**, *30*, 1269–1275. [CrossRef]
69. Opel, D.J.; Taylor, J.A.; Zhou, C.; Catz, S.; Myaing, M.; Mangione-Smith, R. The relationship between parent attitudes about childhood vaccines survey scores and future child immunization status: A validation study. *JAMA Pediatr.* **2013**, *167*, 1065–1071. [CrossRef]
70. Reñosa, M.D.C.; Landicho, J.; Wachinger, J.; Dalglish, S.L.; Bärnighausen, K.; Bärnighausen, T.; McMahon, S.A. Nudging toward vaccination: A systematic review. *BMJ Glob. Health* **2021**, *6*, e006237. [CrossRef] [PubMed]
71. Opel, D.J.; Omer, S.B. Measles, mandates, and making vaccination the default option. *JAMA Pediatr.* **2015**, *169*, 303–304. [CrossRef]
72. Malo, T.L.; Hall, M.E.; Brewer, N.T.; Lathren, C.R.; Gilkey, M.B. Why is announcement training more effective than conversation training for introducing HPV vaccination? A theory-based investigation. *Implement. Sci.* **2018**, *13*, 57. [CrossRef] [PubMed]
73. Blumenthal-Barby, J.; Opel, D.J. Nudge or Grudge? Choice Architecture and Parental Decision-Making. *Hastings Cent. Rep.* **2018**, *48*, 33–39. [CrossRef]
74. Kornides, M.L.; McRee, A.L.; Gilkey, M.B. Parents Who Decline HPV Vaccination: Who Later Accepts and Why? *Acad. Pediatr.* **2018**, *18*, S37–S43. [CrossRef] [PubMed]
75. Margolis, M.A.; Brewer, N.T.; Boynton, M.H.; Lafata, J.E.; Southwell, B.G.; Gilkey, M.B. Provider response and follow-up to parental declination of HPV vaccination. *Vaccine* **2022**, *40*, 344–350. [CrossRef]
76. Miller, W.R. Motivational interviewing: Research, practice, and puzzles. *Addict. Behav.* **1996**, *21*, 835–842. [CrossRef]

77. Miller, W.R.; Rollnick, S. *Preparing People to Change Addictive Behavior*; The Guilford Press: New York, NY, USA, 1991.
78. Dempsey, A.F.; Pyrznawoski, J.; Lockhart, S.; Barnard, J.; Campagna, E.J.; Garrett, K.; Fisher, A.; Dickinson, L.M.; O'Leary, S.T. Effect of a Health Care Professional Communication Training Intervention on Adolescent Human Papillomavirus Vaccination: A Cluster Randomized Clinical Trial. *JAMA Pediatr.* **2018**, *172*, e180016. [CrossRef] [PubMed]
79. Gagneur, A. Motivational interviewing: A powerful tool to address vaccine hesitancy. *Can. Commun. Dis. Rep.* **2020**, *46*, 93–97. [CrossRef] [PubMed]
80. Lemaitre, T.; Carrier, N.; Farrands, A.; Gosselin, V.; Petit, G.; Gagneur, A. Impact of a vaccination promotion intervention using motivational interview techniques on long-term vaccine coverage: The PromoVac strategy. *Hum. Vaccin. Immunother.* **2019**, *15*, 732–739. [CrossRef] [PubMed]
81. Glanternik, J.R.; McDonald, J.C.; Yee, A.H.; Howell Ba, A.; Saba, K.N.; Mellor, R.G.; Fireman, B.; Klein, N.P. Evaluation of a Vaccine-Communication Tool for Physicians. *J. Pediatr.* **2020**, *224*, 72–78.e71. [CrossRef] [PubMed]
82. Opel, D.J.; Robinson, J.D.; Spielvogle, H.; Spina, C.; Garrett, K.; Dempsey, A.F.; Perreira, C.; Dickinson, M.; Zhou, C.; Pahud, B.; et al. 'Presumptively Initiating Vaccines and Optimizing Talk with Motivational Interviewing' (PIVOT with MI) trial: A protocol for a cluster randomised controlled trial of a clinician vaccine communication intervention. *BMJ Open* **2020**, *10*, e039299. [CrossRef] [PubMed]
83. O'Leary, S.T.; Spina, C.I.; Spielvogle, H.; Robinson, J.D.; Garrett, K.; Perreira, C.; Pahud, B.; Dempsey, A.F.; Opel, D.J. Development of PIVOT with MI: A motivational Interviewing-Based vaccine communication training for pediatric clinicians. *Vaccine* **2023**, *41*, 1760–1767. [CrossRef] [PubMed]
84. Szilagyi, P.G.; Humiston, S.G.; Stephens-Shields, A.J.; Localio, R.; Breck, A.; Kelly, M.K.; Wright, M.; Grundmeier, R.W.; Albertin, C.; Shone, L.P.; et al. Effect of Training Pediatric Clinicians in Human Papillomavirus Communication Strategies on Human Papillomavirus Vaccination Rates: A Cluster Randomized Clinical Trial. *JAMA Pediatr.* **2021**, *175*, 901–910. [CrossRef] [PubMed]
85. Andersson, N.; Cockcroft, A.; Ansari, N.M.; Omer, K.; Baloch, M.; Ho Foster, A.; Shea, B.; Wells, G.A.; Soberanis, J.L. Evidence-based discussion increases childhood vaccination uptake: A randomised cluster controlled trial of knowledge translation in Pakistan. *BMC Int. Health Hum. Rights* **2009**, *9* (Suppl. S1), S8. [CrossRef]
86. Lewandowsky, S.; Cook, J.; Ecker, U.K.H.; Albarracín, D.; Amazeen, M.A.; Kendeou, P.; Lombardi, D.; Newman, E.J.; Pennycook, G.; Porter, E.; et al. *The Debunking Handbook 2020*; Skeptical Science: Lake City, FL, USA, 2020.
87. Cataldi, J.R.; Kerns, M.E.; O'Leary, S.T. Evidence-based strategies to increase vaccination uptake: A review. *Curr. Opin. Pediatr.* **2020**, *32*, 151–159. [CrossRef]
88. Cataldi, J.R.; O'Leary, S.T. Parental vaccine hesitancy: Scope, causes, and potential responses. *Curr. Opin. Infect. Dis.* **2021**, *34*, 519–526. [CrossRef]
89. Glanz, J.M.; Wagner, N.M.; Narwaney, K.J.; Pyrzanowski, J.; Kwan, B.M.; Sevick, C.; Resnicow, K.; Dempsey, A.F. Web-Based Tailored Messaging to Increase Vaccination: A Randomized Clinical Trial. *Pediatrics* **2020**, *146*, e20200669. [CrossRef] [PubMed]
90. Atkinson, K.M.; Westeinde, J.; Ducharme, R.; Wilson, S.E.; Deeks, S.L.; Crowcroft, N.; Hawken, S.; Wilson, K. Can mobile technologies improve on-time vaccination? A study piloting maternal use of ImmunizeCA, a Pan-Canadian immunization app. *Hum. Vaccines Immunother.* **2016**, *12*, 2654–2661. [CrossRef] [PubMed]
91. Glanz, J.M.; Wagner, N.M.; Narwaney, K.J.; Kraus, C.R.; Shoup, J.A.; Xu, S.; O'Leary, S.T.; Omer, S.B.; Gleason, K.S.; Daley, M.F. Web-based Social Media Intervention to Increase Vaccine Acceptance: A Randomized Controlled Trial. *Pediatrics* **2017**, *140*, e20171117. [CrossRef]
92. O'Leary, S.T.; Narwaney, K.J.; Wagner, N.M.; Kraus, C.R.; Omer, S.B.; Glanz, J.M. Efficacy of a Web-Based Intervention to Increase Uptake of Maternal Vaccines: An RCT. *Am. J. Prev. Med.* **2019**, *57*, e125–e133. [CrossRef]
93. Dempsey, A.F.; Maertens, J.; Beaty, B.; O'Leary, S.T. Characteristics of users of a tailored, interactive website for parents and its impact on adolescent vaccination attitudes and uptake. *BMC Res. Notes* **2015**, *8*, 739. [CrossRef]
94. Fadda, M.; Galimberti, E.; Fiordelli, M.; Romanò, L.; Zanetti, A.; Schulz, P.J. Effectiveness of a smartphone app to increase parents' knowledge and empowerment in the MMR vaccination decision: A randomized controlled trial. *Hum. Vaccines Immunother.* **2017**, *13*, 2512–2521. [CrossRef]
95. Dudley, M.Z.; Omer, S.B.; O'Leary, S.T.; Limaye, R.J.; Ellingson, M.K.; Spina, C.I.; Brewer, S.E.; Bednarczyk, R.A.; Chamberlain, A.T.; Malik, F.; et al. MomsTalkShots, tailored educational app, improves vaccine attitudes: A randomized controlled trial. *BMC Public Health* **2022**, *22*, 2134. [CrossRef]
96. Bednarczyk, R.A.; Frew, P.M.; Salmon, D.A.; Whitney, E.; Omer, S.B. ReadyVax: A new mobile vaccine information app. *Hum. Vaccin. Immunother.* **2017**, *13*, 1149–1154. [CrossRef] [PubMed]
97. Montagni, I.; Mabchour, I.; Tzourio, C. Digital Gamification to Enhance Vaccine Knowledge and Uptake: Scoping Review. *JMIR Serious Games* **2020**, *8*, e16983. [CrossRef]
98. Nyhan, B.; Reifler, J.; Richey, S.; Freed, G.L. Effective messages in vaccine promotion: A randomized trial. *Pediatrics* **2014**, *133*, e835–e842. [CrossRef]
99. Puri, N.; Coomes, E.A.; Haghbayan, H.; Gunaratne, K. Social media and vaccine hesitancy: New updates for the era of COVID-19 and globalized infectious diseases. *Hum. Vaccines Immunother.* **2020**, *16*, 2586–2593. [CrossRef] [PubMed]
100. World Health Organization. *Fifth Virtual WHO Infodemic Management Conference, 2, 4, 9 and 11 November 2021: Meeting Report. Steps towards Measuring the Burden of Infodemics*; World Health Organization: Geneva, Switzerland, 2022.

101. Murthy, V. *Confronting Health Misinformation: The U.S. Surgeon General's Advisory on Building a Healthy Information Environment*; Office of the Surgeon General: Washington, DC, USA, 2021.
102. Wilhelm, E.; Ballalai, I.; Belanger, M.E.; Benjamin, P.; Bertrand-Ferrandis, C.; Bezbaruah, S.; Briand, S.; Brooks, I.; Bruns, R.; Bucci, L.M.; et al. Measuring the Burden of Infodemics: Summary of the Methods and Results of the Fifth WHO Infodemic Management Conference. *JMIR Infodemiology* **2023**, *3*, e44207. [CrossRef] [PubMed]
103. Rodewald, L.E.; Szilagyi, P.G.; Humiston, S.G.; Barth, R.; Kraus, R.; Raubertas, R.F. A randomized study of tracking with outreach and provider prompting to improve immunization coverage and primary care. *Pediatrics* **1999**, *103*, 31–38. [CrossRef] [PubMed]
104. Lieu, T.A.; Capra, A.M.; Makol, J.; Black, S.B.; Shinefield, H.R. Effectiveness and cost-effectiveness of letters, automated telephone messages, or both for underimmunized children in a health maintenance organization. *Pediatrics* **1998**, *101*, E3. [CrossRef] [PubMed]
105. Lemstra, M.; Rajakumar, D.; Thompson, A.; Moraros, J. The effectiveness of telephone reminders and home visits to improve measles, mumps and rubella immunization coverage rates in children. *Paediatr. Child. Health* **2011**, *16*, e1–e5. [CrossRef] [PubMed]
106. Bordley, W.C.; Chelminski, A.; Margolis, P.A.; Kraus, R.; Szilagyi, P.G.; Vann, J.J. The effect of audit and feedback on immunization delivery: A systematic review. *Am. J. Prev. Med.* **2000**, *18*, 343–350. [CrossRef] [PubMed]
107. Shaw, J.S.; Samuels, R.C.; Larusso, E.M.; Bernstein, H.H. Impact of an encounter-based prompting system on resident vaccine administration performance and immunization knowledge. *Pediatrics* **2000**, *105*, 978–983. [CrossRef] [PubMed]
108. Burns, I.T.; Zimmerman, R.K.; Santibanez, T.A. Effectiveness of chart prompt about immunizations in an urban health center. *J. Fam. Pract.* **2002**, *51*, 1018.
109. Fiks, A.G.; Hunter, K.F.; Localio, A.R.; Grundmeier, R.W.; Bryant-Stephens, T.; Luberti, A.A.; Bell, L.M.; Alessandrini, E.A. Impact of electronic health record-based alerts on influenza vaccination for children with asthma. *Pediatrics* **2009**, *124*, 159–169. [CrossRef]
110. Center for Disease Control and Prevention. About the Vaccines for Children Program (VFC). Available online: https://www.cdc.gov/vaccines/programs/vfc/about/index.html (accessed on 1 April 2024).
111. *Measles and Rubella Strategic Framework 2021–2030*; World Health Organization: Geneva, Switzerland, 2020.
112. Levin, A.; Burgess, C.; Shendale, S.; Morgan, W.; Cw Hutubessy, R.; Jit, M. Cost-effectiveness of measles and rubella elimination in low-income and middle-income countries. *BMJ Glob. Health* **2023**, *8*, e011526. [CrossRef]
113. Yokley, J.M.; Glenwick, D.S. Increasing the immunization of preschool children; an evaluation of applied community interventions. *J. Appl. Behav. Anal.* **1984**, *17*, 313–325. [CrossRef] [PubMed]
114. Banerjee, A.V.; Duflo, E.; Glennerster, R.; Kothari, D. Improving immunisation coverage in rural India: Clustered randomised controlled evaluation of immunisation campaigns with and without incentives. *BMJ* **2010**, *340*, c2220. [CrossRef] [PubMed]
115. Gibson, D.G.; Kagucia, E.W.; Were, J.; Obor, D.; Hayford, K.; Ochieng, B. Text Message Reminders and Unconditional Monetary Incentives to Improve Measles Vaccination in Western Kenya: Study Protocol for the Mobile and Scalable Innovations for Measles Immunization Randomized Controlled Trial. *JMIR Res. Protoc.* **2019**, *8*, e13221. [CrossRef] [PubMed]
116. Seth, R.; Akinboyo, I.; Chhabra, A.; Qaiyum, Y.; Shet, A.; Gupte, N.; Jain, A.K.; Jain, S.K. Mobile Phone Incentives for Childhood Immunizations in Rural India. *Pediatrics* **2018**, *141*, e20173455. [CrossRef]
117. Vanderslott, S.; Marks, T. Charting mandatory childhood vaccination policies worldwide. *Vaccine* **2021**, *39*, 4054–4062. [CrossRef]
118. World Health Organization. Social Determinants of Health. Available online: https://www.who.int/health-topics/social-determinants-of-health#tab=tab_1 (accessed on 30 March 2024).

*vaccines*

MDPI

*Review*

# Challenges for Sustaining Measles Elimination: Post-Verification Large-Scale Import-Related Measles Outbreaks in Mongolia and Cambodia, Resulting in the Loss of Measles Elimination Status

**José Hagan [1], Otgonbayar Dashpagma [2], Ork Vichit [3], Samnang Chham [1], Sodbayar Demberelsuren [1], Varja Grabovac [1], Shafiqul Hossain [1], Makiko Iijima [1], Chung-won Lee [1], Anuzaya Purevdagva [1], Kayla Mariano [1], Roger Evans [1], Yan Zhang [1,†] and Yoshihiro Takashima [1,*,‡]**

1 World Health Organization, 1211 Geneva, Switzerland; haganj@who.int (J.H.)
2 National Immunization Program, Ministry of Health, Ulaanbaatar 14210, Mongolia
3 National Immunization Program, Ministry of Health, Phnom Penh 12151, Cambodia
* Correspondence: yoshi_takashima@cider.osaka-u.ac.jp
† Current address: WHO Western Pacific Regional Measles/Rubella Reference Laboratory, National Institute for Viral Disease Control and Prevention, Chinese Center for Disease Control and Prevention, Beijing 102206, China.
‡ Current address: Center for Infectious Disease Education and Research, Osaka University, Osaka 565-0871, Japan.

**Abstract:** The Western Pacific Region's pursuit of measles elimination has seen significant progress and setbacks. Mongolia and Cambodia were the first two middle-income countries in the Western Pacific to be verified as having eliminated measles by the Western Pacific Regional Verification Commission for Measles and Rubella Elimination, in March 2014 and 2015, respectively. However, both countries experienced large-scale or prolonged importation-related measles outbreaks shortly afterwards, leading to the re-establishment of endemic transmission. We describe the path to initial elimination in both countries and explore these outbreaks' characteristics, factors contributing to the loss of elimination status, and implications for broader elimination efforts. Data sources include case-based epidemiological and laboratory surveillance reports, historical immunization coverage, genotype data, and published reports of in-depth outbreak investigations. In Mongolia, a single prolonged and large-scale outbreak revealed a hidden immunity gap among young adults and was driven in part by nosocomial transmission, leading to significant morbidity and mortality and loss of elimination status. Cambodia suffered multiple importations from neighboring endemic countries during the global measles resurgence in 2018–2019, complicated by cross-border mobility and significant nosocomial amplification, and the country was ultimately unable to sufficiently distinguish independent chains of transmission, leading to loss of elimination status. Our findings highlight the importance of broadening population immunity assessments beyond children to include adults and specific high-risk groups. Robust routine immunization programs, supplemented by tailored SIAs, are crucial for preventing and managing outbreaks. Additionally, strong outbreak preparedness plans, rapid response strategies, and cross-border collaboration and the global effort to prevent multiple resurgences and large-scale importation-induced outbreaks are vital for maintaining elimination status. The experiences of Mongolia and Cambodia underscore the challenges of sustaining measles elimination in the face of importation risks, shared borders with endemic countries, healthcare system gaps, and population movements. Strengthening the global coordination and synchronization of measles elimination activities is imperative to protect the gains achieved and prevent future setbacks.

**Keywords:** measles elimination; outbreak investigation; vaccine-preventable diseases; Mongolia; Cambodia; Western Pacific Region

## 1. Introduction

In 2003, the World Health Organization (WHO) Regional Committee for the Western Pacific resolved to eliminate measles and concurrently strengthen routine immunization [1] and, in 2005, established 2012 as the target year for measles elimination [2]. In 2010 and 2012, the Regional Committee urged the WHO Regional Director for the Western Pacific and Member States to establish independent national and regional verification mechanisms for measles elimination, including the creation of national verification committees (NVCs) and the Regional Verification Commission (RVC) [3,4].

The verification of measles elimination (defined as the absence of endemic measles virus transmission in a region or country for ≥12 months, in the presence of a well-performing surveillance system) addresses three criteria supported by indicators within the five lines of evidence. These three criteria include the following: (1) documentation of the interruption of endemic measles virus transmission for a period of at least 36 months from the last known endemic case; (2) the presence of verification standard surveillance; (3) genotyping evidence that supports the interruption of endemic measles virus transmission [5]. Mongolia and Cambodia were the first two middle-income countries in the Western Pacific to be verified as having eliminated measles by the RVC; however, both countries experienced large-scale or prolonged importation-related measles outbreaks shortly afterwards. The RVC ultimately determined that endemic transmission had been re-established in Mongolia and Cambodia and the criteria for sustained measles elimination could no longer be demonstrated.

In this manuscript, we describe the characteristics of these measles outbreaks in Mongolia and Cambodia after the verification of measles elimination. We review the factors that led to the outbreaks and to the loss of elimination status and consider implications for the broader measles elimination effort.

## 2. Data Sources

This report references data routinely reported to WHO from Mongolia and Cambodia from case-based epidemiological and laboratory surveillance and historical immunization coverage of routine immunization (via WHO–UNICEF joint estimates of national immunization coverage (WUENIC) [6] and supplemental immunization activities (SIAs) by year of activity and by targeted birth cohort. Genotype data were directly reported to the WHO through the Measles–Rubella Regional Reference Laboratory Network, and accessed through the WHO Measles Virus Nucleotide Surveillance genetic database MeaNS [7]. Additional published data are referenced directly from relevant sources related to in-depth outbreak investigation.

## 3. Mongolia

### 3.1. Path to Measles Elimination in Mongolia

Mongolia is a large and sparsely populated Central Asian country bordering the Russian Federation and the People's Republic of China. Administratively, it is divided into 21 provinces ("Aimags") and the capital city, Ulaanbaatar. In the decade following the fall of the Soviet Union in 1990, Mongolia underwent rapid and dramatic social, economic, and political transformations. This period was marked by severe challenges as the country transitioned from a socialist state to a multiparty democratic system and a market economy and experienced sharp drops in foreign aid, causing economic contraction, inflation, and unemployment. Government spending on healthcare significantly reduced, and programmatically the health system shifted from a centrally planned, fully state-funded model to a mixed financing model with the introduction of user fees, leading to a crisis in the provision of health services, including immunization [8]. During this period, intensive urban migration occurred, which among other impacts led to an increase in children living in urban centers but registered for immunization services in their home region and therefore excluded from immunization planning and service delivery.

The measles vaccine was introduced in the national immunization program in 1973, targeting 10–13-month-olds [9], prior to the 1974 World Health Assembly resolution calling for establishment of national immunization programs. The second dose of measles-containing vaccine (MCV) was introduced in 1989 for children 12–18 months, with an updated target age for MCV first dose at 9–12 months. In place of monovalent MCV, the measles–mumps–rubella (MMR) vaccine was introduced in 2009, targeting 9-month-olds for the first dose (MMR1) and 2-year-olds for the second dose (MMR2).

Following the introduction of MCV2 in 1989, there was a decline in measles cases from 1990 to 2002, with periodic relatively small-scale measles outbreaks occurring during 1992 and 1995, and a large outbreak in the capital city in 2001 that affected infants below one year of age and young adults aged 15–24 years [9]. Beginning in 1994, a series of wide age-range supplemental immunization activities were conducted, targeting all birth cohorts born since 1986 at least once and achieving high administrative coverage. Immunization coverage with two doses of measles vaccine has generally been at or above 95% since 2001 [10] (Figure 1). A nationwide serosurvey conducted in 2004 estimated 12–17% measles susceptibility among children who would be aged 13–21 years during the 2015 outbreak [11]. This cohort was partially included in a nationwide SIA conducted in 2007 that achieved 97% administrative coverage, targeting children aged 2–10 years of age (aged 10–18 during the 2015 outbreak).

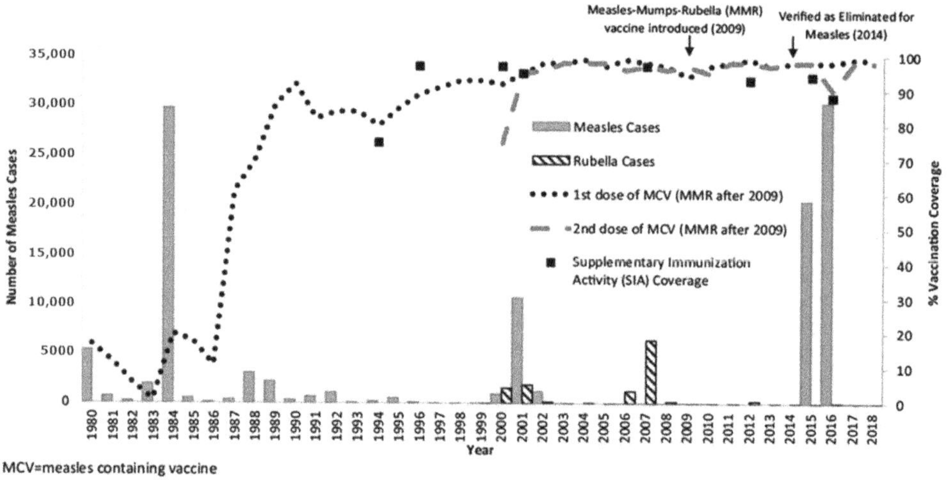


**Figure 1.** Measles and rubella morbidity and measles-containing vaccination coverage by year—Mongolia, 1980–2018. Reprinted from Ref. [10] with permission from Elsevier.

From 2011 to 2014, no confirmed measles cases were reported in Mongolia. The National Verification Committee of Mongolia submitted documentation that endemic measles transmission had been interrupted for 36 months in the presence of elimination-standard surveillance and convincing evidence of high population immunity from routine and supplemental immunization (Figure 1). In March 2014, Mongolia, together with Australia, Macau, and the Republic of Korea, was in the first cohort of countries to be verified by the RVC to have interrupted endemic measles transmission and achieved measles elimination.

### 3.2. *Epidemiology of the Outbreak in Mongolia and Response Measures*

Less than one year after being verified to have achieved elimination, in March 2015 it was confirmed that multiple measles cases were simultaneously detected in several districts in Ulaanbaatar City. By June 2015, cases had been reported from all 21 provinces. In total during an outbreak lasting 24 months, a total of 49,185 cases and at least 115 deaths were confirmed from January 2015 to December 2016 (Figure 2). This was the first and still the largest outbreak to occur in a post-elimination setting; the second-largest post-elimination outbreak occurred in Brazil during 2019, with 15,598 confirmed measles cases [12].

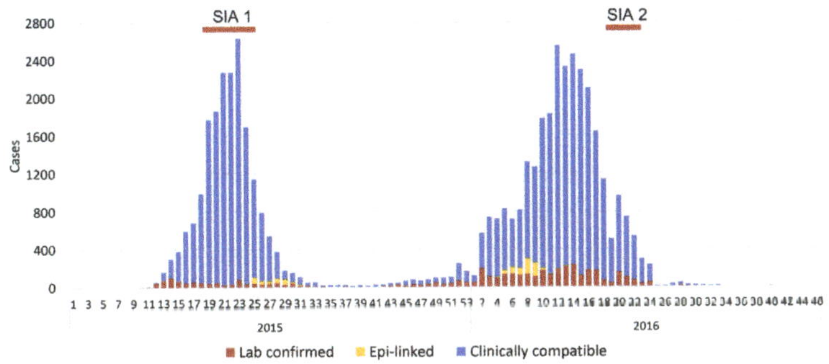


**Figure 2.** Epidemic curve of confirmed measles cases by epidemic week of rash onset—Mongolia, January 2015–December 2016. Data source: case-based measles surveillance data officially reported to the WHO. N = 49,185 cases.

This prolonged period of measles virus transmission in Mongolia had two peaks, one during March–August 2015, and a second peak during October 2015–July 2016; the final measles cases were detected in December 2016. Documentation of measles vaccination among cases was very low. The vast majority of cases reported to the WHO had unknown vaccination status; only 2% had documentation of one or two doses. The most affected age groups overall were infants under 2 years and young adults, with a peak at age 18–22 (Figure 3).

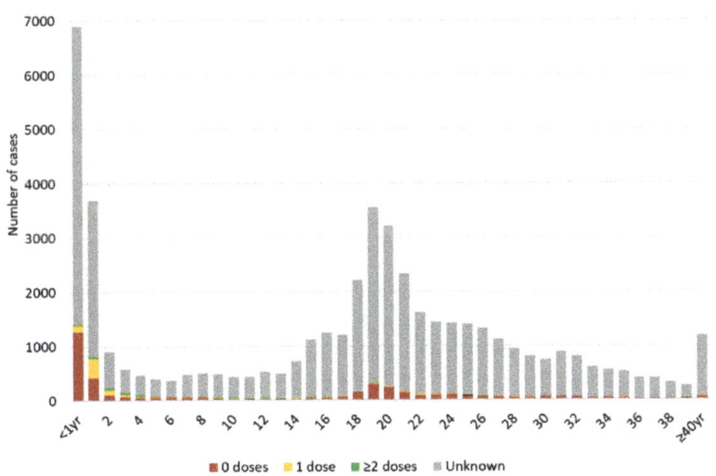


**Figure 3.** Age distribution of confirmed measles cases and reported immunization status—Mongolia, January 2015–December 2016. Data source: case-based measles surveillance data officially reported to the WHO. N = 49,185.

The highest attack rate occurred among young adults aged 15–24 years. This age cohort had been understood to be highly vaccinated through a combination of routine immunization and multiple supplemental immunization campaigns, each achieving at least 96% administrative coverage [13] (Table 1). In addition, people born to these birth cohorts had low incidence during the large outbreak in Ulaanbaatar during 2001 [9], suggesting adequate immunity in those exposed to measles during that period. During outbreak investigations, a small percentage (7%) of adults aged 15–24 years had records of vaccination against measles, but in a published case-control study using reported vaccination status by recall, 23% of cases reported they had received at least one dose of measles vaccine in childhood. That study determined that vaccine effectiveness in this group may be as low as 20–70%, which may have contributed to the high attack rate among young adults [13].

**Table 1.** Supplementary immunization activities (SIA) using measles-containing vaccine—Mongolia, 1994–2016 *.

| Year of SIA | Vaccine Used | Location | Age Group Targeted | Reported Administrative Coverage (%) |
|---|---|---|---|---|
| 1994 | Measles | National | 3–7 years | 75 |
| 1996 | Measles | National | 9 months–11 years | 97 |
| 2000 | Measles | National | 9 months–7 years | 97 |
| 2001 | Measles–Rubella | Ulaanbaatar | 6 months–30 years | 95 |
| 2007 | Measles | National | 2–10 years | 97 |
| 2012 | Measles–Rubella | National | 3–14 years | 93 |
| 2015 | Measles | National | 6 months–<6 years | 94 |
| 2016 | Measles–Rubella | National | 18–<30 years | 88 |

* Reprinted from Ref.[10] with permission from Elsevier.

Most cases were reported from Ulaanbaatar (33,760, 69%), but all 21 Aimags were affected. During the initial peak, transmission appeared to be most concentrated in the southern Aimag of Umnugovi, bordering China; the most intense transmission then spread north through the central Aimags of Dundgovi, Khentii, Tuv, and the capital, Ulaanbataar. During the second peak, intense transmission was initially more concentrated in western (Bayan-Ulgii, Khovd, Uvs) and northern Aimags (Selenge), but rapidly spread nationwide [14].

In 2015 and 2016 (up to August) a total of 14,462 samples were tested for measles IgM and 6962 (48%) were confirmed positive by laboratory criteria. The genotype of the infection was H1; sequencing data indicated a single importation of the MVs/Hong Kong.CHN/49.12/strain that had been circulating predominantly in China since 2012, which was endemic for measles and had been experiencing a large nationwide outbreak during that time [13]. The outbreak timing coincided with the end of the Tsaagansar Mongolian New Year holiday, during which extensive cross-border travel to China and other countries to visit relatives is common.

This outbreak was characterized by a relatively high morbidity and mortality rate. In total, there were 115 deaths officially attributed to measles, and a published manuscript described a number of severe outcomes including encephalitis or meningitis (38 cases) and pneumonia (334 cases) [14]. The overall case-fatality rate was 0.23%; in the capital city, where the majority of cases were registered, case fatality was low (0.1%), but in many rural Aimags, where medical resources were scarcer, case fatality was near or exceeded 1%, up to 1.4% in Khuvsgul Aimag. Severe outcomes were most commonly reported among infants and adults above 25 years of age [14].

Overall, 33% of measles cases were hospitalized [14], which may have contributed to hospital-associated transmission, which was an epidemiological feature of this outbreak [13,15]. This was an important route of exposure for infants and a driver of mortality during the outbreak. Nosocomial infection was a risk factor for death [14,15]. Most officially reported deaths (111, 97%) occurred during the second wave of the outbreak in 2016; this second peak coincided with a peak of seasonal influenza, and a study suggested that co-infection with other respiratory viruses may have led to the significant increase in mortality, especially among young children during this second phase of the outbreak [15].

In response to the initial cases, Mongolia mounted immediate emergency response measures. These included the following: enhancing measles surveillance and public awareness activities; providing vaccination with measles–mumps–rubella vaccine to close contacts of suspected measles cases; conducting a nationwide non-selective (i.e., regardless vaccination history) outbreak response immunization (ORI) campaign with the measles monovalent vaccine. The nationwide non-selective ORI campaign targeted 371,971 children aged six months to five years of age during May 2015–June 2015, achieving 94% administrative coverage nationwide. Following the ORI, measles incidence decreased to a low level during the early winter months, particularly in young children, until the second peak of transmission beginning early 2016 [14]. During the second outbreak period in 2016, there was a slight decrease in the proportion of cases among children aged 1–6 years (12% in 2016 compared to 15% in 2015), but there was a large increase in transmission among infants not targeted by the immunization response in 2015 and not eligible for routine immunization (18% of cases under age 1 year during 2016 compared to 7% during 2015). After the second outbreak peak, a second ORI was conducted during May 2016, targeting 549,846 adults aged 18–30 years, achieving 88% coverage.

Following the second ORI targeting young adults, measles cases rapidly diminished and the final case was reported in December 2016, marking a total of 22 months of transmission without any epidemiological or genotype evidence to suggest multiple independent importations. In September 2016, the Regional Verification Commission determined that measles transmission had continued uninterrupted for greater than 12 months and that measles elimination could no longer be verified [16].

### 3.3. *Root Causes of the Prolonged Outbreak in Mongolia*

Mongolia was verified as having eliminated measles in 2014, but subsequently experienced a prolonged period of nationwide measles transmission that led to loss of measles elimination status in 2016. This unexpected event was the result of several factors.

The outbreak revealed a previously unappreciated large immunity gap among young adults aged 15–24 years, born during the highly unstable decade following the fall of the Soviet Union (1990–2000). This "hidden" immunity gap among young adults may have occurred as a result of mass urban migration in the 1990s, potentially concentrating people from remote areas where historical program gaps may have occurred, or leading to an accumulation of unregistered children and missed vaccinations. In addition, published reports suggest the that waning vaccine field effectiveness in this age group may have occurred as a result of compromised vaccination quality or potency during the 1990s, when infrastructure and public services including public health may have been inconsistent [13]. This multifactorial "hidden" immunity gap among young adults was an unrecognized significant threat to the sustainability of measles elimination. Despite serological evidence of an adult immunity gap in 2004 that was not targeted by the nationwide SIA in 2007, the scale of this gap was not fully understood, and its potential impact was not heavily weighted by the National Verification Committee or the Regional Verification Commission in their determination that Mongolia had achieved measles elimination in 2014. The role of this immunity gap in driving transmission was also not addressed during the initial outbreak response immunization campaign in May–June 2015, which was high quality and achieved high coverage but followed a "traditional" measles outbreak response strategy and targeted young children aged 6 months to 5 years. This led to a further shift of measles epidemiology towards adults and infants below the age of vaccination and wider geographic dissemination of the virus, and this set the conditions for the second wave of transmission during the first quarter of 2016.

Hospital-associated transmission was another major contributor to the scale and duration of the outbreak, particularly at the beginning, when multiple local outbreaks simultaneously occurred in Ulaanbaatar City during the second quarter of 2015, and weak hospital infection prevention and control practices related to measles and other respiratory viruses was another important threat to the sustainability of measles elimination in Mongolia. Healthcare exposure during the incubation period was a significant risk factor for measles infection [13] and measles death [14,15]. Improved infection prevention measures could have prevented the amplification of measles transmission in the healthcare setting, particularly in the early stages of the outbreak, and potentially could have limited the extent of the outbreak after importation. Initial cases were simultaneously detected in several district hospitals before being detected in Ulaanbaatar, suggesting that low-level transmission had already been occurring before the outbreak was detected and that hospital-associated amplification of transmission after importation likely was an important factor in the early spread of the outbreak.

## 4. Cambodia

### *4.1. Path to Measles Elimination in Cambodia*

Cambodia is a lower middle-income country in the Greater Mekong Delta, divided into 25 Provinces, including the Phnom Penh Municipality, and 103 "operational districts" (ODs) (during 2016–2019, there were between 98 and 100 ODs). Cambodia shares porous land borders with three countries that remain endemic for measles: Thailand, Lao People's Democratic Republic, and Vietnam. There is significant mobility across these borders, resulting in distinct challenges for immunization planning and disease surveillance. Several cities in Cambodia are major international tourist destinations, drawing 6.2 million visitors from within the region and beyond in 2018 [17]. Within the Greater Mekong Delta, which includes these neighboring countries, along with Yunnan Province of China and Myanmar, there are an estimated 3–5 million migrant workers supporting generally low-skilled work on an irregular, seasonal, or short-term basis. High-traffic crossing points into Cambodia, including Poipet on the Thai border, Bavet on the Vietnamese border, and Tropaeng Kreal on the Lao PDR border, among many others, are important routes for the potential importation of the measles virus. In addition, there is very easy movement across borders in some parts of the country from village to village, and these countries share a number of cross-border populations and ethnic groups maintaining family ties across national boundaries, including the Khmer Krom, Hmong, and various hill tribes such as Lamam, Brao, Kravet, Jarai, and Chong. In some cases, these populations may lack a sense of specific national identity, remain unregistered in any country, and maintain a highly mobile style of living, creating conditions that lead to the virus being systematically missed by both routine and supplemental immunization planning and implementation.

Following the end of the Khmer Rouge period in 1979, Cambodia underwent significant political and economic transformations, including rebuilding a health sector that had been devastated by the dismantling of medical facilities, systematic targeting of skilled healthcare workers and national resources, and policies focused nearly exclusively on agricultural labor. The government of Cambodia established the expanded program on immunization (EPI) in 1986, and program activities reached all provinces of the country by 1988. The Cambodian Ministry of Health (MOH) established the National Immunization Program (NIP) in 2000. The measles monovalent vaccine was introduced into routine immunization in Cambodia in 1986 at 9 months of age. Reported coverage of the first dose of measles-containing vaccine (MCV1) has trended upward since 2004, with consistently high coverage (over 90%) since 2009 and reaching 95% in 2015 (Figure 4). In 2015, out of 25 provinces in the country, 13 provinces reported >100% (100–122%) MCV1 coverage, while 10 provinces reported <90% (73–89%) (Figure 5). The Cambodia MOH introduced the second routine dose of MCV at 18 months of age in late 2012. The first routine dose of MCV given at 9 months of age was replaced with the measles–rubella vaccine (MR) in late 2013; MCV2 was switched to MR during 2015. Coverage with MCV2 slowly progressed from 63% in 2013 to 72% in 2015, with only two provinces (8%) in 2013 and one province (4%) in 2015 meeting the 95% coverage target.

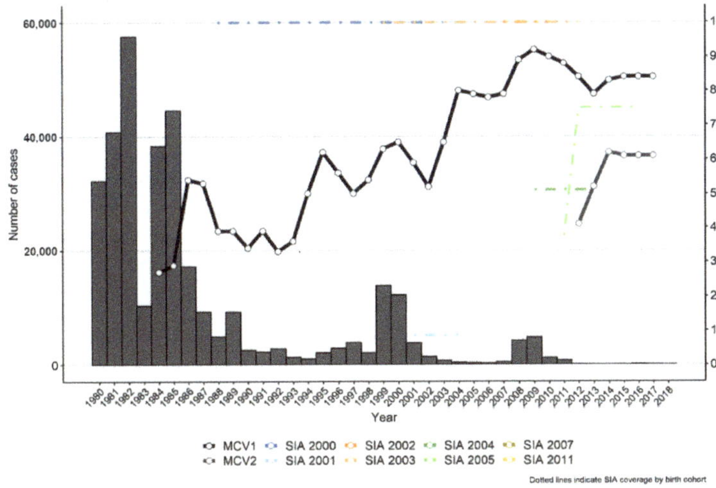


**Figure 4.** Measles morbidity and measles-containing vaccination coverage by year—Cambodia, 1980–2018. Dotted lines indicate SIA coverage by birth year. Data source: case-based surveillance data reported to WHO, WHO-UNICEF Estimates of National Immunization Coverage, and national estimates of SIA coverage by birth cohort, from Cambodia MOH reported to the WHO.

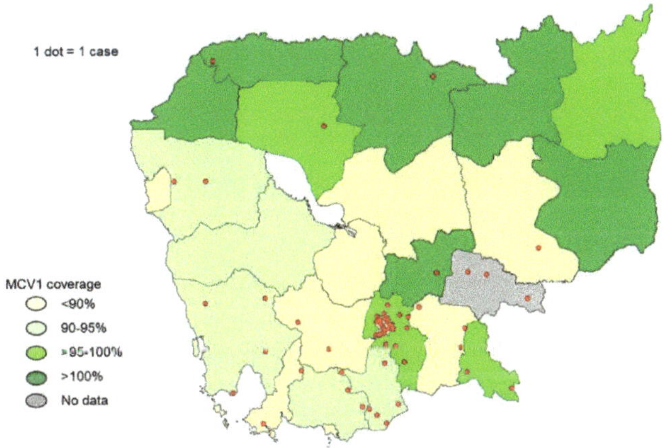


**Figure 5.** Geographic distribution of confirmed measles cases—Cambodia, 2016–2017, and reported Provincial MCV1 coverage in 2015. Source: Case-based surveillance data and immunization coverage data reported to the WHO.

Cambodia conducted six large-scale mass vaccination campaigns with MCV from 2000 to 2014, achieving very high reported coverage (Figure 4). A nationwide measles catch-up SIA, targeting 4.5 million children aged 9 months to 14 years, achieved 98% and 103% during two different phases between October 2001 and April 2003. In 2005, high-risk areas were selected, comprising approximately 10% of the total population, such as mobile Vietnamese villages and boat dwellers along the Tonlesap river and lake, Muslim communities, Khmer and Vietnamese slum areas in Phnom Penh, and migrating Khmer groups at the Thailand border for a mass vaccination campaign targeting 134,067 children aged 9 to 59 months and achieving 86% coverage. During 2007, a nationwide follow-up measles SIA targeted 1,457,235 children from 9 to 59 months of age, achieving 105% coverage. In 2011, a nationwide follow-up measles SIA achieved 105% coverage of 1.5 million children aged 9 months to 59 months. In 2013–2014, a wide age range nationwide SIA targeted 4,345,392 children aged 9 months to 14 years, achieving 105% coverage. This was followed in 2014 by selective catch-up activities in high-risk communities in 23 provinces, vaccinating 11,115 children with MR1 and 21,158 children with MR2.

Measles case-based surveillance was started in 1999. In 2014, a broader case definition for suspected measles cases was updated to include fever and maculopapular rash. The last laboratory confirmed case was detected in November 2011; in March 2015, the Regional Verification Commission for Measles Elimination in the Western Pacific (RVC) verified that Cambodia had interrupted endemic measles transmission for a period of at least 36 months since 2011. Beginning January 2016, Cambodia experienced a series of importations of measles virus that led to a prolonged outbreak until June 2017, and from December 2018 to December 2020 (Figure 6).

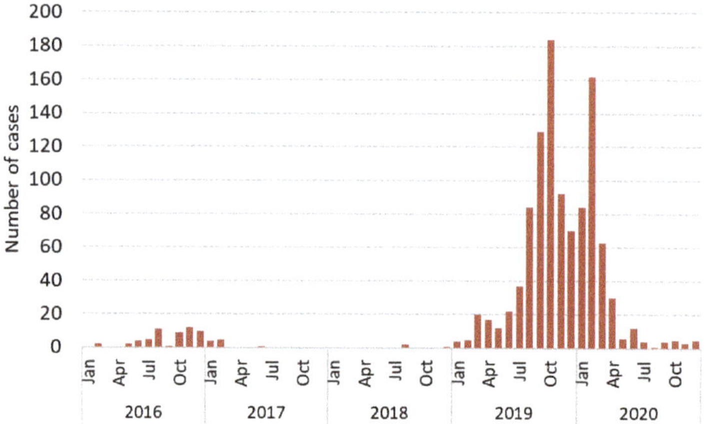


**Figure 6.** Epidemic curve of laboratory-confirmed measles cases by month of rash onset—Cambodia, 2016–2020. Data source: case-based measles surveillance data officially reported to the WHO. N = 1056 cases.

### *4.2. Outbreaks, Root Causes and Loss of Elimination Status in Cambodia*

#### 4.2.1. January 2016–June 2017

Beginning in January 2016, less than one year after achieving measles elimination, Cambodia began detecting laboratory-confirmed cases of measles. In total during January 2016–June 2017, a total of 66 lab-confirmed cases were reported from 33 operational districts in 16 provinces (Figure 5). There were no reported deaths.

A robust outbreak investigation and response was initiated, including local outbreak response immunization, nationwide inclusion of a zero-dose MR vaccine to children aged 6 months–<9 months and an extra vaccination opportunity offered to children aged 24 months to <59 months, and catch-up vaccination in affected ODs. A scheduled Japanese Encephalitis immunization campaign was broadened to include the MR vaccine, non-selectively targeting children aged 9 months to 59 months in 11 provinces and achieving 91% coverage. Finally, a nationwide preventive supplemental immunization campaign that had been previously scheduled for October 2017 was conducted early, during March–April 2017, achieving 90% administrative coverage, but post-survey coverage was 75%. Mop-up activities targeted areas with lower coverage and delivered an additional 103,056 doses. Vitamin A and Mebendazole were also provided as part of this activity. The last case of lab-confirmed measles in 2017 occurred on 8 June. Intensive case investigation and case finding determined that 3 cases were classified as imported, 54 were import-related, and 9 were unknown. During the 17-month duration of the outbreak, there were four gaps longer than 30 days, despite active case finding and surveillance meeting key performance indicators for sensitivity. In two instances, the gap was followed by new importations identified by case investigation; in two instances, the gap was interrupted by cases with no epidemiological link, no travel history, and an unknown source.

There were two genotypes detected during the 2016–2017 outbreak: D8 and B3. B3 had never been detected in Cambodia before 2016, but the B3 genotype detected during this outbreak also had no identical match in MeaNS [7]. Among the B3 and unknown genotype cases, 7 cases had unknown source of infection; 15 cases had contact with a hospital, there were 37 secondary cases in five clusters, and 4 cases that could not be assigned to a cluster. There were three clusters of D8 cases and transmission chains: two unlinked cases in different provinces, with a history of travel to Thailand; one case from Phnom Penh with no history of travel and contact with a hospital during the incubation period; and a cluster of four cases linked to history of travel to Thailand. Genetic sequencing data supported repeated importation from Thailand as the likely source.

To guide RVC deliberations, the WHO conducted an analysis to reassess discarded cases to determine whether true measles cases potentially testing false negative for measles IgM due to timing of specimen collection might have occurred during the gaps in transmission that might indicate uninterrupted transmission exceeding 12 months. The analysis found a total of 342 IgM-negative discarded cases where the specimen was collected <4 and >28 days after rash onset. Of these, 221 had a documented history of vaccination, leaving 121 cases potentially erroneously discarded. All 121 had at least one of the classic symptoms of measles (cough, coryza, conjunctivitis). Cases were reviewed in detail to identify "probable" false negative cases by epidemiological or clinical criteria, yielding 30 such cases: 6 cases had contact with a confirmed measles case during the incubation period, 23 cases had Koplik's sign (a clinical finding highly associated with measles infection) and were from an OD where confirmed cases had been reported, and 1 case met all these criteria. Including these additional probable false negative cases indicated that the maximum duration of continuous transmission may have been 47 weeks, including a 35-day gap in transmission during weeks 37–39, 2017 (Figure 7).

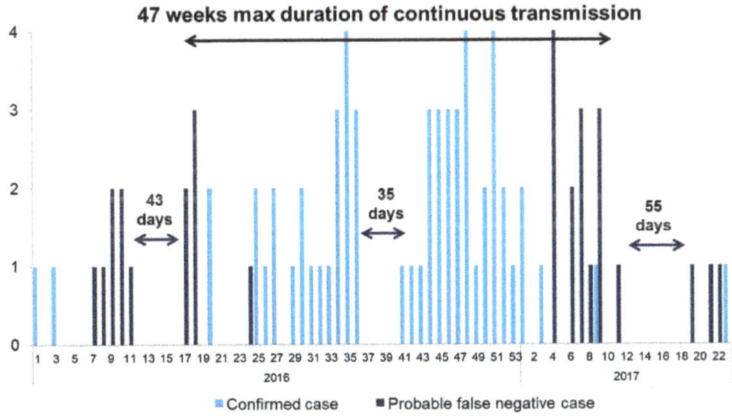


**Figure 7.** Epidemic curve of confirmed (n = 66) and probable (n = 30) measles cases—Cambodia, 2016–2017. "Probable false-negative cases" include cases that were not lab-confirmed but that had epidemiological or clinical characteristics compatible with a potential false negative laboratory result. Source: Case-based surveillance data reported to the WHO.

The RVC determined that the data indicated that the 2016–2017 outbreak was the result of multiple independent importations and low-level transmission sustained largely by nosocomial transmission. Due to aggressive outbreak response and intensive case investigation, the outbreak was contained with a maximum duration of uninterrupted transmission of less than 12 months, and the RVC verified that measles elimination had been sustained.

4.2.2. December 2018–December 2020

During December 2018–December 2020, Cambodia experienced a second, larger outbreak after achieving elimination. A total of 1056 confirmed measles cases and no deaths were reported to the WHO during this period. Most cases were reported from major reference hospitals throughout Cambodia; only 12% of cases were reported from community health facilities. The majority of cases (835, 79%) were among children aged 6 months to 10 years, but 7% of cases occurred among infants below the age of eligibility for MCV1 at 9 months. Most cases were unvaccinated (723, 68%) or had only one dose (172, 16%).

Initially in 2019, the outbreak was concentrated in Siem Reap district, Cambodia's most important area for national and international tourism and the location of a major children's referral hospital. Overall, the capital, Phnom Penh, was the most affected (23% of cases), but there was widespread geographic distribution; cases were reported from 24 of 25 (96%) provinces and 77 of 103 (75%) ODs. During this outbreak, B3 and D8 genotypes were again detected. Detailed genetic characterization of the B3 viruses, detected from Siem Reap OD, indicated one distinct sequence identification (DSID 5937). According to data in MeaNS, globally this DSID has only been identified once before in the Philippines, one month (January 2019) before first detection in Cambodia [7]. The rash onset dates of the B3 cases ranged over 23 weeks from 18 February until 27 July 2019. No cases selected for testing with rash onset after 21 November 2019 resulted in a B3 genotype. It is highly likely that the B3 transmission within Cambodia ended in late July or August 2019. Intensive case investigation indicated multiple independent chains of transmission of the same B3 measles strain, resulting from multiple importations to this major international tourism center. Genotype lineage D8-2019B was the most common in 2019 and 2020. Epidemiological investigation identified at least three independent importations from Vietnam and at least eight independent importations from Thailand. There were four other lineage clusters epidemiologically linked to repeated introductions into the country and 13 other genotype lineages with sporadic detection during the outbreak period.

Epidemiological investigation indicated that nosocomial transmission played a much more important role in the spread of this outbreak and wide geographic distribution than community-based transmission. Medical care in Cambodia is often sought in referral hospitals at great distances from home. From a subset of 1047 cases reported to the WHO between December 2018 and October 2020, 854 (82%) cases were admitted at a hospital for treatment before, during, or after rash onset while symptomatic. Of cases without direct epidemiological linkage to a confirmed case, 58% reported healthcare facility exposure during the incubation period. Of 145 cases with probable nosocomial infection during this period, 125 (86%) exposures occurred in one of five major referral children's hospitals. Table 2 illustrates the large number of measles cases admitted for care in these hospitals, and that cases linked to these hospitals were detected across a wide geographical area within Cambodia. Figure 8 visualizes the exposure patterns of a subset of these cases. Of 590 individual cases with available contact-tracing data during 1 January 2019 to 29 December 2019, 579 (98%) reported hospitalization during the symptomatic period, 139 (24%) reported they had been exposed to a measles case in a hospital prior to symptom onset, and 81 cases (14%) reported exposure to a symptomatic measles case outside of the hospital setting. Of these 81 cases, 38 (47%) reported person–person exposure to contacts who had themselves been previously exposed to measles in a hospital. The investigation determined that, despite efforts to strengthen hospital infection prevention and control measures, healthcare-acquired infections were propagating continuous measles virus transmission and seeding measles virus across a wide geographic area through patients returning to their home province after infection during hospitalization.

**Table 2.** Cases linked to healthcare exposure—Cambodia, December 2018–October 2020. Source: case-based surveillance data reported to the WHO.

| Hospital | Cases Admitted to Hospital (# of Unique Provinces) | Cases Linked to Hospital Exposure | Provinces with Cases Linked to Hospital Exposure | Districts with Cases Linked to Hospital Exposure |
|---|---|---|---|---|
| A | 290 (21) | 51 | 9 | 27 |
| B | 71 (16) | 22 | 8 | 12 |
| C | 40 (1) | 28 | 4 | 8 |
| D | 64 (8) | 21 | 4 | 10 |
| E | 13 (2) | 3 | 1 | 3 |
| Other HCF | 101 (19) | 20 | 11 | 17 |

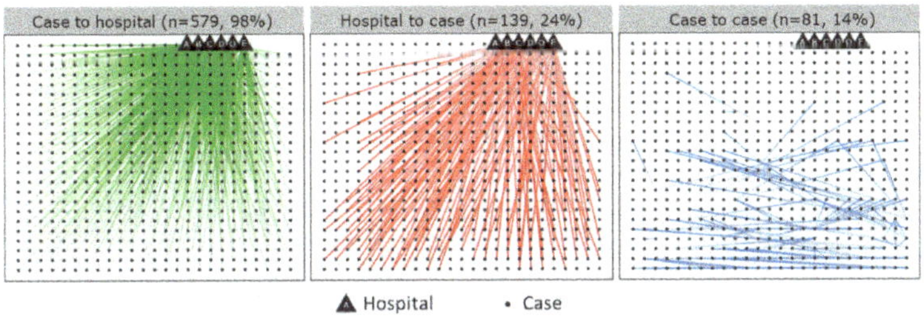


**Figure 8.** Contact tracing indicating the role of nosocomial transmission in the amplification of measles spread—Cambodia, January–December 2019. The dots in each panel represent N = 590 individual cases for which contact-tracing information was available, epidemiologically linking each case to one or more cases or to exposure to a healthcare facility, or who visited a healthcare facility while symptomatic. The same cases are represented in each panel. Each triangle represents a different hospital indicated by letters A–E. Hospital "O" represents any healthcare facility besides the five largest referral hospitals in Cambodia. Green lines indicate cases that were hospitalized during the infectious period (n = 579, 98%). Red lines indicate cases with documented exposure to a measles case at a hospital (n = 139, 24%). Blue lines indicate epidemiological linkage between individual cases (n = 81, 14%).

Following initial detection of confirmed measles cases in December 2018, Cambodia mounted an urgent outbreak response, including intensive case investigation and contact tracing, sensitization of local health authorities, rapid routine coverage assessment at the village level (Figure 9), and local outbreak response immunization, which vaccinated a total of 158,189 children aged 6 months to less than 15 years. A nationwide catch-up campaign vaccinated an additional 102,804 children aged 6 months to 15 years, and in Siem Reap district, a sub-national non-selective campaign vaccinated 96,893 children aged 6 months to 15 years during April–May 2019, achieving 89.3% coverage.

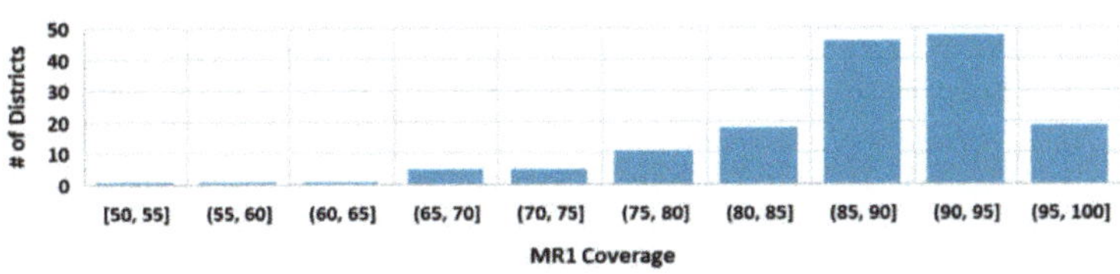


**Figure 9.** Histogram of average village-level routine MR1 coverage by district from rapid coverage assessments during case investigation—Cambodia, 2019–2020.

The endemicity of measles virus transmission in both Thailand and Vietnam and the pressure of imported viruses from these countries was low from 2015 to the first half of 2018, but significantly increased in Thailand from the second half of 2018 to the first quarter of 2020 (D8 and B3) and in Vietnam from early 2018 to the first quarter of 2020 (D8). This resulted in the increased importation of measles into Cambodia from early 2019 to the first quarter of 2020. Epidemiological case investigation and genotyping sequence data indicated numerous independent measles importations of predominantly the D8 virus during this prolonged period of transmission (Figure 10). As case counts increased and public health resources became strained towards the end of 2019, the capacity for intensive case investigation and genotyping to identify independent chains of importation was reduced. From October 2019, most lab-confirmed cases lacked information on epidemiological linkage, and most cases lacked serological samples for laboratory case confirmation or virological samples to facilitate genotyping; as a result, until the end of the outbreak, Cambodia was unable to differentiate independent importations or unlinked chains of transmission.

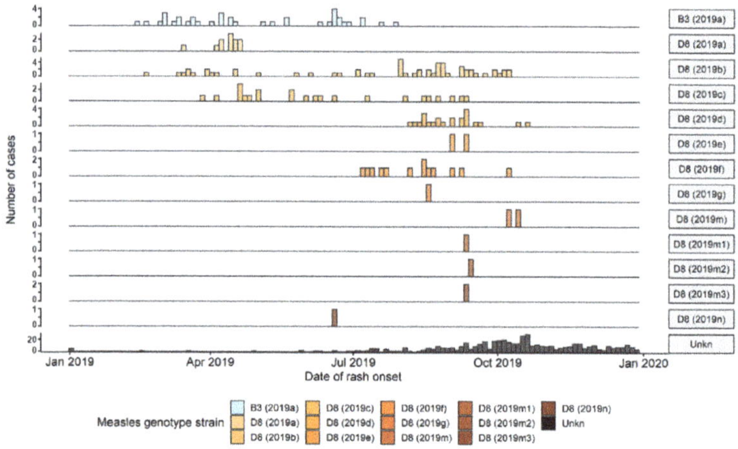


**Figure 10.** Epidemic curve by genotype strain and date of rash onset—Cambodia, January 2019–December 2019. Source: Case-based surveillance and laboratory data officially reported to the WHO.

During its 2021 meeting, the RVC concluded that "[a] D8 lineage, detected between February 2019 and April 2020, has a 15-month period of likely transmission that included many sporadic measles cases of unknown genotype and origin" and determined that measles elimination status had not been sustained.

## 5. Conclusions and Implications for the Global Measles Elimination Effort

The achievement of measles elimination in Mongolia and Cambodia illustrated the success that is possible by a strong national commitment to the regional public health goal and strong immunization program focused on a national goal. The path to achieving elimination in these countries reflected decades of intensive investment by the countries and partners to achieve the highest possible vaccination coverage among children through routine immunization program and supplementary immunization activities targeting young birth cohorts, and to implement high-quality, sensitive, and representative surveillance. The prolonged outbreaks in these countries following the importation of the virus from neighboring endemic countries, which led to loss of elimination so soon after this impressive achievement, revealed vulnerabilities that had been previously unrecognized during the lead-up to achieving elimination.

The experiences of Mongolia and Cambodia provide several important lessons for the global initiative to eliminate measles from all six WHO regions. First, these events underscore the need for National Verification Committees (NVCs) and Regional Verification Commissions (RVCs) to consider additional issues when assessing the elimination status of countries, with particular attention on the "sustainability" criteria. First, these bodies should extend their assessment and evaluation of population immunity beyond the traditional focus on children. It is essential that these bodies consider a wider age demographic, including adults, as well as high-risk groups within the population in their efforts to understand the risk of large outbreaks after future importation, and sustainability of measles elimination. NVCs should collaborate closely with National Immunization Programs (NIPs) to identify subpopulations with significant immunity gaps who may be left out of routine immunization programming, such as young adults and migrant workers. These are often the segments of the population that fuel outbreaks due to their mobility and concentration in certain employment sectors. Collaboration of the NIP with non-traditional sectors such as the Ministries of Labor or Immigration may be required in order to develop strategies for the vaccination of groups normally excluded from routine immunization programming. Proactive identification and vaccination of these groups can significantly reduce the risk of outbreaks. In addition, this may include advocating for countries to take steps to address threats to sustainability that are outside the immunization program, such as poor hospital infection prevention and control practices, and cross-border movement.

Countries that have interrupted endemic transmission and achieved measles elimination status continue to be vulnerable to the importation of the measles virus from other endemic countries, particularly if they share porous borders with these countries, and be at risk for losing elimination status if the imported virus finds a significant population immunity gap, leading to prolonged transmission. The large outbreak in Mongolia is one example of the risk that, even in countries with high estimated vaccine coverage among children, significant but unknown immunity gaps might exist or emerge in the population. This may result from undocumented or under-appreciated historical disruptions to the immunization program (e.g., cold chain failures) and other events such as mass population movement or temporary immigration such as labor migration, that might impact coverage estimates or immunization program planning. Countries at particular risk of frequent importation of the measles virus from neighboring endemic countries, as exemplified by the experience of Cambodia during 2016–2020, may have the additional burden of needing to invest significant resources and effort into both epidemiological investigation and the collection of virological samples for genotyping in order to distinguish independent importations and limited chains of transmission from continuous re-establishment of endemic measles transmission. Differentiating endemic transmission from frequent importation–elimination cycles will remain difficult while there is endemic transmission across porous borders and state-less populations are accounted for in no country's denominator.

Cambodia's experience in particular highlights that hospital-associated amplification of measles transmission is a serious potential threat to countries working to achieve or sustain measles elimination. During the 2019–2020 outbreak in Cambodia, an overwhelming majority of cases either visited healthcare facilities during their symptomatic period or were exposed to hospital facilities during the incubation period, and confirmed exposures in a small number of referral hospitals were linked to cases with widespread geographic distribution within the country. This experience illustrates the importance of strengthening infection prevention and control practices within healthcare settings (including strict isolation of measles cases in hospitals and clinics where possible), to prevent such facilities from becoming epicenters for disease spread, and is a reminder that sustaining elimination requires investment in health system resilience, inter-sectoral collaboration, and community engagement.

Strong political support for and a proactive attitude towards prevention and preparedness are therefore required in order to sustain elimination status. Strong routine immunization programs that aim to ensure equitable delivery of immunization through strategic and high-quality micro-planning, outreach, and catch-up vaccinations should be the backbone of outbreak prevention. Outbreaks and individual cases should be carefully investigated to identify root causes for lack of vaccination and risks for virus importation. This use of measles cases as a "tracer" may identify systematic issues related to routine immunization strategy and implementation, can guide broader immunization systems strengthening, and focus surveillance efforts. Supplemental immunization activities (SIA) should be implemented to close immunity gaps before an imported case leads to a large outbreak and potential loss of elimination status. SIAs, tailored to the needs of specific at-risk groups, are vital for maintaining the hard-won gains against measles. Development of and regularly updating national outbreak preparedness plans is critically important to ensure that the impact of potential outbreaks can be minimized. This includes meticulous and timely investigation of measles cases and outbreaks to identify and disrupt all chains of virus transmission through enhanced surveillance and contact tracing, and to understand the transmission dynamics and root causes of outbreaks to guide both the immediate response as well as programmatic changes or strengthening.

Stronger coordination and synchronized operations should be established and promoted at the global level to achieve and sustain measles elimination. Cambodia and Mongolia invested significant effort and resources towards achieving measles elimination, but they had neighboring countries still experiencing large-scale endemic transmission with frequent cross-border importation of the virus. The WHO and the global community must intensify their promotion of coordinated and synchronized activities towards measles elimination. The vulnerability of countries (particularly lower- and middle-income countries) who have achieved measles elimination to repeated importation of the measles virus from endemic countries highlights the need for greater collaboration and coordination across neighboring countries and regions. This includes the sharing of best practices, alignment of messaging to shared special populations, sharing of surveillance and epidemic intelligence data in a systematic and standardized manner between countries and across regions, and synchronization of activities targeting highly mobile groups that may span borders and which may not otherwise be included in routine national planning. This synergy is essential for the efficient use of resources and for effectively managing cross-border disease threats.

## 6. Conclusions

These experiences of Mongolia and Cambodia demonstrate that the asynchronous and uncoordinated pursuit of measles elimination in individual countries can ultimately create a vulnerability in those countries that do invest effort and resources towards achieving that goal. While countries and regions have made great progress towards the goal of measles elimination, without a global measles eradication goal and accelerated efforts coordinated at the regional and global level some of these successes have become Pyrrhic victories. Countries that have made substantial progress towards or have reached elimination should not be penalized by their successes by the burden of preventing re-establishment in the face of the continued regional and global circulation of measles. A global measles eradication goal is not merely aspirational but would be an essential step in safeguarding the investments and public health triumphs of countries that have achieved elimination status, and ultimately lead to a legacy of enhanced global health security and a healthier world.

**Author Contributions:** Conceptualization, J.H. and Y.T.; methodology, J.H., V.G. and Y.T.; formal analysis, J.H., O.D., O.V., S.C., S.D., V.G., S.H., K.M., R.E. and Y.T.; investigation, J.H., O.D., O.V., S.C., S.D., V.G., S.H., R.E., Y.Z. and Y.T.; data curation, J.H., V.G. and K.M.; writing—original draft preparation, J.H., A.P., C.-w.L., V.G. and Y.T.; writing—review and editing, J.H., O.D., O.V., S.C., S.D., V.G., S.H., M.I., C.-w.L., A.P., K.M. and Y.T.; visualization, J.H., K.M. and V.G.; supervision, Y.T. All authors have read and agreed to the published version of the manuscript.

**Funding:** This research received no external funding.

**Conflicts of Interest:** The authors declare no conflicts of interest.

## Abbreviations

The following abbreviations are used in this manuscript:

| | |
|---|---|
| WHO | World Health Organization |
| RVC | Regional Verification Commission |
| MCV | Measles-Containing Vaccine |
| SIA | Supplemental Immunization Activities |
| MR | Measles–Rubella (vaccine) |
| NVC | National Verification Committee |
| EPI | Expanded Program on Immunization |
| NIP | National Immunization Program |
| MOH | Ministry of Health |
| OD | Operational District |
| MeaNS | Measles Virus Nucleotide Surveillance |
| WUENIC | WHO–UNICEF Estimates of National Immunization Coverage |
| MMR | Measles–Mumps–Rubella (vaccine) |
| ORI | Outbreak Response Immunization |
| IgM | Immunoglobulin M |
| DSID | Distinct Sequence Identification |

## References


1. WHO Regional Office for the Western Pacific. *WPR/RC54.R3 Expanded Programme on Immunization: Measles and Hepatitis B (Resolution)* ; Regional Committee for the Western Pacific: Manila, Philippines , 2003.
2. WHO Regional Office for the Western Pacific. *WPR/RC56.R8 Measles Elimination, Hepatitis B Control and Poliomyelitis Eradication (Resolution)*; Regional Committee for the Western Pacific: Manila, Philippines, 2005.
3. WHO Regional Office for the Western Pacific. *WPR/RC61.R7 Vaccine Preventable Diseases: Measles Elimination, Hepatitis B Control and Poliomyelitis Eradication (Resolution)*; Regional Committee for the Western Pacific: Manila, Philippines, 2010.
4. WHO Regional Office for the Western Pacific. *WPR/RC63.R5 Elimination of Measles and Acceleration of Rubella Control (Resolution)*; Regional Committee for the Western Pacific: Manila, Philippines, 2012.
5. World Health Organization Regional Office for the Western Pacific. *Guidelines on Verification of Measles and Rubella Elimination in the Western Pacific Region*, 2nd ed.; World Health Organization Regional Office for the Western Pacific: Manila, Philippines, 2019.
6. World Health Organization; United Nations Children's Fund. *WHO/UNICEF Estimates of National Immunization Coverage*; Technical Report; World Health Organization: Geneva, Switzerland, 2022.
7. Public Health England; World Health Organization. *Measles Nucleotide Surveillance Database (MeaNs) [Online Database]*; Technical Report; Public Health England: London, UK; World Health Organization: Geneva, Switzerland, 2020.
8. Tsilaajav, T.; Ser-Od, E.; Baasai, B.; Byambaa, G.; Shagdarsuren, O. *Mongolia Health System*; Chapter Historical Background; World Health Organization: Geneva, Switzerland, 2013.
9. Rentsen, T.; Enkhtuya, B.; Nymadawa, P.; Kobune, F.; Suzuki, K.; Yoshida, H.; Hachiya, M. Measles outbreak after a post-honeymoon period in Mongolia, 2001. *Jpn. J. Infect. Dis.* **2007**, *60*, 198–199. [CrossRef]
10. Nogareda, F.; Gunregjav, N.; Sarankhuu, A.; Munkhbat, E.; Ichinnorov, E.; Nymadawa, P.; Wannemuehler, K.; Mulders, M.N.; Hagan, J.; Patel, M.K. Measles and Rubella IgG Seroprevalence in Persons 6 Month-35 Years of Age, Mongolia, 2016. *Vaccine* **2020**, *38*, 4200–4208. [CrossRef] [PubMed]
11. Gantulga, D.; Tuul, R.; Anand, S. *Determination of Immunity Level against Vaccine-Preventable Diseases among General Population of Mongolia*; Technical Report; National Center for Communicable Diseases, Ministry of Health: Mongolia, Ulaanbaatar, 2005.
12. Makarenko, C.; San Pedro, A.; Paiva, N.S.; Santos, J.P.C.D.; Medronho, R.A.; Gibson, G. o Paulo. *Rev. Saude Publica* **2022**, *56*, 50. [CrossRef] [PubMed]
13. Hagan, J.E.; Takashima, Y.; Sarankhuu, A.; Dashpagma, O.; Jantsansengee, B.; Pastore, R.; Nyamaa, G.; Yadamsuren, B.; Mulders, M.N.; Wannemuehler, K.A.; et al. Risk Factors for Measles Virus Infection Among Adults During a Large Outbreak in Postelimination Era in Mongolia, 2015. *J. Infect. Dis.* **2017**, *216*, 1187–1195. [CrossRef] [PubMed]
14. Orsoo, O.; Saw, Y.M.; Sereenen, E.; Yadamsuren, B.; Byambaa, A.; Kariya, T.; Yamamoto, E.; Hamajima, N. Epidemiological characteristics and trends of a Nationwide measles outbreak in Mongolia, 2015–2016. *BMC Public Health* **2019**, *19*, 201. [CrossRef] [PubMed]
15. Lee, C.T.; Hagan, J.E.; Jantsansengee, B.; Tumurbaatar, O.E.; Altanchimeg, S.; Yadamsuren, B.; Demberelsuren, S.; Tserendorj, C.; Munkhtogoo, O.; Badarch, D.; et al. Increase in Infant Measles Deaths During a Nationwide Measles Outbreak-Mongolia, 2015–2016. *J. Infect. Dis.* **2019**, *220*, 1771–1779. [CrossRef] [PubMed]

16. WHO Regional Office for the Western Pacific. *Fifth Annual Meeting of the Regional Verification Commission for Measles Elimination in the Western Pacific, Sydney, Australia, 20–23 September 2016: Meeting Report*; WHO Regional Office for the Western Pacific: Manila, Philippines, 2016.
17. Cambodia Ministry of Tourism. *Tourism Statistics Report*; Technical Report; Cambodia Ministry of Tourism: Phnom Penh, Cambodia, 2018.

*vaccines*

MDPI

*Article*

# Congenital Rubella Syndrome Does Not Increase with Introduction of Rubella-Containing Vaccine

**Kurt Frey**

Institute for Disease Modeling, Bill and Melinda Gates Foundation, Seattle, WA 98109, USA;
kurt.frey@gatesfoundation.org

**Abstract:** Rubella infection is typically mild or asymptomatic except when infection occurs during pregnancy. Infection in early pregnancy can cause miscarriage, stillbirth, or congenital rubella syndrome. Only individuals that are still susceptible to rubella infection during child-bearing age are vulnerable to this burden. Rubella-containing vaccine (RCV) is safe and effective, providing life-long immunity. However, average age-at-infection increases with increasing vaccination coverage, which could potentially lead to increased disease burden if the absolute risk of infection during child-bearing age increases. The dynamics of rubella transmission were explored using EMOD, a software tool for building stochastic, agent-based infection models. Simulations of pre-vaccine, endemic transmission of rubella virus introduced RCV at varying levels of coverage to determine the expected future trajectories of disease burden. Introducing RCV reduces both rubella virus transmission and disease burden for a period of around 15 years. Increased disease burden is only possible more than a decade post-introduction, and only for contexts with persistently high transmission intensity. Low or declining rubella virus transmission intensity is associated with both greater burden without vaccination and greater burden reduction with vaccination. The risk of resurgent burden due to incomplete vaccination only exists for locations with persistently high infectivity, high connectivity, and high fertility. A trade-off between the risk of a small, future burden increase versus a large, immediate burden decrease strongly favors RCV introduction.

**Keywords:** rubella; congenital rubella syndrome; vaccine introduction; agent-based model

## 1. Introduction

Infection by the rubella virus is typically mild [1], with symptoms that are often subclinical or absent [2]. However, infection in early pregnancy can cause miscarriage, stillbirth, or congenital rubella syndrome (CRS) [3]. Only individuals that are still susceptible to rubella infection during child-bearing age are vulnerable to this burden.

A single dose of rubella-containing vaccine (RCV) induces high seroconversion rates (≥95%) and provides long-term immunity, like that produced by natural infection. In most countries, RCV is administered along with the measles vaccine and follows the two-dose schedule for measles. Rubella control efforts benefit from established measles control programs; RCV introduction is typically achieved by switching from monovalent measles-containing vaccine (MCV) to bivalent measles–rubella (MR) vaccine. This switch leverages established delivery modes and avoids many logistical challenges associated with new vaccine introduction. Switching to a bivalent vaccine leads to around a two-fold increase in its cost, but the vaccine cost is a minority component in the total cost of delivery [4].

The global incidence of rubella and the burden of CRS has decreased significantly since the introduction of a rubella-containing vaccine in 1969. A majority of the remaining burden is in countries that do not routinely vaccinate for rubella [5,6]. At the end of 2023, nineteen countries had yet to introduce RCV into their recommended schedule for vaccination. As shown in Figure 1, these countries are predominantly in sub-Saharan Africa. While the economic benefits of rubella vaccination are large [7], resource constraints in low- and lower-middle-income countries are also substantial. Operational considerations may limit the reach of health services and result in incomplete vaccination, which has the potential to lead to an increase in disease burden [8].

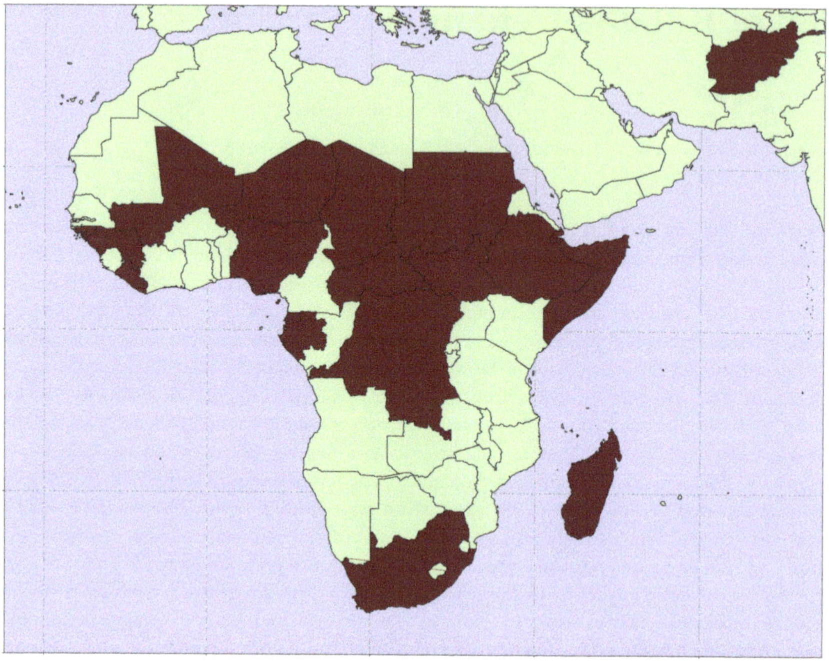

**Figure 1.** Map showing the locations of nineteen countries yet to introduce RCV [9].

The average age-at-infection increases with increasing vaccination coverage, which has the potential to increase the disease burden if the absolute risk of rubella infection during child-bearing age increases. The primary consideration when deciding to introduce RCV is ensuring that the burden of disease will go down. Current guidance from the World Health Organization suggests that countries planning to introduce RCV should have at least 80% coverage with the first dose of the measles vaccine [10]. This level of coverage was established to support the control of rubella in very-high-transmission settings [11] and is sufficient for elimination in nearly all contexts.

Sustained rubella transmission tends to occur only in large populations, with interruption of transmission occurring during epidemic troughs in smaller communities [12]. Local extinction will tend to increase average age-at-infection by allowing individuals to remain susceptible for longer, possibly extending into child-bearing age. Outbreaks following re-introduction of the pathogen have the potential for elevated burden because of this accumulation of susceptibility.

Any approach to vaccination that ensures immunity before child-bearing age will lead to a reduced burden. Historically, two primary approaches were considered: selective vaccination of girls and young women, and universal vaccination of infants [8]. Selective vaccination aims to reduce burden without interrupting transmission, but can still result in an accumulation of susceptibility leading to severe outbreaks [13]. Universal vaccination leading to the interruption of transmission is the preferred strategy for controlling the rubella burden [10], although selective vaccination can be a useful supplement when infant vaccination rates are low.

After RCV introduction, population immunity for rubella continues to be supported through supplemental immunization activities (SIAs), although the schedule for these activities is dictated by needs for measles control [14].

This study explores the dynamics of rubella virus transmission and rubella burden following RCV introduction at various levels of coverage. Simulations explore the implications of declining fertility (an expected part of demographic transition), incomplete population mixing, and heterogeneous infectivity. Constant birth rates, well-mixed connectivity, and homogeneous infectivity are all useful approximations for modeling pathogen transmission in a population, but will have a tendency to bias outcomes. This bias may result in incorrect, unnecessarily conservative policy guidance.

## 2. Materials and Methods

The dynamics of rubella transmission were explored using EMOD, a software tool for building stochastic, agent-based infection models [15]. Details of the rubella model have been described previously [16]. That model has been generalized by applying population, fertility, and mortality estimates for sub-Saharan Africa from the United Nations World Population Prospects (WPP) [17].

New agents are added on each time step, and start as either maternally protected or susceptible. Mortality is possible for all conditions and is unrelated to infection. Vaccination that occurs while an agent is maternally protected, exposed, or infected is assumed to not provide immunity. Maternal protection ends after a mean duration of three months. Immunity to rubella was assumed to be binary (i.e., either present or absent). Immunity from infection or vaccination was assumed to provide life-long protection and did not wane.

The simulations are initialized in the year 2000 starting with a population of 1 million; outcomes from the first 20 years are ignored as endemic pathogen transmission is established. The results for the subsequent 40 years, from 2020 to 2060, are depicted for a variety of scenarios. In each scenario, RCV is introduced in 2025 at several levels of coverage. All scenarios include 0% coverage as a reference to illustrate continued endemic transmission without vaccination. The use of a stochastic, agent-based model allows for exploring the dynamics of interruption and re-introduction.

The rubella burden includes miscarriage, stillbirth, and CRS. This study groups those outcomes together. The likelihood of burden associated with a rubella infection was approximated as 80% if infection occurs during the first trimester of pregnancy, and 50% if infection occurs in the four weeks prior to conception or in the first four weeks of the second trimester of pregnancy [18,19]. The estimated burden scales linearly with these probabilities, which multiply age-structured infection rates and age-structured fertility rates. The relative burden with respect to baseline scenarios without vaccination is independent of these probabilities.

Infectivity has been assumed to be uniform over all age groups. Other investigators [6,20,21] consider age-structure in the force of infection in order to more closely match the observed serological profiles for rubella seronegativity (e.g., <13 years, and 13+ years; <3 years, 3–15 years, and 15+ years). Uniform infectivity was selected as the best representation for about half of the countries examined [6]. Data quality is a significant consideration in those estimates, and a moderate reduction in infectivity for older age groups seems to be the most likely case. Uniform infectivity is a simplifying assumption as well as a conservative one from the perspective of risk associated with incomplete vaccination. Reduced infectivity in older cohorts would lead to lower rubella burden and lower risk of resurgent burden.

## 3. Results

The modeled results depict a mean rate of infection and burden for the various scenarios; each trajectory is averaged over ten-thousand stochastic outcomes. Individual timeseries are highly variable and include both outbreaks and periods of elimination.

Persistent importation of rubella virus ensures that elimination only occurs when simulated immunity levels exceed the threshold for herd immunity (i.e., $1 - 1/R_0$). Above this threshold, infections still occur because of importations, but they do not lead to sustained chains of transmission.

### 3.1. Representative Timeseries for Rubella Burden

The outcomes depicted in Figure 2 are of RCV introduction in 2025 through the routine immunization system only. The recommended vaccine introduction strategy is to simultaneously implement a wide age range (9 months–15 years) vaccination campaign as well [10]. That approach leads to a step-change decrease in both infections and burden, with probable (although potentially impermanent) elimination of rubella. The catch-up campaign has been omitted in these scenarios to more clearly illustrate the dynamics of infection and burden. The age structure of the population is held constant at 2020 levels so that clearly defined equilibrium rates exist.

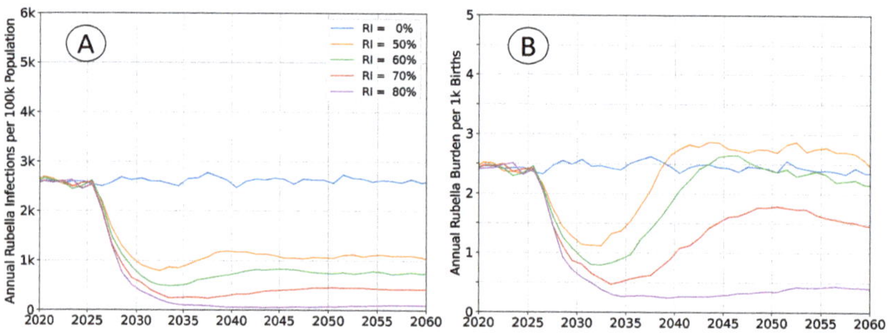


**Figure 2.** Average simulation outcomes for a steady-state population. (**A**) Mean annual incidence of rubella virus infections per 100 k total population as a function of time following RCV introduction through routine immunization only. (**B**) Mean annual burden of rubella virus infection per 1 k births.

Following vaccine introduction, a new equilibrium infection rate is established within a period of about 5 years. However, the rate of disease burden equilibrates over a period of 15 to 20 years. Time scales for infection are more rapid because they depend only on virus transmission. The burden of rubella infection depends on age-structured susceptibility, which is a demographic process that changes more slowly.

All rates of vaccination initially reduce burden. The absence of a wide age range vaccine introduction campaign, or mediocre rates of vaccination cannot lead to an immediate burden increase. The potential for increased burden exists only around 15 years post-vaccine introduction as a new, potentially susceptible cohort of individuals reaches child-bearing age.

The average timeseries depicted in Figure 2 incorporate large and potentially increasing levels of variance. As vaccination coverage increases, the variability of outbreaks also increases [22]. For simulations with steady-state populations, the average burden levels over the period 2050 to 2060 are near their long-term equilibrium values. Histograms of annual burden during this decade for the no vaccination and 60% vaccination scenarios are shown in Figure 3.

Although the mean value of both histograms in Figure 3 is around 2.2 per thousand births per year, the median annual burden in scenarios with 60% vaccination is lower, and the 95% bounds on the annual burden span a larger interval: no vaccination = $(0.3, 4.7)$ and 60% vaccination = $(0.0, 8.2)$. The interruption of transmission becomes more likely in scenarios with vaccination, but persistent elimination is not possible because of pathogen importation.

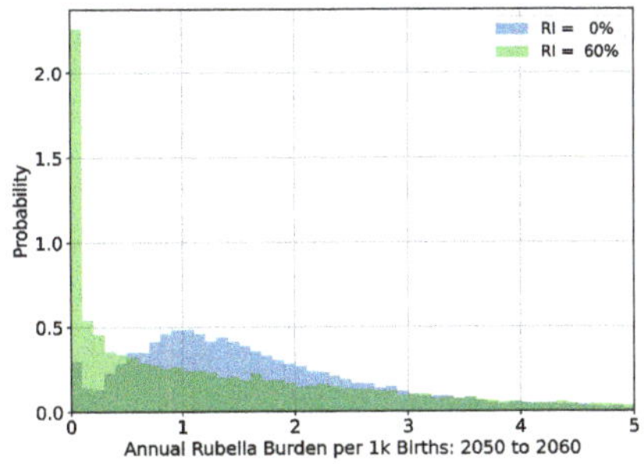


**Figure 3.** Histograms of annual rubella burden estimated over the period 2050 to 2060 for simulations of steady-state populations with no vaccination and with 60% vaccination. Average burden for both distributions is around 2.2 per thousand births per year.

### 3.2. *Impact of a Demographic Transition*

The outcomes depicted in Figure 4 reproduce those in Figure 2, but do not enforce a constant population pyramid. The age structure of the population evolves as described by medium forward projections from the UN WPP for sub-Saharan Africa. Declining fertility affects infection rates in a manner that is analogous to moderately increasing rates of vaccination.

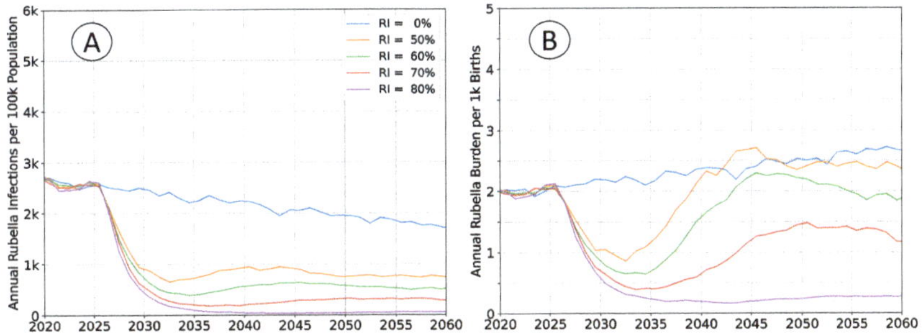


**Figure 4.** Average simulation outcomes incorporating a changing population structure. (**A**) Mean annual incidence of rubella virus infections per 100 k total population as a function of time following RCV introduction through routine immunization only. (**B**) Mean annual burden of rubella virus infection per 1 k births.

Absent vaccination, rubella incidence will trend downward, and burden will trend upward. Any non-zero rate of RCV use will lead to greater reductions in burden than would be estimated when assuming a steady-state population structure.

### 3.3. *Population Connectivity Considerations*

The outcomes depicted in Figure 5 reproduce those in Figure 2, but subdivide the population into four non-interacting, but otherwise identical sub-populations. The total simulated population remains unchanged, and the rate of pathogen importation events also remains unchanged.

The equilibrium infection rates are similar to simulations with a well-mixed population, although the time scale for attaining that equilibrium increased. The birth rates and vaccination rates are the same in both scenarios; outbreaks are limited by the size of the sub-population, leading to overall slower dynamics and an accumulation of susceptible agents. The equilibrium annual burden is elevated, around 3.0 per thousand births, compared to 2.2 in well-connected simulations, which aligns with the accumulation of susceptibility and an increased average age-at-infection.

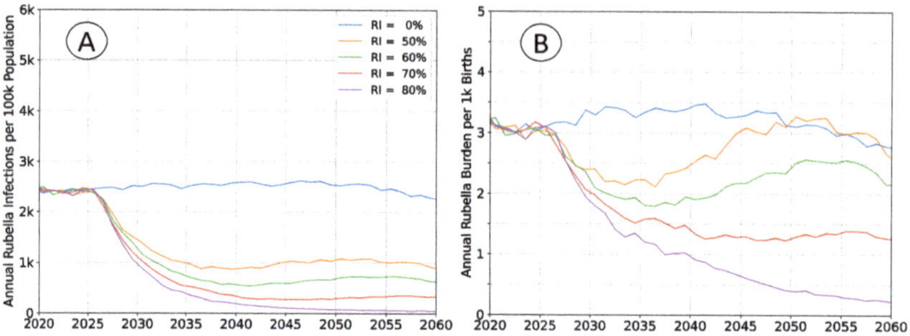


**Figure 5.** Average simulation outcomes for a steady-state population, divided into multiple non-interacting sub-populations. (**A**) Mean annual incidence of rubella virus infections per 100 k total population as a function of time following RCV introduction through routine immunization only. (**B**) Mean annual burden of rubella virus infection per 1 k births.

### *3.4. Variability of Transmission Intensity*

Assumptions regarding the intensity of pathogen transmission have the largest effect on the estimated rubella burden. The simulations examining demographics and connectivity assumed a transmission intensity such that the mean $R_0$ value was 5.0, near the middle of the typical range of 3.0 to 8.0 [23]. The outcomes when assuming $R_0$ is 3.0 are presented in Figure 6; the outcomes when assuming $R_0$ is 7.0 are presented in Figure 7.

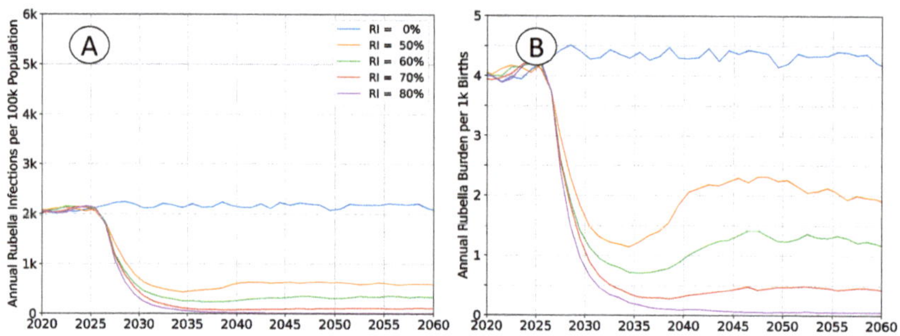


**Figure 6.** Average simulation outcomes assuming $R_0 = 3.0$. (**A**) Mean annual incidence of rubella virus infections per 100 k total population as a function of time following RCV introduction through routine immunization only. (**B**) Mean annual burden of rubella virus infection per 1 k births.

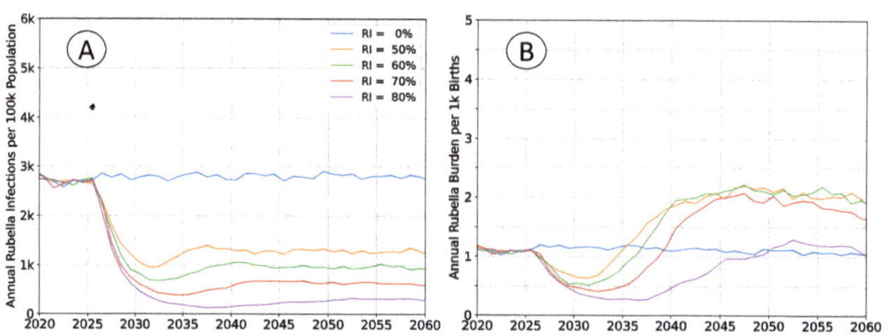


**Figure 7.** Average simulation outcomes assuming $R_0 = 7.0$. (**A**) Mean annual incidence of rubella virus infections per 100 k total population as a function of time following RCV introduction through routine immunization only. (**B**) Mean annual burden of rubella virus infection per 1 k births.

The infection rates absent vaccination are roughly equivalent in both scenarios. Rubella infection provides lifelong immunity, and almost all susceptible individuals will eventually be infected, even at lower transmission intensity. However, an individual's expected age-at-infection increases in the low transmission scenarios, leading to an elevated burden. This effect is non-linear over the range illustrated. Increasing $R_0$ from 5.0 to 7.0 halves the burden in the no-vaccine scenarios, while reducing $R_0$ from 5.0 to 3.0 nearly doubles the burden.

At lower transmission intensity, vaccination decreases the rubella burden relative to baseline at all levels of coverage. At higher transmission intensities, intermediate levels of vaccination have elevated levels of equilibrium burden, and higher coverage is required to ensure a decrease in burden.

## 4. Discussion

The outcomes are presented using mean trajectories, which do not highlight important differences in the distribution of burden. The likelihood of interruption increases with increasing vaccination, with more frequent periods of local extinction and zero infection. Endemic transmission at low vaccination coverages transitions into long periods of interruption, where importation can lead to a large outbreak. At intermediate vaccination coverages, where the long-term average rubella burden may appear comparable to scenarios without vaccination, the median burden will still have decreased. With increasing vaccination coverage, the total burden is concentrated into fewer, larger outbreaks.

The omission of a wide age range catch-up campaign in these examples is only to emphasize the disease dynamics. The introduction of RCV without a campaign is associated with a potential resurgence in rubella burden [24,25]. The introduction of RCV initially leads to declining incidence across all age groups, but many individuals <15 years old at the time of introduction are still susceptible and would be ineligible for vaccination through routine services. Accumulation of susceptibility increases outbreak risk, and vaccinating these individuals at the time of RCV introduction via a wide age range campaign should be a priority.

The baseline scenarios depict a setting with $R_0 = 5.0$, where a 60% rate of vaccination is sufficient to avoid a long-term increase in the average burden. These scenarios were selected for demonstration purposes. Not all levels of rubella infectivity are equally likely, and values $R_0 < 5.0$ are more probable [23,26].

Accurately incorporating the expected demographic transition into baseline scenarios reduces the rate of vaccination that avoids a long-term increase in the average burden to 50%. All simulations leverage demographics for sub-Saharan Africa, which are generally appropriate for countries that have not yet introduced the vaccine, but are not specific to any individual country. Above average fertility rates would be expected to decline more rapidly, and below average rates would be expected to decline more slowly. Both variations, either fertility declining more rapidly than average, or starting at a lower level than average, reduce the likelihood of increased burden due to incomplete vaccination.

Disconnected sub-populations result in slower dynamics than the well-mixed populations in the baseline scenario. These outcomes emphasize the value of implementing wide-age range vaccination campaigns concurrent to vaccine introduction through the routine immunization system. Vaccination campaigns lead to step-change decreases in both infection rate and burden, which provide the greatest benefit to disconnected sub-populations, such as those that may be geographically remote or rural locations. Reduced connectivity also elevates burden with respect to the baseline scenario, which again corresponds to greater reductions in burden when vaccinating.

Rubella infectivity is uncertain for most settings, and sub-national variation is expected in large, heterogeneous countries, such as Nigeria [21] or the Democratic Republic of the Congo [16]. Neglecting demographic effects and connectivity effects, the demonstration outcomes show a vaccination rate of 60% would decrease the equilibrium rate of burden for $R_0 = 3.0$ (from 4 to 2), increase the equilibrium rate of burden for $R_0 = 7.0$ (from 1 to 2), and not change the equilibrium rate for $R_0 = 5.0$. If all levels of infectivity were equally likely, the average outcome for these three scenarios would be to reduce the overall burden. That result contrasts with the outcome for the average scenario ( $R_0 = 5.0$), which is no reduction in burden. Heterogeneity in infectivity leads to greater burden reduction when vaccinating.

The outcomes presented here are not intended to identify appropriate vaccination thresholds for RCV introduction; they emphasize that a fixed, generally applicable threshold is inappropriate. The risk for increased rubella burden associated with incomplete vaccination occurs decades in the future and only for settings with persistently high fertility, high connectivity, and high infectivity. It is not a hypothetical risk, but it is especially unlikely. A focus on mitigating that risk accepts the certainty of increasing rubella burden absent vaccination.

This study is not specific to any particular country. It uses demographics that are an average for sub-Saharan Africa and infectivity ( $R_0 = 5.0$) that is also an average for the region [27]. Each country that has not yet introduced RCV will have individual needs that are not average. However, all countries do feature the same overall trends. All countries have declining birth rates, all have regions that are less than completely well mixed, and all have some degree of heterogeneity in infectivity.

After RCV introduction, ongoing control efforts will be driven by measles considerations because of that virus' greater infectiousness and the combined formulation of the vaccine. Declining overall rubella incidence and a tendency toward greater variability in that incidence will require increased emphasis on surveillance to identify any sporadic transmission and ensure that it does not lead to an outbreak of disease.

## 5. Conclusions

The guidance that 80% coverage of measles-containing vaccine is a necessary prerequisite for rubella vaccine introduction was created to ensure against any possibility of a future resurgence in burden. That guidance is unnecessarily conservative. It does not account for the continuously increasing current rate of burden that exists absent vaccination, which is a consequence of falling birth rates.

Rubella vaccine introduction supported by a wide age range vaccination campaign will lead to a large decrease in burden for a period of at least 15 years. The risk of a future burden resurgence due to incomplete vaccination only exists for communities with persistently high infectivity, high connectivity, and high fertility. After vaccine introduction, an emphasis on surveillance will help identify any sporadic transmission and support communities that may be at risk of outbreaks.

**Funding:** This work is based on research conducted by the Institute for Disease Modeling, a research group within, and solely funded by, the Bill and Melinda Gates Foundation.

**Institutional Review Board Statement:** Not applicable.

**Informed Consent Statement:** Not applicable.

**Data Availability Statement:** Source code for EMOD is available on GitHub: https://github.com/InstituteforDiseaseModeling/EMOD-Generic, accessed on 1 July 2024. Implementation of the rubella model and configurations for the simulations presented here are hosted in a separate repository: https://github.com/InstituteforDiseaseModeling/EMOD-Generic-Scripts, accessed on 1 July 2024.

**Acknowledgments:** Many thanks to Kari Hanson and the Xplore research program at Stanford's Institute for Computational and Mathematical Engineering. Development of these scenarios was supported by several student research groups: Fan Liu, Helen Gu, and Xiaoying Shi (demographic trends); Weian Yin (immunization trends); Nina Cruz (immunization disruptions); Benson Zu and Maximilian Sabayev (connectivity and population size effects).

**Conflicts of Interest:** The funders had no role in the analysis, or interpretation of the data; the preparation, review, or approval of the report; or the decision to submit the manuscript for publication. All authors are employees of the Bill and Melinda Gates Foundation; however, this study does not necessarily represent the views of the Bill and Melinda Gates Foundation.

## References


1. Lambert, N.; Strebel, P.; Orenstein, W.; Icenogle, J.; Poland, G.A. Rubella. *Lancet* **2015**, *385*, 2297–2307. [CrossRef]
2. Centers for Disease Control and Prevention. *Epidemiology and Prevention of Vaccine-Preventable Diseases*; Public Health Foundation: Washington, DC, USA, 2021.
3. Boshoff, L.; Tooke, L. Congenital rubella—Is it nearly time to take action? *S. Afr. J. Child Health* **2012**, *6*, 106–108. [CrossRef]
4. Zimmermann, M.; Frey, K.; Hagedorn, B.; Oteri, A.J.; Yahya, A.; Hamisu, M.; Mogekwu, F.; Shuaib, F.; McCarthy, K.A.; Chabot-Couture, G. Optimization of frequency and targeting of measles supplemental immunization activities in Nigeria: A cost-effectiveness analysis. *Vaccine* **2019**, *37*, 6039–6047. [CrossRef]
5. Vynnycky, E.; Knapp, J.K.; Papadopoulos, T.; Cutts, F.T.; Hachiya, M.; Miyano, S.; Reef, S.E. Estimates of the global burden of Congenital Rubella Syndrome, 1996–2019. *Int. J. Infect. Dis.* **2023**, *137*, 149–156. [CrossRef]
6. Vynnycky, E.; Adams, E.J.; Cutts, F.T.; Reef, S.E.; Navar, A.M.; Simons, E.; Yoshida, L.M.; Brown, D.W.J.; Jackson, C.; Strebel, P.M.; et al. Using Seroprevalence and Immunisation Coverage Data to Estimate the Global Burden of Congenital Rubella Syndrome, 1996–2010: A Systematic Review. *PLoS ONE* **2016**, *11*, 1–20. [CrossRef] [PubMed]
7. Levin, A.; Burgess, C.; Shendale, S.; Morgan, W.; Hutubessy, R.; Jit, M. Cost-effectiveness of measles and rubella elimination in low-income and middle-income countries. *BMJ Glob. Health* **2023**, *8*, e011526. [CrossRef]
8. Knox, E.G. Strategy for Rubella Vaccination. *Int. J. Epidemiol.* **1980**, *9*, 13–23. [CrossRef] [PubMed]
9. ESRI. World Countries—Generalized. Available online: https://hub.arcgis.com/datasets/esri::world-countries-generalized/explore (accessed on 31 December 2023).
10. World Health Organization. Rubella vaccines: WHO position paper—July 2020. *Wkly. Epidemiol. Rec.* **2020**, *95*, 306–324.
11. Cutts, F.T.; Abebe, A.; Messele, T.; Dejene, A.; Enquselassie, F.; Nigatu, W.; Nokes, D.J. Sero-epidemiology of rubella in the urban population of Addis Ababa, Ethiopia. *Epidemiol. Infect.* **2000**, *124*, 467–479. [CrossRef] [PubMed]
12. Rozhnova, G.; Metcalf, C.J.E.; Grenfell, B.T. Characterizing the dynamics of rubella relative to measles: The role of stochasticity. *J. R. Soc. Interface* **2013**, *10*, 20130643. [CrossRef]
13. Ujiie, M.; Nabae, K.; Shobayashi, T. Rubella outbreak in Japan. *Lancet* **2014**, *383*, 1460–1461. [CrossRef]
14. Cutts, F.T.; Danovaro-Holliday, M.C.; Rhoda, D.A. Challenges in measuring supplemental immunization activity coverage among measles zero-dose children. *Vaccine* **2021**, *39*, 1359–1363. [CrossRef]
15. Bershteyn, A.; Gerardin, J.; Bridenbecker, D.; Lorton, C.W.; Bloedow, J.; Baker, R.S.; Chabot-Couture, G.; Chen, Y.; Fischle, T.; Frey, K.; et al. Implementation and applications of EMOD, an individual-based multi-disease modeling platform. *Pathog. Dis.* **2018**, *76*, fty059. [CrossRef]
16. Cheng, A.; Frey, K.; Mwamba, G.N.; McCarthy, K.A.; Hoff, N.A.; Rimoin, A.W. Examination of scenarios introducing rubella vaccine in the Democratic Republic of the Congo. *Vaccine X* **2021**, *9*, 100127. [CrossRef]
17. United Nations Department of Economic and Social Affairs, Population Division. *World Population Prospects 2022: Summary of Results*; United Nations Department of Economic and Social Affairs, Population Division: New York, NY, USA, 2022.
18. Miller, E.; Cradock-Watson, J.E.; Pollock, T.M. Consequences of Confirmed Maternal Rubella at Successive Stages of Pregnancy. *Lancet* **1982**, *320*, 781–784. [CrossRef]
19. Thompson, K.M.; Simons, E.A.; Badizadegan, K.; Reef, S.E.; Cooper, L.Z. Characterization of the Risks of Adverse Outcomes Following Rubella Infection in Pregnancy. *Risk Anal.* **2016**, *36*, 1315–1331. [CrossRef] [PubMed]
20. Rodríguez-Cartes, S.A.; Zhang, Y.; Mayorga, M.E.; Swann, J.L.; Allaire, B.T. Evaluating the potential impact of rubella-containing vaccine introduction on congenital rubella syndrome in Afghanistan, Dem. Republic of Congo, Ethiopia, Nigeria, and Pakistan: A mathematical modeling study. *PLoS Glob. Public Health* **2024**, *4*, 1–14. [CrossRef] [PubMed]
21. Nakase, T.; Brownwright, T.; Okunromade, O.; Egwuenu, A.; Ogunbode, O.; Lawal, B.; Akanbi, K.; Grant, G.; Bassey, O.O.; Coughlin, M.M.; et al. The impact of sub-national heterogeneities in demography and epidemiology on the introduction of rubella vaccination programs in Nigeria. *Vaccine* **2024**, in press. [CrossRef]
22. Graham, M.; Winter, A.K.; Ferrari, M.; Grenfell, B.; Moss, W.J.; Azman, A.S.; Metcalf, C.J.E.; Lessler, J. Measles and the canonical path to elimination. *Science* **2019**, *364*, 584–587. [CrossRef]
23. Edmunds, W.J.; Gay, N.J.; Kretzschmar, M.; Pebody, R.G.; Wachmann, H. The pre-vaccination epidemiology of measles, mumps and rubella in Europe: Implications for modelling studies. *Epidemiol. Infect.* **2000**, *125*, 635–650. [CrossRef]
24. Panagiotopoulos, T.; Berger, A.; Antoniadou, L.; Valassi-Adam, E. Increase in congenital rubella occurrence after immunisation in Greece: Retrospective survey and systematic review. How does herd immunity work? *BMJ* **1999**, *319*, 1462–1467. [CrossRef] [PubMed]
25. US Center for Disease Control. Nationwide Campaign for Vaccination of Adults Against Rubella and Measles—Costa Rica, 2001. *Morb. Mortal. Wkly. Rep.* **2021**, *50*, 976–979.
26. Papadopoulos, T.; Vynnycky, E. Estimates of the basic reproduction number for rubella using seroprevalence data and indicator-based approaches. *PLoS Comput. Biol.* **2022**, *18*, 1–21. [CrossRef]
27. Lessler, J.; Metcalf, C.J.E. Balancing Evidence and Uncertainty when Considering Rubella Vaccine Introduction. *PLoS ONE* **2013**, *8*, e67639. [CrossRef]

*vaccines*

MDPI

*Article*

# Estimates of Potential Demand for Measles and Rubella Microarray Patches

**Lidia K. Kayembe *, Leah S. Fischer, Bishwa B. Adhikari, Jennifer K. Knapp, Emily B. Khan, Bradford R. Greening, Mark Papania * and Martin I. Meltzer ***

The U.S. Centers for Disease Control and Prevention, 1600 Clifton Rd NE, Atlanta, GA 30329, USA; wvj1@cdc.gov (L.S.F.); bia6@cdc.gov (B.B.A.); emilysbkahn@gmail.com (E.B.K.); kax9@cdc.gov (B.R.G.)
* Correspondence: yfv9@cdc.gov (L.K.K.); myp7@cdc.gov (M.P.); qzm4@cdc.gov (M.I.M.)

**Abstract:** Global measles vaccine coverage has stagnated at approximately 85% for over a decade. By simplifying vaccine logistics and administration, the measles and rubella microarray patch (MR-MAP) may improve coverage. Clinical trials have demonstrated similar safety and immunogenicity in 9-month-old infants for MR-MAPs compared with syringe-and-needle vaccination. To aid commercialization, we present estimates of MR-MAP demand. We created a spreadsheet-based tool to estimate demand for MR-MAPs using data from 180 WHO countries during 2000–2016. Five immunization scenarios were analyzed: (1a) Supplementary Immunization Activities (SIAs) in Gavi, the Vaccine Alliance (Gavi)-eligible countries and (1b) WHO countries where preventive SIAs are routinely conducted; (2) SIAs and outbreak response immunization in all WHO countries; (3) routine immunization (RI) and SIAs in six high-burden measles countries (the Democratic Republic of the Congo, Ethiopia, India, Indonesia, Nigeria, and Pakistan); (4) RI and SIAs in six high-burden countries and Gavi-eligible countries; and (5) hard-to-reach populations. MR-MAP demand varied greatly across scenarios. Forecasts for 2025–2034 estimate from 137 million doses in hard-to-reach populations (scenario 5) to 2.587 billion doses for RI and SIAs in six high-burden countries and Gavi-eligible countries (scenario 4). When policymakers and manufacturers assess MR-MAP demand, they may consider multiple scenarios to allow for a complete consideration of potential markets and public health needs.

**Keywords:** transdermal patch; vaccination; microneedle; health service needs and demand; measles vaccine; rubella vaccine

## 1. Introduction

Measles remains one of the leading causes of childhood morbidity and mortality worldwide, and rubella is the leading cause of preventable severe birth defects, despite the availability of a safe and effective vaccine against these diseases since the 1960s [1]. Global measles routine immunization coverage has stagnated at around 85% for over a decade. Coverage declined to approximately 81% during the COVID-19 pandemic, increasing to 83% in 2022 1]. Coverage levels falling short of 95% are insufficient to stop ongoing transmission. In 2022, there were 9,232,300 estimated measles cases worldwide [2] and 17,407 rubella cases reported to the World Health Organization [3]. In 2022, measles killed an estimated 136,200 people—mostly children under five years of age [1]. Additionally, worldwide, 117 million children currently are at risk for measles due to weakened immunization systems, delayed campaigns, and a decline in disease surveillance caused by the COVID-19 pandemic and response [4].

Increasing global immunization coverage among children in resource-constrained settings is challenging for many reasons, including the characteristics of the existing syringe-and-needle (S/N) vaccination technology. Current S/N technology requires all measles-containing vaccines (MCVs) to be consistently stored between 2 °C and 8 °C until the point of delivery. This storage requirement can be difficult to maintain in many settings. In low- and middle-income countries (LMICs), MCVs are typically procured in 10-dose vials to minimize costs due to packaging and storage requirements. The vaccine is shipped and stored in two parts (a lyophilized powder and sterile water), reconstituted at the point of delivery, and must be used within 6 h [5]. Onsite reconstitution and multidose withdrawal from the vial may create risks for contamination and diluent errors. Challenges of syringe- and needle (S/N) administration include the need for highly trained immunization staff (who are in short supply in many LMICs), disposal of sharps, risk of needle stick injury to healthcare workers, and the pain associated with injection, which might limit potential demand for vaccination. To overcome these barriers to increasing immunization coverage, alternative vaccine technologies are needed that have less strict cold chain requirements (especially at the point of delivery), require no reconstitution, are made in a single-dose format, and can be delivered without S/N.

An existing technology, the measles–rubella vaccine microarray patch (MR-MAP), can potentially address the key logistical barriers to immunization delivery in resource-constrained settings. MAPs consist of multiple microprojections (<1 mm tall) mounted on a small coin-sized patch applied to the skin by thumb pressure or with an applicator [6–8]. Because the penetration of the projections into the skin does not reach the nerve layer, the application of MAPs is often painless. MR-MAPs are more thermostable than the lyophilized vaccine, and no diluent or reconstitution is needed. They do not require highly trained personnel for administration, are needle-free, and do not have the risk of needle reuse. There is also the potential that MR-MAPs may not need to be kept in the cold chain, unlike the current measles vaccine technology. Recent phase 2 clinical trials have shown similar immunogenicity and safety results when comparing MR-MAPs with S/N MR vaccination in subjects as young as 9 months [8]. In those trials, there were no acute allergic reactions in either toddlers or adults. The most common vaccine-related reaction among toddlers was a mild local reaction at the MR-MAP application site, with 50 toddlers (83%) having such a mild local reaction, compared with 18 toddlers (30%) at the placebo-MAP application site. Adults in the MR-MAP group had almost the same rate of local solicited adverse events as adults in the placebo-MAP group. There were no related severe or serious adverse events [8]. In infants, vaccination with MR-MAPs resulted in 93% (95% CI 83.0–97.2) seroconverting to measles and 100% (93.8–100) seroconverting to rubella. Among infants vaccinated with S/N technology, 90% (79.2–95.2) and 100% (93.9–100) seroconverted to measles and rubella, respectively [8]. The WHO has produced a MR-MAP target product profile to document the desired features for use in LMICs [9].

While the potential public health benefit of MR-MAPs is clear, the business case for commercializing MR- MAPs is less so, especially for vaccine manufacturers who already have MCV products on the market. We present ten-year estimates of potential demand for MR-MAPs in five scenarios, each of which includes a different mix of countries and vaccination scenarios. These scenarios and the spreadsheet-based tool used to produce them can aid policymakers, donors, and vaccine manufacturers in making crucial decisions regarding investment in the commercialization of MR-MAPs. Our estimates extend previous work [10] by using a methodology for estimating future potential demand by statistical, regression-based extrapolation. We used country-specific coverage rates of growth, stagnation, or decline, based on historical data trends. Further, we provide a spreadsheet tool allowing users to update the data included and examine potential demand under alternate scenarios of their choosing.

## 2. Methods

### 2.1. Tool Overview

We developed a spreadsheet-based "Tool for Estimating the Potential Demand of Measles and Rubella Microarray Patches" (hereafter, "the Tool") to estimate MR-MAP potential demand (see the Spreadsheet Tool as a Supplement.). Potential demand estimates were based on data from 180 WHO countries with the necessary data variables (14 WHO member states for which there were no data available to complete the analysis were omitted from the list (Andorra, Antigua and Barbuda, Cook Islands, Dominica, Kiribati, Marshall Islands, Monaco, Nauru, Niue, Palau, Saint Kitts and Nevis, San Marino, Seychelles, and Tuvalu)). The list of variables used in the Tool is provided in Table 1 (including where country-specific values can be found).

**Table 1.** Variables used to estimate measles and rubella microarray patch (MR-MAP) potential demand.

| Variable * | Description | Location of Values in the Tool † |
|---|---|---|
| MR-MAP wastage rate | Vaccine wastage rate by scenario, 15–30%, scenario-dependent ‡ | MAP characteristics tab |
| Global annual MAP potential demand for outbreak responses | Baseline value of global annual MR-MAP potential demand for outbreak response used in Scenario 2, assumed: 10 million | Adjusting MAP demand tab |
| Adoption rate of MR-MAPs | MR-MAP assumed estimated potential demand adjusted for partial adoption of the new technology; assumed baseline range: 50%, 75%, 90% | Adjusting MAP demand tab |
| MCV1 | Estimated future coverage for the first dose of measles-containing vaccine (180 country-specific; 2025–2055) | MCV1 tab |
| MCV2 | Estimated future coverage for the second dose of measles-containing vaccine (180 country-specific; 2025–2055) | MCV2 tab |
| Historical MCV1 | Coverage for the first dose of measles-containing vaccine (WUENIC country-specific estimates, for 180 countries, 2000–2016) ** | Historical MCV1 tab |
| Historical MCV2 | Coverage for the second dose of measles containing vaccine (WUENIC country-specific estimates, for 180 countries, 2000–2016) ** | Historical MCV2 tab |
| SIAs | Tool-estimated historical and future coverage of MR Supplementary Immunization Activities (SIAs) (180 country-specific; 2025–2055) †† | SIA tab |
| SIA age | Upper age limit of 5 years for SIAs | SIA age tab |
| Surviving infants | Number of surviving infants by year per country, for 180 countries (UNDESA; 2025–2035) | SurvInf tab |
| Under 12 months population | Number of children under 12 months of age by year per country, for 180 countries (UNDESA; 2025–2055) | Population < 12 mo tab |
| Under 5 years population | Number of children under 5 years of age by year per country, for 180 countries (UNDESA; 2025–2055) | Population < 59 m tab |
| Gavi countries | List of 54 Gavi-eligible countries in 2024 | Gavi countries tab |
| WHO countries | List of 180 WHO countries | WHO states tab |
| Six countries | The six high-burden countries are the DRC, Ethiopia, Nigeria, India, Indonesia, and Pakistan, selected by the Measles and Rubella Partnership (M&RP) | MRI tab |

* MR-MAP = measles and rubella microarray patch; MCV1 = measles-containing vaccine first dose; MCV2 = measles-containing vaccine second dose; WUENIC = WHO/UNICEF Estimates Of National Immunization Coverage; SIA = supplementary immunization activity; UNDESA = The United Nations Department of Economic and Social Affairs; Gavi = Gavi, the Vaccine Alliance; WHO = World Health Organization; DRC = Democratic Republic of the Congo. † "Tool" refers to the Excel spreadsheet Tool provided as Supplementary Information. The "Location in Tool" column refers to specific sheets ("Tabs") in the Tool. Each Tab in the Tool contains the values used and the source of such values. ‡ See "Data sources" in the main text for an explanation of the source of these wastage rates. References [11–14]. ** Available online: https://www.who.int/teams/immunization-vaccines-and-biologicals/immunization-analysis-and-insights/global-monitoring/immunization-coverage/who-unicef-estimates-of-national-immunization-coverage (accessed on 19 July 2024). †† Available online: WHO/IVB Database workbook containing summary of Supplementary Immunization Activities (SIAs). https://immunizationdata.who.int/global?topic=Additional-datasets&location= (accessed on 19 July 2024).

The Tool includes five population-level immunization scenarios for routine immunization (RI) and Supplementary Immunization Activities (SIAs), as follows (see Appendix A for the list of countries by scenario):

(1a) Supplementary Immunization (SIAs) in the Gavi, the Vaccine Alliance (Gavi)-eligible countries as listed in 2024 (inclusive of countries in transition phases).
(1b) WHO countries routinely holding large-scale SIAs.
(2) SIAs and outbreak response immunization in all WHO countries.
(3) SIAs and routine immunization in six high-burden measles countries (the Democratic Republic of the Congo, Ethiopia, India, Indonesia, Nigeria, and Pakistan) (the six high-burden countries were selected by the then Measles and Rubella Initiative (M&RI) formed by the American Red Cross, CDC, United Nations Foundation, UNICEF and WHO; the M&RI was replaced, in 2023, by the Measles and Rubella Partnership (M&RP) which includes new partners, Gavi and the Bill and Melinda Gates Foundation, and is under the umbrella of the Immunization Agenda 2030).
(4) SIAs and routine immunization in six high-burden countries and Gavi-eligible countries.
(5) Hard-to-reach (hard-to-reach populations of any given country are defined as the population represented by the difference between the coverage needed to attain measles herd immunity (95%) and the WHO/UNICEF National Immunization Coverage Estimates for the first dose of measles-containing vaccine in a given year) populations (niche market).

### 2.2. Base Case and Alternate Adoption Scenarios

For the base case, for each scenario it is assumed that MAPs will replace all MCV1 and MCV2 doses forecasted to be administered by the existing S/N technology (i.e., 100% adoption of all vaccinations administered). Note that for Scenario 5 (the hard-to-reach populations), because there are no existing coverage data, we assume in the base case that 100% of this population will be vaccinated with MAPs. For a variety of reasons, including price and production capacity constraints, it is likely that there will not be an instantaneous replacement of S/N by MR-MAPs. Therefore, we estimated the partial adoption of the technology in 50% and 90% of the estimated baseline potential demand of MR-MAPs over 10 years for each scenario. These estimates do not represent a confidence interval but alternate outcomes of the degree of acceptance of the new vaccination technology.

### 2.3. Adjusting the Scenarios

A user of the Tool can adjust almost all the input values (Table 1) and other aspects. For example, a user can select the starting year of the forecast (2025 to 2030) and the duration (5 or 10 years) and adjust the vaccine wastage rate for routine immunization and Supplementary Immunization Activities in each scenario. The user can also change the historical and projected MCV coverage of RI and SIAs for each of the 180 countries (see Appendix F).

### 2.4. Data Sources

For the 180 countries included in the Tool, we used historical routine immunization coverage data from 2000 to 2016 on measles-containing vaccines/rubella-containing vaccines (MCVs/RCVs) from the WHO UNICEF Estimates of National Immunization Coverage (WUENIC) database (Table 1).

We used historical data on MR SIAs from the WHO SIA database (2000–2016), and we complemented these data with country-specific Expanded Programme on Immunization (EPI) data when needed. Countries were categorized using the 2017 World Bank per capita Gross National Income classification system [15]. Country-specific demographic information was taken from the World Population Prospects 2017, published by the United Nations Department of Economic and Social Affairs (UNDESA) [16]. Vaccine wastage rates for routine immunization and SIAs came from data from various WHO countries [11–14].

*2.5. Forecast of RI Demand*

We assume that the rubella-containing vaccine (RCV) will be introduced with an MR SIA for children under 15 in all countries prior to the public availability of MR MAPs; in this study, this was assumed to occur by 2025, the first year of estimates in the vaccine potential demand forecasting Tool. Countries introduce the rubella vaccine in a combined measles–rubella formulation, which is then used for all MR vaccination activities. Therefore, the estimated RCV coverage equals the MCV coverage for both the first and second doses.

Following the methodology of Winter et al. [17], we estimated the potential demand for MR-MAP for each country, using country-specific historical coverage data of measles and rubella RI and SIAs. We first used natural logarithmic regression to fit the 2000–2016 historical MCV1 coverage data for each country. We then estimated future potential demand year by year (2017–2055), using the equation set out in Appendix E. For each country and each future year, the equation combines the target population, the extrapolated MCV1 coverage, and the wastage rate. For each country, for each year (both historical and estimates of future coverage), the data are available in the Tool (see Table labeled "Contents Variables List"). Figure 1 provides four country-specific examples of estimates of future MCV routine immunization coverage based on historical MCV coverage data. As shown in Figure 1, using the regression equations to extrapolate forward resulted in estimates of future coverage increasing at a decreasing rate (i.e., diminishing returns). For 22 (European region: Georgia, Kyrgyzstan, Moldova, Italy, Malta, Russian Federation, Serbia, Slovenia, Spain, Macedonia; Eastern Mediterranean region: Djibouti, Jordan, Pakistan, Yemen, Libya, Oman, Saudi Arabia, UAE; Western Pacific region: Mongolia, Philippines, Fiji, Malaysia) of the 180 countries, MCV1 coverage did not follow a natural logarithmic function, and we averaged their most recent coverage data. We extrapolated forward by holding each respective average coverage rate constant. A user of the Tool can adjust the estimates of potential future coverage (and thus automatically update or alter estimates of demand) by adding in their own estimates of future coverage (Appendix F).

We used several approaches to estimate the future coverage of the second dose of the measles-containing vaccine (MCV2). For countries with 4 or more years of MCV2 coverage data, we applied the natural logarithmic function process as described for the MCV1 doses. For countries with 0 to 3 years of MCV2 data, we used the average fit (slope) from similar countries, as classified by the World Bank's income classification [18]. For example, for an African country in the low-income World Bank classification group, we used the slope derived from all countries in the same category with 4 or more years of MCV2 data.

We then estimated MCV2 coverage as a fixed percentage of MCV1 coverage. The fixed percentage of MCV1 coverage percentage difference was calculated based on region-income level-specific MCV1-MCV2 differences in countries with at least 4 years of MCV2 data (Appendix B). For example, a low- or middle-income country in the Africa region had MCV2 coverage 32% lower than its MCV1 value in the year of MCV2 introduction.

Forecasted coverage levels were used to estimate future doses needed. We set the upper limit of future MR coverage estimates to 99% and further assumed that MCV2 could not exceed MCV1 (detailed explanation in Appendix C). In total, 360 individual equations were created to estimate MCV coverage (one equation per country for each MCV dose provided through routine immunization).

*2.6. Forecast of SIA Demand*

The timing of future SIAs (2017 onward) was set as the year when the number of measles-susceptible individuals reached the size of a birth cohort in a particular country (the susceptibility threshold) or four years since the last SIA, whichever occurred first. All preventive SIAs target children under five years of age, with a lower bound age of nine months. Future SIA coverage is based on the country's average historical coverage. To account for potential improvement in the planning and implementation of SIAs, SIA coverage was increased by 10% of the difference between the previous SIA coverage estimate and 100% for three subsequent SIAs and held constant through 2055.

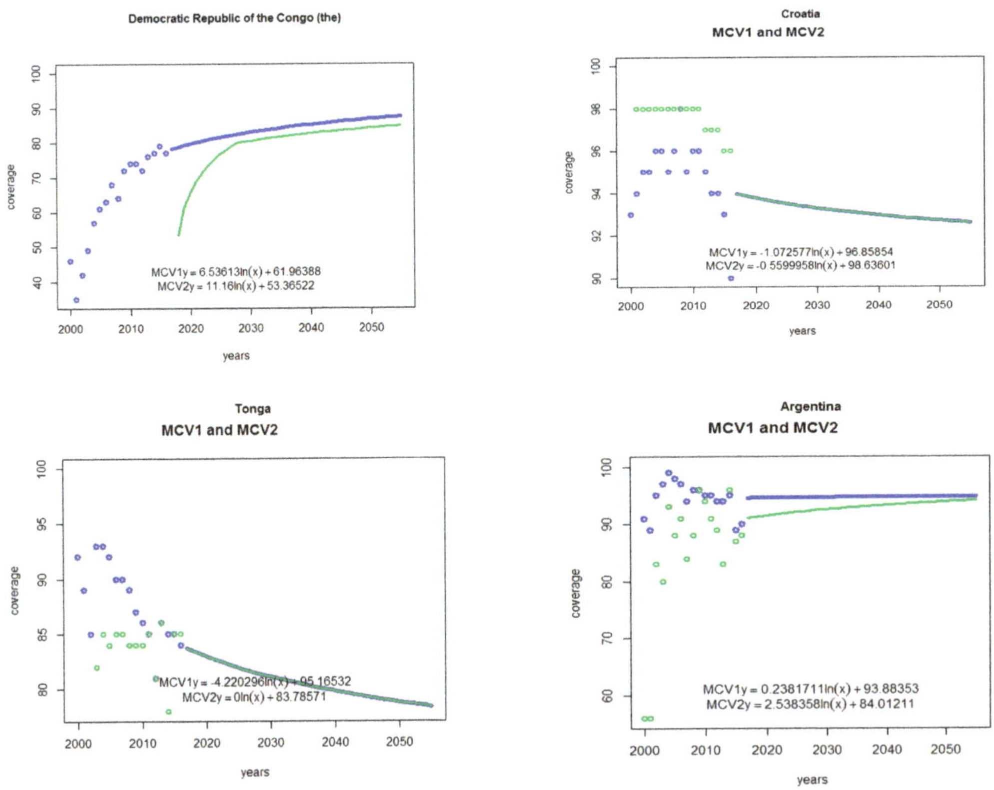


**Figure 1.** Examples of MCV1 and MCV2 historical coverage and estimated future coverage (2000–2055) Notes: Blue and green dots represent the historical coverage rates for the measles-containing vaccine first dose (MCV1) and measles-containing vaccine second dose (MCV2), respectively. The solid blue and green lines represent the future estimates of such coverage based on extrapolations from regression analyses. See text for additional details. The equations in each graph are logistic regressions used to fit the historical data and subsequently used to estimate future potential demand by extrapolating forward, producing the solid line shown.

To ensure the reality of SIA implementation, we added a cessation rule aligning with the measles vaccines WHO position paper [19] "Cessation of SIAs should be considered only when >90–95% immunization coverage has been achieved at the national level for both MCV1 and routine MCV2 as determined by the most accurate means available for a period of at least 3 consecutive years".

The following additional three criteria had to be met for a country to stop SIAs:

1. Two doses of MCVs were part of the national EPI schedule for more than 5 years;
2. RCVs were introduced with an MR SIA for those under 15 years and at least one additional follow-up campaign; and
3. The susceptibility threshold was not reached within 8 years after the previous SIA.

### *2.7. Potential Total Demand Estimation*

For each of the 180 countries included in the Tool, we estimated future MCV1 and MCV2 coverage and future SIA timing and coverage. Examples of future SIA timing and coverage are shown in Appendix D.

RI and SIA coverage were converted into MR doses needed by multiplying these values by the size of the target population while accounting for vaccine wastage rates (Appendix E). These calculations were applied to all countries of each of the five scenarios for 10 years, from 2025 to 2034, and the number of doses needed was summed by scenario.

## 3. Results

### 3.1. Base Case

The base case results represent the estimated MR-MAP potential demand when MAPs fully replace S/N technology (i.e., 100% adoption). As shown in Table 2, MR-MAP potential demand varies from 137 million doses (Scenario 5: hard-to-reach populations) to 2587 million doses (Scenario 4: SIAs and routine immunization in six high-burden countries and Gavi-eligible countries). As shown in Figure 2, MR-MAP potential demand varies over time for any given scenario (Table 2 contains the 10-year cumulative totals for each scenario). The driving factor behind the year-to-year fluctuations shown in Figure 2 is the occurrence of SIAs in countries with large under-five populations (e.g., Ethiopia, the Democratic Republic of the Congo, Indonesia, Nigeria and Pakistan). For example, for Ethiopia, we assumed SIAs would take place in the years 2027 and 2031, which would consume 23,505,000 and 24,028,000 MR-MAP doses, respectively, compared to the years between 2025 and 2039 when SIAs do not take place and when annual potential demand varies between 7,042,000 and 7,396,000 doses. Note that for Scenario 5 (hard-to-reach populations), in the absence of historical coverage data for this group, we assumed in the base case that 100% of this population will be vaccinated with MAPs, with no SIAs. This results in a steady year-to-year demand, with no fluctuations.

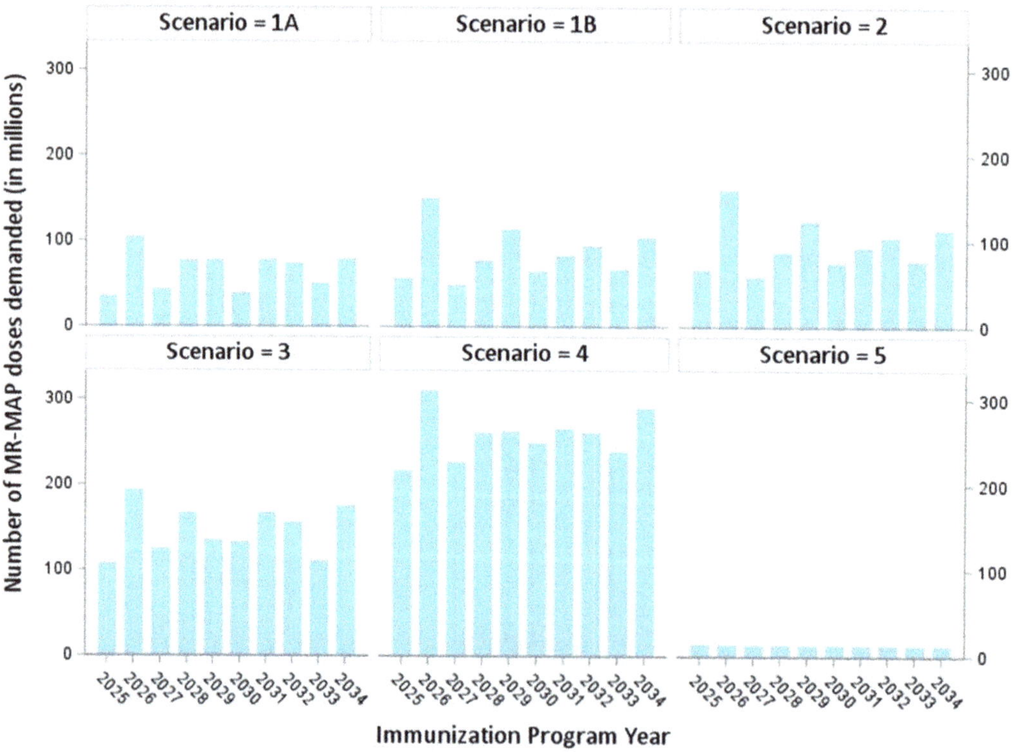


**Figure 2.** MR-MAP potential demand by estimation scenario and by year (2025–2034) Notes: The measles–rubella microarray patch potential demand scenarios are for (1A) SIAs in Gavi, the Vaccine

Alliance (Gavi)-eligible countries; (1B) SIAs in all WHO countries; (2) SIAs and outbreak response immunization; (3) SIAs and routine immunization in six high-burden measles countries: the Democratic Republic of the Congo, Ethiopia, India, Indonesia, Nigeria, and Pakistan; (4) SIAs and routine immunization in six high-burden countries and in Gavi countries; and (5) hard-to-reach populations. Note that for Scenario 5, because there are no existing coverage data, we assume in the base case that 100% of this population will be vaccinated with MAPs.

**Table 2.** Estimates of potential demand for measles and rubella microarray patches (MR-MAPs) in millions of doses for 10 years, 2025 to 2034.

| Adoption Scenarios * | MR-MAP Usage | Target Population: Cumulative Population over 10 Years (in Millions) † | Cumulative Estimated Potential Demand of MR-MAPs, 2025–2034 (Millions of Doses) | |
|---|---|---|---|---|
| | | | Base Case (Assuming 100% Adoption) ‡ | Assuming Lower Levels of Adoption (50% to 90% Transition from S/N to MAPs) ¶ |
| Scenario 1A | Supplementary Immunization Activities in Gavi-eligible countries | 2341 | 663 | 331–596 |
| Scenario 1B | Supplementary Immunization Activities in WHO countries | 2653 | 866 | 433–779 |
| Scenario 2 | Supplementary Immunization Activities and outbreak responses-WHO countries | 2653 + 10 million doses § | 966 | 483–869 |
| Scenario 3 | Supplementary Immunization Activities and routine immunization in six high-burden countries | 2651 | 1471 | 736–1324 |
| Scenario 4 | Supplementary Immunization Activities and routine immunization in six high-burden countries and GAVI-eligible countries | 4421 | 2587 | 1294–2328 |
| Scenario 5 | Hard-to-reach populations | 137 | 137 | 68–123 |

Notes: * Description of scenarios: (1a) supplementary immunization activities (SIAs) in Gavi, The Vaccine Alliance (Gavi)-eligible countries (inclusive of countries in transition phases in 2018 and (1b) in WHO countries routinely holding large-scale SIAs; (2) in SIAs and outbreak response immunization in all WHO countries; (3) in SIAs and routine immunization in six countries with high measles burden (Democratic Republic of the Congo, Ethiopia, India, Indonesia, Nigeria, and Pakistan); (4) in SIAs and routine immunization in six high-burden countries and Gavi-eligible countries; (5) and in hard to reach populations. Scenario 5 represents the additional population of the 180 WHO countries needing to be vaccinated to reach 95% MCV1 coverage for each of the countries in the analysis. Note that for Scenario 5, because there are no existing coverage data, we assume in the base case that 100% of this population will be vaccinated with MAPS. † The total target population represents the cumulative population targeted for RI (MCV1 and MCV2) and SIAs from 2025 to 2034. ‡ 100% adoption here means microarray patches are assumed to replace all MCV1 and MCV2 doses forecasted to be administered by the existing needles-and-syringe technology. ¶ Estimates of MR MAPs potential demand if MR-MAPs replace 50% and 90% of MCV doses currently administered by the existing needles-and-syringe technology (routine immunization and SIAs). § Scenario 2 includes an estimate of 10 million doses of MR-MAP needed for outbreak response at the global level.

### 3.2. *Alternate Estimates*

Table 2 shows the base case estimation and alternate results for 50% and 90% adoption of the new technology. When considering lower levels of adoption, such as assuming 50% of MCV1 and MCV2 doses are administered by MR-MAP technology, the 10-year estimates of MR-MAP potential demand declines to between 68 and 123 million doses (Scenario 5: hard-to-reach populations) and between 1294 and 2328 million doses (Scenario 4: SIAs and routine immunization in six high-burden countries and Gavi-eligible countries).

## 4. Discussion

Our 10-year estimates of potential demand for MR-MAPS, assuming a 100% replacement of S/N technology, ranged from 137 million doses in hard-to-reach populations to

2.587 billion doses for RI and SIAs (Table 2). Reducing the assumption to 50% replacement of doses administered by S/N yielded 10-year estimates of MR-MAP potential demand ranging from 137 million doses to 1294 million doses. Of potentially equal importance when considering potential demand over 10 years is the estimated year-to-year fluctuations in potential demand. In some scenarios, such as Scenario 2 (SIAs and outbreak responses in WHO countries), potential demand in a given year can almost double or be halved compared to the previous year. The scenarios with larger 10-year total potential demands (e.g., Scenarios 3 and 4) show less frequent large year-to-year fluctuations.

The WHO estimated MR-MAP potential demand and presented three eleven-year estimates of potential demand for 2030 to 2040, ranging from 1.2 million doses (regional MR-MAP pilots) to 4.05 billion doses (for RI and SIAs) [10]. The latter was revised to 1.46 billion doses when the WHO applied assumptions of country adoption and market penetration, which are lower than our MAP demand estimates for RI and SIAs but are within the range of our five scenarios. The main reason for the difference between our estimates is that the WHO estimates were produced assuming a uniform annual growth of 3% in MCV coverage in each country. As noted earlier, we used country-specific coverage growth rates, with some countries growing at faster rates than others, others having a declining growth rate over time, and others having stagnated. Our methodology also included, for those estimated to have growth over time, a decreasing rate of increase over time. Further, unlike the WHO estimates, we did not have any scenario in which all countries simultaneously adopted MR-MAPs, which limited our estimates of potential demand. We excluded an all-countries-simultaneously-adopt scenario because we think there may be both notable lags in willingness to adopt MR-MAPs and delays in building production capacity to achieve such a scenario realistically.

Our estimates of MR-MAP potential demand are limited in a few ways. We did not include the COVID-19 pandemic-related reductions in coverage in our models (Figure 1). We considered such reductions in coverage to be anomalies not indictive of non-pandemic demand. While universal rubella vaccine introduction may not be complete by 2025, the vast majority of the global population should have the rubella vaccine prior to the public availability of MR-MAPs; by the end of 2022, 175 of 194 countries were already using MR vaccines [3], with additional countries already preparing for rubella vaccine introduction. Our estimates also do not incorporate the effects of the cost of MR-MAPs, because reliable product costs are not yet readily available. Two papers report the cost-effectiveness of MR-MAPs. One paper [20] used a range of USD 0.95 to 1.19 (2010 USD)/per MR-MAP. Another paper [21] used, for low-income countries, costs adjusted for wastage ranging from USD 1.30 to 2.95 (2020 USD). This latter range was compared to the USD 0.86 for the Gavi-priced 5-dose vials for the MR vaccine [21]. For both papers, however, MR-MAP costs are speculative, as there are no published costs for MR-MAP production and marketing.

Two companies, one in Australia and one in the U.S., are setting up pilot production lines which may each produce up to 10 million MR-MAP doses/year [22,23]. Reaching such a production goal may be some years in the future, as both companies need to conduct safety-and-efficacy Phase III trials and have their facilities inspected and certified. Creelman et al. have detailed the barriers and problems which must be overcome to achieve full-scale production of MR-MAPs [24]. In the initial years of MR-MAP production and use, S/N is likely to be less expensive per dose administered. The impact on the potential demand for MR-MAPs caused by higher prices than S/N technology can be examined by considering the 50% and 90% demand forecasts presented in Table 2, as well as using the Tool to further examine additional alternative adoption rates. An additional important limitation is, from the vaccine manufacturer's business perspective, the potential demand for MR-MAPs essentially replacing the existing demand for MCVs administered via S/N. Thus, from the vaccine manufacturer's point of view, much of the estimated MR-MAP demand presented here represents a "cannibalization" of an existing market. Such cannibalization may reduce existing MR vaccine producers' interest in adopting the MAP technology. Finally, we did not allow for the fact that it may take time for production capacity to grow to the levels needed to meet some of the calculated potential demand estimates. Allowing for such production constraints would require currently unavailable data on production capacities and the growth of such capacities. In the Tool, the estimates presented here can be adjusted downward to account for the assumed impact of these limitations.

## 5. Conclusions

MR-MAPs could revolutionize vaccine delivery, making MR vaccines more accessible to the approximately 22 million children who missed their first measles vaccine dose in 2022 [25]. The large-scale adoption of MR-MAPs, however, may need to overcome the already noted potential problems of price differentials (i.e., existing vaccination technologies may be notably cheaper, at least initially) and "market cannibalization". Policymakers may wish to use our estimates to help consider various options to spur potential demand for MR-MAPs. Such "market-enhancing" options might include strategies such as purchase orders guaranteeing the purchase of a minimum number of MR-MAPs and/or agreements to subsidize the purchase of a given number of MR-MAPs. Such strategies would likely require building a consensus between potential users (e.g., Ministries of Health), regulatory authorities, manufacturers, and donor organizations. Considerations and estimates provided by the Tool may help build a global consensus regarding the benefits of producing large numbers of MR-MAPs to improve global MCV coverage and the public health of tens of millions of children and adults around the world.

**Supplementary Materials:** The following supporting information can be downloaded at: https://www.mdpi.com/article/10.3390/vaccines12091083/s1. The Spreadsheet Tool as a Supplement.

**Author Contributions:** Conceptualization, M.I.M. and M.P.; Methodology, B.B.A., B.R.G., E.B.K., J.K.K., L.K.K. and M.I.M.; Validation, B.B.A., B.R.G., L.K.K. and M.I.M.; Formal Analysis, B.B.A., B.R.G., L.K.K. and M.I.M.; Resources, B.B.A. and M.I.M.; Data Curation, J.K.K. and L.K.K.; Writing—Original Draft Preparation, B.B.A., L.S.F., L.K.K., M.I.M. and M.P.; Writing—Review and Editing, B.B.A., B.R.G., E.B.K., J.K.K., L.S.F., L.K.K., M.I.M. and M.P.; Visualization, B.B.A., J.K.K., L.S.F., L.K.K. and M.I.M.; Supervision, M.I.M.; Project Administration, J.K.K., L.S.F. and L.K.K. All authors have read and agreed to the published version of the manuscript.

**Funding:** This research received no external funding.

**Institutional Review Board Statement:** Not relevant. This study only accessed and used published aggregated secondary data that contains no personal identifying information. That is, there were no human subjects involved.

**Data Availability Statement:** Publicly available data sources are cited in the manuscript and references. Archived versions of the data and additional calculated projection data are included in the Tool.

**Conflicts of Interest:** The authors declare no conflicts of interest.

## Appendix A. Cumulative 10-Year Target Population Size by Country by Scenario

| Country | Scenario 1A Population (In 000) | Scenario 1B Population (In 000) | Scenario 3 Population (In 000) | Scenario 4 Population (In 000) | Scenario 5 Population (In 000) |
|---|---|---|---|---|---|
| Afghanistan | 50,306 | 50,306 | | 61,583 | 2605 |
| Albania | | | | | |
| Algeria | | | | | |
| Angola | | 64,743 | | | 4764 |
| Argentina | | | | | 22 |
| Armenia | | | | | |
| Australia | | | | | |
| Austria | | | | | 20 |

| Country | Scenario 1A Population (In 000) | Scenario 1B Population (In 000) | Scenario 3 Population (In 000) | Scenario 4 Population (In 000) | Scenario 5 Population (In 000) |
|---|---|---|---|---|---|
| Azerbaijan | | | | | |
| Bahamas | | | | | 2 |
| Bahrain | | | | | |
| Bangladesh | 122,479 | | | 148,775 | 9 |
| Barbados | | | | | 2 |
| Belarus | | | | | |
| Belgium | | | | | |
| Belize | | | | | |
| Benin | 20,094 | 20,094 | | 24,845 | 1144 |
| Bhutan | | | | | |
| Bolivia | | | | | |
| Bosnia and Herzegovina | | | | | 14 |
| Botswana | | | | | |
| Brazil | | | | | |
| Brunei Darussalam | | | | | |
| Bulgaria | | | | | 10 |
| Burkina Faso | 36,846 | 36,846 | | 45,560 | 523 |
| Burundi | 21,658 | 21,658 | | 26,795 | |
| Cambodia | 15,022 | 15,022 | | 18,338 | 431 |
| Cameroon | 40,951 | 40,951 | | 50,526 | 1006 |
| Canada | | | | | 196 |
| Cape Verde | | | | | |
| Central African Republic | 7795 | 7795 | | 9622 | 744 |
| Chad | 30,524 | 30,524 | | 37,767 | 2531 |
| Chile | | | | | 76 |
| China | | | | | |
| China, Hong Kong Special Administrative Region | | | | | 675 |
| China, Macao Special Administrative Region | | | | | 68 |
| Colombia | | | | | 149 |
| Comoros | 1195 | 1195 | | 1470 | 19 |
| Congo | 11,352 | 9194 | | 11,352 | 219 |
| Costa Rica | | | | | 20 |
| Côte d'Ivoire | 44,133 | 44,133 | | 54,533 | 2725 |
| Croatia | | | | | 5 |
| Cuba | | | | | |
| Cyprus | | | | | 8 |
| Czech Republic | | | | | |
| Democratic People's Republic of Korea | 15,183 | | | 18,467 | |
| Democratic Republic of the Congo | 171,096 | 171,096 | 211,750 | 211,750 | 4938 |
| Denmark | | | | | 30 |
| Djibouti | 906 | 906 | | 1105 | 30 |
| Dominican Republic | | 8835 | | | 185 |

| Country | Scenario 1A Population (In 000) | Scenario 1B Population (In 000) | Scenario 3 Population (In 000) | Scenario 4 Population (In 000) | Scenario 5 Population (In 000) |
|---|---|---|---|---|---|
| Ecuador | | 14,280 | | | 183 |
| Egypt | | | | | 407 |
| El Salvador | | | | | 25 |
| Equatorial Guinea | | 2152 | | | 285 |
| Eritrea | 7533 | | | 9277 | |
| Estonia | | | | | 2 |
| Ethiopia | 149,947 | 149,947 | 183,748 | 183,748 | 6279 |
| Federated States of Micronesia | | | | | 3 |
| Fiji | | | | | 2 |
| Finland | | | | | 0 |
| France | | | | | 242 |
| Gabon | | 2571 | | | 146 |
| Gambia | 4016 | | | 4959 | |
| Georgia | | | | | 6 |
| Germany | | | | | |
| Ghana | 40,232 | 40,232 | | 49,481 | 250 |
| Greece | | | | | |
| Grenada | | | | | |
| Guatemala | | 18,939 | | | 440 |
| Guinea | 22,103 | 22,103 | | 27,273 | 1718 |
| Guinea-Bissau | 2986 | 2986 | | 3683 | 95 |
| Guyana | | | | | |
| Haiti | 10,663 | 10,663 | | 13,023 | 793 |
| Honduras | | 8582 | | | 196 |
| Hungary | | | | | |
| Iceland | | | | | 1 |
| India | | | 1,290,390 | 1,290,390 | 6528 |
| Indonesia | | 204,516 | 249,566 | 249,566 | 7025 |
| Iran (Islamic Republic of) | | | | | |
| Iraq | | 63,688 | | | 5151 |
| Ireland | | | | | |
| Israel | | | | | |
| Italy | | | | | 313 |
| Jamaica | | | | | 12 |
| Japan | | | | | 23 |
| Jordan | | | | | |
| Kazakhstan | | | | | |
| Kenya | 74,170 | 74,170 | | 91,239 | 2081 |
| Kuwait | | | | | |
| Kyrgyzstan | 5696 | | | 6960 | |
| Lao People's Democratic Republic | 7833 | 6422 | | 7833 | 194 |
| Latvia | | | | | 3 |
| Lebanon | | 3183 | | | 83 |
| Lesotho | 2571 | 2571 | | 3143 | 21 |

| Country | Scenario 1A Population (In 000) | Scenario 1B Population (In 000) | Scenario 3 Population (In 000) | Scenario 4 Population (In 000) | Scenario 5 Population (In 000) |
|---|---|---|---|---|---|
| Liberia | 7999 | 7999 | | 9870 | 350 |
| Libyan Arab Jamahiriya | | | | | |
| Lithuania | | | | | 4 |
| Luxembourg | | | | | |
| Madagascar | 43,214 | 43,214 | | 53,262 | 2900 |
| Malawi | 33,943 | 33,943 | | 41,864 | 493 |
| Malaysia | | | | | |
| Maldives | | | | | |
| Mali | 39,296 | 39,296 | | 48,681 | 1852 |
| Malta | | | | | 4 |
| Mauritania | 7149 | 7149 | | 8818 | 305 |
| Mauritius | | | | | 0 |
| Mexico | | | | | 0 |
| Mongolia | | | | | 0 |
| Montenegro | | | | | 19 |
| Morocco | | | | | 0 |
| Mozambique | 57,737 | 57,737 | | 71,429 | 1061 |
| Myanmar | 40,055 | 40,055 | | 48,884 | 553 |
| Namibia | | 3296 | | | 84 |
| Nepal | 23,477 | 23,477 | | 28,480 | 178 |
| Netherlands | | | | | |
| New Zealand | | | | | |
| Nicaragua | | | | | |
| Niger | 59,118 | 59,118 | | 73,808 | 2185 |
| Nigeria | 439,216 | 355,901 | 440,357 | 440,357 | 31,743 |
| Norway | | | | | |
| Oman | | | | | |
| Pakistan | 224,766 | 224,766 | 274,998 | 274,998 | 15,720 |
| Panama | | | | | 17 |
| Papua New Guinea | 12,941 | 10,544 | | 12,941 | 294 |
| Paraguay | | | | | 43 |
| Peru | | 25,283 | | | 378 |
| Philippines | | 108,950 | | | 1971 |
| Poland | | | | | |
| Portugal | | | | | |
| Puerto Rico | | | | | 322 |
| Qatar | | | | | |
| Republic of Korea | | | | | |
| Republic of Moldova | | | | | 6 |
| Romania | | | | | 98 |
| Russian Federation | | | | | |
| Rwanda | 16,751 | | | 20,587 | |
| Saint Lucia | | | | | |
| Saint Vincent and the Grenadines | | | | | |

| Country | Scenario 1A Population (In 000) | Scenario 1B Population (In 000) | Scenario 3 Population (In 000) | Scenario 4 Population (In 000) | Scenario 5 Population (In 000) |
|---|---|---|---|---|---|
| Samoa | | | | | 8 |
| Sao Tome and Principe | 323 | 323 | | 399 | 0 |
| Saudi Arabia | | | | | |
| Senegal | 27,320 | 27,320 | | 33,701 | 475 |
| Serbia | | | | | 39 |
| Sierra Leone | 11,277 | 11,277 | | 13,853 | 302 |
| Singapore | | | | | |
| Slovakia | | | | | 0 |
| Slovenia | | | | | 1 |
| Solomon Islands | 988 | | | 988 | |
| Somalia | 32,045 | 32,045 | | 39,759 | 3388 |
| South Africa | | 49,049 | | | 2406 |
| South Sudan | 21,361 | 21,361 | | 26,337 | 3732 |
| Spain | | | | | |
| Sri Lanka | | | | | |
| Sudan | 65,013 | 65,013 | | 80,216 | 677 |
| Suriname | | | | | 4 |
| Swaziland | | 1644 | | | 12 |
| Sweden | | | | | |
| Switzerland | | | | | |
| Syrian Arab Republic | 27,545 | 22,468 | | 27,545 | 1690 |
| Tajikistan | 10,594 | | | 12,978 | |
| Thailand | | | | | |
| The former Yugoslav Republic of Macedonia | | | | | 1 |
| Timor-Leste | | 2209 | | | 69 |
| Togo | 12,612 | 12,612 | | 15,568 | 278 |
| Tonga | | | | | 4 |
| Trinidad and Tobago | | | | | 6 |
| Tunisia | | | | | |
| Turkey | | | | | |
| Turkmenistan | | | | | |
| Uganda | 91,863 | 91,863 | | 113,665 | 1735 |
| Ukraine | | | | | 1153 |
| United Arab Emirates | | | | | |
| United Kingdom | | | | | |
| United Republic of Tanzania | 113,951 | | | 141,069 | |
| United States of America | | | | | 1302 |
| Uruguay | | | | | |
| Uzbekistan | | | | | |
| Vanuatu | | 350 | | | 34 |
| Venezuela (Bolivarian Republic of) | | 25,643 | | | 310 |
| Viet Nam | | | | | |
| Yemen | 38,249 | 38,249 | | 46,795 | 2308 |

| Country | Scenario 1A Population (In 000) | Scenario 1B Population (In 000) | Scenario 3 Population (In 000) | Scenario 4 Population (In 000) | Scenario 5 Population (In 000) |
|---|---|---|---|---|---|
| Zambia | 34,112 | 34,112 | | 42,213 | 511 |
| Zimbabwe | 23,410 | 23,410 | | 28,748 | 132 |

## Appendix B. Average Percentage Difference between MCV1 and MCV2 Coverage at the Year of Introduction of MCV2

| WHO Region Countries | Low- and Lower-Middle Income Countries | Upper-Middle- and High-Income Countries |
|---|---|---|
| AFR | 32.2% | 16.1% |
| AMR | 10.8% | 24.4% |
| EMR | 20.3% | N/A |
| SEAR | 40.1% | N/A |
| WPR | 22.3% | N/A |

The work of LK Kayembe and JL Kriss derived from the 2016 revision of the WHO/UNICEF Estimates Of National Immunization Coverage and the corresponding historical World Bank Country and Lending Groups can be found at https://datahelpdesk.worldbank.org/knowledgebase/articles/906519-world-bank-country-and-lending-groups (accessed on 5 September 2024). Data file is: https://datacatalogfiles.worldbank.org/ddh-published/0037712/DR0090754/OGHIST.xlsx (accessed on 5 September 2024).

## Appendix C. Relative Future MCV1 and MCV2 Coverage Estimation Methodology

At any given coverage level, the difference between MCV1 and MCV2 is subject to capping; in other words, the minimum difference between MCV1 and MCV2 varies depending on the value of MCV1 coverage. All coverage caps were determined by the median of minimum differences between MCV1 and MCV2 coverage of countries in each World Bank income group. For low- and middle-income countries with MCV1 coverage below 80%, the minimum difference is 4%; for countries with MCV1 coverage from 80% to 89%, the value is 3%. MCV2 coverage could equal MCV1 coverage when the latter is 90% or higher. Similarly, for high-income countries, MCV1 and MCV2 coverages could be equal.

## Appendix D. Supplemental Immunization Activity (SIA) Interval and Estimated Coverage for Select Countries

| Country | SIA interval | SIA Coverage |
|---|---|---|
| DRC | 4-year interval | 95.3 (2028) to 95.7 (2032) |
| Guinea | 3-year interval | 95.9 (2026), 95.9 (2029), 95.9 (2032) |
| CAR | 2-year interval | 93.7 (2026), 93.7 (2028), 93.7 (2030), 93.7 (2032) |

## Appendix E. Example of Estimation of Future Potential Demand for Measles Vaccine (Detailed Calculation)

Data for the DRC for the year 2028:

MCV1: 82.5%; RI wastage rate: 30%; surviving infant population size of 3,896,524.

MCV1 doses needed for 2028 for DRC (MAP1):

$$\begin{aligned} MAP1 &= Target\ population \times MCV1\ coverage \times wastage\ rate \\ &= 3,896,524 \times 82.5\% \times \frac{100}{100-30} \\ &= 4,592,332 \end{aligned}$$

## Appendix F. Notes on Altering Estimates of Future Potential Demand

As described in the main text, we estimated future potential demand by extrapolating historical measles vaccination coverage for each of the 180 countries included in our estimations. We first used natural logarithmic regression to fit the 2000–2016 historical measles-containing vaccine first dose (MCV1) coverage data for each country. The results of such estimations are available in the Tool, in the Tabs labeled "MCV1" and "MCV2".

The calculated future demand was then estimated, year by year, using the equation set out in Appendix E. For each country and each future year, the equation combines the target population, the extrapolated MCV1 coverage and the wastage rate. For each country, for each year (both historical and estimates of future coverage), the data are available in the tool (see Table labeled "Contents Variables List" for guidance as to where each dataset is in the tool).

## Appendix G. Altering the Estimates of Future Potential Demand

The Tool (MR MAP tool v1.0 FINAL.xlsm) can be accessed at www.mdpi.com/xxx/s1. Users of the tool can adjust the estimates of potential future coverage (and thus automatically update/alter estimates of demand) by adding in their own estimates of future coverage. Such estimates need to be performed "on the sides", with the results being placed in the appropriate country and year (in the Tab labeled "MCV1").

Estimations of future potential demand for MCV2 can be similarly altered (but attention needs to be paid to the "Cessation Rules"—as described in the main text).

## References


1. Measles & Rubella Initiative. The Problem. Available online: https://measlesrubellainitiative.org/learn/the-problem/ (accessed on 12 February 2024).
2. Minta, A.A.; Ferrari, M.; Antoni, S.; Portnoy, A.; Sbarra, A.; Lambert, B.; Hatcher, C.; Hsu, C.H.; Ho, L.L.; Steulet, C.; et al. Progress Toward Regional Measles Elimination—Worldwide, 2000–2022. *MMWR Morb. Mortal. Wkly. Rep.* **2023**, *72*, 1262–1268. [CrossRef] [PubMed]
3. Ou, A.C.; Zimmerman, L.A.; Alexander, J.P., Jr.; Crowcroft, N.S.; O'Connor, P.M.; Knapp, J.K. Progress Toward Rubella and Congenital Rubella Syndrome Elimination—Worldwide, 2012–2022. *MMWR Morb. Mortal. Wkly. Rep.* **2024**, *73*, 162–167. [CrossRef] [PubMed]
4. United Nations International Children's Emergency Fund (UNICEF). More than 117 Million Children at Risk of Missing out on Measles Vaccines, as COVID-19 Surges. Available online: https://www.unicef.org/press-releases/more-117-million-children-risk-missing-out-measles-vaccines-covid-19-surges (accessed on 5 September 2024).
5. World Health Organization. Measles vaccines: WHO position paper—April 2017. *Wkly. Epidemiol. Record* **2017**, *92*, 205–228.
6. Korkmaz, E.; Balmert, S.C.; Sumpter, T.L.; Donahue Carez, C.; Erdos, G.; Falo, L.D. Microarray patches enable the development of skin-targeted vaccines against COVID-19. *Adv. Drug Deliv. Rev.* **2021**, *171*, 164–186. [CrossRef] [PubMed]
7. VAXXAS. Technology Platform. 2023. Available online: https://www.vaxxas.com/technology-platform/ (accessed on 12 February 2024).
8. Adigweme, I.; Yisa, M.; Ooko, M.; Akpalu, E.; Bruce, A.; Donkor, S.; Jarju, L.B.; Danso, B.; Mendy, A.; Jeffries, D.; et al. A measles and rubella vaccine microneedle patch in The Gambia: A phase 1/2, double-blind, double-dummy, randomised, active-controlled, age de-escalation trial. *Lancet* **2024**, *403*, 1879–1892. [CrossRef] [PubMed]
9. World Health Organization; UNICEF. Measles-Rubella Microarray Patch (MR–MAP) Target Product Profile. June 2019. Available online: https://apps.who.int/iris/bitstream/handle/10665/330394/9789240000209-eng.pdf (accessed on 12 February 2024).
10. Ko, M.; Malvolti, S.; Cherian, T.; Mantel, C.; Biellik, R.; Jarrahian, C.; Menozzi-Arnaud, M.; Amori, J.-P.; Christiansen, H.; Papania, M.J.; et al. Estimating the future global dose demand for measles-rubella microarray patches. *Front. Public Health* **2023**, *10*, 1037157. [CrossRef] [PubMed]
11. Nkenyi, R.; Pak, G.D.; Tonga, C.; Chon, Y.; Park, S.E.; Kang, S. A retrospective review of vaccine wastage and associated risk factors in the Littoral region of Cameroon during 2016–2017. *BMC Public Health* **2022**, *22*, 1956. [CrossRef] [PubMed]
12. Mvundura, M.; Ng, J.; Reynolds, K.; Ng, Y.; Bawa, J.; Bambo, M.; Bonsu, G.; Payne, J.; Chua, J.; Guerette, J.; et al. Vaccine wastage in Ghana, Mozambique, and Pakistan: An assessment of wastage rates for four vaccines and the context, causes, drivers, and knowledge, attitudes and practices for vaccine wastage. *Vaccine* **2023**, *41*, 4158–4169. [CrossRef] [PubMed]
13. Bol, K.; Atem Anyuon, N.; Nyasimi Mokaya, E. Assessment of vaccine wastage in South Sudan. *Pan Afr. Med. J.* **2021**, *40*, 114. [CrossRef] [PubMed]
14. Dadari, I.; Ropiti, L.; Patson, A.; Okia, P.; Narasia, J.; Hare'e, T.; Namohunu, S.; Ogaoga, D.; Gaiofa, J.; Usuf, E. An assessment of vaccine wastage in the Solomon Islands. *PLOS Glob. Public Health* **2022**, *2*, e0000572. [CrossRef] [PubMed]
15. World Bank Open Data. 2017. Available online: https://data.worldbank.org/ (accessed on 15 May 2018).

16. United Nations Department of Economic and Social Affairs. World Population Prospects 2024. Available online: https://population.un.org/wpp/ (accessed on 4 September 2024).
17. Winter, A.K.; Lambert, B.; Klein, D.; Klepac, P.; Papadopoulos, T.; Truelove, S.; Burgess, C.; Santos, H.; Knapp, J.K.; Reef, S.E.; et al. Feasibility of measles and rubella vaccination programmes for disease elimination: A modelling study. *Lancet Glob. Health* **2022**, *10*, e1412–e1422. [CrossRef] [PubMed]
18. World Bank Data Team. New Country Classifications by Income Level: 2017–2018. 1 July 2017. Available online: https://blogs.worldbank.org/en/opendata/new-country-classifications-income-level-2017-2018 (accessed on 5 September 2024).
19. World Health Organization. Measles vaccines: WHO position paper. *Wkly. Epidemiol. Rec.* **2009**, *84*, 349–360.
20. Adhikari, B.B.; Goodson, J.L.; Chu, S.Y.; Rota, P.A.; Meltzer, M.I. Assessing the Potential Cost-Effectiveness of Microneedle Patches in Childhood Measles Vaccination Programs: The Case for Further Research and Development. *Drugs R D* **2016**, *16*, 327–338. [CrossRef] [PubMed]
21. Fu, H.; Abbas, K.; Malvolti, S.; Gregory, C.; Ko, M.; Amorij, J.P.; Jit, M. Impact and cost-effectiveness of measles vaccination through microarray patches in 70 low-income and middle-income countries: Mathematical modelling and early-stage economic evaluation. *BMJ Glob. Health* **2023**, *8*, e012204. [CrossRef] [PubMed]
22. Lohmann Therapie-Systeme AG Press Release. LTS to Support Micron Biomedical as Strategic CDMO Partner to Scale Up Micron's Microarray Patch Technology. 15 January 2024. Available online: https://www.ltslohmann.com/en/press-releases/lts-to-support-micron-biomedical-as-strategic-cdmo-partner-to-scale-up-microns-microarray-patch-technology/ (accessed on 25 April 2024).
23. Nelson, M.; Vaxxas Opens Needle-Free Vax Patch Plant Down under. BioProcess Insider. 20 June 2023. Available online: https://www.bioprocessintl.com/facilities-capacity/vaxxas-opens-needle-free-vax-patch-plant-down-under (accessed on 25 April 2024).
24. Creelman, B.; Frivold, C.; Jessup, S.; Saxon, G.; Jarrahian, C. Manufacturing readiness assessment for evaluation of the microneedle array patch industry: An exploration of barriers to full-scale manufacturing. *Drug Deliv. Transl. Res.* **2022**, *12*, 368–375. [CrossRef] [PubMed]
25. World Health Organization. Global Measles Threat Continues to Grow as Another Year Passes with Millions of Children Unvaccinated. Available online: https://www.who.int/news/item/16-11-2023-global-measles-threat-continues-to-grow-as-another-year-passes-with-millions-of-children-unvaccinated#:~:text=Of%20the%2022%20million%20children,,%20Nigeria,%20Pakistan%20and%20Philippines (accessed on 26 February 2024).

*vaccines* MDPI

*Article*

# Exploring Important Attributes, the Potential Use Cases and Feasibility of Introduction of Measles and Rubella Microarray Patches (MR-MAPs): Insights from Nine Countries

**Mateusz Hasso-Agopsowicz [1,*], Dijana Spasenoska [1], Maarten Paul Maria Jansen [1], Balcha Girma Masresha [2], Desiree Pastor [3], Abay Hagos Gebrekidan [4], Olivi Silalahi [5], Janice Woolford [6], Annet Kisakye [7], Anna-Lea Kahn [1] and Birgitte Giersing [1]**

1 Vaccine Product & Delivery Research, Department of Immunization, Vaccines & Biologicals, World Health Organization, 1211 Geneva, Switzerland
2 Vaccine Preventable Diseases, World Health Organization Regional Office for Africa (AFRO/WHO), Harare P.O. Box CY 348, Zimbabwe
3 Immunization Unit, Pan American Health Organization (PAHO), Washington, DC 20037, USA
4 WHO Ethiopia Country Office, Addis Ababa P.O. Box 3069, Ethiopia
5 WHO Indonesia Country Office, Jakarta 12940, Indonesia
6 Family and Community Health-Immunization Focal Point, PAHO/WHO Guyana Country Office, Georgetown P.O. Box 10969, Guyana
7 WHO Uganda Country Office, Kampala P.O. Box 24578, Uganda
* Correspondence: hassoagopsowiczm@who.int

**Abstract: Background**: Microarray patches (MAPs) are innovative, needle-free vaccine delivery systems, suitable for administration by minimally trained health care workers or trained community health workers. Their introduction may transform immunization programmes, particularly for vaccines where high coverage is required for population immunity, such as measles, and where vaccine delivery is challenging, such as in low- and middle-income countries. Recognizing the need to understand how best to tailor these products to reflect country priorities, workshops on measles and rubella MAPs (MR-MAPs) were conducted in multiple regions to collect insights on needs and preferences from relevant stakeholders at country level. **Methods**: The CAPACITI Innovation Framework was used to structure stakeholder discussions in nine countries in the period from August 2022 to July 2023. The discussions, building on the findings from a situation analysis on the barriers related to measles and rubella vaccine delivery, followed the four-step process outlined in the framework. **Results**: Key barriers hindering delivery of measles and rubella vaccines across the countries were in the categories of human resource management, service delivery, and demand generation. MR-MAP attributes that stakeholders believed would reduce or eliminate these barriers included ease of preparation and administration, improved thermostability, fewer (ancillary) components, and single-dose presentation. Some attributes such as the site of administration, wear time, and storage volume could exacerbate certain barriers. Based on an understanding of key barriers, product attributes, and underserved populations, stakeholders identified several potential use cases for MR-MAPs: (i) delivery at a fixed health post, (ii) delivery through outreach sessions conducted by health workers, and (iii) administration by community health workers. To enable robust national decision making about the introduction of MR-MAPs and successful implementation, global and national evidence on feasibility and acceptability of MR-MAPs should be generated. To prepare for the potential introduction of MR-MAPs, immunization programmes should evaluate their immunization policies based on their preferred use cases and modify them if needed, for example, to enable community health workers to administer vaccines, along with making programmatic adjustments to waste management and training. **Conclusions**: MR-MAPs have the potential to reduce key barriers to MR delivery. Yet, their future impact depends on the ability of global stakeholders to steer the development of MR-MAPs to be responsive to country needs and preferences. The generation of evidence to enable robust decision making, timely modification of vaccine policies, and addressing programmatic considerations will be key to successful uptake.

**Keywords:** microarray patches; measles; rubella; vaccine

## 1. Introduction

Microarray patches (MAPs) are anticipated to become a transformative, needle-free vaccine delivery innovation. Comprised of micro-projections on a 'patch' laden with a dried vaccine, these patches, when applied to the skin, directly deliver the vaccine into the dermis and/or epidermis. MAPs remove the need for vaccine reconstitution, thereby improving safety during administration, enabling administration by minimally trained personnel, and removing sharps waste. They also appear to be less painful than injectable vaccines which could increase the willingness to be vaccinated among those for whom fear of needles or pain is a significant issue. Currently, MAPs are under development for various vaccines, including measles and rubella (MR) vaccines. The latter receive a significant focus due to the need for high coverage to establish and maintain herd immunity and achieve the global goal of eliminating MR. Yet, 22 million children in 2022 did not receive their first dose of measles containing vaccine, and the number of measles cases increased to 9.2 million [1]. Hence, innovations in delivering vaccines are needed to improve access, increase vaccination coverage, and reduce inequity. MR-MAPs have been identified by WHO's Strategic Advisory Groups of Experts on Immunization (SAGE) as a priority innovation to help eliminate measles and rubella [2].

The single-dose format of MR-MAPs eliminates the hesitancy to open multi-dose vials when only a few children are present at the vaccination session. This reduces missed opportunities for vaccination (MOVs) and vaccine wastage. Importantly, MAPs could also offer improved thermostability, which could reduce the need for cold chain during vaccine delivery in outreach or campaigns [3]. Given these operational advantages, MAPs have the potential to increase equitable coverage and facilitate vaccine administration in inaccessible areas, playing a pivotal role in reducing the disease burden [4]. MAPs were prioritized by the Gavi, World Health Organization (WHO), and UNICEF-led Vaccine Innovation Prioritisation Strategy (VIPS) in 2020 to advance development of vaccine innovations with expected impact on equity and coverage [5].

Significant work has been conducted to advance MR-MAP development. Examples include development of a target product profile for MR-MAPs [6]; identification and validation of use cases [7]; acceptability and human factor studies [8,9]; evaluation of thermostability [10,11]; impact and cost-effectiveness study [4]; and estimation of MR-MAP demand [12]. A phase I/II trial in nine-month-old infants in the Gambia has shown that safety and immunogenicity of MR vaccines delivered by a MAP is comparable to MR vaccines delivered by needle and syringe (N/S) [13]. Despite these efforts, it is unlikely that MR-MAPs will become available before 2029. Broad-scale and early availability requires substantial at-risk investment in manufacturing for MAP developers, MR manufacturers, and partners, as there are uncertainties in MR-MAP demand [14,15].

Historical trends have shown that a lack of understanding regarding the specific needs and preferences of low- and middle-income countries (LMICs) often culminates in vaccine products that are ill suited for these settings [16]. In the context of MR-MAPs, it is paramount to gain a clear understanding of countries' viewpoints on several issues: the potential use cases of MR-MAPs, important MAP attributes for priority use cases, and the evidence countries deem essential to confidently decide on the introduction of MR-MAPs. Gaining insights into these issues is instrumental to understand the demand for MR-MAPs, guide investments in their production, ensure the developed products are tailored to countries' requirements, and facilitate their rapid uptake into national immunization programmes. Given the ongoing investments in manufacturing facility, these questions need to be answered now to influence the finalization of the MAP design. Furthermore, the insights will chart the course for decision-making pathways, ensuring that the right evidence to enable robust decision making is collected during development, and appropriate guidance is on hand to aid countries in adopting and using MR-MAPs [3].

Recognizing the importance of country-level perspectives to evaluate the product innovation, we have conducted consultations with national stakeholders from nine countries to (1) determine and prioritize immunization barriers specific to MR vaccines which can be impacted by changing the way vaccines are delivered; (2) identify critical attributes of MR-MAPs to reduce or eliminate these prioritized barriers; (3) understand and validate potential use cases for MR-MAPs; (4) identify likely data and evidence needed for the eventual introduction of MR-MAPs before they are approved for use, but not yet deciding whether to introduce the product; (5) familiarize stakeholders with MR-MAPs, their attributes, and status of development. In this paper we report the findings from these consultations.

## 2. Methodology

### 2.1. The CAPACITI Innovation Framework

The CAPACITI Innovation Framework, developed by WHO, was used as a methodology for conducting the workshops. The CAPACITI Innovation Framework is a tailored process, which facilitates discussion, deliberation, and communication between stakeholders from diverse levels and disciplines within the immunization system to agree on potential programmatic implications of an innovation. Furthermore, it guides discussions around perceived value and acceptability requirements of the innovation in comparison with the current practice and seeks to identify important decision criteria and the evidence needed for eventual robust decisions on the introduction of the innovation. The Innovation Framework is available in an Excel workbook, which has been adapted with specific questions for MR-MAPs. The outcomes of each of the workshops have been systematically documented in separate, dedicated workbooks. Figure 1 shows the steps of the framework, which are further described below. A full methodology of the CAPACITI Innovation Workshops is described elsewhere [17].

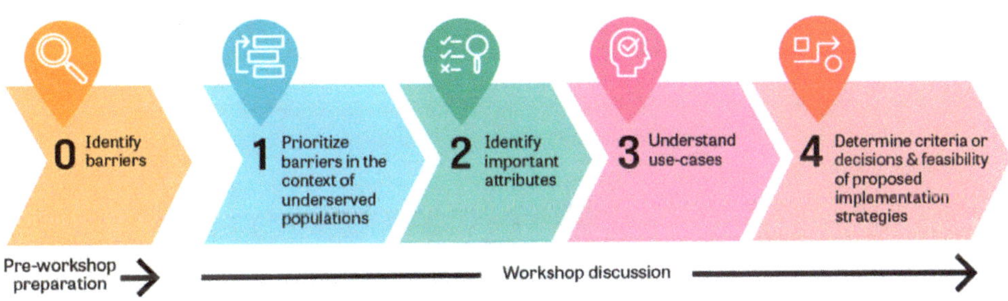


**Figure 1.** The methodology of the Innovation Framework workshops.

### 2.2. Step 0: Identifying Barriers

To understand the country context, a comprehensive evidence-based situation analysis of the national immunization programme performance was conducted [18]. Existing documents on immunization programme performance were reviewed and evidence around barriers was documented, for each of the seven EPI categories: programme management; human resources management; vaccine supply, quality and logistics; service delivery; immunization coverage and adverse events following immunization (AEFI); disease surveillance; and demand generation. The outcome of the situation analysis was a list of programmatic barriers undermining high and equitable vaccine coverage. The list of identified barriers was validated by national stakeholders.

### 2.3. Step 1: Prioritizing Barriers in the Context of Underserved Populations

The list of programmatic barriers to equitable and high vaccination coverage was reduced to barriers relevant to MR vaccine coverage and equity, through a discussion with participants. The relevance of barriers and their impact on coverage of MR vaccines varies at sub-national level depending on the context of the underserved and unvaccinated populations. Thus, each country defined their own specific sub-national settings based on specific characteristics (e.g., geography, socio-economic, and cultural context). For instance, in Ethiopia, the stakeholders specified agrarian, pastoralist, and urban settings, while in Indonesia, the settings were grouped based on their socio-economic development. In Uganda, the settings reflected the diverse terrains and communities–mountainous regions, conflict-prone areas and islands, inhabited by nomadic and fishing communities, as well as refugees and displaced populations. Stakeholders discussed a comprehensive list of barriers within the identified settings and determined the highest priority barriers for each. They then finalized a combined list of the highest priority barriers by automatically including those that are cross-cutting across settings and debating the inclusion of additional high-priority barriers relevant only to specific underserved populations.

### 2.4. *Step 2: Identifying Important Attributes of MR-MAPs*

For each of the high-priority barriers identified in Step 1, stakeholders were asked to evaluate whether MR-MAP attributes, identified in the WHO/UNICEF Target Product Profile (TPP) for MR-MAPs [6], could have an effect on the barrier. An attribute could reduce or eliminate the barrier, increase the barrier, have an indirect benefit, impose indirect challenges, or it might not have any effect. More than one attribute and effect could be selected per barrier.

### 2.5. *Step 3: Understanding the Potential Use of MR-MAPs*

To effectively guide MR-MAP product development, it is essential to anticipate how this innovation would be used by immunization programmes. Identifying the likely use cases will further validate the importance of critical product attributes, help to understand the feasibility and acceptability of MR-MAPs, and inform introduction strategies. Prior studies have explored MR-MAPs' use based on the service provider (health worker, community health worker, or self-administration) and delivery location (fixed health post, outreach, other setting) (Supplementary Figure S1) [7]. The six distinct use cases that emerged from the prior studies were consolidated into four use cases considered during the workshops. Participants discussed whether these use cases could be feasible and desirable in their country and reflected appropriate and desired applications of MR-MAPs to reduce the identified barriers.

### 2.6. *Step 4: Understanding Decision Pathways and Decision Criteria for Decision Making About the Introduction of MR-MAPs in the Immunization Programme at the National Level*

To understand the introduction decision pathway at the national level, stakeholders were asked to describe the steps required for decision making about the potential introduction of MR-MAPs in the immunization programme.

Focusing on the potential decision to introduce MR-MAPs, stakeholders were asked to agree on important decision-making criteria and key evidence needed to ensure robust decision making, drawing on their previous discussions throughout the workshop. The design of this group discussion was informed by the CAPACITI decision-support tool guidance [19], in particular, regarding part 2 identifying decision criteria, and part 3 evidence assessment, which provides guidance on the development of an evidence assessment plan. Finally, stakeholders were asked about the perceived feasibility of delivering two MR vaccine presentations in a country: a mixed delivery of MAP and needle and syringe (N/S).

### 2.7. *Selection of Countries for Engagement*

To capture multiple and varied national contexts, a long list of target countries was developed. Key considerations for choosing the countries included geographic diversity, number of zero-dose children, sub-national variation in vaccination coverage, and unique features (e.g., local production of vaccines, large number of special populations such as refugees). Focal points in the identified countries were contacted through official communication channels by WHO and partner organizations. Following initial discussions around the feasibility of conducting such workshop (e.g., elections preventing workshops to take place, stakeholders busy responding to an outbreak or conducting a vaccination campaign), and in consultation with WHO Regional Offices, nine countries were identified.

Between August 2022 and July 2023, four workshops were conducted with a total of nine countries, and three WHO regions, through single-country and multi-country engagements. Single country workshops were conducted in Ethiopia, Indonesia, and Uganda, while Guyana, Belize, Trinidad, and Tobago, Suriname, Jamaica, and Barbados were engaged in a multi-country workshop.

### *2.8. Selection of Workshop Stakeholders*

The list of participants for each workshop was developed in consultation with the respective Ministry of Health, WHO headquarters, Regional Offices, or Country Offices. The general guidance for each country was to nominate 30 to 50 participants who are relevant to the measles and rubella vaccination in the country. They were encouraged to include a wide range of stakeholders, for instance various departments within the ministry, sub-national focal points, health workers, national immunization technical advisory groups, academia, implementing partners, and civil society organizations. The list of organizations represented varied between countries, although the general profile was within the suggested guidelines. The details of the workshop logistics are listed in the Supplementary Material Table S1.

## 3. Results and Discussion

### *3.1. Step 1: Identification and Prioritisation of Barriers to Measles and Rubella Immunization*

In each country, the situation analysis revealed 30-40 barriers of the national immunization programme performance across all seven EPI categories. The list was narrowed to 15–18 barriers through a prioritization discussion during the workshop. Some of the prioritized barriers hindering MR vaccination coverage and equity included an inadequate supply of health staff coupled with a high turn-over of staff, and inadequate training. Furthermore, the transport of vaccines to remote delivery settings was a big challenge, together with inadequate cold chain quality and inappropriate monitoring of heat or freeze exposure during transport. The logistics were further challenged by long distance and travel time, and the need for intensified outreach to special and remote populations. Challenges around data quality and accuracy of denominators for calculating target populations were prevalent across the majority of settings. Lastly, demand-related barriers were prevalent such as fear of multiple injections, cultural and religious concerns, and lack of confidence and trust in vaccines. The full list of prioritized barriers is available in the Supplementary Material.

### *3.2. Step 2: Identification of Important Attributes of MR-MAPs*

Most of the positive effects of MR-MAPs on barriers were associated with ease of preparation and administration, single-dose presentation, improved thermostability, and fewer ancillary components required for vaccination (Figure 2). There is variability across countries in the number of barriers that stakeholders believed a specific attribute could impact, and there are differences across countries regarding which attributes were perceived as having the potential to impact the widest range of barriers. For instance, in Ethiopia, the attribute around reduced clinical training requirements could address only four barriers, while in Uganda, it could positively impact nine barriers. Moreover, there were some attributes that could negatively affect barriers, such as the site of administration, the required wear time of up to five minutes, and the relatively bulkier volume of MR-MAPs as compared to a single MR dose within a multi-dose vial. The nuanced discussions about the impact of specific MR-MAP attributes on the immunization barriers are further explained below.

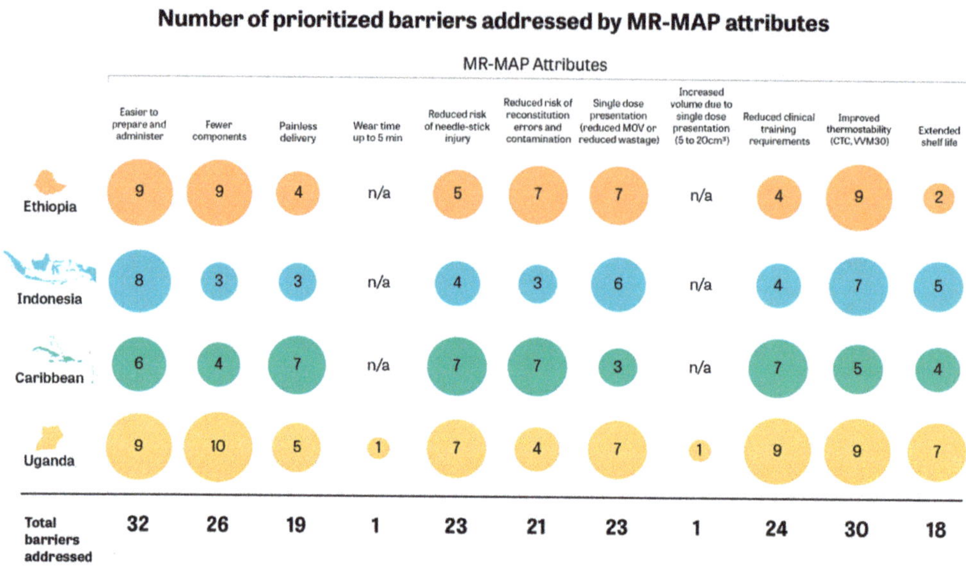


**Figure 2.** Number of prioritized barriers addressed by MR-MAP attributes. CTC (controlled temperature chain), VVM30 (vaccine vial monitor 30), MOV (missed opportunities for vaccination), n/a (not applicable).

3.2.1. Focus on Specific Attributes: Thermostability

Improved thermostability of MR-MAPs is seen as a significant leap towards ensuring broader vaccine access, especially in areas where maintaining a cold chain is difficult. This can particularly aid in reaching vulnerable or hard-to-reach populations. The WHO/UNICEF TPP for MR-MAPs stipulates that vaccine stability should surpass that of the current MR vaccines. MAPs should have vaccine vial monitors (VVMs)—small temperature-sensitive indicators that gradually darken as the vaccine is exposed to cumulative heat. The range of acceptable VVMs consists of those with a 14-day maximum cumulative heat exposure (VVM14), and ideally those with a 30-day threshold (VVM30) or more, allowing for greater and longer exposures to temperatures beyond the standard 2 to 8 °C cold chain. MR-MAPs should also be compatible with use in a controlled temperature chain (CTC), tolerating a single excursion out of the standard cold chain of at least three days at 40 °C [6].

The positive impact of potentially enhanced thermostability resonated with all national immunization programme stakeholders. This attribute could reduce logistical challenges in transporting vaccines over long distances to remote sites, reaching currently underserved populations. Moreover, it could reduce the risk of closed vial wastage due to heat or freeze damage, which may occur with inadequate maintenance of the cold chain or mishandling of the vaccine, challenges that are currently not well documented.

However, it is essential to also recognize the new challenges MR-MAPs might introduce. Implementing vaccine delivery under CTC conditions would necessitate initial specialized training. Furthermore, concerns were raised about potential wastage; poor microplanning could lead to an excessive number of vaccines being taken out of the cold chain into CTC and as they cannot then be returned to the cold chain, they must be discarded if they are unused at the end of the specified number of days. This is a particularly important consideration in the context of identified challenges around accurate estimates of the size of populations who need to be vaccinated.

### 3.2.2. Focus on Specific Attributes: Wear Time

The WHO/UNICEF TPP states that the acceptable wear time for MR-MAPs is up to five minutes and optimally less than one minute. A MAP should be worn for the specified time, observed and removed by an HCW, trained lay health worker, or caregiver [6]. Among workshop stakeholders and those familiar with MAPs, there was a shared concern that a duration up to five minutes might extend the immunization sessions.

However, stakeholders in the workshops argued that with some adjustments, the five-minute wear time could be accommodated into routine immunization sessions. Generally, caregivers spend about 30 min at vaccination points for the monitoring of AEFIs. Additionally, the time spent in a clinic often exceeds an hour, to include activities such as health measurements, vitamin administration, and informational discussions about vaccines, nutrition, and more. As such, accommodating a five-minute wear time during standard immunization sessions appears feasible. The challenges might differ for immunization campaigns or house-to-house delivery, where the five minute wear time could exceed the length of a contact point during vaccine delivery. The challenges associated with the five-minute wear time could potentially be reduced by planning the order of administered vaccines—starting with the MR-MAP and then proceeding with other injectable vaccines.

Stakeholders expressed the need for additional data on the consequences of wearing the MAP for too long, and on the protocol to supervise a child and ensure that the MAP stays at the site of administration. They emphasized that if a MAP needs to be held in place for the duration of wear time, it would be preferred for caregivers to do so rather than health workers, to avoid increasing the time burden and reducing session quality.

In conclusion, there is preference for wear time of up to one minute over five minutes, and caregivers to hold the child's body part still during application and wear time over health workers.

### 3.2.3. Focus on Specific Attributes: Site of Administration

The WHO/UNICEF TPP specifies that the site of application should not impede efficacy of vaccination, however, it does not specify the exact site. The noted preferable locations on infants and toddlers are those that are less likely to be disturbed and/or removed (such as the scapula) or the upper arm in older children. However, some of the MAPs in development are being tested on other anatomical sites such as the wrist. Hence, during the discussions in Uganda, the feasibility and desirability of the wrist as a delivery site was explored.

Stakeholders expressed preference for the flexibility to apply the MR-MAP at various anatomical sites. There were some concerns around the wrist as a delivery site. Some argued that children could remove the patch, while others proposed that with robust adhesion, this issue could be mitigated. In other countries, marking of the wrist might have some negative cultural and religious connotation, so appropriate communication strategies must be in place to avoid significant challenges around community acceptance. However, despite some reservations, participants agreed that the delivery site is not a critical concern that would significantly impede introduction of MR-MAPs.

Furthermore, participants expressed a desire for more evidence on how different skin factors, such as moisture levels, thickness, and external factors like air humidity, could affect effectiveness of MR-MAPs.

### 3.2.4. Focus on Specific Attributes: Increased Volume

The minimal acceptable target for MR-MAPs cold chain storage volume per dose is specified as no greater than a single-dose vial of injectable MR vaccine (21.09 $cm^3$). Yet, given that the current practice is the use of a five or ten multi-dose vial, with volumes ranging between 5.5 $cm^3$/dose and 2.1 $cm^3$/dose in secondary packaging, the single-dose presentation of MR-MAPs would inevitably lead to increased cold chain volume, bringing a set of direct and indirect challenges. Directly, the larger volume could result in larger cold chain space requirements prior to the final stages of vaccine delivery, thereby putting a strain on existing infrastructure, especially in regions where cold chain systems might already be at capacity. Indirectly, this increased volume implies a surge in needed financial resources for the necessary cold chain enhancements and other logistical considerations. However, the impact of MAPs on cold chain requires further evaluation as it depends on the final MAP attributes, available cold chain equipment, and capacity in countries.

While the MR-MAPs could offer thermostability benefits, these might not be enough to entirely counterbalance the cold chain constraints associated with their increased volume. The CTC advantage, though significant, is only available as an option during the final stages of vaccine delivery, also referred to as the "last mile", and it typically applies for only a few days just prior to administration.

Given these concerns, participants specified that before any widespread introduction of MR-MAPs, a thorough assessment of their impact on existing cold chain systems would be needed. Such evaluations could be conducted before or integrated into pilot studies, ensuring that countries are adequately prepared to handle the logistical demands of these patches.

#### 3.2.5. Acceptability of MR-MAPs

The introduction of MR-MAPs into immunization programmes may impact vaccine acceptance. It could alleviate barriers associated with fear or dislike of multiple injections during a single visit, often a concern for both caregivers and health workers. The trust in the immunization process could be further bolstered if community health workers or caregivers were trained to administer these patches, increasing ownership of the vaccination process, and reducing distrust in the health system. Additionally, workshop participants acknowledged that by eliminating vaccine reconstitution errors, MR-MAPs can reduce the occurrence of adverse effects post-immunization, alleviating concerns that caregivers might have around vaccine safety.

However, the novel vaccine presentation might also exacerbate some demand barriers. If communication and community sensitization prior to introduction of MR-MAPs is inadequate, hesitancy might be observed. Doubts might arise around the novel presentation of the vaccine both among caregivers and health workers, as it is different from the current practice a needle and syringe.

### 3.3. *Step 3: Understanding the Potential Use Cases of MR-MAPs*

All use cases discussed during the workshops, and their anticipated adoption and rationale, are shown in Figure 3. Delivery of MR-MAPs at a *fixed post by health or community health workers*, where fixed health post is defined as a permanent structure which has full cold chain capabilities, was deemed attractive for stakeholders from across the participating countries. MR-MAPs, with their ease of administration and potential to reduce injection fear, can benefit immunization programmes by easing the task of vaccination and reducing training needs. For delivery of MR-MAPs *by health workers in settings with limited or no health services* (including delivery in areas that do not have access to fixed health posts and have reduced or no cold chain capacities), workshop participants attributed the value of MR-MAPs to their improved thermostability, making the devices apt for challenging terrains and able to improve reach, which could augment MR vaccine coverage. Provided sufficient CTC time allowances and appropriate demand forecasting, the flexibility afforded by removing cold chain constraints was cited as making MR-MAPs a desirable option not only for routine vaccination but also for targeted campaigns and situations like humanitarian disasters and outbreaks catering to remote populations.

| Use case | Delivery in a **fixed post by health worker or community health worker** | Delivery by **health worker** in settings with limited or no health services | Outreach or campaign delivery by **community health worker** | **Self-administration** with or without health worker or community health worker assistance |
|---|---|---|---|---|
| Adoption | Likely, but requires policy changes | Likely | Likely, but requires policy changes | Challenging, but interested to explore |
| Why? | • Easier to prepare and administer<br>• Less resources needed (e.g. time)<br>• Useful in outbreak settings<br>• Policy change required for community health worker | • Potential to improve coverage<br>• Thermostability key attribute for excursions of cold chain<br>• Easy transport as no need to maintain cold chain<br>• Useful for campaigns, natural disasters, outbreaks, hard to reach populations, surveillance response | • Community trust can decrease hesitancy<br>• Requires less resources and is non-invasive, would lead to greater reach<br>• Alleviates human resources/logistics burden as it is easier to prepare and administer<br>• Useful for high-risk groups, outreach, school-based immunization, outbreak response, natural disasters, mop up campaigns and case surveillance<br>• Requires policy change to allow community health worker to administer<br>• Required conditions: proper training and supervision | • Encourages ownership of care by caregivers and reduces anxiety related to vaccines<br>• Could be used in campaigns<br>• Need more research and policy considerations<br>• Difficulties in disposing biohazard, documenting coverage and monitoring adverse events following immunisation<br>• Policy change required to allow self-admin or community health worker assistance |

**Figure 3.** Use cases to understand the potential use of MR-MAPs. HW, health worker; CHW, community health worker; SIAs, supplementary immunization activities; MR-MAP, measles and rubella microarray patch.

The use of MR-MAPs in *outreach or campaign delivery by community health care workers* was perceived as highly favourable by workshop participants. The foundation of this preference is the belief that vaccinations offered by community health workers operating in settings where they are well known and respected can elevate trust in vaccines, fostering higher acceptance. Deploying MR-MAPs through these workers was viewed as resource efficient, promising a more extensive outreach strategy. Additionally, since MR-MAPs are easier to prepare and administer, their use could significantly lessen the human resource training needs. Such an approach was considered particularly beneficial for targeting high-risk groups, facilitating outreach, initiating school-based immunizations, responding to outbreaks, addressing natural disasters, conducting mop-up campaigns, and strengthening case surveillance. Ensuring the success of these use cases would also hinge on providing these workers with proper training and consistent supervision.

The ability for the *self-administration of MR MAPs with or without health worker or community health worker assistance* offers promising prospects, but their implementation poses notable challenges. The potential for caregivers to administer the vaccines themselves can promote a sense of responsibility towards personal health and possibly diminish anxieties associated with vaccines. These use cases could be especially beneficial during mass vaccination campaigns. However, it was highlighted that several factors need addressing before such use cases can be broadly adopted. Concerns were raised around the documentation of vaccination coverage and ensuring compliance, as well as the monitoring of AEFIs caused mainly by programmatic errors. Similar concerns were shared by stakeholders who contributed to the development of the initial use cases. Moreover, operating procedures for waste management and proper disposal need to be explored. While stakeholders did not rule out these use cases, they noted that significant evidence on the feasibility needs to be generated that would support potential policy and programmatic changes to enable such use.

### 3.3.1. The Ability of Community Health Workers (CHWs) to Deliver Vaccines

As discussed above, workshop participants confirmed the desirability of Community Health Workers (CHWs) to deliver MR vaccines using MAPs which could potentially extend vaccination to underserved populations and alleviate barriers around the shortage of health workers. However, significant policy and programmatic changes are needed to allow for the uptake through these use cases.

CHWs typically reside within the communities they serve, often receiving lower levels of formal education and clinical training than professional healthcare personnel, specifically nurses and doctors. They are either paid community health workers, or volunteers, and they play a key role in supporting and extending health care services to vulnerable and difficult-to-reach populations. Their role in administering vaccines varies across countries and some national policies prevent CHWs from delivering vaccines [20]. From the countries participating in the workshops, some could be categorized as more permissive for the CHW delivery of vaccines (Ethiopia), those that permit vaccine delivery with CHWs in special situations, such as hard-to-reach populations or conflict zones (Indonesia, Uganda), and those that do not permit vaccine delivery with CHWs (Jamaica).

Thus, policy change is needed to allow CHWs to administer vaccines in certain countries. Participants from all countries, except Jamaica, expressed an openness to revising their policies, especially given the MR-MAP is a non-injectable vaccine. Second, a programmatic change is needed to further formalize the role of CHWs and ensure adequate financial compensation for their extended services. The opinions between participants differed about the feasibility of including the CHWs' salaries in the budget, and they highlighted that this would require additional advocacy.

#### 3.3.2. Implications of Integrating MR-MAPs Delivery with Other Non-MAP Vaccines

In Uganda, as well as in several other countries, the potential co-administration of MR-MAPs with other non-MAP vaccines during routine immunization has been discussed. Currently, the MR vaccine is co-administered with yellow fever vaccine in some countries, and there is potential to co-administer it with typhoid, malaria, and other vaccines. However, there is a concern that the unique advantages of MR-MAPs might be reduced when administered alongside other vaccines. For instance, the significant benefit of MR-MAPs' increased thermostability might not be fully appreciated if the cold chain during outreach or campaigns must be maintained for other co-delivered vaccines. Conversely, co-administering MR-MAPs with other vaccines or health interventions could introduce operational efficiencies, such as freeing up cold chain space for the last mile of vaccine delivery or optimizing session time. Importantly, key MR-MAP attributes such as ease of preparation and administration, and non-injectable delivery, were perceived as sufficient advantages for the immunization program to justify MR-MAP use even without enjoying the full advantages.

### *3.4. Step 4: Understanding Decision Pathways and Criteria for Decision Making About the Introduction of MR-MAPs in the Immunization Programme*

Understanding the criteria for decision making about the introduction of MR-MAPs in countries and the evidence needs to inform that process is important for the optimal design of phase III clinical trials, identification of key implementation research, development of financing plans, and introduction and communication strategies.

Countries expressed that the typical decision-making process is expected to be employed to determine whether to introduce and integrate an MR-MAP. With political interest and commitment to measles and rubella elimination, Ministries of Health would likely request a recommendation from National Immunization Technical Advisory Groups (NITAGs) about if and how to introduce MR-MAPs.

As part of the discussion, countries deliberated on a hypothetical potential full switch from MR needle and syringe vaccines to MR-MAPs or a partial switch designated only for certain hard-to-reach populations or limited to delivery strategies such as campaigns. The discussion included the assumption that MR-MAPs will be more expensive than N/S vaccines; however, with growing demand, the price of MAPs should decrease, hopefully making the innovation financially sustainable for countries. Stakeholders identified a wide range of decision criteria, beyond just the cost of the product, such as impact on coverage and equity, waste management implications, and measles elimination targets that would be considered during decision making. Budget impact, cold chain requirements, and vaccine acceptability also featured prominently in countries' considerations. A consolidated list of the evidence required to consider the introduction of MR-MAPs by the participating countries is available in the Supplementary Material, Table S2. It was further suggested that adoption of MR-MAPs would be unlikely if MR-MAPs are not prequalified by WHO.

Ahead of broad-scale implementation, the preference of the nine participating countries leant towards generating local evidence. This might take the form of feasibility studies aimed at addressing vital implementation questions, pilot projects, or subsequently, phased introductions.

#### 3.4.1. Understanding the Feasibility of Mixed Delivery

The feasibility of implementing mixed delivery, where MR vaccines are delivered via MAPs in certain sub-national settings or delivery strategies and through needle and syringe in others, would be influenced by an array of factors that span policy, programmatic, and procurement domains. Countries highlighted that lessons learned from the switch from 10 to 5 dose vials of measles containing vaccine (MCV) should be leveraged to inform the mixed use of MR vaccines delivered by N/S and MAP.

A standard pathway to introduce a new vaccine into a country immunization programme is expected to be followed for MR-MAPs. In addition, inclusion of MAPs into an immunization programme for delivery alongside N/S would also necessitate guidance from technical agencies (e.g., WHO), development of standard operating procedures, and financial backing.

From a programmatic perspective, there are training requirements to facilitate the delivery of mixed presentations of vaccines. Workshop participants expressed that particular attention should be given to training focusing on handling different thermostability profiles, administration routes, and vaccine presentations. Appropriate training would need to be developed and implemented to enable safe and effective administration of MR-MAPs by CHWs—if countries' policies permit. Training and guidance to inform and sensitize communities about MR-MAPs and prevent concerns about different presentations of MR vaccines would be required. Additional training and guidance priorities that were expressed by participating countries included assessment of cold chain capacity coupled with appropriate microplanning for campaigns and outreach immunization to reduce vaccine wastage. Furthermore, effective waste management protocols and updates to the existing information systems are imperative to accommodate mixed delivery, as the waste disposal procedures for the two presentations might differ.

The feasibility of mixed delivery is also underpinned by supply chain considerations. For countries procuring through UNICEF, it is important to understand whether differentiated supply chains are feasible. Additionally, factors such as supply availability, cost per dose, and minimum order requirements might affect the country decision for a mixed-delivery strategy.

#### 3.4.2. The Impact of Cost on the Decision to Introduce MR-MAPs

The price of MR-MAPs is central to considerations for the introduction of MR-MAPs. While the precise price of MR-MAPs remains uncertain, it is anticipated that they will be more expensive than MR vaccines delivered by N/S. During the workshop in Uganda, different cost scenarios were discussed by stakeholders to identify criteria and incremental impact that would justify the increased price. The discussion was conducted under the assumption that the immunogenicity and safety of MR-MAPs will be non-inferior to N/S delivery.

A substantial price disparity between MR-MAPs and conventional MR vaccines could significantly hinder their inclusion in vaccine programmes. Crucially, before considering broader introduction, countries emphasized the importance of undertaking cost–benefit analyses in pilot evaluations, and considering the results in a broader context of the financial challenges and limited budgets facing countries. Nuanced perspectives emerged from different countries. For instance, participants from Uganda underscored the necessity of a comprehensive evaluation of immunization costs. They believe it is essential to consider costs of MR-MAP delivery and introduction in relation to MR-MAPs' impact on wastage, health worker time, and the consequences of inaction, such as the continued prevalence of measles and rubella cases, deaths, and cost of outbreak response. Likewise, in the Caribbean and Guyana, there was a strong regional commitment towards MR elimination. The consensus was that if MR-MAPs could more effectively contribute towards and maintain MR elimination, they should be considered, even if the price were to be higher. However, middle-income countries procuring through the PAHO Revolving Fund have stressed the importance of securing fair pricing for MR-MAPs. In Indonesia, the position was more pragmatic; increased cost would be considered as long as it remained within the pre-determined immunization budget. Overall, gaining a comprehensive understanding of the broader impacts and benefits of MR-MAPs is essential for countries to make informed decisions about their potential adoption.

#### 3.4.3. Considerations for Countries Using MMR in Routine Immunization

The introduction of MR-MAPs in regions where Measles, Mumps, and Rubella (MMR) vaccines are in use, such as the American Region, comes with its own challenges and advantages. Although participating PAHO countries acknowledged the benefits of MR-MAPs, they would be unlikely to replace an MMR vaccine for routine immunization with one effective only against MR, losing the mumps protection. Still, participants expressed that the high cost associated with maintaining measles elimination makes MR-MAPs attractive for strategies other than routine immunization, including follow-up campaigns, mop-up activities especially targeting older groups, outbreak responses, and reaching difficult areas. However, if supplementary immunization activities were to be phased out, the comparative advantage of MR-MAPs will likely diminish. Future deliberations in this context should focus on the investment case for an MMR-MAP.

#### 3.4.4. Evidence Generation and Pilot Programmes Ahead of Wide MR-MAP Implementation

Stakeholders in the workshops acknowledged the need for evidence generation ahead of the introduction of MR-MAPs. Indonesia, Ethiopia, Uganda, and Guyana were interested in participating in clinical trials, conducting feasibility or pilot studies to answer outstanding MR-MAP questions and assumptions and contribute to global evidence generation.

In addition, the majority of countries said that successful implementation of MR-MAPs is likely to require introduction pilots in areas with well-functioning immunization programmes before a wider introduction. These pilot programmes serve a dual purpose: First, they aim to test key assumptions associated with the implementation of MR-MAPs, such as their impact on the cold chain, and impact on vaccine wastage, potential budgetary implications, the quality and effectiveness of health worker training, the acceptability by caregivers and the capability of community health workers to effectively administer MAPs. Second, they are an avenue to curate communication and training materials anchored in local data and perspectives. Engaging local community and religious leaders in this process ensures that the introduction of MR-MAPs resonates with the community and facilitates a smoother, broader rollout in the rest of the country.

## 4. Recommendations

The below recommendations, based on the findings from these workshops, should not supersede those found in the WHO/UNICEF MR-MAP TPP and are intended to complement or highlight attributes that need particular focus during the product development, on the basis of country stakeholder feedback.

On MR-MAP attributes, the following recommendations can be made:

- **Easy Preparation and Administration**: Ensure that the MR-MAP operation is intuitive and straightforward, minimizing requirements for training, as well as steps for vaccine preparation and administration, thereby simplifying the process and minimizing potential errors or challenges in the field. Accompany the product with clear, easy-to-understand instructions, potentially augmented by visual aids or digital tutorials, ensuring that even those with minimal training can administer the vaccine effectively.
- **Thermostability Compliant with VVM14 and CTC Indications**: Dedicate efforts to ensure the MR-MAPs meet at least the VVM14, and ideally VVM30 targets, and are compatible with CTC indications for as long a duration as the stability permits, as outlined in the MR-MAP TPP. Ensure sufficient cold chain capacity to accommodate increased volume for MR-MAPs, if needed.
- **Fewer Components**: Strive for a minimalist design that reduces the volume of a MAP, and the number of ancillary devices (including applicators) required for delivering a vaccine dose.
- **Wear Time**: Given the preference for shorter wear time across use cases, developers should aim for MR-MAPs with no higher than one-minute wear time, ensuring the efficacy or thermostability are not compromised. Provide clear information to vaccinators and caregivers about the consequences of wear time of the MR-MAP beyond the stated duration, improving confidence and ensuring safe application during both routine immunization sessions and campaigns.
- **Site of administration**: Evaluate flexibility in the MR-MAP application site given cultural and programmatic challenges and sensitivities. Undertake studies to evaluate the impact of various skin factors and conditions on MR-MAP efficacy, to ensure broad acceptability and generalizability of their use.

On MR-MAP use cases:

- **Study on Caregiver Involvement**: Conduct studies to assess the feasibility and acceptability of having caregivers hold the child's arm during MR-MAP application, if not already evaluated in trials and if arm restraint is required.
- **Prioritization of Use Cases**: Given the high favourability and potential for broad use of MR-MAPs, should there be financial or supply constraints, prioritize the implementation and scaling of use of MAPs in outreach immunization and campaigns, leveraging community health care workers for effective MR-MAP deployment.
- **Policy and Training**: Develop policies allowing community health workers to administer MR-MAPs and invest in their training.

On MR-MAP introduction and integration, the following recommendations can be made:

- **Research and Feasibility**: In addition to confirmation of safety and immunogenicity of MR-MAPs in clinical trials, conduct operational studies to understand the implementation and integration of MR-MAPs with the immunization programmes in the context of priority use cases.
- **Price Equivalence**: Strive to ensure that the overall cost to immunize a child with MR-MAPs is not significantly higher than MR delivery in multi-dose vials via needle and syringe to encourage widespread adoption.
- **Cold chain assessment**: Conduct comprehensive cold chain impact assessments for MR-MAPs, factoring in volume requirements and thermostability attributes, to inform effective and resource-efficient integration into national immunization programmes.
- **Guidance on CTC**: Develop and support the implementation of clear guidance on CTC for MR-MAPs in countries and regions, as part of the MR-MAP training.
- **Microplanning Tools**: Highlight the need for microplanning tools to account for conditions specific to MR-MAPs, such as CTC, wear time, and way of administering a MAP, to ensure optimized distribution and minimal wastage.

- **Communication**: Prioritize the development of a comprehensive communication strategy to prevent increased hesitancy and concerns stemming from using different vaccine presentations in various populations.
- **Support for pilot studies**: Assist countries expressing interest in MR-MAP pilot programmes to evaluate MAP integration with immunization programmes and measuring impact on MR coverage. Such support should encompass training and communication material development, stakeholder engagement, and evidence generation.

**Supplementary Materials:** The following supporting information can be downloaded at: https://www.mdpi.com/article/10.3390/vaccines12091084/s1. Figure S1: List of six use-cases for MR-MAPs identified through previous analyses (7); Table S1: Overview of types of workshop participants per country; Table S2: A list of the identified criteria required by countries to consider the introduction of MR-MAPs.

**Author Contributions:** M.H.-A. and B.G. secured the funding; M.H.-A., D.S., M.P.M.J. and A.-L.K. designed the study; all authors were involved in the preparation and running of the workshops; M.H.-A., D.S., M.P.M.J., A.-L.K. and B.G. wrote the first draft. All authors have read and agreed to the published version of the manuscript.

**Funding:** This work was funded by a Bill and Melinda Gates Foundation grant (INV-005318) and a grant from the Foreign, Commonwealth & Development Office (FCDO), (award HQUHL2221008/1.2.1/68566) to the World Health Organization.

**Institutional Review Board Statement:** Ethical review and approval was not required for this study because interviews were conducted with experts about their field of expertise.

**Informed Consent Statement:** Informed consent was obtained from all subjects involved in the study.

**Data Availability Statement:** The original contributions presented in the study are included in the article and the Supplementary Material; further inquiries can be directed to the corresponding authors.

**Acknowledgments:** The authors would like to acknowledge the participation of workshop attendees and their contribution to the discussion. The authors would like to also thank the MR-MAP developers for providing MAP samples. We extend our thanks to colleagues who reviewed the article: Natasha Crowcroft (WHO), Philipp Lambach (WHO), Jean-Pierre Amorij (UNICEF), Marion Menozzi-Arnaud (Gavi), Tiziana Scarna (Gavi), and Jarrahian Courtney (PATH).

**Conflicts of Interest:** None of the authors declare a conflict of interest.

**Author Disclaimer:** The findings and conclusions in this article are those of the authors and do not represent the official position of the participating countries, the World Health Organization, Pan American Health Organization or other institutions with which they are affiliated.

## References

1. Minta, A.A.; Ferrari, M.; Antoni, S.; Portnoy, A.; Sbarra, A.; Lambert, B.; Hatcher, C.; Hsu, C.H.; Ho, L.L.; Steulet, C.; et al. Progress Toward Measles Elimination—Worldwide, 2000–2022. *MMWR Morb. Mortal. Wkly. Rep.* **2023**, *72*, 1262–1268. [CrossRef] [PubMed]
2. World Health Organization (WHO). Measles vaccines: WHO position paper April 2017. *Wkly. Epidemiol. Rec.* **2017**, *92*, 205–228.
3. Hasso-Agopsowicz, M.; Crowcroft, N.; Biellik, R.; Gregory, C.J.; Menozzi-Arnaud, M.; Amorij, J.-P.; Gilbert, P.A.; Earle, K.; Frivold, C.; Jarrahian, C.; et al. Accelerating the Development of Measles and Rubella Microarray Patches to Eliminate Measles and Rubella: Recent Progress, Remaining Challenges. *Front. Public Health* **2022**, *10*, 809675. [CrossRef] [PubMed]
4. Fu, H.; Abbas, K.; Malvolti, S.; Gregory, C.; Ko, M.; Amorij, J.-P.; Jit, M. Impact and cost-effectiveness of measles vaccination through microarray patches in 70 low-income and middle-income countries: Mathematical modelling and early-stage economic evaluation. *BMJ Glob. Health* **2023**, *8*, e012204. [CrossRef] [PubMed]
5. Gavi. The Vaccine Innovation Prioritisation Strategy (VIPS). 2020. Available online: https://www.gavi.org/our-alliance/market-shaping/vaccine-innovation-prioritisation-strategy (accessed on 20 April 2021).
6. World Health Organization (WHO). Measles-Rubella Microarray Patch (MR-MAP) Target Product Profile. 2019. Available online: https://www.who.int/publications/i/item/9789240000209 (accessed on 17 June 2024).
7. Malvolti, S.; Ko, M.; Menozzi-Arnaud, M.; Mantel, C.; Jarrahian, C.; Amorij, J.P.; Giersing, B.; Hasso-Agopsowicz, M. Exploring potential applications of measles and rubella microarray patches (MR-MAPs): Use case identification. *Front. Public Health* **2023**, *11*, 1165110. [CrossRef] [PubMed]

8. Guillermet, E.; Alfa, D.A.; Phuong Mai, L.T.; Subedi, M.; Demolis, R.; Giersing, B.; Jaillard, P. End-user acceptability study of the nanopatch$^{TM}$; a microarray patch (MAP) for child immunization in low and middle-income countries. *Vaccine* **2019**, *37*, 4435–4443. [CrossRef] [PubMed]
9. PATH. The PATH Center of Excellence for Microarray Patch Technology. 2019. Available online: https://www.path.org/our-impact/resources/path-center-excellence-microarray-patch-technology/ (accessed on 22 May 2024).
10. Baker, B.; Bermingham, I.M.; Leelasena, I.; Hickling, J.; Young, P.R.; Muller, D.A.; Forster, A.H. Safety, Tolerability, and Immunogenicity of Measles and Rubella Vaccine Delivered with a High-Density Microarray Patch: Results from a Randomized, Partially Double-Blinded, Placebo-Controlled Phase I Clinical Trial. *Vaccines* **2023**, *11*, 1725. [CrossRef] [PubMed]
11. Joyce, J.C.; Collins, M.L.; Rota, P.A.; Prausnitz, M.R. Thermostability of Measles and Rubella Vaccines in a Microneedle Patch. *Adv. Ther.* **2021**, *4*, 2100095. [CrossRef] [PubMed]
12. Ko, M.; Malvolti, S.; Cherian, T.; Mantel, C.; Biellik, R.; Jarrahian, C.; Menozzi-Arnaud, M.; Amorij, J.P.; Christiansen, H.; Papania, M.J.; et al. Estimating the future global dose demand for measles-rubella microarray patches. *Front. Public Health* **2022**, *10*, 1037157. [CrossRef] [PubMed]
13. Adigweme, I.; Yisa, M.; Ooko, M.; Akpalu, E.; Bruce, A.; Donkor, S.; Jarju, L.B.; Danso, B.; Mendy, A.; Jeffries, D.; et al. A measles and rubella vaccine microneedle patch in The Gambia: A phase 1/2, double-blind, double-dummy, randomised, active-controlled, age de-escalation trial. *Lancet* **2024**, *403*, 1879–1892. [CrossRef] [PubMed]
14. Scarnà, T.; Menozzi-Arnaud, M.; Friede, M.; DeMarco, K.; Plopper, G.; Hamer, M.; Chakrabarti, A.; Gilbert, P.A.; Jarrahian, C.; Mistilis, J.; et al. Accelerating the development of vaccine microarray patches for epidemic response and equitable immunization coverage requires investment in microarray patch manufacturing facilities. *Expert Opin. Drug Deliv.* **2023**, *20*, 315–322. [CrossRef] [PubMed]
15. Forster, A.; Junger, M. Opportunities and challenges for commercializing microarray patches for vaccination from a MAP developer's perspective. *Hum. Vaccines Immunother.* **2022**, *18*, 2050123. [CrossRef] [PubMed]
16. Giersing, B.; Shah, N.; Kristensen, D.; Amorij, J.-P.; Kahn, A.-L.; Gandrup-Marino, K.; Jarrahian, C.; Zehrung, D.; Menozzi-Arnaud, M. Strategies for vaccine-product innovation: Creating an enabling environment for product development to uptake in low- and middle-income countries. *Vaccine* **2021**, *39*, 7208–7219. [CrossRef] [PubMed]
17. TechNet-21. Tools and Platforms that Support Selection, Access, and Service Strategies (17th TechNet Conference). 2023. Available online: https://www.youtube.com/watch?v=hsdQfBbVtLk (accessed on 5 June 2024).
18. World Health Organization (WHO). Guide for Conducting a Situation Analysis of Immunization Programme Performance. 2021. Available online: https://www.who.int/publications/m/item/guide-and-workbook-for-conducting-a-situation-analysis-of-immunization-programme-performance (accessed on 17 June 2024).
19. World Health Organization. CAPACITI Decision Support Tool Manual. 2020. Available online: https://www.who.int/publications/m/item/capaciti-decision-support-tool-manual (accessed on 17 June 2024).
20. Gibson, E.; Zameer, M.; Alban, R.; Kouwanou, L.M. Community Health Workers as Vaccinators: A Rapid Review of the Global Landscape, 2000–2021. *Glob. Health Sci. Pract.* **2023**, *11*, e2200307. [CrossRef] [PubMed]

*vaccines*

MDPI

*Article*

# Measles Population Immunity Profiles: Updated Methods and Tools

**Xi Li *, James L. Goodson and Robert T. Perry**

Accelerated Disease Control Branch, Global Immunization Division, Centers for Disease Control and Prevention, Atlanta, GA 30329, USA
* Correspondence: oql9@cdc.gov; Tel.: +1-(404)-431-1586

**Abstract:** Measles is a highly contagious disease and remains a major cause of child mortality worldwide. While measles vaccine is highly effective, high levels of population immunity are needed to prevent outbreaks. Simple but accurate tools are needed to estimate the profile of population measles immunity by age to identify and fill immunity gaps caused by low levels of vaccination coverage. The measles immunity profile estimates and visualizes the percentage of each birth cohort immune or susceptible to measles based on measles vaccination coverage. Several tools that employed this approach have been developed in the past, including informal unpublished versions. However, these tools used varying assumptions and produced inconsistent results. We updated the measles population immunity profile methodology to standardize and better document the assumptions and methods; provide timely estimates of measles population immunity; and facilitate prompt actions to close immunity gaps and prevent outbreaks. We recommend assuming that the second dose of the measles-containing vaccine (MCV2) and doses given during supplementary immunization activities (SIAs) first reach children who have been previously vaccinated against measles, so that previously unvaccinated children are reached only when the coverage of MCV2 or SIA is higher than the coverage achieved by all previous measles vaccination opportunities. This updated method provides a conservative estimate of immunization program impact to assess measles outbreak risk and to facilitate early planning of timely preventive SIAs to close population immunity gaps.

**Keywords:** measles; vaccination; immunity; risk assessment; coverage; mathematical model

## 1. Introduction

Measles remains a major cause of child mortality, despite being preventable by vaccination: in 2022, an estimated 136,200 measles deaths occurred worldwide, mostly among children less than 5 years of age [1]. The measles virus is one of the most contagious human pathogens known with a basic reproductive number ($R_0$) of 9–18 [2,3]. As a consequence of high transmissibility of the measles virus, high population immunity (estimated to be 89–94%) is needed in order to achieve herd immunity and prevent large and disruptive outbreaks of measles [4]. The exact threshold for herd immunity varies depending on context-specific determinants, such as birth rate, population density, age-specific contact rates, and population mixing. Measles can be prevented by using measles-containing vaccines (MCVs), which are safe and effective. The World Health Organization (WHO) recommends that all countries provide two doses of a measles-containing vaccine (MCV) in their national immunization schedule during infancy and early childhood [5]. Implementing periodic mass vaccination campaigns, also referred to as supplementary immunization activities (SIAs), is an effective strategy to close population immunity gaps by delivering the second dose (if not already introduced into the routine schedule), catching up children missing the first or second dose, and reaching hard-to-reach children. WHO recommends that countries conduct SIAs until >90–95% coverage has been achieved for both the first and second dose of a measles-containing vaccine (MCV1 and MCV2, respectively) in the national routine immunization schedule [5]. Nationwide preventive SIAs aim to vaccinate all children in the country in the target age group, regardless of their previous vaccination history. SIAs should be conducted regularly when the number of measles-susceptible children less than 5 years of age approaches the size of one birth cohort [5].

Global progress has been made toward reducing measles incidence and mortality and achieving measles elimination. During 2000–2022, global measles mortality was reduced by 82% and measles incidence decreased by 75% [1]. In 2010, at the World Health Assembly (WHA), countries endorsed the target to increase MCV1 to ≥90% at national level and ≥80% in every district, reduce global annual measles incidence to less than 5 cases per million population, and reduce global measles mortality by 95% from the 2000 estimate by 2015 [6]. In 2012, the WHA endorsed a resolution to eliminate measles in five of the six WHO regions by 2020 [7]. As of the end of 2022, 83 (43%) countries have achieved measles elimination [1]. However, in recent years, there have been large measles upsurges. In 2019, the global measles incidence was 120 cases per million population, representing a 567% increase compared to 18 cases per million in 2016, the year with the lowest incidence during 2000–2019 [1]. By 2021, global measles incidence decreased by 86% from 2019 to 17 cases per million population, but increased 71% to 29 cases per million population in 2022, although only 43% of countries reported an adequate incidence of febrile rash illness for which measles has been ruled out by laboratory testing, indicating inadequate surveillance sensitivity globally [1]. Global MCV1 coverage decreased from 86% in 2019 to 81% in 2021, and then increased to 83% in 2022 [1]. As a result of immunization service interruptions due to the COVID-19 pandemic, 41 SIAs were delayed; of these, 35 had been completed by the end of 2022 [1].

Estimating measles population immunity gaps can help guide immunization program managers using data to monitor program performance, identify the timing for the next SIAs, and identify age groups with large measles immunity gaps that need to be included in the SIA target age group. Serosurveys provide direct estimates of measles immunity through the collection of biological specimens such as blood and saliva from participants and testing for measles-specific immunoglobulin G (IgG) levels; the percentage of a population susceptible to measles is defined by the percentages of persons negative for measles IgG by age group. If serosurveys are geographically representative and well implemented, then they provide a valid empirical measurement of the population immunity gaps. However, serosurveys are costly and conducted infrequently, only provide a cross-sectional snapshot of measles immunity at the time when conducted, and often do not provide timely results for programmatic decision-making given the time for specimen collection, transport to the lab, testing, and statistical analysis. Estimating population immunity using readily available data, namely, MCV1, MCV2, and SIA coverage, can provide more timely estimates on measles population immunity gaps. Measles immunity profiles show the percentage of persons immune as a result of routine immunization with MCV1, routine immunization with MCV2, and vaccination through SIAs, and the percentage of persons susceptible to measles by each year's birth cohort based on the analysis of vaccination coverage data that are publicly available, including the WHO and United Nations Children's Fund (UNICEF) Estimates of National Immunization Coverage (WUENIC).

Several tools have been previously developed to generate measles immunity profiles. Since the 1990s, multiple informal tools have been developed using different versions of Microsoft Excel and used by countries and partners. These spreadsheets included varying assumptions and formulas, did not clearly document the methods and assumptions, and often generated inconsistent results. Analytical results of these previously existing informal tools, named susceptibility profiles, have been used for programmatic decision-making and occasionally were included in published articles [8,9]. To provide a more standardized and documented approach, WHO joined with PATH and Stanford University to develop the Measles Strategic Planning (MSP) tool. This tool was designed to show the impact on immunity, cases, and deaths of various options to accelerate measles control effort [10]. The MSP tool provides measles immunity profiles for the baseline and final year of the modeled period and shows the percentage of persons immune as a result of routine immunization with MCV1 and MCV2, and vaccination through SIAs and measles infection, and the percentage of persons who remain susceptible for each birth cohort. One key assumption of the MSP tool was independence between MCV1 and SIA doses, which meant that every child in a country had the equal chance to be vaccinated with each SIA dose regardless of whether they had been previously reached by immunization services. This approach predicted small immunity gaps in age groups that contributed significant numbers of cases according to surveillance data. As detailed below, we recommend using the assumption that children who have been previously vaccinated have higher chances of being reached by routine immunization with MCV2 and by SIAs in order to provide a conservative estimate of immunization program impact, which aids early and timely planning of SIAs. We have developed a set of tools based on Microsoft Excel and a program written in the R programming language with the following objectives: (1) standardize and better document assumptions and methods; (2) provide timely estimates of population measles immunity levels to facilitate prompt actions to close immunity gaps and prevent outbreaks.

## 2. Method

### 2.1. Tool Development Process

We reviewed the methods, assumptions, and input parameters for several informal versions of measles immunity profile tools and the MSP tool. Subject matter experts were consulted to gain consensus on choices of methods and parameters that were then presented to the WHO Immunization and Vaccines Related Implementation Research Advisory Committee for review in August 2021 [11].

### 2.2. Input Data

The input data of the immunity profiles include coverage of MCV1, MCV2, and SIAs, the target population is relevant for SIAs, and population size by age. For MCV1 and MCV2, we used WUENIC as they are based on administrative data, surveys, and information on routine immunization program performance (strikes, stockouts, etc.) and updated annually for all WHO member states. Estimates of coverage reached by SIAs were based on post-campaign coverage surveys (PCCSs) whenever available, or if a survey coverage estimate was not available, then they were based on estimates from administrative data. Administrative coverage for SIAs was capped at 95% if not supported by a PCCS, as very high administrative coverage is usually an indication of poor data quality and to avoid coverages greater than 100%.

We used population estimates of the number of persons by each one-year of age (i.e., <1 year, 1 year to less than 2 years, etc.) from the World Population Prospects, 2019 Revision published by United Nations Population Division.

### 2.3. Key Assumptions and Formulas

#### 2.3.1. Association between Doses

WHO recommends that an administered dose of MCV should be recorded as MCV2 only if the child has the documented first dose of MCV1 [12,13]. In an ideal routine immunization services delivery program, all children coming for measles vaccination will be screened and receive MCV1 or MCV2 based on information in the clinic's vaccination register or the home-based record. Therefore, the formulas use the assumption that the children receiving the second dose would only be those who have already received the first dose; that is, MCV2 is dependent on MCV1. However, in the real world, some children coming for the MCV2 visit may not have received MCV1 but may be accidently recorded as having received MCV2 during the visit, not MCV1, because the child's age is at or past the age when they were expected to receive MCV2. MCV1 coverage may be lower than MCV2 in some situations, for example, when doses given at an older age are recorded as MCV2 without checking the child's MCV1 status. Furthermore, MCV1 and MCV2 reported in the same year are often given to different birth cohorts, so for some years in some countries, the MCV2 estimate is higher than that for MCV1.

During each SIA, if the chance of being vaccinated is the same both for children who have previously received an MCV and for children who have not received an MCV, then the chance of vaccination is independent of the vaccination status before the SIA (the "independent scenario"). This assumption contrasts with the common observation that vaccinated children have better access to health services and these children are generally more reachable by subsequent SIAs. In addition, SIAs will also reach some previously unvaccinated children because of SIA strategies such as increased outreach, social mobilization, communications, and resources designed to reach previously unvaccinated children. To better capture the dependency between vaccination opportunities, we assumed that each vaccination opportunity reaches all children who have been vaccinated before, and then, only if the vaccination coverage is higher than previous vaccination opportunities, will the SIA reach and vaccinate previously unvaccinated children (the "dependent scenario"). The "independent scenario" and "dependent scenario" represent the boundaries of a range where the real-world association between previous vaccination status and the probability of receiving a subsequent dose lies. As noted below, some previously vaccinated children may still not be immune, and we assume that revaccination will provide these children with a second opportunity for immunity.

We recommend using the "dependent scenario" to provide a conservative estimate of immunization program impact, and to reduce the chance of overestimating population immunity and delaying vaccination activities. Formulas using the dependent assumption are shown in Figure 1.

$$\%\ of\ persons\ immune\ from\ MCV1 = MCV1 * MCV1\ VE$$

$$\%\ of\ additional\ persons\ immune\ from\ MCV2 = \begin{cases} (MCV1 - MCV1 * MCV1\ VE) * \dfrac{MCV2}{MCV1} * MCV2\ VE, & when\ MCV2 < MCV1, \\ (MCV1 - MCV1 * MCV1\ VE) * MCV2\ VE + (MCV2 - MCV1) * MCV2\ VE, & when\ MCV2 \geq MCV1 \end{cases}$$

$$Cumulative\ percentage\ vaccinated\ after\ SIA_n = \begin{cases} cumulative\ percentage\ vaccinated\ with\ any\ MCVs\ before\ SIAn, when\ SIA_n\ coverage < cumulative\ \%\ vaccinated\ with\ any\ MCVs\ before\ SIA_n \\ SIA_n\ coverage * \%\ population\ targeted + cumulative\ precentage\ vaccinated\ with\ any\ MCVs\ before\ SIA_n * (1 - \%\ population\ targeted) \\ when\ SIA_n\ coverage \geq cumulative\ \%\ vaccinated\ with\ any\ MCVs\ before\ SIA_n \end{cases}$$

$$\%\ of\ additional\ persons\ immune\ from\ SIA_n = \begin{cases} (cumulative\ \%\ vaccinated\ before\ SIA_n - cumulative\ \%\ immune\ before\ SIA_n) * \dfrac{SIA_n\ coverage}{cumulative\ \%\ vaccinated\ before\ SIA_n} * SIA\ VE * \%\ population\ targted, \\ when\ SIA_n\ coverage < cumulative\ \%\ vaccinated\ before\ SIA_n, \\ (SIA_n\ coverage - cumulative\ \%\ immune\ before\ SIA_n) * SIA\ VE * \%\ population\ targeted, when\ SIA_n \geq cumulative\ \%\ vaccinated\ before\ SIA_n \end{cases}$$

**Figure 1.** Measles population immunity profile method formulas using the dependent assumption that previously vaccinated children are first reached by a subsequent vaccine dose. Notes—MCV: measles-containing vaccine. MCV1: coverage of the first dose of MCV delivered through routine immunization; MCV2: coverage of the second dose of MCV delivered through routine immunization; SIA: supplementary immunization activity; VE: vaccine effectiveness.

### 2.3.2. Impact of Subnational SIAs

To account for subnational SIAs, we estimated the additional percentage of the national population immune to measles by multiplying the additional percentage of children who gained measles immunity through the SIA in the targeted subnational area by the estimated proportion of the country's population living in that same subnational area.

#### 2.3.3. Vaccine Effectiveness

The vaccine effectiveness (VE) of a measles vaccine dose is dependent on the age of administration and is measured by comparing disease rates in vaccinated vs. unvaccinated people, as compared to the proportion of previously seronegative people with adequate immunity after vaccination [14]. A literature review suggested the median VE of a single dose of MCV1 to be 84% if administered at 9–11 months of age, and 92.5% if administered at 12 months and above [15]. Among children who do not develop immunity after MCV1, approximately 95% will develop immunity with a second dose [5]. A second literature review estimated the MCV1 VE for children vaccinated before 9 months of age to be 58% [16]. Our assumptions of the VE of MCV1 and MCV2 were based on the recommended age of vaccine administration in the national immunization schedule. For routine immunization, vaccines were assumed to be given at the earliest ages in the national immunization schedule. SIAs provide vaccinations for people of a defined age range, typically children, based on the rate of accumulation of measles-susceptible persons to prevent outbreaks, or to respond to outbreaks. Age-specific estimates of vaccine effectiveness were applied to SIA doses and age-disaggregated SIA vaccination coverage data were used whenever available.

#### 2.3.4. Cohort Granularity

In previous Excel-based measles population immunity profile tools, calculations were limited to whole calendar year birth cohorts, which means that the entire yearly cohort is either covered or not covered by an SIA. In the R-based measles immunity profile tool, cohorts were constructed based on the exact dates of SIAs and each cohort has unique experiences of MCV1 coverage, MCV2 coverage, SIA coverage, and vaccine effectiveness at the time of vaccine administrations. The percentage of persons immune to measles is calculated for each birth cohort and the results could be aggregated by age in years or by calendar year. This approach allows more accurate estimates of the youngest and oldest age groups in cohorts covered by an SIA, and more accurate calculations using age-specific vaccine effectiveness inputs.

#### 2.3.5. Date of the Profile

The profiles may be constructed at any date, as long as input data are available. When constructed for a future date, the profile could show the immunity gaps by cohort before a planned SIA, or the increase in population immunity after a planned SIA.

## 3. Results

We developed a set of tools to generate and visualize measles population immunity profiles to suit the needs of users with different software skill levels. The calculations were implemented through either a Microsoft Excel 365 spreadsheet or a program written in the R language. The calculations using R generate more accurate estimates than the calculations possible in Excel as more granular analyses could be performed in R, whereas in the Excel spreadsheet, one row represents each whole calendar year birth cohort. The key assumptions and characteristics for the calculations in Microsoft Excel and in R are shown in Table 1. A Power BI dashboard was developed to visualize the results of the R programs and an online, web-based Shiny R dashboard was developed for users to review and revise the input data and perform the calculations based on the formulas in R codes. The codes were annotated in a Jupyter notebook.

National-level measles immunity profiles have been developed for global, regional, and national partners and programs. A few examples of use cases are listed below.

**Table 1.** Assumptions and methods of previous measles population immunity profiles and the updated the Microsoft Excel 365 and R versions of the tool.

| | Previous Tools | | Tools Described in this Manuscript | |
|---|---|---|---|---|
| | **Informal versions of Excel tools** | **Measles strategic planning tool** | **Excel version** | **R version** (in Shiny R app and Jupyter notebook, Microsoft Power BI dashboard) |
| Main considerations | Easy to understand calculations in an Excel workbook that allows users to estimate the number of susceptible individuals in each birth cohort. | Estimate effectiveness and cost-effectiveness of vaccination strategies. | Calculations laid out, allowing the average Microsoft Excel user to follow them. | Provide profiles more accurately reflecting the timing of vaccination opportunities and age-specific SIA VE compared to the Excel version. Possible to rapidly generate profiles for all countries. |
| **Assumptions and methods** | | | | |
| Correlation between doses | Independence between campaign and routine immunization doses. | MCV2 reaches 25% of children who missed MCV1 if MCV2 is given before 3 years of age in the national schedule, and 75% of children who missed MCV1 if it is given after 3 years of age. SIA and MCV2 are independent of each other. | Only the dependence assumption is implemented in this version; that is, MCV2 and SIA doses are given first to children who have been previously vaccinated, and when coverage is higher than the coverage of all previous MCV vaccination opportunities, then doses are given to previously unvaccinated children. | Dependence or independence options are available, allowing users to see and compare profiles calculated using either assumption. The total dependence is the recommended default assumption. |
| Temporal granularity | Routine and SIA coverage applied to whole year birth cohorts. For example, an SIA in 2020 with a target age range of 9–59 months would cover 2016–2019 birth cohorts. | Routine and SIA coverage applied to whole year birth cohorts. | Routine and SIA coverage applied to whole year birth cohorts. | Routine and SIA coverage applied to the number of children born each day that are eligible for vaccination, based on the routine immunization schedule and SIA implementation dates and target age group. |
| Vaccine effectiveness (VE) | Non-standardized, depending on the user input. | 85% for ages < 1 year, 95% for ages ≥ 1 year. | VE is dependent on age of administration: 58% for MCV1 given at 6–8 months of age or earlier, 84% at 9–11 months, 92.5% at ≥12 months of age, and 95% for MCV2 given at ≥12 months of age. For SIAs, the same VE (95%) is used for all age groups targeted by the SIA. | VE for MCV1 and MCV2: same as the Excel version. Age-specific VE estimates used for SIAs: 58% for children 6–8 months of age, 84% for children 9–11 months of age, and 95% for children ≥12 months of age. |

**Table 1.** *Cont.*

| | Previous Tools | | | Tools Described in this Manuscript |
|---|---|---|---|---|
| Sequence of routine and SIA doses | Assumes SIA doses are always given after MCV1 and MCV2. | Assumes SIA doses are always given after MCV1 and MCV2. | Assumes SIA doses are always given after MCV1 and MCV2. | Routine doses and SIA doses are put in sequence according to age of administration for each birth cohort at the time of SIA implementation. For example, SIA targeting 6–59 months of age will deliver vaccine to some children before MCV1, between MCV1 and MCV2, or after MCV2 based on age of eligibility according to the national immunization schedule. |
| Subnational SIAs and phased SIAs | Subnational SIAs in the same year are combined to calculate the average coverage in the proportion of the country that is covered. Phased SIAs over multiple years are combined into one entry, and the year when the greatest proportion of target population is reached is assigned as the year of implementation for the combined SIA. | Subnational SIAs in the same year are combined to calculate the average coverage in the proportion of the country that is covered. Phased SIAs over multiple years are combined into one entry, and the year when the greatest proportion of the total target population is reached is assigned as the year of implementation for the combined SIA. | Subnational SIAs in the same year are combined to calculate the average coverage in the proportion of the country that is covered. Phased SIAs over multiple years are combined into one entry, and the year when the greatest proportion of the total target populations is reached is assigned as the year of implementation for the combined SIA. | The percentage of additional children reached is calculated for each subnational area covered based on the exact dates when the subnational/phased SIAs were conducted, and then aggregated at the national level for a national profile. |
| Immunity acquired through natural infection | Focused on immunity among younger children. The method does not estimate immunity acquired through natural infection, although assumptions may be made on the percentage of older populations immune through natural infection. | A dynamic transmission model was used to estimate immunity acquired through natural infections. Profiles with and without immunity through natural infection are generated. | Focused on immunity among younger children. The method does not estimate immunity acquired through natural infection. | Focused on immunity among younger children. The method does not estimate immunity acquired through natural infection. |

Notes—MCV1: the first dose of measles-containing vaccines; MCV2: the second dose of measles-containing vaccines; SIA: supplementary immunization activity; VE: vaccine effectiveness.

### *3.1. Identify Birth Cohorts with Measles Immunity Gaps*

The measles population immunity profile graph visualizes immunity by birth cohort. Figure 2 shows an example of an immunity profile as of 31 December 2020 in a hypothetical country with an annual birth cohort of 1 million infants. The immunization coverage data for MCV1 and MCV2 delivered by routine immunization and data for MCVs delivered by SIA in this hypothetical country are shown in Tables 2 and 3. The profile indicates that among children born since 2014, >10% of children in each birth cohort are not protected against measles by vaccination, as a result of suboptimal routine immunization coverage and the suboptimal coverage of the last SIA. Achieving higher coverage through routine immunization and a high-quality SIA among the cohorts with large population immunity gaps would be needed to close the immunity gaps.

**Table 2.** Annual coverage of the first and second dose of measles-containing vaccine (MCV1 and MCV2, respectively) in a hypothetical country, 2000–2020.

| Year of Vaccine Administration | MCV1 | MCV2 |
|---|---|---|
| 2020 | 82 | 70 |
| 2019 | 81 | 68 |
| 2018 | 79 | 65 |
| 2017 | 85 | 60 |
| 2016 | 82 | 54 |
| 2015 | 80 | 23 |
| 2014 | 82 | 0 |
| 2013 | 80 | 0 |
| 2012 | 76 | 0 |
| 2011 | 75 | 0 |
| 2010 | 80 | 0 |
| 2009 | 81 | 0 |
| 2008 | 85 | 0 |
| 2007 | 84 | 0 |
| 2006 | 82 | 0 |
| 2005 | 81 | 0 |
| 2004 | 80 | 0 |
| 2003 | 75 | 0 |
| 2002 | 74 | 0 |
| 2001 | 74 | 0 |
| 2000 | 72 | 0 |

Notes—MCV1: the first dose of measles-containing vaccines; MCV2: the second dose of measles-containing vaccines.

**Table 3.** Supplementary immunization activities using measles-containing vaccines since 2000 in a hypothetical country.

| Year | Intervention | Start Date | End Date | Age Group | Extent | Status | Target Population | Reached Population | % Reached | Survey Results |
|---|---|---|---|---|---|---|---|---|---|---|
| 2007 | Measles | 4/1/2007 | 4/8/2007 | 6–59 M | National | Completed | 4,500,000 | 4,140,000 | 92 | |
| 2010 | Measles | 8/12/2010 | 8/20/2010 | 9–59 M | National | Completed | 4,250,000 | 4,037,500 | 95 | 86 |
| 2012 | Measles | 8/21/2012 | 9/4/2012 | 6–59 M | Subnational | Completed | 2,390,000 | 2,103,200 | 88 | |
| 2014 | MR | 12/31/2014 | | 9 M–14 Y | Rollover-National | Completed | 10,260,000 | 9,336,600 | 91 | |
| 2015 | MR | 5/18/2015 | | 9 M–14 Y | Rollover-National | Completed | 3,990,000 | 3,710,700 | 93 | |
| 2016 | MR | 2/21/2016 | 3/5/2016 | 6–59 M | Subnational | Completed | 1,090,000 | 1,079,100 | 99 | |
| 2018 | MR | 4/1/2018 | 4/10/2018 | 6–59 M | National | Completed | 4,500,000 | 4,050,000 | 90 | 82 |
| 2021 | MR | 12/1/2021 | 12/15/2021 | 9–59 M | National | Planned | 4,250,000 | | | |

Notes—M: months; Y: years. Date format: MM/DD/YYYY.

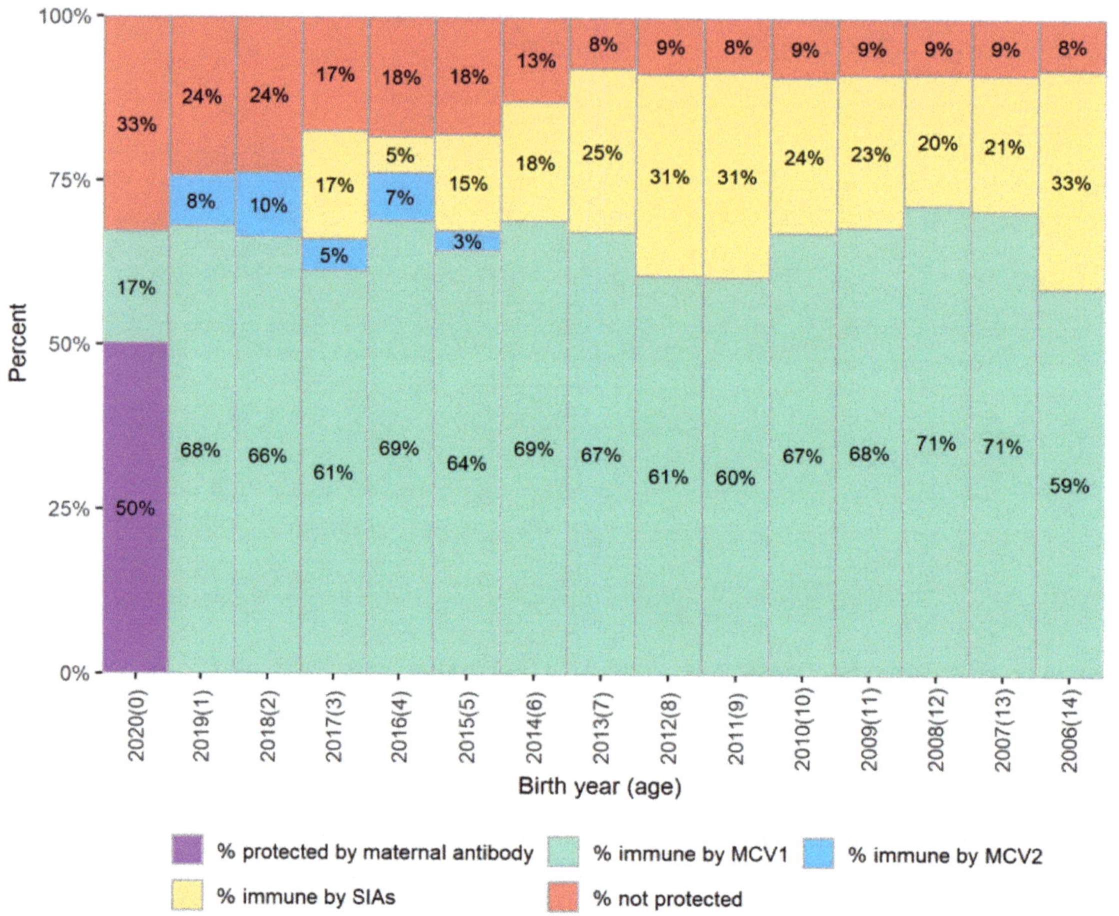


**Figure 2.** The measles population immunity profile as of 31 December 2020 showing estimated measles immunity gaps in red vertical bars for each birth cohort in a hypothetical country. Notes—MCV1: the first dose of measles-containing vaccines; MCV2: the second dose of measles-containing vaccines; SIA: supplementary immunization activity.

### *3.2. Estimate Impact of a Planned SIA or Change in Routine Immunization Coverage*

The population immunity profiles can also be generated based on projections of routine immunization coverage and assumptions on the coverage and target age groups of proposed SIAs. Figure 3 shows an example of the hypothetical country planning to conduct an SIA among children aged 9–59 months in December 2021 that should reach 95% coverage. This SIA should close the immunity gap among children less than 5 years of age. However, children born in 2014 and 2016, aged 5–7 years by the end of 2021, will still have persistent immunity gaps and will likely contribute to the risk of measles outbreaks. An expanded SIA target age group or additional vaccination activities would be needed to reduce immunity gaps among these birth cohorts.

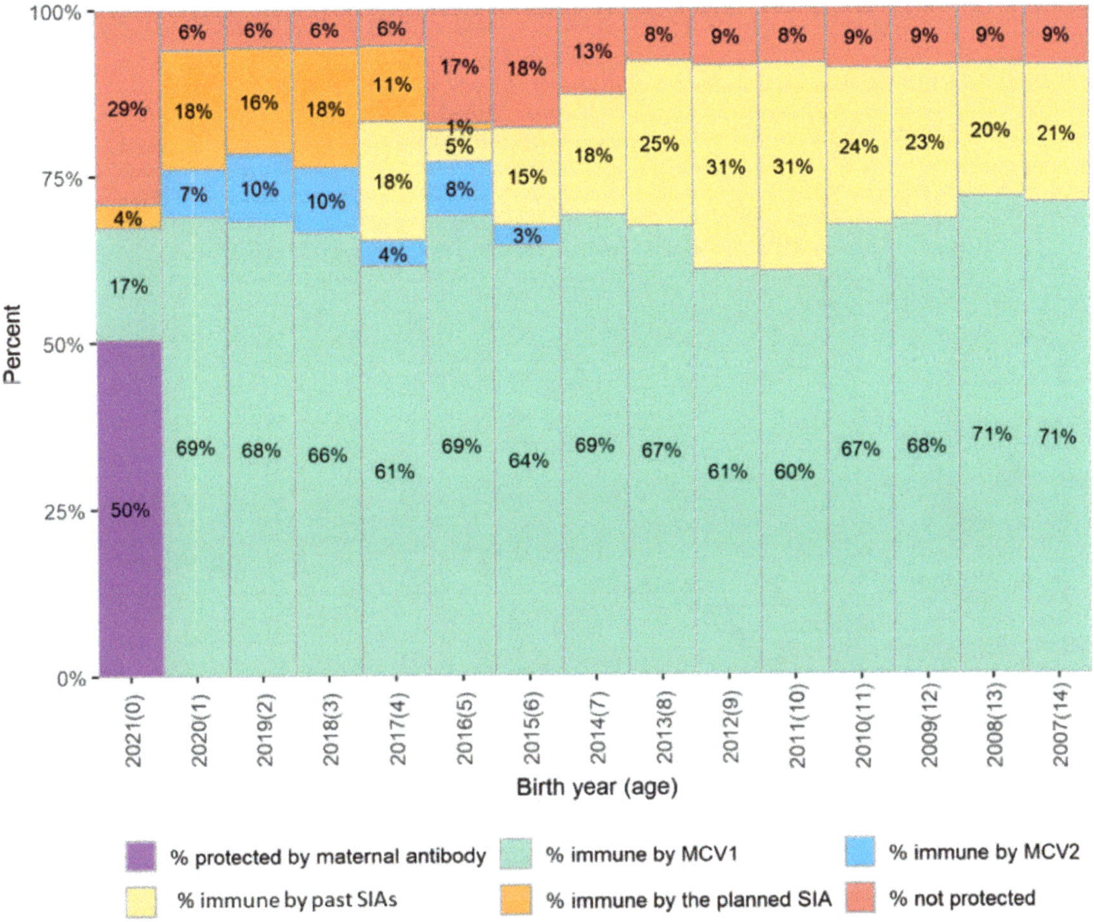


**Figure 3.** The measles population immunity profile as of 31 December 2021 showing projections of estimated measles immunity gaps in red vertical bars for each birth cohort in a hypothetical country if a proposed SIA targeting children aged 9–59 months was to be conducted during 1–15 December 2021 and reach 95% coverage. Notes—MCV1: the first dose of measles-containing vaccines; MCV2: the second dose of measles-containing vaccines; SIA: supplementary immunization activity.

### *3.3. Monitor the Timing of Preventive SIAs*

The measles immunity profile method can be used to estimate the number of measles-susceptible children less than 5 years of age at different time points and under different scenarios of coverage assumptions. Figure 4 shows the estimated number of measles-susceptible children under 5 years of age and the ratio of it to the size of one birth cohort during 2016–2022 in the hypothetical country. In this country, the number of measles-susceptible children under 5 years of age exceeded the number of one birth cohort in the first quarter of 2017. A national SIA was conducted in 2018, and the post-campaign coverage survey showed that the SIA reached 82% coverage among the target population. The ratio of the number of measles-susceptible children under five years old to the number of children in the youngest one-year birth cohort, that is, children under 1 year of age, decreased to 0.78 right after the SIA in 2018 but increased steadily because of suboptimal routine immunization coverage. The ratio exceeded 1 again in the last quarter of 2018. By the end of 2020, the ratio increased to 1.16, indicating elevated risk of measles outbreaks. If MCV1 and MCV2 coverage in 2021 remains at the same level as in 2020 and a national SIA was to be conducted in December 2021 with 95% coverage, then the number of measles-susceptible children would be reduced to about half the size of one birth cohort (best-case scenario). If the SIA reaches 80% coverage, then the number of measles-susceptible children less than 5 would remain above the size of one birth cohort (intermediate scenario). If MCV1 and MCV2 decreases by 25% in 2021 compared to 2020 (i.e., possibly due to vaccine stockout or service interruptions related to the COVID-19 pandemic) and no SIA was conducted (worst-case scenario), then the number of measles-susceptible children less than 5 years of age would increase to 1.6 million, 1.6 times the size of one birth cohort, by the end of 2022. This demonstrates the increased risk if no SIA is conducted or if an SIA is of suboptimal quality.

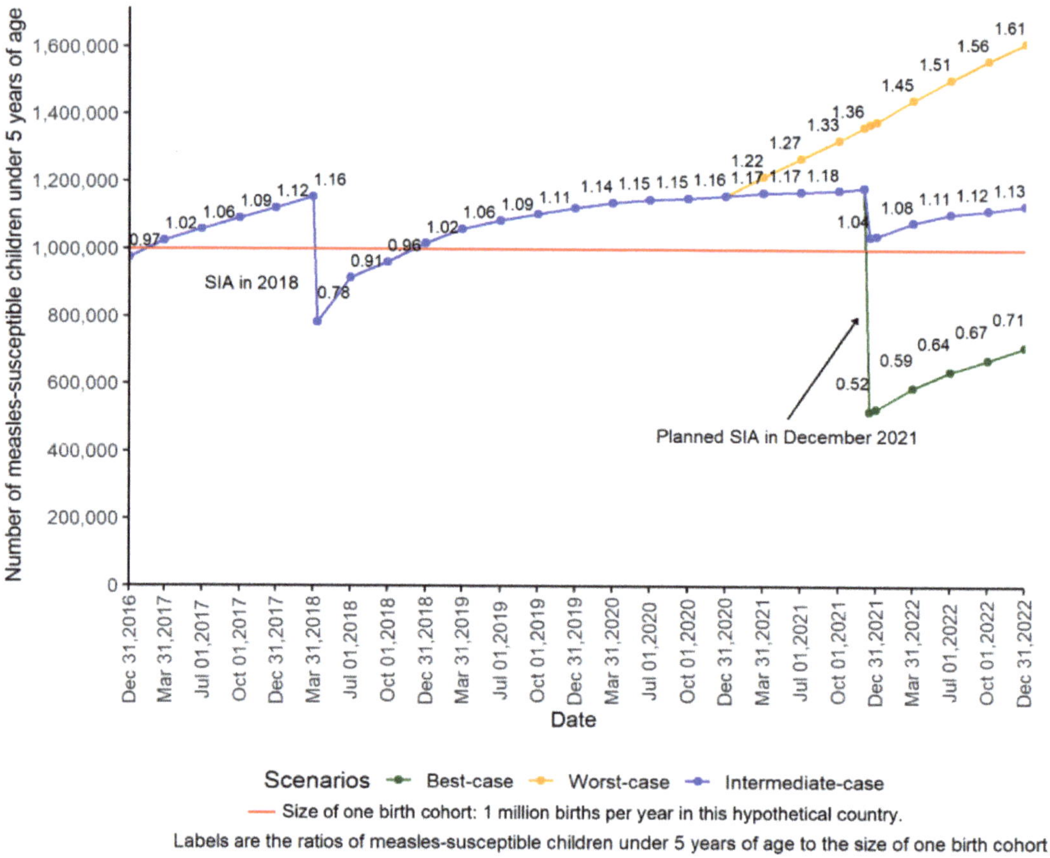


**Figure 4.** Estimates of the number of measles-susceptible children less than 5 years of age under different projected scenarios in a hypothetical country, 2016–2022. Notes—MCV1: the first dose of measles-containing vaccines; MCV2: the second dose of measles-containing vaccines; SIA: supplementary immunization activity. Best-case scenario: MCV1 and MCV2 coverage in 2021 remained the same as in 2020, and an SIA was conducted in December 2021, reaching 95% coverage. Intermediate scenario: MCV1 and MCV2 coverage in 2021 remained the same as in 2020, and an SIA was conducted in December 2021, reaching 80% coverage. Worst-case scenario: MCV1 and MCV2 coverage in 2021 decreased by 25% compared to 2020, and no SIA is conducted in 2021.

## 4. Discussion

We developed a measles population immunity profile tool set that builds on previous efforts by the public health community to analyze measles immunity gaps by birth cohort. The tool set promotes a standard way of analyzing measles immunity with documented methods and assumptions. Users may choose from the set of tools using different platforms, including R codes embedded in a Shiny R dashboard, or calculations in Microsoft Excel spreadsheets, based on the appropriate use case scenarios and their software skills. The profiles could be made available to partners and program managers through a web-based data visualization platform such as Power BI, helping them to identify cohorts at high risk of measles outbreaks, and to plan for preventive actions. The tool has been used to support multiple countries in the assessment of the risk of measles outbreaks, to forecast optimal timing of the next preventive SIA, and to demonstrate the needs for SIAs to prevent outbreaks. Early planning of the timely preventive SIA is critical in preventing measles outbreaks as it allows countries and donors to have sufficient lead time to allocate, approve, and secure in-country funds and to conduct micro-planning and readiness assessments to ensure quality of the SIAs. Profiles are also used to help justify to donor organizations the need for funding to support preventive SIAs.

Using our recommended assumption that MCV2 doses delivered through routine immunization and MCV doses administered during SIAs are primarily given to persons who have been previously vaccinated provides a conservative estimate of population immunity. This approach avoids overestimates that could lead to complacency, delays in vaccination activities, and preventable outbreaks and deaths. The identification of population immunity gaps allows for early planning of immunization activities to close immunity gaps. Previous research has proposed ways to quantify the efficiency of immunization activities in reaching additional children, or the percentage of zero-dose children reached based on empirical data [17,18]. The assumption on the overlap between routine doses and SIAs will be informed by additional data collected during SIAs and surveys.

The results of the measles immunity profile should be interpreted along with other information, such as measles surveillance data, to provide stronger evidence to guide programmatic decisions. The measles immunity profiles analyze susceptibility by birth year in the time dimension. It is complementary to the Measles Programmatic Risk Assessment tool, which aims to identify subnational areas at risk of measles outbreaks in the geographical dimension based on administrative coverage data only from the past three years [19]. Subnational profiles can also be constructed, provided that the required input data are available for the subnational unit(s). The tool could be used to evaluate the options on when to conduct an SIA to reduce the risk of measles outbreaks through estimating the build-up of measles-susceptible children based on projected future coverage. The tool could also be used to estimate the impact of immunization programs, such as estimating the number of additional persons immune from an SIA.

One limitation of the measles population immunity profile is that most profiles are generated for the national level and do not account for geographical variations within a country. While immunity profiles could be developed for subnational areas, such analyses are often not feasible because of the unavailability of coverage estimates validated by surveys for routine immunization or SIAs and population data at subnational levels. Because of the lack of reliable coverage and population data at subnational levels, the impact of each SIA is averaged at the national level, which is equivalent to assuming a complete mixing of the population in the country after each immunization opportunity, whether it is routine immunization or SIAs. This assumption may not hold in countries with large disparities in immunization program performance at subnational levels. Furthermore, our methods to produce an immunity profile do not consider immunity acquired through natural measles infection, likely a significant source of immunity in older age groups that were born when measles was highly endemic. The accuracy of the analysis also relies on the quality of input data. Investing in activities to obtain more accurate data, such as strengthening the availability and retention of home-based immunization records, frequent population-based health surveys including immunization indicators, and timely implementation of PCCSs, will help to improve the accuracy of the estimation of measles susceptibility.

Future development of this tool may include linking the measles population immunity profiles with measles dynamic models to account for the proportion of persons immune from natural measles infection and validating if the population immunity gaps estimated using this method are predictive of measles outbreaks detected through surveillance. More training materials and training opportunities will be provided to build capacity among immunization program managers and technical partners to use the tool for programmatic purposes. Feedback from the users will be gathered to improve the usability and performance of the tools.

## 5. Conclusions

The updated methods and tools to develop the measles immunity profiles promote a standard approach of analyses with the transparent documentation of methods and assumptions. The R version of the tool generates more granular profiles. The tools can be used to identify the cohorts with large immunity gaps and at risk of measles outbreaks and demonstrate the needs for SIAs.

**Author Contributions:** Conceptualization, methodology, writing: X.L., J.L.G. and R.T.P.; formal analysis, visualization: X.L. All authors have read and agreed to the published version of the manuscript.

**Funding:** This research received no external funding.

**Institutional Review Board Statement:** This analysis does not require Institutional Review Board reviews.

**Informed Consent Statement:** Not applicable.

**Data Availability Statement:** Vaccination coverage and population data presented in this study were hypothetical. When developing national level profiles, we typically use WHO-UNICEF Estimates of National Immunization Coverage (available at https://immunizationdata.who.int/, accessed 16 August 2024), population data from United Nations Population Division (available at https://population.un.org/wpp/, accessed 8 August 2024), or data provided by national governments.

**Conflicts of Interest:** The authors declare no conflicts of interest. The findings and conclusions in this report are those of the authors and do not necessarily represent the official position of the U.S. Centers for Disease Control and Prevention.

## References

1. Minta, A.A. Progress toward measles elimination—Worldwide, 2000–2022. *MMWR. Morb. Mortal. Wkly. Rep.* **2023**, *72*, 1262–1268. [CrossRef] [PubMed]
2. Rota, P.A.; Moss, W.J.; Takeda, M.; de Swart, R.; Thompson, K.M.; Goodson, J.L. Measles. *Nat. Rev. Dis. Primers* **2016**, *2*, 16049. [CrossRef] [PubMed]
3. Guerra, F.M.; Bolotin, S.; Lim, G.; Heffernan, J.; Deeks, S.L.; Li, Y.; Crowcroft, N.S. The basic reproduction number (R 0 ) of measles: A systematic review. *Lancet Infect. Dis.* **2017**, *17*, e420–e428. [CrossRef] [PubMed]
4. Thompson, K.M. Evolution and use of dynamic transmission models for measles and rubella risk and policy analysis. *Risk Anal.* **2016**, *36*, 1383–1403. [CrossRef] [PubMed]
5. World Health Organization. Measles vaccines: WHO position paper–April 2017. *Wkly. Epidemiol. Rec.* **2017**, *92*, 205–227.
6. World Health Organization. *Global Eradication Of Measles: Report by the Secretariat*; WHO: Geneva, Switzerland, 2010.
7. World Health Organization. *Global Vaccine Action Plan 2011–2020*; WHO: Geneva, Switzerland, 2013.
8. Goodson, J.L.; Perry, R.T.; Mach, O.; Manyanga, D.; Luman, E.T.; Kitambi, M.; Kibona, M.; Wiesen, E.; Cairns, K.L. Measles outbreak in Tanzania, 2006–2007. *Vaccine* **2010**, *28*, 5979–5985. [CrossRef] [PubMed]
9. Sugerman, D.E.; Fall, A.; Guigui, M.-T.; N'dolie, M.; Balogun, T.; Wurie, A.; Goodson, J.L. Preplanned National Measles Vaccination Campaign at the Beginning of a Measles Outbreak—Sierra Leone, 2009–2010. *J. Infect. Dis.* **2011**, *204* (Suppl. S1), S260–S269. [CrossRef] [PubMed]
10. Simons, E.; Mort, M.; Dabbagh, A.; Strebel, P.; Wolfson, L. Strategic planning for measles control: Using data to inform optimal vaccination strategies. *J. Infect. Dis.* **2011**, *204* (Suppl. S1), S28–S34. [CrossRef] [PubMed]
11. World Health Organization. Meeting of the Immunization and Vaccine-related Implementation Research Advisory Committee (IVIR-AC), September 2021. *Wkly. Epidemiol. Rec.* **2021**, *96*, 569–578.

12. World Health Organization. *A Guide to Introducing a Second Dose of Measles Vaccine into Routine Immunization Schedules*; WHO: Geneva, Switzerland, 2013.
13. World Health Organization. *Establishing and Strengthening Immunization in the Second Year of Life: Practices for Vaccination beyond Infancy*; WHO: Geneva, Switzerland, 2018.
14. Orenstein, W.A.; Bernier, R.H.; Dondero, T.J.; Hinman, A.R.; Marks, J.S.; Bart, K.J.; Sirotkin, B. Field-evaluation of vaccine efficacy. *Bull. World Health Organ.* **1985**, *63*, 1055–1068. [PubMed]
15. Uzicanin, A.; Zimmerman, L. Field effectiveness of live attenuated measles-containing vaccines: A review of published literature. *J. Infect. Dis.* **2011**, *204* (Suppl. S1), S133–S149. [CrossRef] [PubMed]
16. Nic Lochlainn, L.M.; de Gier, B.; van der Maas, N.; Strebel, P.M.; Goodman, T.; van Binnendijk, R.S.; de Melker, H.E.; Hahné, S.J.M. Immunogenicity, effectiveness, and safety of measles vaccination in infants younger than 9 months: A systematic review and meta-analysis. *Lancet Infect. Dis.* **2019**, *19*, 1235–1245. [CrossRef] [PubMed]
17. Lessler, J.; Metcalf, C.J.E.; Grais, R.F.; Luquero, F.J.; Cummings, D.A.T.; Grenfell, B.T. Measuring the performance of vaccination programs using cross-sectional surveys: A likelihood framework and retro-spective analysis. *PLoS Med.* **2011**, *8*, e1001110. [CrossRef] [PubMed]
18. Portnoy, A.; Jit, M.; Helleringer, S.; Verguet, S. Impact of measles supplementary immunization activities on reaching children missed by routine programs. *Vaccine* **2018**, *36*, 170–178. [CrossRef] [PubMed]
19. Lam, E.; Schluter, W.W.; Masresha, B.G.; Teleb, N.; Bravo-Alcántara, P.; Shefer, A.; Jankovic, D.; McFarland, J.; Elfakki, E.; Takashima, Y.; et al. Development of a district-level programmatic assessment tool for risk of measles virus transmission. *Risk Anal.* **2017**, *37*, 1052–1062. [CrossRef] [PubMed]

*vaccines*

MDPI

*Article*

# Measles–Rubella Microarray Patches Phase III Clinical Trial Framework: Proposal and Considerations

**Darin Zehrung [1], Bruce L. Innis [2], Auliya A. Suwantika [3], Mahmoud Ameri [4], Robin Biellik [5], James C. Birchall [6], Alejandro Cravioto [7], Courtney Jarrahian [8], Lee Fairlie [9], James L. Goodson [10], Sonali Kochhar [11], Katrina Kretsinger [12], Christopher Morgan [13], Mercy Mvundura [8], Niraj Rathi [14], Edward Clarke [15], Jessica Joyce Mistilis [8], Marie-Chantal Uwamwezi [16], Birgitte Giersing [1] and Mateusz Hasso-Agopsowicz [1,*]**

1 World Health Organization, 1211 Geneva, Switzerland
2 Independent Researcher, Haverford, PA 19041, USA
3 Department of Pharmacology and Clinical Pharmacy, Faculty of Pharmacy, Universitas Padjadjaran, Bandung 45363, Indonesia
4 Independent Researcher, Fremont, CA 9453, USA
5 Independent Researcher, 1278 La Rippe, Switzerland
6 School of Pharmacy and Pharmaceutical Sciences, Cardiff University, Cardiff CF10 3NT, UK
7 Departamento de Salud Pública, Facultad de Medicina, National Autonomous University of Mexico, Mexico City 04510, Mexico
8 PATH, Seattle, WA 98121, USA
9 Wits RHI, University of Witwatersrand, Johannesburg 2001, South Africa
10 Centers for Disease Control and Prevention, Atlanta, GA 30333, USA
11 Department of Global Health, University of Washington, Seattle, WA 98105, USA
12 Independent Researcher, Decatur, GA 30033, USA
13 JHPIEGO, Baltimore, MD 21231, USA
14 PATH, New Delhi 110001, India
15 Medical Research Council Unit, The Gambia at the London School of Hygiene and Tropical Medicine, Banjul P.O. Box 273, The Gambia
16 PATH, 1040 Brussels, Belgium
* Correspondence: hassoagopsowiczm@who.int

**Abstract: Background**: The Measles–Rubella Microarray Patch (MR-MAP) is an important technology that is expected to reduce coverage and equity gaps for measles-containing vaccines (MCVs), reach zero-dose children, and contribute to elimination of measles and rubella. MR-MAPs are anticipated to be easier to deploy programmatically and could be delivered by lesser-trained health workers, thereby increasing immunization coverage. The most advanced MR-MAP has reached clinical proof-of-concept through a Phase I/II trial in the target population of infants and young children. The World Health Organization (WHO) and partners have developed the Phase III clinical trial framework for MR-MAPs presented in this article. **Objectives and Methods**: The purpose of such framework is to inform the considerations, design and approach for the pivotal clinical trial design, while considering the anticipated data requirements to inform regulatory approval, WHO prequalification, and policy decision. **Results**: The proposed Phase III trial would compare the immunogenicity and safety of an MR-MAP with MR vaccine delivered subcutaneously in 9- to 10-month-old infants. An analysis of non-inferiority (NI) of immunogenicity would occur six weeks after the first dose. Should regulatory agencies or policy makers require, a proportion of infants could receive a second dose of either the same or alternate MR vaccine presentation six months after the first dose, with those children returning six weeks after the second dose for a descriptive assessment of immunogenicity, and then followed up six months after the second dose for evaluation of safety and immunogenicity. It is anticipated that this proposed pivotal Phase III trial framework would generate the required clinical data for regulatory licensure and WHO prequalification (PQ) of MR-MAPs. However, the trial design would need to be reviewed and confirmed by a national regulatory authority (NRA) that will assess the product for regulatory licensure and the WHO PQ team. Additional research will likely be required to generate data on concomitant vaccine delivery, the safety and immunogenicity of MR-MAPs in other age groups such as children 1–5 years and infants younger than 9 months of age, and the impact of MR-MAPs on coverage and equity. Such studies could be conducted during or after clinical MR-MAP development.

**Keywords:** measles; rubella; vaccines; micropatch; clinical trial

## 1. Introduction

Between 2021 and 2022, modeled global measles cases increased by 18% from 7,802,000 to 9,232,300, and the number of countries facing large or disruptive outbreaks rose from 22 to 37 [1]. In 2023, approximately 35 million children missed their first or second dose of measles-containing vaccine (MCV1 and MCV2), with 83% receiving MCV1 and 74% receiving both doses [2]. The WHO recommends that countries should strive to attain and sustain a minimum of 95% MCV coverage for both doses [3]. While vaccine effectiveness of a single dose rubella-containing vaccine (RCV) is higher than MCV, it is recommended that RCV in a 2-dose schedule be provided in combination with the measles vaccine, and the goal for rubella vaccination coverage should also be >95% given the common presentation for the vaccine [4]. Despite considerable progress incorporating the RCV into routine immunization programs globally, approximately 25 million infants still do not have access to the RCV every year [5]. Modeled estimates show a 66% decrease in the worldwide burden of congenital rubella syndrome (CRS) from 2010 to 2019; however, over 32,000 infants are still born with CRS annually, nearly all in countries that have not introduced a routine dose of the RCV [6].

Currently available MCVs are in a vial presentation and are lyophilized, requiring reconstitution with diluent prior to immunization use. They are reconstituted with a reuse prevention syringe and administered with an auto-disable needle and syringe (N&S). MCVs are often in a multi-dose vial presentation, which can result in vaccine wastage as any remaining doses in reconstituted open vials must be discarded within 6 h of opening. This has led to vaccinator reluctance in opening multi-dose vials, which results in missed opportunities for vaccination [7–9].

There are challenges with N&S-delivered MCV that constrain immunization programs from reaching high vaccine coverage. Examples include the requirements for vaccinators to reconstitute and administer a vaccine, the logistics of reaching remote populations due to limited vaccine thermostability, as well as safe sharps waste disposal [9].

Microarray patches (MAPs) are novel vaccine delivery devices in product development comprising multiple microprojections coated with, or composed of, a vaccine. Upon application to the skin, the vaccine is delivered to the dermis and epidermis in a usually less painful and minimally invasive manner than N&S. This single dose, ready-to-use presentation is expected to be easier to use, will not require vaccine reconstitution, nor require additional supplies such as syringes and, therefore, will reduce open-vial wastage and sharps waste, and is likely to have enhanced thermostability [10,11], when compared to vaccines delivered by N&S. Such attributes are anticipated to bring many opportunities to increase equitable vaccination coverage; for example, a possibility of administration of MR-MAPs by community health workers, immunization of hard-to-reach populations, the potential for partial distribution beyond the cold chain, and fewer missed opportunities for vaccination. The opportunities are likely to translate to public health impact—it has been estimated that between 2030 and 2040, the use of MR-MAPs in routine immunization and supplementary immunization activities (SIAs), partially replacing N&S use, could reduce measles burden by 27–37% in 70 low- and middle-income countries (LMICs) compared to the current N&S-only immunization strategy [12]. The evaluation and further validation of MR-MAP use cases in nine countries highlighted that the use of MR-MAPs in outreach immunization and SIAs would have the highest impact on MR vaccine coverage [9,13]. As such, MR-MAPs are anticipated to play a crucial role in eliminating measles and rubella and have been designated as a priority innovation by global initiatives such as Vaccine

Innovation Prioritization Strategy, global stakeholders [14–16], and the Measles & Rubella Partnership [17].

There are two MR-MAP candidates that are currently in clinical development. A dissolving MAP from Micron Biomedical Inc has recently been evaluated in a Phase I/II trial in 15-month-old MR vaccinated toddlers and 9-month-old MR naïve infants in the Gambia. The trial reported that MR vaccines delivered by a MAP have comparable safety and immunogenicity to MR vaccines delivered by N&S [18,19]. Another candidate, a high-density vaccine-coated microarray patch (HD-MAP) developed by Vaxxas, has been evaluated in a Phase I trial in previously MR vaccinated, healthy Australian young adults. The trial reported that the MR vaccine delivered by a MAP has similar levels of safety and immunogenicity as the MR vaccine delivered by N&S [20]. Other MR-MAP candidates are in preclinical development. In June 2023, the WHO's Product Development for Vaccines Advisory Committee (PDVAC) held a meeting to discuss the Phase I/II proof-of-concept clinical trial results presented by Micron Biomedical and provide recommendations for further clinical development and implementation research for MR-MAPs (Box 1) [21].

**Box 1.** 2023 PDVAC MR-MAP Recommendations [21].

- A regulatory strategy should be developed to allow for the quickest route of product approval and WHO PQ, which would be with WHO prequalified MR vaccines.
- Priority use cases are campaigns and supplementary immunization activities and outbreak response.
- Conduct safety and immunogenicity assessment in naïve 9-month-old infants to optimize dose, wear time and anatomical site.
- Assess an application on the wrist for a 1-min wear time with the dose used in the Phase I/II study, shifting to a 5-min wear time and a different application site out of the reach of the child, depending on the data generated.
- MR-MAP product labeling for a VVM 30 (stability at 37 °C) as well as controlled temperature chain (CTC), which requires thermostability at 40 °C for a minimum of 3 days to allow for the use case in supplemental immunization activities (SIA—campaigns) and outbreak scenarios.
- Evaluate the potential for dose reduction and the possible impact on thermostability.
- In future clinical research, include mild and moderately malnourished infants in a Phase II study and severely malnourished infants in a Phase III study.
- Identify vaccines that could be co-administered with MR-MAPs and related use cases.
- Expanded use/indications for MR-MAPs: inclusion of 6-month old infants, next generation MR vaccines, HIV+ individuals.
- Develop Evidence Considerations for Vaccine Policy (ECVP) for MR-MAPs.

The first MR-MAP for use is anticipated to be available for introduction by 2030, following product design finalization, construction and validation of an initial commercial manufacturing facility, Phase III clinical testing, approval of regulatory applications for marketing authorization, and prequalification (PQ) by the WHO. The initial commercial production lines are anticipated to launch by 2030, with limited supply at product launch until manufacturing scale-up is achieved. Further manufacturing scale-up or scale-out will depend upon demand from end-users and additional investment from vaccine developers.

While the pilot-scale manufacturing facilities are being designed and built, an opportunity exists to refine the MR-MAP design, dose, wear time, and anatomical site for delivery, prepare for future programmatic implementation and to discuss the confirmatory clinical data required to support licensure for MR-MAPs.

Therefore, the purpose of this manuscript is to develop a framework to inform considerations, design, and approach for the Phase III trial for MR-MAPs. Through such framework, this manuscript helps ensure that data on MR-MAPs required to inform regulatory and policy decisions are available, limiting the delay in introducing this important innovation to the immunization programs of countries. To support such goal, the WHO, with support from partners, organized a Global Convening of measles and rubella experts, regulators, policymakers, MAP developers, and vaccine manufacturers on MR-MAPs that occurred in April 2024 in New Delhi, India. Here, we report on the background work, discussions, and recommendations and propose an approach for a pivotal MR-MAP Phase III clinical trial.

## 2. Phase III Trial Framework—Methods

The following methods and approaches were implemented to develop a Phase III trial framework that describes parameters intended to inform marketing application approval by regulatory authorities and WHO policy and prequalification requirements.

### 2.1. Desk-Based Research and Stakeholder Interviews

Between November 2023 and February 2024, the WHO team conducted a desk-based review of published literature accessed through PubMed, determined to be relevant to the design of a pivotal Phase III trial for MR-MAPs. The review also included published strategy and policy documents, guidelines, reports, and other grey literature documents (see Table 1): the WHO position papers on measles and rubella, the Technical Report Series on the requirements for measles, mumps, and rubella vaccines and combined vaccine as well as clinical trials for vaccines, the WHO/UNICEF MR-MAP Target Product Profile, the PDVAC report from the MR-MAP meeting held June 2023, past published research on MCV and alternative delivery technologies, studies that led to MCV licensure, MCV indications for use and labeling, with emphasis on WHO PQ MR vaccines, regulatory guidance documents (African Vaccine Regulatory Forum (AVAREF), Central Drugs Standard Control Organization (CDSCO), Drugs Controller General of India (DCGI), European Medicines Agency (EMA), United States Food and Drug Administration (USFDA), WHO) and MR-MAP-related research and strategic documents.

**Table 1.** Desk-based Review Documents.

| **Global Guidelines** | **Summary** |
|---|---|
| WHO Position papers on Measles and Rubella [3,4] | Provide the WHO's official recommendations and guidance on measles and rubella vaccines, including vaccination schedules, target groups, and strategies for global immunization efforts. |
| WHO/UNICEF MR-MAP Target Product Profile [10] | Defines the desired characteristics of MR-MAPs, outlining the requirements for product development to meet global public health needs. |
| PDVAC MR-MAP meeting report [21] | Summarizes the discussions and outcomes from a meeting of the WHO's Product Development for Vaccines Advisory Committee (PDVAC) regarding the development of MR-MAPs |
| WHO Technical Report Series for MMR, clinical trials and prequalification requirements [22–26] | Technical guidelines and standards issued by the WHO covering the clinical trials, manufacturing, and prequalification criteria for measles, mumps, and rubella (MMR) vaccines. |
| WHO prequalified MR vaccine package inserts [27,28] | Official package inserts for measles–rubella vaccines that have been prequalified by the WHO, detailing the vaccine's composition, usage, and safety information. |
| WHO strategy, policy and programmatic requirements [29,30] | Documents detailing the methods and processes used by the WHO's Strategic Advisory Group of Experts on Immunization (SAGE) to develop evidence-based immunization policies, along with a generic framework for considering evidence in vaccine and monoclonal antibody policy development. |
| WHO PQ and product testing [31–34] | Guidelines and procedures for the WHO prequalification of vaccines, including testing methods and quality assurance processes. |
| **National guidelines** | |
| National regulatory authority guidance documents for clinical trials and non-inferiority margin [35–48] | Guidelines from various national regulatory authorities on conducting clinical trials, with a focus on determining non-inferiority margins in vaccine studies. |

**Table 1.** *Cont.*

| **Research studies** | |
|---|---|
| MR-MAP published research, study protocols and strategic documents [9,14,18,19,49,50] | Collection of research papers, study protocols, and strategic documents focused on the development, testing, and implementation of MR-MAP technology. |
| Alternative delivery technology published research [51–63] | Compilation of research on various innovative vaccine delivery technologies beyond traditional injection methods, including needle-free devices and other novel approaches. |
| Measles containing vaccine research, including studies that led to regulatory licensure or WHO PQ [64–68] | Research studies and clinical trials that have contributed to the licensure and WHO prequalification of measles-containing vaccines. |

In parallel to the desk-based research review, experts in the fields of measles and rubella vaccination, vaccine product development, and in the development of MR microarray patches, were interviewed on the potential design of a Phase III trial, regulatory licensure strategies, and potential programmatic introduction strategies.

For the desk review and the interviews, the information sources were selected based on their relevance, completeness, and quality to identify data to inform regulatory and policy decisions for MR-MAPs. The review focused on peer-reviewed literature published in reputable journals and incorporated positions, strategies, and guidance from leading international organizations. Additionally, interviews were conducted with top experts in measles, rubella, vaccination, and microarray patches to ensure the accuracy and breadth of data. Although a comprehensive desk review was performed, it is acknowledged that this method could have been strengthened by conducting a systematic review. However, given the limited data published on MR-MAPs, the available information was likely already familiar to the authors, who are experts in the field. Factors beyond the scope of informing regulatory and policy decisions were not included in the review.

### *2.2. MR-MAP Global Convening*

During 16–17 April 2024, a global convening was held in New Delhi, India by the WHO Immunization Vaccines and Biologicals Department, WHO India Country Office, and WHO South-East Asia Regional Office. The convening brought together experts and researchers in measles and rubella vaccines and microarray patches; regulatory representatives from the European Medicines Agency (EMA), United States Food and Drug Administration (USFDA), African Vaccine Regulatory Forum (AVAREF), and Drug Controller General of India (DCGI); global experts including from UNICEF, Gavi, PATH, Médecins Sans Frontières, US Centers for Disease Control and Prevention, and Coalition for Epidemic Preparedness Innovations; funders including the Bill & Melinda Gates Foundation and the RIGHT Foundation; vaccine manufacturers; MAP developers; representatives from the Indian Council of Medical Research; and the WHO HQ, Regional (WPRO, SEARO, AFRO, EMRO), and India Country office. The data obtained from desk-based research and stakeholder interviews were presented at the global convening and discussed in six breakout groups focused on (1) Phase III trial design and appropriate primary endpoint(s); (2) appropriate non-inferiority (NI) margin; (3) priority target populations; (4) concomitant vaccine delivery; (5) manufacturing strategy and shelf life; and (6) evaluation of immune responses. The recommendations reported here were formulated based on the presentations and discussions of the stakeholders and finalized during a closed meeting of the WHO Technical Advisory Group on MR-MAPs and the WHO Secretariat, which was held in April 2024.

## 3. Phase III Trial Framework—Recommendations

This framework is structured to include key elements required to inform the protocol design of a pivotal Phase III clinical trial for MR-MAPs. The national regulatory authorities (NRAs) and the WHO PQ team will need to define key aspects of a proposed study protocol. The data collected during the pivotal Phase III clinical trial should fulfill the regulatory and WHO PQ requirements and, to the extent feasible, generate evidence that is anticipated to inform a policy decision. The additional policy-related data and evidence that are expected to be needed for an MR-MAP, beyond the clinical outcomes and the chemistry, manufacturing and controls (CMC) data required for regulatory marketing authorization approval, will be described in future guidance in the form of WHO Evidence Considerations for Vaccine Policy (ECVP) [30]. The Phase III clinical trial framework will also inform the development of implementation plans for priority use cases of MR-MAPs. Such an approach, along with potential Phase IV "post-marketing" studies aimed at updating the product label or informing policy decisions (such as use in special populations or co-administration), could accelerate the pathway to programmatic introduction, uptake, and public health impact.

The following Phase III clinical trial framework considers the appropriate comparator arms within the trial design (Table 2) and considerations for non-inferiority (NI) margin (Tables 3 and 4) for the selected primary endpoint, both of which are critical components that inform the clinical trial study arms, number of participants, and complexity of a clinical trial. The priority populations in which the immunogenicity and safety of MR-MAPs should be evaluated are discussed in Table 5. In Table 6, the administration of non-MR vaccines and other health interventions is discussed. The manufacturing considerations that could impact the design of a Phase III clinical trial are discussed in Table 7. Lastly, the appropriateness and selection of immune assays to be included in a clinical trial are covered in Table 8.

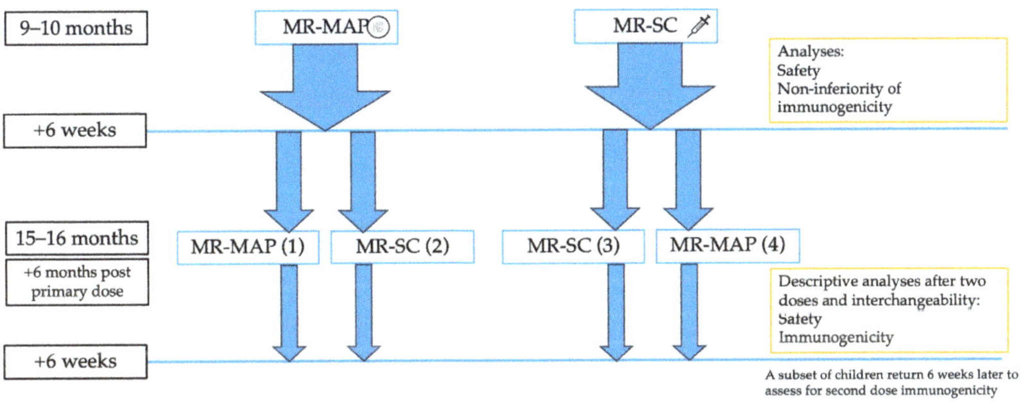


Notes:
- Infants will receive 2 doses of MR vaccine (MR-MAP or MR-SC)
- Infants will be vaccinated at 9–10 months (primary dose), followed by half receiving MR-MAP or MR-SC at 15–16 months (secondary dose – 6 months post primary dose).
- This design will allow for NI analysis of the primary dose between MR-MAP and MR-SC (6 weeks post primary dose).
- Secondary dose safety and immunogenicity (not powered for NI, a descriptive analysis of immunogenicity), which will provide evidence for the interchangeability of vaccine presentations (MAPs and SC), which are important considerations for programmatic use (6 weeks post-secondary dose).
- Potential 6 month follow up post-secondary dose – dependent upon NRA and WHO PQ team opinion.

**Figure 1.** Proposed Phase III Trial Design.

**Table 2.** Clinical Trial Design.

| |
|---|
| The proposed design for a pivotal Phase III clinical trial includes 9–10 month-old MR naïve infants, immunized with two doses of MR SC or/and MR-MAP vaccines, administered six months apart, to assess immunogenicity and safety after the first dose, and provide a descriptive analysis of safety, immunogenicity, and interchangeability of vaccine presentations (MAP then N&S, or the converse) after the second dose of an MR vaccine. |
| **Question** |
| • Is the proposed design appropriate for a pivotal Phase III clinical trial? |

**Table 2.** *Cont.*

| |
|---|
| **Discussion** |
| • The WHO position paper on measles notes that a single dose of the MCV will provide long-term protection for healthy vaccinees, with measles virus antibodies detected throughout the life of the individual. Research indicates that waning immunity may be a contributing factor in some cases of secondary vaccination failures; however, it does not seem to have a significant epidemiological impact on the transmission of the measles virus. The WHO recommends two doses for primary immunization and notes that measles vaccines are safe and effective, and vaccines from different suppliers may be used interchangeably within immunization programs [3]. Based upon this information, some regulatory authorities and WHO SAGE may require safety and immunogenicity data for two doses of the MR-MAP, including demonstrating interchangeability with the existing MCV and an MR-MAP to inform consideration of a policy recommendation.<br>• Measurement of immunogenicity after the last dose of a vaccination series is noted as the standard approach, be it the evaluation of seroresponse rate (SRR) or a geometric mean concentration (GMC) of neutralizing antibodies (see Table 3 for further information). However, if primary vaccination elicits immune memory in naïve vaccinees, post-primary doses may not allow for detecting differences and may be more appropriate as a secondary endpoint [37].<br>• Given that a single dose of the MCV is highly immunogenic with seroprotection rates consistently above 90% in >9 M old infants, the primary endpoint for a pivotal Phase III trial of MR-MAPs could be assessed six weeks after the first dose of an MR vaccine.<br>• A six-week follow-up after receiving the second dose of the MR vaccine (either MR-MAP or MR-SC) should be sufficient to assess immunogenicity in a subset of trial participants. Per the WHO guideline on clinical evaluation of vaccines, reports of SAEs should be collected for all trial participants 6 months post final dosing [23]. The trial sponsor and/or market authorization holder (MAH) should confirm the adequacy of this approach as part of pre-Phase III consultations with regulatory authorities.<br>• The evaluation of the relative persistence of antibody responses one or two years after one or two vaccinations, however, could be conducted either in a sub-study to the pivotal Phase III trial or in a separate study. This will be considered after the MR-MAP is licensed and utilized programmatically. |
| **Recommendations** |
| • A primary consideration should be given to a pivotal Phase III trial (Figure 1), which would be an individually randomized (1:1), open-label NI trial to receive an MR-MAP or MR-SC at 9–10 months of age (measles–rubella naïve infants) to assess non-inferiority of immunogenicity and safety (primary endpoints) of MR vaccines delivered by a MAP.<br>• The primary NI analysis of safety and immunogenicity of the MR-MAP could be conducted at six weeks after the first dose of the MR vaccine [19,68].<br>• As a secondary consideration, should regulatory agencies and policy makers require, the trial should continue in a subset of children who would be randomized to receive either the same vaccine presentation or a different vaccine presentation (those who received an MR-MAP would receive MR-SC and vice versa) 6 months after the first MR dose, at 15–16 months of age. Consequently, the trial would include four arms: primary and secondary doses of an MR-MAP (arm 1); primary dose of an MR-MAP followed by a secondary dose of an MR-SC (arm 2); primary and secondary doses of an MR-SC (arm 3); and primary dose of an MR-SC followed by a secondary dose of an MR-MAP (arm 4)–see Figure 1.<br>• Data from children who were vaccinated with the second dose of the MR vaccine at 15–16 months old could be descriptively evaluated six weeks after the second dose of the MR vaccine to assess the immunogenicity and safety of using two MR-MAP doses, as well as using two MR vaccine presentations (MAP and SC) interchangeably. However, the sample size of a trial needs not be powered for a formal NI analysis of immunogenicity after the second dose of an MR vaccine (see Figures 1 and 2).<br>• To address potential ethical concerns, all trial subjects should receive two doses of the MR vaccine (MR-MAP or MR-SC) to complete their vaccination series, as well as other co-administered vaccines, depending upon local immunization program requirements.<br>• Safety would be assessed immediately after each vaccination and likely for all vaccinated infants, and the extent of the safety endpoint data required is dependent upon NRA and WHO PQ team agreement. The number, severity, and relatedness of solicited local and systemic adverse events (AEs) should be collected on the day of MR vaccine administration and daily until two weeks post-vaccination, as per the Division of AIDS (DAIDS) Table for Grading the Severity of Adult and Pediatric Adverse Events [69]. Skin discoloration is an expected event in dark-skinned individuals and should be specifically assessed [19].<br>• The number, severity, and relatedness of all unsolicited (AE) should be assessed six weeks after each vaccination, and unsolicited serious adverse events (SAEs) for the duration of the clinical trial (potentially up to 6 months post-second dose for SAEs dependent upon NRA and the WHO PQ team opinion).<br>• Prior to the Phase III pivotal trial, it is recommended that the anatomical application site or sites be determined to be safe, immunogenic, have suitable biomechanical properties to enable efficient MAP delivery, and must be acceptable by health workers and caregivers. The MR-MAP application sites could be the wrist, anterolateral thigh, and/or the deltoid, for example; however, this must be confirmed in prior studies. Optimally, the wear time would be under one minute. The leading MR-MAP developers are working to determine the wear time in upcoming research studies.<br>• The NRA(s) considered for initial marketing authorization application will need to confirm if the proposed trial design would be acceptable for licensure and, therefore, should be consulted as part of pre-Phase III regulatory consultations. Justification for and nature of a descriptive analysis post-secondary dose will need to be presented by the trial sponsor to the NRA. |

**Table 3.** Non-inferiority margin for seroresponse rates comparison.

When designing a vaccine clinical trial, determining an appropriate NI margin is crucial for ensuring the trial's validity and reliability. The non-inferiority margin defines the acceptable difference in immunogenicity or efficacy between the new vaccine and the established reference vaccine, indicating that the new vaccine is not significantly worse than the reference within a pre-specified limit. Selecting this margin impacts several key aspects of the trial, including the sample size needed to achieve the required statistical power and the likelihood of trial success or failure. A narrower margin always demands a larger trial to achieve sufficient power, increasing costs and complexity, while a wider margin may raise concerns about the use of a less immunogenic or efficacious vaccine. Moreover, the choice of NI margin can directly influence the probability of the new vaccine's introduction into the market, as it determines the threshold at which the vaccine is deemed effective enough for licensure and widespread use. This discussion will explore these factors and their implications for vaccine approval and public health.

**Questions**

- Given the safety and effectiveness of the current MR vaccines, should the commonly used margins of 5 or 10% be used to demonstrate non-inferiority of immunogenicity between the two vaccine presentations?
- What are the considerations for the non-inferiority margin from a policy perspective?

**Discussion**

- There are two assessments to consider in selecting primary endpoints to assess immunogenicity NI for MR-MAPs relative to MR-SC: seroresponse rate (SRR) difference and Geometric Mean Concentration (GMC) ratio. The SRR difference relates to the proportion of trial subjects in which a minimum protective antibody level is induced six weeks after vaccination (for measles $\geq$ 200 mIU/mL, for rubella $\geq$ 10 IU/mL ref). The GMC ratio is the geometric mean magnitude of the immune response relative to the comparator (MR-MAP compared to MR-SC).
- A published meta-analysis of any vaccine NI randomized clinical trials indicated that most NI margins were 10%, although some vaccine NI studies had a lower NI margin such as 5% [70]. Based on such analysis, the study identified general considerations for selection of NI margins [70].
- MCV products have been licensed and prequalified by the WHO based on clinical trials with a 5 and 10% NI margin difference in SRR [28,52,66–68].
- There are advantages and disadvantages for each of the NI margins, which are presented in Table 4.
- As per the US FDA, the NI margin is usually determined by what would be clinically acceptable in terms of loss of effect [43]. The agency notes that planning for an NI study tends to be conservative, often confirmed by ensuring that the upper bound of the 95% confidence interval is less than the NI margin.
- Per the EMA, guidance on the NI margin should be sought from the Committee for Medicinal Products for Human Use (CHMP) through scientific advice. Mortality rate and disease risk are clinical considerations that should be referenced when determining the NI margin, and it was noted that sample size should not be a consideration [36,43].
- Per the CDSCO, pivotal clinical trials should use a predetermined and justifiable NI margin. The determination of a NI margin should consider the clinical significance of the endpoint, the severity of the disease, target population susceptibility, the availability of an established immune correlate of protection (ICP), and the assay performance characteristics. A more stringent NI margin may be suitable when the vaccine aims to prevent severe or life-threatening diseases and/or will be used in particularly vulnerable populations, such as infants. The use of a stricter NI margin might be suitable in cases where there is a chance of reduced immunogenicity, such as when comparing a new vaccine only with those approved based on NI trials. On the other hand, if a new vaccine is recognized to provide substantial safety advantages or better coverage, the agency states that less strict NI margins could be considered [41].

**Recommendations**

- As international standards for defining measles and rubella seroprotection exist, the primary endpoint should be NI of the SRR (MR-MAP relative to MR-SC) [3,4].
- The NI analysis can be conducted six weeks after receipt of the first dose of an MR vaccine. Should all children be vaccinated with two doses, the NI analysis can be conducted six weeks after receiving the second dose of the MR vaccine. A comparison of an incremental increase in immunogenicity between the first and second vaccine dose would be challenging given the expected marginal increases in the proportion of seroconverted individuals compared to when measured six weeks after the first dose of an MR vaccine.
- Analyses of immunogenicity and safety after the second dose of an MR vaccine could be a secondary endpoint based on descriptive statistics. Figure 2 illustrates an example of a trial protocol.
- Ultimately, the appropriateness of the proposed NI analysis should be confirmed with the relevant NRAs during end-of-Phase II/pre-Phase III consultations.

**Table 4.** NI Margin—Advantages and Disadvantages.

| Non-Inferiority Margin | Advantages | Disadvantages |
| --- | --- | --- |
| 5% | • High immunogenicity with minimum or no inferiority to current vaccines is desired, given the high transmission of measles and need for a high proportion of seroprotected individuals.<br>• Highly effective vaccines exist, are routinely implemented and are an important reference point for countries—generating data at 5% NI will provide greater confidence to countries to introduce MR-MAPs into programmatic use.<br>• A WHO Listed Authority (WLA) may require a 5% NI for the pivotal Phase III trial [71]. | • Very stringent success criterion for a Phase III trial—failing to meet the NI threshold, even marginally, may delay and/or prevent the technology from moving forward into programmatic use and reaching public health impact.<br>• If potency variability of released MR-MAPs or MR-SC products exists, this may result in variations in immunogenicity and increase the potential for the product to fail at 5% NI. |
| 10% | • Reduces costs and accelerates potential time to product licensure, while meeting select NRA recommendations that led to MCV product licensure and WHO PQ.<br>• The potential decrease in immunogenicity could be offset by an increase in vaccine coverage, with important public health implications such as reaching zero-dose children.<br>• Published results comparing MCVs (single dose) with 10% NI margin led to successful product licensure and use.<br>• A 10% non-inferiority margin could accommodate greater variability in immunogenicity within the trial, which, in turn, may allow for the inclusion of broader and more diverse populations (HIV+, malnourished children, broad age range 9–12 months), increasing the generalizability of the trial results to a wider population. | • A highly effective vaccine exists—there is the potential that as a novel delivery technology MR-MAPs may be perceived as a less effective and will negatively impact acceptability, product uptake and use in countries.<br>• The use of MR-MAPs may fail to translate to increased vaccine coverage, and coupled with decreased immunogenicity it may lead to increased MR incidence. |

**Table 5.** Vaccinated Populations.

In the context of clinical trials, the inclusion of additional populations, such as those with underlying health conditions or diverse demographic groups, is crucial for ensuring that the trial's findings are applicable to real-world scenarios. Ideally, data collected from a trial should support the expected use of a vaccine in various contexts, such as during public health campaigns or outbreak responses. However, achieving this ideal can be challenging due to pragmatic considerations, such as limitations in resources, ethical concerns, and logistical constraints. Expanding the trial population to include groups like HIV-positive individuals, malnourished children, or broader age ranges can enhance the generalizability of the results and provide valuable insights into the vaccine's efficacy and safety across different subgroups. This discussion will explore the key factors that must be considered when deciding whether to include additional populations in the pivotal Phase III trial for MR-MAPs.

**Questions**

- In addition to the 9–10-, and 15–16-month-old children, what (if any) other age groups or priority populations should be included in the Phase III trial and required for a policy decision?
- Should malnourished and HIV+ children be included in the Phase III trial?
- What is the minimum level of country, population, and regional diversity needed to be considered in the Phase III trial and required for policy decision?

**Table 5.** *Cont.*

**Discussion**

- From a Phase III trial implementation perspective, the enrollment of 9–10-month-old infants for the primary dose (and not 9–12 month olds), who six months later at age 15–16 months (and not 15–18 months) would receive their second dose in alignment with the current schedule, will allow for a more focused implementation of the trial, marginal expected differences in immunogenicity, and higher chance of reaching the NI margin while broadly supporting use in children less than two years of age.
- In addition to routine immunization, MCVs are used in supplementary immunization activities, measles outbreak response, and other delivery strategies, often extending the vaccine use to older populations [3,72]. As such, additional data indicating safety and immunogenicity in older children is likely to be required to inform regulatory and policy decisions. This could be achieved in pre- or post-licensure studies.
- PDVAC has recommended that moderately-to-severely malnourished infants should be included in the pivotal clinical trial; however, their inclusion in a pivotal licensure trial presents a challenge to the trial, as malnourished children, especially those with vitamin A deficiency, have an increased risk of developing severe or fatal measles [21]. Using stratified randomization to allocate malnourished infants equally to the MR-MAPs or MR SC trial arms will minimize trial bias when evaluating NI.
- PDVAC has recommended that infants living with HIV should be included in the clinical development, either during Phase II, III, or in additional studies that run parallel to Phases II–III. The limited evidence available indicates that measles vaccines are safe in HIV-infected children who are not severely immunocompromised, and measles vaccines are recommended for use in that population [3,21]. The immunogenicity of MCVs in children living with HIV and on antiretroviral therapy appears to be similar to the immunogenicity in children without HIV [73,74].
- MR-MAPs could play an important role in the response to measles outbreaks, including in infants younger than 9 months. However, the inclusion of 6-month-old infants in a pivotal Phase III trial risks extending the timeline and increasing the costs and complexity of the trial.
- In countries with high incidence of measles and HIV infection, a zero dose of measles at 6 months (MCV0) is recommended [3]. This recommendation will need to be considered in the context of enrolling measles–rubella vaccine (MRV) naïve infants in the pivotal Phase III trial and selecting the countries to conduct the trial.

**Recommendations**

- In the pivotal Phase III trial, the decision to include moderately to severely malnourished or HIV+ infants who are on anti-retroviral therapy should consider the incidence of malnutrition and HIV at a site of the trial, the NI margin (a higher margin is more permissive of differences in immunogenicity between vaccines), logistical and operational challenges associated with recruiting and retaining HIV+ and malnourished infants in the trial, including coordinating with HIV and nutritional treatment regimens and programs, and implications of including these populations on the generalizability of the trial results.
- If moderately to severely malnourished or HIV+ infants are included in a trial, they should be evenly assigned to treatments by stratified randomization to either the MR-MAP or MR-SC trial arms, to ensure balanced enrollment. Their data can be part of the full analysis set; however, they may be excluded from the per-protocol analysis, meaning the data would not be part of the analysis to determine comparability in immunogenicity and safety between the MR-MAP or MR-SC. There is a risk of increasing the heterogeneity of the immune response and the chances of not meeting the NI margin. Although these infants may comprise a small proportion of the trial's participants, their responses are likely to be carefully assessed by NRAs and the WHO PQ team due to their vulnerable status.
- Should the moderately-to-severely malnourished or HIV+ infants not be included in the Phase III trial, a separate study should be conducted to collect data on safety and immunogenicity of MR-MAPs, which may be required to inform a policy decision.
- 6-month-old infants should not be included in the Phase III trial but rather be evaluated post-licensure to simplify the pivotal Phase III trial.
- Data describing immunogenicity and safety in older children up to 5 years old should be evaluated in a separate descriptive trial, ideally pre-licensure upon consultation with relevant NRAs. Such data are likely to be required for a policy decision and sufficient to inform the use of MR-MAPs in children older than 5 years old and adults.
- The trial should be conducted in multiple countries that appropriately represent those populations where MR-MAPs will be used, accounting for HIV status, malnutrition, and other factors that may influence the safety/reactogenicity and immunogenicity of MR-MAPs.

**Table 6.** Concomitant delivery of vaccines, vitamins, and micronutrients.

| |
|---|
| Measuring the concomitant delivery of vaccines in clinical trials is crucial for ensuring the safety and immunogenicity of vaccines and the effectiveness of immunization programs. When vaccines are administered together, there is potential for interactions that could impact their vaccine's immunogenicity, effectiveness, or safety profiles. Understanding these interactions is essential to confirm that co-administration does not compromise the immune response or increase the risk of adverse effects. |
| **Questions**<br>• Should data demonstrating the safety and immunogenicity of the MR-MAP delivered concomitantly with other vaccines and supplementation with vitamins and micronutrients that are typically administered at the 9–12 month and 15–18-month timepoints be collected in the Phase III trial? Which vaccines should be considered and why?<br>• Are data demonstrating safety and immunogenicity of the MR-MAP delivered concomitantly with other vaccines ("co-administration") required to inform the policy decision? If yes, what are the recommended vaccines that should be considered? |
| **Discussion**<br>• The standard approach is to design dedicated NI trials and confirm non-interference for novel vaccines targeted for infant use by comparing co-administration versus staggered administration of the new vaccine with licensed vaccines given at the same age [23].<br>• However, the pivotal Phase III trial may not need to be powered to evaluate interference with concomitantly delivered vaccines, vitamins and micronutrients, and inclusion of additional trial arms to evaluate the impact of concomitant vaccines will significantly complicate and increase the cost of the Phase III trial.<br>• Live vaccines should be delivered concurrently with MCVs or at 4-week intervals. The oral poliovirus vaccine (OPV) is one exception, which can be delivered without interference before, at the same time, or after measles immunization [3]. For delivery of the MCV aligned with the EPI schedule (9–12 and 15–18 months), some vaccines need to be delivered concomitantly and are standard of care, which are region- and context-specific: Yellow Fever Vaccine (YFV), Meningococcal (A, C, Y, W, X) Polysaccharide Conjugate Vaccine (MenFive™), polio (IPV/bOPV2), Typhoid Conjugate Vaccine (TCV), Malaria, Diphtheria-Tetanus-Pertussis, Hepatitis A, Japanese Encephalitis (JE), and Pneumococcal Conjugate Vaccine (PCV). Notably, MMR and YF vaccine co-administration may result in interference in children under 2 years of age [3].<br>• Concomitant delivery of the RCV can occur with inactivated and live virus vaccines; the RCV should be delivered concurrently with the MCV. In studies of co-administration of the RCV with the YF vaccine, lower GMCs for both antigens were observed; however, the values were well above the threshold necessary for seroconversion [4]. The WHO recommends co-administration of the RCV and the YFV despite the potential lower titers of rubella and YF antibodies. The rationale for this recommendation is that the potential reduction in immune response (lower titers) is outweighed by programmatic implications of delaying vaccinations, and the potential for a more significant impact on population immunity with co-administration [4].<br>• Vitamin A, Vitamin D, and iron supplements could be provided to infants as needed in the Phase III trial per WHO guidelines and country health status (high rates of Vitamin A deficiency, malnutrition, anemia) and local programmatic practice [75,76]. |
| **Recommendations**<br>• If other vaccines are given at the same age as MR in an immunization program setting, then during the Phase III trial such vaccines could be given concomitantly or within one month, dependent upon consultation with NRA and the WHO PQ team. The immune response of other vaccines could potentially be evaluated, and comparisons made between MAP and N&S SC groups using the same co-administered vaccines for dose 1 and then for dose 2 (separate comparisons).<br>• Data showing concomitant delivery of live vaccines such as YF, JE, or polio are likely to be required due to potential for interference. The delivery of dietary supplements should also be considered when designing the pivotal Phase III trial. Alternatively, such data could be collected through other studies completed prior to regulatory and policy review [77].<br>• The inclusion of concomitant vaccines in the Phase III trial will require discussions with relevant NRAs and the WHO PQ team to obtain agreement. |

**Table 7.** Manufacturing and Shelf Life.

It is essential to evaluate manufacturing consistency before licensure as a critical aspect of vaccine product development and manufacturing in the initial launch facilities. For MCV product lot release, virus concentration and thermostability per the specified shelf life must be assessed [22]. The assessment of consistency should be conducted on successive lots [25]. Such an approach allows for the assessment of any potential differences in immunogenicity between MCVs at the beginning and end of their shelf life, ensuring that the vaccine remains effective throughout its intended use period. This approach helps to identify any potential discrepancies or variations that could affect the overall effectiveness and safety of MCVs when administered to the broader population.

**Questions:**

- Should a comparison of immunogenicity between MR-MAPs lots (lot-to-lot (L2L)) be included in the pivotal Phase III trial? If so, how would that impact the design of the trial?
- Will it be required to generate safety data for a high-dose MR-MAP (maximum possible production dose, given the variations in MAP delivery at different points of MAP shelf-life and the associated dose)?

**Discussion**

- The WHO recommends that assays to identify and determine viral concentrations should be used for MCVs. Such assays are required due to the potential impact of diluents and stabilizers on the potency and stability of the individual antigens. Given that the MR vaccine given by a MAP will have a modified formulation to MR-SC, such tests will need to be conducted for the measles and for the rubella vaccine that are given via the MAP [22].
- For each vaccine, live virus concentration of the individual antigens for an individual lot should be determined by cell culture during vaccine manufacturing. For both measles and rubella, a minimum of 1000 viral infective units measured by a 50% cell culture infectious dose (CCID50) has been demonstrated to be immunogenic in MR SC trials. "At least three" containers (such as individual vials) randomly selected would be assessed individually from at least three consecutive Drug Product production lots. The geometric mean infectious virus titer of each container should meet the minimum requirements after incubation, with the virus titer decrease not exceeding 1.0 log.
- Thermostability testing should also occur with the selected containers at 37 °C for seven days [22]. Another consideration related to the thermostability testing described in Technical Report Series (TRS) No. 840 is the MR-MAP TPP recommendation [10] to conduct testing for VVM 30 (37 °C for 30 days at the beginning of shelf life) [33] and CTC (40 °C for three days at the end of shelf life) for product labeling [34].
- The formulations being tested in pivotal trials are typically manufactured using validated processes and go through lot release per NRA and WHO TRS requirements just like they would for the commercial product [23]. WHO TRS states that one batch of vaccine produced through each method might be enough for the comparison; however, data from multiple lots might be required. In vaccine development, typically, three lots are utilized when conducting lot-to-lot consistency in a clinical trial.
- Previous MCV trials have included at least three lots of the MCV and the estimated NI of immunogenicity as well as the reactogenicity and safety between the evaluated arms while combining the evaluated lots [78]. Some studies have also analyzed the immunogenicity between the MCV lots within the same arm; however, the trial was not powered to evaluate non-inferiority between each MCV lot [64].
- The evaluation of a maximum production dose (high potency) for an MR-MAP product may not be required for the pivotal Phase III trial; however, this could be addressed in upcoming Phase II or non-pivotal Phase III studies. Similarly, the lowest acceptable levels of potency at end of shelf life may need to be evaluated in an appropriately designed trial to demonstrate acceptable clinical performance [23,79]. The NRAs for the initial marketing authorization application (MAA) and the WHO PQ team, which will likely need assurance that the proposed potency specifications for lot release, have been demonstrated to be acceptable during clinical development. These considerations should also be addressed during end-of-Phase II/pre-Phase III regulatory consultations [35].

**Recommendations**

- Manufacturing and analytical L2L consistency from a CMC perspective must be demonstrated prior to the pivotal Phase III trial and at the time of authorization of commercial lots.
- MR-MAP thermostability and potency (high and low doses related to manufacturing and product shelf life) testing should be conducted prior to the pivotal Phase III trial.
- To ensure representativeness, three production lots of MR-MAPs with similar expiry dates should be included in the pivotal Phase III trial.
- NRAs and/or the WHO PQ team may require clinical data demonstrating the comparison of equivalent immunogenicity among three production lots of MAP. If so, the sample size for the pivotal Phase III trial will need to be adjusted to assure adequate statistical power and control of the Type I error.
- Owing to the unique nature of the MR-MAP, including both a biological and a device component, MR-MAP developers should seek guidance from NRAs including WLAs and from the WHO PQ tean regarding their proposed CMC and device data package for licensure. Such consultations should ideally be initiated after successful Phase II completion.

**Table 8.** Evaluation of Immune Responses.

Evaluation of immune responses is essential in measuring immunogenicity between different MCVs. Both humoral and cellular immune responses could be included in such evaluation; however, it is recognized that humoral responses, typically measured through assays that detect specific antibodies, play a major role in protection against measles and rubella. To ensure the accuracy and reliability of these measurements, it is imperative that the assays used to evaluate immune responses are rigorously validated. Validation ensures that these assays are precise, reproducible, and suitable for establishing the immunogenicity and non-inferiority of MCVs in clinical trials. This section will explore the recommended assays and approaches for evaluating immune responses to MCVs, drawing on established guidelines and recent advancements in the field.

**Question:**

- What immunological and functional assays should be used to evaluate the immune response to MR-MAPs?

**Discussion**

- Neutralizing antibodies targeting the H antigen play a crucial role in preventing measles virus infection. However, once an individual is infected, cell-mediated immunity becomes essential for clearing the virus. Post wild-type viral infection, the presence of both circulating measles virus-specific CD4+ and CD8+ T cells, as well as the continuous production of measles virus-specific antibodies, contributes to the establishment of a long-term, potentially lifelong, immune memory. Protection from infection is sustained through the rapid development of secondary humoral and cellular immune responses, even as the levels of anti-measles virus antibodies may diminish over time [3].
- For rubella, the RA27/3 strain develops antibody levels that closely mimic those generated by natural infection. During clinical trials, a single dose of the vaccine led to the development of rubella antibodies in 95–100% of susceptible individuals aged ≥9 months. A meta-analysis of 26 clinical trials revealed that 99% (95% CI, 98–99%) of children aged 9–18 months produced antibodies after receiving a single dose of the rubella vaccine containing the RA27/3 strain. Administering a second dose of the rubella vaccine with the RA27/3 strain resulted in 100% seroconversion (99–100%) [4,80].
- Per the EMA, assays used for measurement of primary or secondary endpoints are required to be validated and calibrated to relevant international standards. Immune response characterization for a new vaccine can include functional and/or binding antibody determination, immune response kinetics, immune memory induction, or humoral immune response-related aspects such as previous vaccination or natural infection/exposure or cross-reactive antibody, cross-priming or correlation between cytokine/gene expression profile, or an ICP. CMI assessment is also encouraged [37].
- Per the CDSCO, reference to existing immune response information related to similar, approved vaccines may be suitable for characterization of a new vaccine. The past preclinical and clinical research conducted will inform the CDSCO regarding what will be required for a Phase III trial. In the case of measles and rubella, an ICP for each has been established. Assessment of the humoral response (functional antibody and/or total antibody) after vaccination may be sufficient. Total immunoglobulin (IgG) can be suitable for clinical trials if a correlation between functional and total antibody responses exists. However, in specific age groups and target populations the functional immune response might need to be determined. Per the CDSCO, Cellular Mediated Immunity (CMI) is highlighted as a potential area of investigation for new vaccines to support research conducted on the humoral immune response and could provide useful information to compare between treatment groups [41].

**Recommendations**

- Serum neutralizing antibody assays (SNAs) were proposed to measure immunogenicity endpoints (measles and rubella). Measles seroprotection would be defined, based on current international standards as ≥200 mIU/mL, and rubella seroprotection would be defined as a standardized titer of ≥10 IU/mL. The acceptability of these cutoff values, as well as the appropriateness of the associated immunological assays, however, will need to be confirmed by the NRAs and the WHO PQ team. Other endpoints would include the seroresponse rate (% attaining or exceeding the minimum protective threshold) and GMCs.
- The microbead assay (MBA) is being validated and could be ready for the Phase III trial as a potential alternative or used in addition to the SNAs [18,19,81]. The MBA could allow for rapid immunogenicity testing for both antigens in a centralized laboratory with harmonized protocols. The regulatory authorities and the WHO PQ team would need to confirm the suitability of that assay in MR-MAP clinical development.
- CMI assessment could be an exploratory objective in earlier phase trials or potentially the Phase III trial (subset of samples); however, concerns were raised about increasing the complexity of the trial—which likely will not be required from a regulatory licensure perspective.

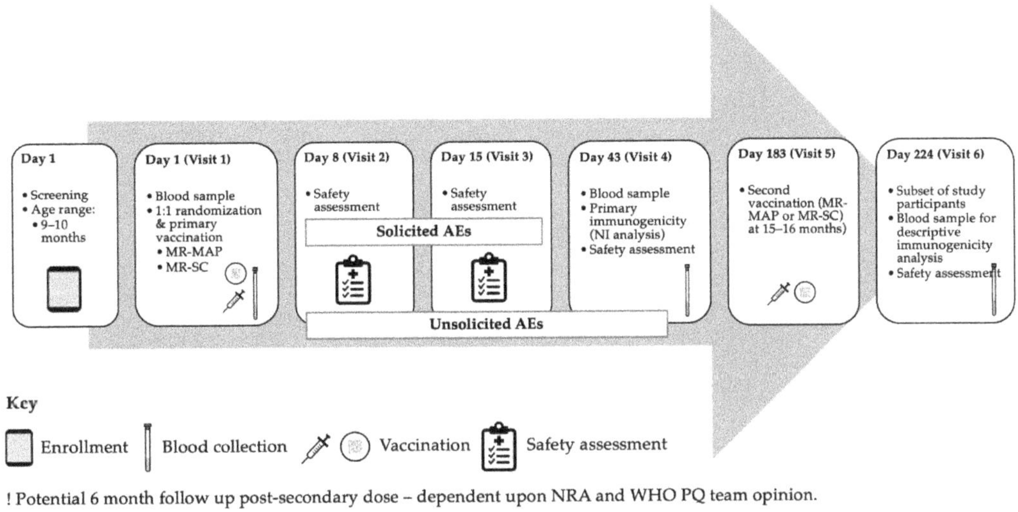


**Figure 2.** Illustrative Phase III Trial Flowchart.

## 4. Additional Recommendations to Support the MR-MAP Pathway to Policy Recommendation and Programmatic Use

Additional data and evidence were identified during the stakeholder discussions on the pivotal Phase III trial design. Such evidence would inform and then expand policy recommendations and support programmatic implementation post initial regulatory licensure and policy.

### *4.1. Other Studies (Descriptive/Post-Market/Implementation)*

Given that at least initially, MR-MAPs are expected to be used in outreach delivery and supplementary immunization activities, data pertaining to older ages, beyond 15–18 months, are likely to be required for licensure and policy decisions. Upon agreement with NRAs and WHO PQ, descriptive analyses of safety and immunogenicity in children up to five years of age could be sufficient to inform MR-MAP use in outreach and campaigns for this age range and older and could be added to the product label. After product licensure, safety and immunogenicity data could also be collected in infants younger than nine months or to evaluate interference with concomitantly delivered vaccines (with emphasis on live vaccines such as YF, polio, and JE). As such, MR-MAP developers and global health stakeholders should consider conducting additional informative clinical studies outside of the pivotal Phase III trial. In addition, if moderately to severely malnourished and HIV+ children are excluded from the trial, data demonstrating safety and immunogenicity of MR-MAPs should be collected in parallel research studies to inform a policy decision.

From a programmatic implementation perspective, it is vital to engage with Gavi-supported, self-procuring countries, other countries utilizing MRV, or those interested in the use of MR-MAP early to design and conduct implementation studies (both pre- and post-licensure) to evaluate MR-MAP's ability to reach zero-dose children and reach other programmatic benefits, key elements of the value proposition. Prior to the Phase III pivotal trial, it is recommended to conduct research studies to evaluate that the anatomical application site or sites are safe, immunogenic, have suitable biomechanical properties to enable efficient MAP delivery, and are acceptable by health workers and caregivers. The MR-MAP application sites could be the wrist, anterolateral thigh, and/or the deltoid, for example. However, this must be confirmed in prior studies. Implementation research in parallel to the Phase III trial is required to provide program design learnings, prospective impact assessment, and other evidence required to inform integration of MR-MAPs into countries' immunization programs. The completed, ongoing, and planned evaluations of the switch to 5-dose MRV will be an important reference for planning such research for MR-MAPs [82–84]. The WHO is leading the work in identifying and prioritizing implementation research questions, which will further enrich the existing knowledge and prepare for programmatic introduction [85].

*4.2. Manufacturing, Regulatory and Policy Considerations*

Defining the MAHs will be critical to advancing the timeline to regulatory submission, licensure, and commercial manufacture to generate supply for programmatic introduction. The MAH should engage with regulatory authorities and policymakers to align the regulatory and clinical strategies. The MR-MAP is a novel vaccine product, with its unique biologic-device combination configuration, and there are no existing specific guidelines from regulators or from the WHO, which is an important implication for a regulatory pathway.

The WHO Technical Report Series (TRS) includes guidelines about vaccine quality assurance and inform WHO prequalification of vaccines [24], which is required for the use of vaccines in LMICs, financed by Gavi, or procured by UNICEF. There are two WHO TRS documents relevant to the MR-MAP: TRS 840 [22] and TRS 1004 [23]. TRS 840's manufacturing requirements sections for measles (pages 105–121) and rubella (pages 137–152) may need to be edited to accommodate the different manufacturing processes and platforms for MR-MAPs. Ideally, such revision would occur before manufacturing of Phase III clinical material, to ensure compliance with proposed standards for both the drug product and the device components, as Phase III clinical material are expected to be representative of initial launch material.

Another consideration is the WHO programmatic suitability criteria for the PQ of the vaccine [31], which were developed taking into account vial presentation and syringe reconstitution and delivery. MR-MAP vaccines should meet the mandatory criteria; however, a revision to this document may be valuable in order to take into account specific aspects of MR-MAP devices [31].

The NRAs targeted for initial licensure and for Phase III conduct will need to opine on the overall design of the pivotal Phase III trial, including the critical questions of immunologic endpoints and their NI margins. Those areas not addressed in the Phase III design could be included in additional Phase III studies or research post-licensure as noted above. Discussions with NRAs and WHO PQ need to include aspects related to manufacturing consistency, specifications for lot release, and end-of-shelf life (EOSL) potency. Given that current MR vaccines are primarily produced in India, the CDSCO will likely play a critical role in the regulatory licensure of MR-MAP products. Importantly, if the Phase III trial is conducted in India, a Phase II leading arm might be considered for addition to the trial to address the need for a Phase II/III bridging trial with Indian infants and children for licensure of vaccines imported or from technology transfer (as opposed to domestic development).

After regulatory licensure and pending WHO PQ, MR-MAPs will require a policy recommendation from global or country stakeholders to allow for MR-MAP introduction and use in countries. The WHO, informed by the Strategic Advisory Group of Experts on Immunization (SAGE), can issue a policy decision on MR-MAPs, allowing for their financing by Gavi and procurement by UNICEF. To determine appropriate data to inform policy, SAGE considers the evidence-to-recommendations tables [29] and the ECVP [30]. Data showing MAP impact and cost-effectiveness modeling will likely be required for the policy. However, it is recognized that increased coverage cannot be demonstrated before MAPs are licensed and deployed. Data showing the acceptability and feasibility of health workers' use of MAPs, acceptability in zero-dose populations, other programmatic benefits, and ability to reach remote populations, together with modeling, could be used to inform policy decisions.

## 5. Conclusions

It is anticipated that MR-MAPs will play a vital role in immunization programs, particularly in reaching zero-dose children through outreach and campaign efforts, addressing the coverage gap for MRVs, and contributing to MR elimination. The proposed Phase III trial framework attempts to align regulatory, policy, and immunization program needs and is intended to address the recommendations from the MR-MAP TAG, other key stakeholders, regulatory, and WHO PQ and policy requirements. The proposed framework has also been developed to anticipate and prevent potential challenges associated with the design and running of a clinical trial, particularly in LMICs, such as inclusion of appropriate populations, or ensuring that the non-inferiority margin is appropriately defined and measured. This manuscript focuses on aspects related to the design of the Phase III clinical trial for MR-MAPs and other important considerations common to all vaccine trials, such as regulatory and ethical consultations, site selection, staff training, participant recruitment, and logistics, are addressed through adherence to international guidelines, and not discussed here [86].

The pivotal Phase III trial, which should be an individually randomized (1:1), open-label NI trial to receive an MR-MAP or MR-SC at 9–10 months of age to assess safety and non-inferiority of immunogenicity of MR vaccines delivered by a MAP, six weeks after the first dose of the MR vaccine. Dependent upon the NRA and the WHO PQ team review and agreement of the proposed pivotal Phase III trial framework, the trial could continue in a subset of children who would be randomized to receive either the same vaccine presentation or a different vaccine presentation 6 months after the first MR dose, at 15–16 months of age. The trial should be conducted in countries where MR-MAPs are to be utilized programmatically and in representative populations regarding health status, informed by the use cases and projected demand for the product in LMICs.

The relevant NRAs and WHO PQ should confirm the acceptability of the proposed immunogenicity endpoints and their NI margin as part of the overall clinical data set that will be submitted for regulatory approval and should opine on the overall Phase III trial design. Consultations involving both NRAs and the WHO PQ team concurrently should be favored to minimize delays to Phase III start.

In addition to the pivotal Phase III trial, additional clinical studies may be required to meet regulatory, WHO or programmatic needs for MR-MAPs. Such studies could address different age groups outside of the 9 to 16-month-old age group, such as younger infants (down to 6 months old) or older children and adults. The studies could also address the safety and immunogenicity of MR-MAPs in moderately-to-severely malnourished children, should they be excluded from the Phase III trial. Concomitant vaccine administration, with priority live virus vaccines that may present the potential for interference, may also need to be addressed. Such studies may be possible pre- or post-licensure, depending upon the final clinical and regulatory strategy.

Determination of the MAH and Phase III trial sponsor will be vital to advancing MR-MAPs through the regulatory licensure process and WHO PQ, and eventual commercialization, ensuring sufficient supply for programmatic introduction. Ideally, this responsibility should be taken on by a manufacturer of prequalified MR vaccines. The NRAs for initial licensure and WHO PQ team will need to address outstanding questions regarding regulatory requirements for quality aspects (manufacturing, controls) of the biological and the device components of MR-MAPs.

Pathways to facilitate joint NRA and WHO PQ reviews such as the EMA M4-all should be explored to determine alignment with an MR-MAP regulatory and marketing strategy. However, before implementing a pivotal Phase III trial, completing MR-MAP device design development will be critical to address issues such as human factors, application site(s), wear time, and cGMP compliant manufacturing facilities. Validation of manufacturing and controls in such facilities is required to produce the Phase III clinical product and prepare for the regulatory licensure process, WHO PQ, and meeting the initial product demand once it is ready for immunization program use. From a WHO policy perspective, the development of the WHO ECVP should be advanced to identify data and evidence to support policy needs, building upon this Phase III framework that describes the parameters for a pivotal licensure trial.

**Author Contributions:** M.H.-A. and B.G. secured the funding; D.Z., M.H.-A. and B.G. developed the approach to developing the Phase III trial framework; all authors were involved in the preparation and running of the global convening and breakout groups; D.Z., M.H.-A. and B.G. wrote the first draft. All authors reviewed and approved the manuscript. All authors have read and agreed to the published version of the manuscript.

**Funding:** This work was funded by the Bill & Melinda Gates Foundation grant (INV-005318) and a grant from the Foreign, Commonwealth & Development Office (FCDO), (award HQUHL2221008/1.2.1/68566 to the World Health Organization.

**Institutional Review Board Statement:** Under WHO procedures, this study was exempt from ethical review because (1) research activities pose minimal risk to participants and (2) participants were asked to provide only objective information or professional opinion on a topic under their direct responsibility or expertise, with their expressed knowledge and consent, and without providing any private individual opinions or opinions on matters outside their direct expertise.

**Informed Consent Statement:** Not applicable. The study did not involve humans.

**Data Availability Statement:** The data presented in this study are available in this article.

**Acknowledgments:** The authors would like to acknowledge the participation of stakeholders interviewed, the global convening attendees, and the MR-MAP TAG for their contributions to the framework design. The authors would like to particularly acknowledge the experts who have reviewed the article and provided feedback: Jon Abramson, Jean-Pierre Amorij, Ben Baker, Marco Cavaleri, Kristen Earle, Matthew Hanson, Ravi Menon, Parag Nagarkar, Mark Papania, Paul Rota, and Tiziana Scarna.

**Conflicts of Interest:** The authors declare no conflicts of interest.

**Author Disclaimer**: The findings and conclusions in this article are those of the authors and do not represent the official position of the World Health Organization. The findings and conclusions in this report are those of the authors and do not necessarily represent the official position of the US Centers for Disease Control and Prevention.

## References


1. Minta, A.A.; Ferrari, M.; Antoni, S.; Portnoy, A.; Sbarra, A.; Lambert, B.; Hatcher, C.; Hsu, C.H.; Ho, L.L.; Steulet, C.; et al. Progress Toward Measles Elimination—Worldwide, 2000–2022. *MMWR Morb. Mortal Wkly. Rep.* **2023**, *72*, 1262–1268. [CrossRef] [PubMed]
2. WHO. Immunization Coverage. 2024. Available online: https://www.who.int/news-room/fact-sheets/detail/immunization-coverage (accessed on 19 August 2024).
3. WHO. Measles Vaccines: WHO Position Paper—2017. *Wkly. Epidemiol. Rec.* **2017**, *92*, 205–227.
4. WHO. Rubella vaccines: WHO position paper—July 2020. *Wkly. Epidemiol. Rec.* **2020**, *95*, 27.
5. Ou, A.C.; Zimmerman, L.A.; Alexander, J.P., Jr.; Crowcroft, N.S.; O'Connor, P.M.; Knapp, J.K. Progress Toward Rubella and Congenital Rubella Syndrome Elimination—Worldwide, 2012–2022. *MMWR Morb. Mortal Wkly. Rep.* **2024**, *73*, 162–167. [CrossRef]
6. Vynnycky, E.; Knapp, J.K.; Papadopoulos, T.; Cutts, F.T.; Hachiya, M.; Miyano, S.; Reef, S.E. Estimates of the global burden of Congenital Rubella Syndrome, 1996–2019. *Int. J. Infect. Dis.* **2023**, *137*, 149–156. [CrossRef]
7. WHO. *WHO Policy Statement: Multi-Dose Vial Policy (MDVP). Revision 2014*; Handling of Multi-Dose Vaccine Vials After Opening; WHO: Geneva, Switzerland, 2014.
8. Mvundura, M.; Ng, J.; Reynolds, K.; Theng Ng, Y.; Bawa, J.; Bambo, M.; Bonsu, G.; Payne, J.; Chua, J.; Guerette, J.; et al. Vaccine wastage in Ghana, Mozambique, and Pakistan: An assessment of wastage rates for four vaccines and the context, causes, drivers, and knowledge, attitudes and practices for vaccine wastage. *Vaccine* **2023**, *41*, 4158–4169. [CrossRef]
9. Hasso-Agopsowicz, M. Exploring important attributes, the potential use-cases and feasibility of introduction of measles and rubella microarray patches (MR-MAPs): Insights from nine countries. *Vaccines* **2024**, *12*, 1084. [CrossRef]
10. WHO; UNICEF. *Measles-Rubella Microarray Patch (MR–MAP) Target Product Profile*; WHO: Geneva, Switzerland, 2019.
11. Prausnitz, M.R.; Goodson, J.L.; A Rota, P.; A Orenstein, W. A microneedle patch for measles and rubella vaccination: A game changer for achieving elimination. *Curr. Opin. Virol.* **2020**, *41*, 68–76. [CrossRef]
12. Fu, H.; Abbas, K.; Malvolti, S.; Gregory, C.; Ko, M.; Amorij, J.P.; Jit, M. Impact and cost-effectiveness of measles vaccination through microarray patches in 70 low-income and middle-income countries: Mathematical modelling and early-stage economic evaluation. *BMJ Glob. Health* **2023**, *8*, e012204. [CrossRef]

13. Malvolti, S.; Ko, M.; Menozzi-Arnaud, M.; Mantel, C.; Jarrahian, C.; Amorij, J.P.; Giersing, B.; Hasso-Agopsowicz, M. Exploring potential applications of measles and rubella microarray patches (MR-MAPs): Use case identification. *Front. Public Health* **2023**, *11*, 1165110. [CrossRef]
14. Scarnà, T.; Menozzi-Arnaud, M.; Friede, M.; DeMarco, K.; Plopper, G.; Hamer, M.; Chakrabarti, A.; Gilbert, P.A.; Jarrahian, C.; Mistilis, J.; et al. Accelerating the development of vaccine microarray patches for epidemic response and equitable immunization coverage requires investment in microarray patch manufacturing facilities. *Expert Opin. Drug Deliv.* **2023**, *20*, 315–322. [CrossRef] [PubMed]
15. Gavi. *Vaccine Microarray Patches (MAPs): Public Summary of the VIPS Alliance Action Plan*; Vaccine Innovation Prioritisation Strategy: Geneva, Switzerland, 2021.
16. Gavi. Vaccine Innovation Prioritisation Strategy (VIPS). 2020. Available online: https://www.gavi.org/our-alliance/market-shaping/vaccine-innovation-prioritisation-strategy (accessed on 19 August 2024).
17. Measles & Rubella Partnership. *Measles & Rubella Strategic Framework 2021–2030*; Measles and Rubella Partnership: Geneva, Switzerland, 2020.
18. Adigweme, I.; Akpalu, E.; Yisa, M.; Donkor, S.; Jarju, L.B.; Danso, B.; Mendy, A.; Jeffries, D.; Njie, A.; Bruce, A.; et al. Study protocol for a phase 1/2, single-centre, double-blind, double-dummy, randomized, active-controlled, age de-escalation trial to assess the safety, tolerability and immunogenicity of a measles and rubella vaccine delivered by a microneedle patch in healthy adults (18 to 40 years), measles and rubella vaccine-primed toddlers (15 to 18 months) and measles and rubella vaccine-naive infants (9 to 10 months) in The Gambia [Measles and Rubella Vaccine Microneedle Patch Phase 1/2 Age De-escalation Trial]. *Trials* **2022**, *23*, 775. [PubMed]
19. Adigweme, I.; Yisa, M.; Ooko, M.; Akpalu, E.; Bruce, A.; Donkor, S.; Jarju, L.B.; Danso, B.; Mendy, A.; Jeffries, D.; et al. A measles and rubella vaccine microneedle patch in The Gambia: A phase 1/2, double-blind, double-dummy, randomised, active-controlled, age de-escalation trial. *Lancet* **2024**, *403*, 1879–1892. [CrossRef] [PubMed]
20. Baker, B.; Bermingham, I.M.; Leelasena, I.; Hickling, J.; Young, P.R.; Muller, D.A.; Forster, A.H. Safety, Tolerability, and Immunogenicity of Measles and Rubella Vaccine Delivered with a High-Density Microarray Patch: Results from a Randomized, Partially Double-Blinded, Placebo-Controlled Phase I Clinical Trial. *Vaccines* **2023**, *11*, 1725. [CrossRef]
21. WHO. *Meeting Report: WHO PDVAC Meeting on MR-MAPs*; WHO: Geneva, Switzerland, 2023.
22. WHO. *Requirements for Measles, Mumps and Rubella Vaccines and Combined Vaccine (Live)*; Technical Report Series; No. 840, Annex 3; WHO: Geneva, Switzerland, 1994.
23. WHO. *Guidelines on Clinical Evaluation of Vaccines: Regulatory Expectations*; Technical Report Series; No. 1004, Annex 9; WHO: Geneva, Switzerland, 2017.
24. WHO. *Procedure or Assessing the Acceptability, in Principle, of Vaccines for Purchase by United Nations Agencies*; Technical Report Series 978; Annex 6; WHO: Geneva, Switzerland, 2013.
25. WHO. *Guidelines for Independent Lot Release of Vaccines by Regulatory Authorities*; Technical Report Series; No. 978, Annex 2; WHO: Geneva, Switzerland, 2010.
26. WHO. *WHO Expert Committee on Biological Standardization*; 67th Report: WHO TRS No. 1004; WHO: Geneva, Switzerland, 2017.
27. SIIL. Measles and Rubella Vaccine. *Live, Attenuated (Freeze-Dried) Package Insert.* 2021. Available online: https://extranet.who.int/prequal/sites/default/files/vwa_vaccine/pq_138_139_140_141_MR_SII_PI-UNICEF_2022.pdf (accessed on 19 August 2024).
28. BiologicalE. Measles and Rubella Vaccine (Live) (Attenuated, Freeze Dried). *Package Insert.* 2019. Available online: https://extranet.who.int/prequal/sites/default/files/vwa_vaccine/pq_343_344_345_MR_BiolE_PI-2019.pdf (accessed on 19 August 2024).
29. WHO. *Development of WHO Immunization Policy and Strategic Guidance. Methods and Processes Applied by the Strategic Advisory Group of Experts on Immunization (SAGE) to Develop Evidence-based Recommendations*; WHO: Geneva, Switzerland, 2024.
30. WHO. *WHO Evidence Considerations for Vaccine Policy Development (ECVP): Generic Framework for Vaccines/Monoclonal Antibodies in Development*; WHO: Geneva, Switzerland, 2022.
31. WHO. *Assessing the Programmatic Suitability of Vaccine Candidates for WHO Prequalification*; WHO: Geneva, Switzerland, 2014.
32. WHO. Prequalification of Medical Products. *Vaccines. Guidance Documents.* 2024. Available online: https://extranet.who.int/prequal/vaccines/guidance-documents (accessed on 19 August 2024).
33. WHO. *PQS Independent Type-Testing Protocol. Vaccine Vial Monitor*; WHO/PQS/E006/IN05-VP.3; WHO: Geneva, Switzerland, 2018.
34. WHO. *Annex 5. Guidelines on the Stability Evaluation of Vaccines for Use Under Extended Controlled Temperature Conditions*; WHO: Geneva, Switzerland, 2016.
35. EMA. *Public Guidance. Parallel Application for EU-M4all (Article 58) Opinion and Centralised Marketing Authorisation Procedure. Promoting EU-Medicines4all*; EMA/104275/2021; EMA: Amsterdam, The Netherlands, 2021.
36. EMA. *Guideline on the Choice of the Non-Inferiority Margin*; EMA: Amsterdam, The Netherlands, 2005.
37. EMA. *Guideline on Clinical Evaluation of Vaccines*; EMAEMA: Amsterdam, The Netherlands, 2023.
38. EMA. *ICH Topic E9 Statistical Principles for Clinical Trials*; (CPMP/ICH/363/96); EMA: Amsterdam, The Netherlands, 1998.
39. EMA. *ICH Topic E10 Choice of Control Group in Clinical Trials*; (CPMP/ICH/364/96); EMA: Amsterdam, The Netherlands, 2001.
40. EMA. *ICH Guideline E8 (R1) on General Considerations for Clinical Studies*; EMA: Amsterdam, The Netherlands, 2021.

41. CDSCO. *Draft Regulatory Guidelines for Development of Vaccines with Special Consideration for COVID-19 Vaccine*; CDSCO: New Delhi, India, 2023.
42. CDSCO. *The New Drugs and Clinical Trials Rules, 2019*; G.o.I. Ministry of Health and Family Welfare: New Delhi, India, 2023.
43. USFDA. *Non-inferiority Clinical Trials to Establish Effectiveness. Guidance for Industry*; USFDA: Silver Spring, MD, USA, 2016.
44. USFDA. *Application of Human Factors Engineering Principles for Combination Products: Questions and Answers. Guidance for Industry and FDA Staff*; USFDA: Silver Spring, MD, USA, 2023.
45. USFDA. *Bridging for Drug-Device and Biologic-Device Combination Products. Guidance for Industry*; USFDA: Silver Spring, MD, USA, 2019.
46. USFDA. *Guidance for Industry and FDA Staff: Current Good Manufacturing Practice Requirements for Combination Products*; USFDA: Silver Spring, MD, USA, 2015.
47. USFDA. *Demonstrating Substantial Evidence of Effectiveness for Human Drug and Biological Products Guidance for Industry*; USFDA: Silver Spring, MD, USA, 2019.
48. AVAREF. *African Vaccine Regulatory Forum (AVAREF)—Joint Review Process*; AVAREF: Entebbe, Uganda, 2020.
49. Nic Lochlainn, L.M.; de Gier, B.; van der Maas, N.; Strebel, P.M.; Goodman, T.; van Binnendijk, R.S.; E de Melker, H.; Hahné, S.J.M. Immunogenicity, effectiveness, and safety of measles vaccination in infants younger than 9 months: A systematic review and meta-analysis. *Lancet Infect. Dis.* **2019**, *19*, 1235–1245. [CrossRef]
50. Hasso-Agopsowicz, M.; Crowcroft, N.; Biellik, R.; Gregory, C.J.; Menozzi-Arnaud, M.; Amorij, J.P.; Gilbert, P.A.; Earle, K.; Frivold, C.; Jarrahian, C.; et al. Accelerating the Development of Measles and Rubella Microarray Patches to Eliminate Measles and Rubella: Recent Progress, Remaining Challenges. *Front. Public Health* **2022**, *10*, 809675. [CrossRef]
51. Bavdekar, A.; Oswal, J.; Ramanan, P.V.; Aundhkar, C.; Venugopal, P.; Kapse, D.; Miller, T.; McGray, S.; Zehrung, D.; Kulkarni, P.S.; et al. Immunogenicity and safety of measles-mumps-rubella vaccine delivered by disposable-syringe jet injector in India: A randomized, parallel group, non-inferiority trial. *Vaccine* **2018**, *36*, 1220–1226. [CrossRef]
52. Low, N.; Bavdekar, A.; Jeyaseelan, L.; Hirve, S.; Ramanathan, K.; Andrews, N.J.; Shaikh, N.; Jadi, R.S.; Rajagopal, A.; Brown, K.E.; et al. A Randomized, Controlled Trial of an Aerosolized Vaccine against Measles. *N. Engl. J. Med.* **2015**, *372*, 1519–1529. [CrossRef]
53. Henao-Restrepo, A.M.; Greco, M.L.X.; John, O.; Aguado, T. *WHO Product Development Group for Measles Aerosol Project. Measles Aerosol Project*; WHO: Geneva, Switzerland, 2010; Volume 2, pp. 147–150.
54. Castro, J.F.; Bennett, J.V.; Rincon, H.G.; Munoz, M.T.; Sanchez, L.A.; Santos, J.I. Evaluation of immunogenicity and side effects of triple viral vaccine (MMR) in adults, given by two routes: Subcutaneous and respiratory (aerosol). *Vaccine* **2005**, *23*, 1079–1084. [CrossRef]
55. Díaz-Ortega, J.L.; Bennett, J.V.; Castañeda, D.; Martinez, D.; de Castro, J.F. Antibody persistence in young adults 1 year after MMR immunization by aerosol or by subcutaneous route. *Vaccine* **2010**, *28*, 7228–7232. [CrossRef]
56. Diaz-Ortega, J.L.; Bennett, J.V.; Castaneda, D.; Vieyra, J.-R.; Valdespino-Gomez, J.L.; de Castro, J.F. Successful seroresponses to measles and rubella following aerosolized Triviraten vaccine, but poor response to aerosolized mumps (Rubini) component: Comparisons with injected MMR. *Vaccine* **2010**, *28*, 692–698. [CrossRef] [PubMed]
57. Díaz-Ortega, J.-L.; Bennett, J.V.; Castañeda-Desales, D.; Quintanilla, D.-M.A.; Martínez, D.; de Castro, J.F. Booster immune response in children 6–7 years of age, randomly assigned to four groups with two MMR vaccines applied by aerosol or by injection. *Vaccine* **2014**, *32*, 3680–3686. [CrossRef] [PubMed]
58. Wong-Chew, R.M.; García-León, M.L.; Torrija, B.E.-T.; Hernández-Pérez, B.; Cardiel-Marmolejo, L.E.; Beeler, J.A.; Audet, S.; Santos-Preciado, J.I. Increasing the time of exposure to aerosol measles vaccine elicits an immune response equivalent to that seen in 9-month-old Mexican children given the same dose subcutaneously. *J. Infect. Dis.* **2011**, *204*, 426–432. [CrossRef] [PubMed]
59. Wong-Chew, R.M.; Islas-Romero, R.; García-García, M.d.L.; Beeler, J.A.; Audet, S.; Santos-Preciado, J.I.; Gans, H.; Lew-Yasukawa, L.; Maldonado, Y.A.; Arvin, A.M.; et al. Immunogenicity of aerosol measles vaccine given as the primary measles immunization to nine-month-old Mexican children. *Vaccine* **2006**, *24*, 683–690. [CrossRef]
60. Wong-Chew, R.M.; Islas-Romero, R.; García-García, M.d.L.; Beeler, J.A.; Audet, S.; Santos-Preciado, J.I.; Gans, H.; Lew-Yasukawa, L.; Maldonado, Y.A.; Arvin, A.M. Induction of cellular and humoral immunity after aerosol or subcutaneous administration of Edmonston-Zagreb measles vaccine as a primary dose to 12-month-old children. *J. Infect. Dis.* **2004**, *189*, 254–257. [CrossRef]
61. Sepúlveda-Amor, J.; Valdespino-Gómez, J.L.; García-García, M.d.L.; Bennett, J.; Islas-Romero, R.; Echaniz-Aviles, G.; de Castro, J.F. A randomized trial demonstrating successful boosting responses following simultaneous aerosols of measles and rubella (MR) vaccines in school age children. *Vaccine* **2002**, *20*, 2790–2795. [CrossRef]
62. Dilraj, A.; Cutts, F.T.; de Castro, J.F.; Wheeler, J.G.; Brown, D.; Roth, C.; Coovadia, H.M.; Bennett, J.V. Response to different measles vaccine strains given by aerosol and subcutaneous routes to schoolchildren: A randomised trial. *Lancet* **2000**, *355*, 798–803. [CrossRef]
63. Dilraj, A.; Sukhoo, R.; Cutts, F.T.; Bennett, J.V. Aerosol and subcutaneous measles vaccine: Measles antibody responses 6 years after re-vaccination. *Vaccine* **2007**, *25*, 4170–4174. [CrossRef]
64. Klein, N.P.; Abu-Elyazeed, R.; Povey, M.; Parra, M.M.; Diez-Domingo, J.; Ahonen, A.; Korhonen, T.; Tinoco, J.-C.; Weiner, L.; Marshall, G.S.; et al. Immunogenicity and Safety of a Measles-Mumps-Rubella Vaccine Administered as a First Dose to Children Aged 12 to 15 Months: A Phase III, Randomized, Noninferiority, Lot-to-Lot Consistency Study. *J. Pediatr. Infect. Dis. Soc.* **2020**, *9*, 194–201. [CrossRef]

65. Vesikari, T.; Becker, T.; Gajdos, V.; Fiquet, A.; Thomas, S.; Richard, P.; Baudin, M. Immunogenicity and safety of a two-dose regimen of a combined measles, mumps, rubella and varicella live vaccine (ProQuad(®)) in infants from 9 months of age. *Vaccine* **2012**, *30*, 3082–3089. [CrossRef]
66. Sood, A.; Mitra, M.; Joshi, H.A.; Nayak, U.S.; Siddaiah, P.; Babu, T.R.; Mahapatro, S.; Sanmukhani, J.; Gupta, G.; Mittal, R.; et al. Immunogenicity and safety of a novel MMR vaccine (live, freeze-dried) containing the Edmonston-Zagreb measles strain, the Hoshino mumps strain, and the RA 27/3 rubella strain: Results of a randomized, comparative, active controlled phase III clinical trial. *Hum. Vaccin. Immunother.* **2017**, *13*, 1523–1530. [CrossRef] [PubMed]
67. Santos, E.M.D.; Noronha, T.G.; Alves, I.S.; Cruz, R.L.S.; Ferroco, C.L.V.; Brum, R.C.; Oliveira, P.M.N.; Siqueira, M.M.; Lima, M.C.; Ramos, F.L.P.; et al. Immunogenicity and safety of the combined vaccine for measles, mumps, and rubella isolated or combined with the varicella component administered at 3-month intervals: Randomised study. *Mem. Inst. Oswaldo Cruz* **2019**, *114*, e180517. [CrossRef] [PubMed]
68. Thuluva, S.; Gunneri, S.; Turaga, K.; Mogulla, R.R.; Yerroju, V.; Peta, K.; Suneetha, P.V.; Matur, R.V. A phase II/III randomised, comparative study evaluating the safety and immunogenicity of Biological E's live, attenuated Measles-Rubella vaccine in 9–12 month old healthy infants. *Contemp. Clin. Trials Commun.* **2023**, *36*, 101232. [CrossRef] [PubMed]
69. USNIH. *Division of AIDS (DAIDS) Table for Grading the Severity of Adult and Pediatric Adverse Events*; USNIH: Bethesda, MD, USA, 2017.
70. Donken, R.; de Melker, H.; Rots, N.; Berbers, G.; Knol, M. Comparing vaccines: A systematic review of the use of the non-inferiority margin in vaccine trials. *Vaccine* **2015**, *33*, 1426–1432. [CrossRef]
71. Cavaleri, M. MR-MAP considerations. In *WHO Global Convening on Measles-Rubella Microarray Patches (MR-MAPs)*; WHO: Geneva, Switzerland, 2024.
72. WHO. Measles. 2024. Available online: https://www.who.int/news-room/fact-sheets/detail/measles (accessed on 19 August 2024).
73. Mutsaerts, E.A.; Nunes, M.C.; van Rijswijk, M.N.; Klipstein-Grobusch, K.; Grobbee, D.E.; Madhi, S.A. Safety and Immunogenicity of Measles Vaccination in HIV-Infected and HIV-Exposed Uninfected Children: A Systematic Review and Meta-Analysis. *EClinicalMedicine* **2018**, *1*, 28–42. [CrossRef]
74. Seth, A.; Deepa, S.; Dutta, R.; Chandra, J. Evaluation of Immune Response to Measles Component of MMR Vaccine in Children with HIV Infection Receiving Antiretroviral Therapy. *Pediatr. Infect. Dis. J.* **2016**, *35*, e8–e11. [CrossRef]
75. WHO. *Guideline: Vitamin A Supplementation in Infants and Children 6–59 Months of Age*; WHO: Geneva, Switzerland, 2011.
76. WHO. *WHO Recommendations on Child Health. Guidelines Approved by the WHO Guidelines Review Committee*; WHO: Geneva, Switzerland, 2017.
77. WHO. Vitamin A Supplementation. 2024. Available online: https://www.who.int/teams/immunization-vaccines-and-biologicals/essential-programme-on-immunization/integration/linking-with-other-health-interventions/vitamin-a#:~:text=*Vitamin%20A%20can%20be%20stored%20in%20the%20liver,,treat%20clinical%20vitamin%20A%20deficiency%20and%20measles%20cases (accessed on 19 August 2024).
78. MMR-162 Study Group. Safety and immunogenicity of an upper-range release titer measles-mumps-rubella vaccine in children vaccinated at 12 to 15 months of age: A phase III, randomized study. *Hum. Vaccines Immunother.* **2018**, *14*, 2921–2931. [CrossRef]
79. Jarrahian, C. *MR-MAP Phase II*; Zehrung, D., Ed.; WHO: Geneva, Switzerland, 2024.
80. van den Boogaard, J.; de Gier, B.; Lima, P.d.O.B.; Desai, S.; de Melker, H.E.; Hahné, S.J.; Veldhuijzen, I.K. Immunogenicity, duration of protection, effectiveness and safety of rubella containing vaccines: A systematic literature review and meta-analysis. *Vaccine* **2021**, *39*, 889–900. [CrossRef]
81. Coughlin, M.M.; Matson, Z.; Sowers, S.B.; Priest, J.W.; Smits, G.P.; van der Klis, F.R.M.; Mitchell, A.; Hickman, C.J.; Scobie, H.M.; Goodson, J.L.; et al. Development of a Measles and Rubella Multiplex Bead Serological Assay for Assessing Population Immunity. *J. Clin. Microbiol.* **2021**, *59*, 889–900. [CrossRef]
82. Krudwig, K.; Knittel, B.; Karim, A.; Kanagat, N.; Prosser, W.; Phiri, G.; Mwansa, F.; Steinglass, R. The effects of switching from 10 to 5-dose vials of MR vaccine on vaccination coverage and wastage: A mixed-method study in Zambia. *Vaccine* **2020**, *38*, 5905–5913. [CrossRef]
83. Oo, A.N.; Thekkur, P.; Thar, A.M.C.; Htet, K.K.K.; Lin, H.H. Small Session Size and Big Vial Size: Operational Research Assessing Open Vial Vaccine Wastage at the Service Delivery Points in the Mandalay Region of Myanmar During 2018. *Trop. Med. Infect. Dis.* **2020**, *5*, 60. [CrossRef] [PubMed]
84. Wedlock, P.T.; Mitgang, E.A.; Haidari, L.A.; Prosser, W.; Brown, S.T.; Krudwig, K.; Siegmund, S.S.; DePasse, J.V.; Bakal, J.; Leonard, J.; et al. The value of tailoring vial sizes to populations and locations. *Vaccine* **2019**, *37*, 637–644. [CrossRef] [PubMed]
85. Sá Silva, S. MR-MAPs Implementation Research Agenda: A framework to identify priority implementation research questions for MR-MAPs. In *MR-MAP Global Convening*; WHO: Geneva, Switzerland, 2024.
86. Saluja, T.; Giri, B.R.; Chaudhary, S.; Tamrakar, D.; Kanodia, P.; Palkar, S.; Vemula, S.; Chinaworapong, S.; Kim, B.; Gupta, B.P.; et al. Challenges and opportunities in setting up a phase III vaccine clinical trial in resource limited settings: Experience from Nepal. *Hum. Vaccines Immunother.* **2021**, *17*, 2149–2157. [CrossRef] [PubMed]

*vaccines*

MDPI

*Article*

# Progress with the Second Dose Measles Vaccine Introduction and Coverage in the WHO African Region

**Balcha G. Masresha [1,*], Messeret E. Shibeshi [2], Gavin B. Grant [3], Cynthia Hatcher [3] and Charles S. Wiysonge [1]**

1 Vaccine Preventable Diseases Program, World Health Organization, Regional Office for Africa, Brazzaville P.O. Box 06, Congo; sheyc@who.int
2 Vaccine Preventable Diseases Program, World Health Organization, Regional Office for Africa, Inter-Country Support Team, Harare P.O. Box CY 348, Zimbabwe; eshetum@who.int
3 Global Immunization Division, Global Health Center, U.S. Centers for Disease Control and Prevention, Atlanta, GA 30333, USA; gig9@cdc.gov (G.B.G.); ctp0@cdc.gov (C.H.)
* Correspondence: masreshab@who.int

**Abstract:** Introduction: To achieve global and regional measles elimination objectives, the World Health Organization (WHO) recommends coverage of 95% or higher with two doses of measles-containing vaccine. A second dose of measles-containing vaccine (MCV) is typically administered in the second year of life after 12 months of age. Methods: We reviewed WHO-UNICEF estimates of national coverage (WUENIC) for the first and second doses of MCV (MCV1 and MCV2, respectively) and calculated drop-out rates between MCV1 and MCV2 for countries in the WHO African Region. Results: From 2013 to 2023, estimated regional MCV2 coverage increased from 7% to 49%, and at the end of 2023, 43 (91%) countries had introduced MCV2 into their routine immunization programs. Countries with more antigens provided in the second year of life had higher mean and median MCV2 coverage levels, and lower drop-out rates between MCV1 and MCV2, as compared to countries providing only MCV2. Discussion: Despite substantial progress, MCV2 coverage remains below the required levels to achieve and sustain elimination, and many countries have high drop-out rates between MCV1 and MCV2 coverage, indicating challenges in reaching children over 12 months of age. Increasing coverage of MCV2 and other vaccines in the second year of life is essential to achieving higher and equitable routine immunization coverage. This will require continued efforts to understand and mitigate barriers to reaching children after 12 months of age and accelerated implementation of available tools.

**Keywords:** measles; elimination; measles second dose; routine immunization; second-year of life; Africa

## 1. Introduction

The African Regional Immunisation Strategic Plan 2021–2030 aims to achieve measles and rubella elimination in at least 80% of the countries by 2030 [1]. To achieve this goal, the World Health Organization (WHO) recommends reaching all susceptible persons with two doses of measles-containing vaccine (MCV) [2]. The routine administration of a second dose of measles-containing vaccine (MCV2), usually in the second year of life (2YL) between 15 and 18 months of age, reduces susceptibility in up to 15% of individuals who do not seroconvert after the first dose of MCV (MCV1) at 9 months of age [2]. MCV2 was originally recommended for countries with MCV1 coverage at or above 80%, but WHO guidance was updated in 2017 to recommend MCV2 introduction, regardless of MCV1 coverage [2]. In addition to MCV2, the 2YL platform provides a scheduled vaccination opportunity to administer MCV1 to unvaccinated children to reach the high population immunity levels needed to prevent measles transmission and integrate with other immunizations and health services [3].

One of the Immunization Agenda 2030 (IA2030) strategic priorities is for all people to benefit from recommended immunizations throughout the life course, effectively integrated with other essential health services [1,4]. MCV2 coverage is one of the critical indicators used to monitor progress towards the Sustainable Development Goals (SDGs) [4]. As of 2023, 190 (98%) of 194 member states have introduced MCV2, and the estimated global MCV2 coverage was 74% [5]. However, an estimated 11 million children did not receive MCV2 in routine immunization in 2022, and global and regional MCV2 coverage remains below the target of 95% or higher [6].

Operational guidelines are available to assist countries to plan and prepare for MCV2 introduction, and countries are encouraged to conduct post-introduction evaluation (PIE) exercises within the first few months of new vaccine introduction to assess roll-out and address any gaps as early as possible [7] [AFRO guidelines].

This paper describes the progress in introducing a second dose of measles vaccination in the WHO African Region (AFR) more than a decade after the global push for introduction with support from Gavi, the Vaccine Alliance (Gavi). We reviewed the vaccination coverage levels attained within the context of the broader vaccination initiative in the second year of life platform.

## 2. Methods

Every year, all countries report to WHO and UNICEF their national MCV1 and MCV2 administrative coverage (as calculated by dividing the total number of doses administered to children by the number of children in the respective target age groups), as well as the national vaccination schedule. WHO and UNICEF generate estimates of coverage for key antigens, including first and second doses of measles-containing vaccines, based on the reported data, as well as national coverage estimates, data from vaccination coverage surveys, and other sources of data validation [5,8]. For the status regarding the introduction of MCV2, we reviewed the program information as of the end of 2023. Using the officially published WHO-UNICEF estimates of national immunization coverage (WUENIC) for MCV1 and MCV2, we examined the MCV2 coverage rates over the ten-year period from 2013 to the latest available coverage estimate data from 2023. For the year 2023, using the WUENIC estimates, we calculated the drop-out rates between MCV1 and MCV2 and the ratio of MCV2 coverage to the MCV1 coverage for the countries in the AFR region that have had MCV2 in their routine immunization schedules for at least three years. To evaluate the role of the health system strength in countries introduced prior to 2022, we correlated MCV2 coverage to the universal health coverage (UHC) service index and general domestic general health expenditures (GGHEs) (as a percent of Gross Domestic Product) [9].

## 3. Results

MCV2 introduction in AFR has accelerated from 2013, when only 11 (24%) of 46 countries had introduced MCV2, to 43 (92%) of 47 countries having introduced MCV2 by the end of 2023. At the end of 2023, only Benin, Central African Republic (CAR), Gabon, and South Sudan had not introduced MCV2.

Nearly all AFR countries schedule the MCV2 dose at 15 or 18 months, except for South Africa, which provides MCV2 at 12 months of age, Mauritius at 17 months of age, and Cape Verde and Seychelles at 6 years of age. Mauritius only shifted to 17 months of age from 5 years of age in 2023 to ensure the early protection of children.

The MCV1 and MCV2 WUENIC coverage estimates for AFR from 2013 to 2023 are given in Figure 1. As of December 2023, the estimated regional MCV2 coverage reached 49%, a substantial increase from the 7% coverage documented in 2013. Only three countries had ≥90% MCV2 coverage in 2023: Algeria (93%), Mauritania (94%), and Sao Tome and Principe (90%). Eleven countries had MCV2 coverage levels of ≥80%, while 14 countries had coverage of less than 50% (Angola, Cameroon, Central African Republic, Chad, Republic of Congo, Cote d'Ivoire, DR Congo, Equatorial Guinea, Gabon, Guinea, Guinea-Bissau, Madagascar, Mauritania, Mozambique, Nigeria, South Sudan, and Uganda) (Table 1).

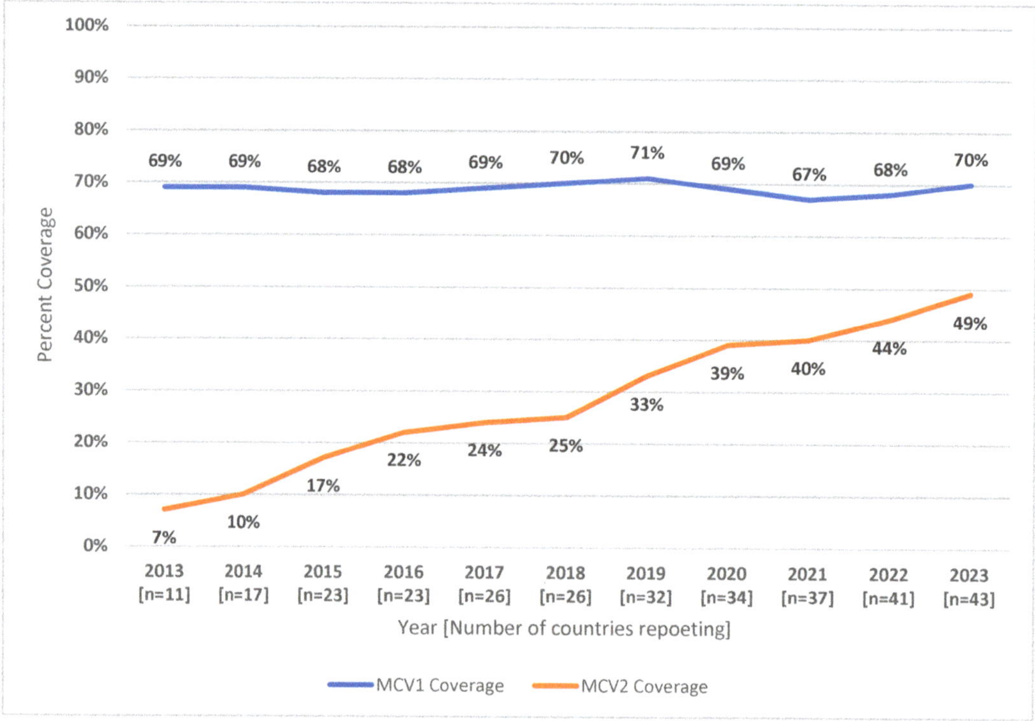


**Figure 1.** MCV1 and MCV2 estimated coverage (WUENIC estimates)—World Health Organization African Region, 2013–2023. Abbreviations: MCV1 = first dose of measles-containing vaccine; MCV2 = second dose of measles-containing vaccine; WUENIC = WHO and UNICEF estimates of national immunization coverage.

**Table 1.** MCV1 and MCV2 estimated coverage (WUENIC estimates), drop-out rates, vaccine type and year of MCV2 introduction—World Health Organization African Region, 2022.

| Country | Type of Vaccine Used | Year MCV2 Introduced | MCV1 Coverage (WUENIC 2023) | MCV2 Coverage (WUENIC 2023) | Drop-Out Rate [1] |
|---|---|---|---|---|---|
| Algeria | MMR | Pre-2000 | 99 | 93 | 6% |
| Angola | MR | 2015 | 50 | 35 | 30% |
| Benin | M | N/A | 52 | 0 | N/A |
| Botswana | MR | 2011 | 97 | 79 | 19% |
| Burkina Faso | MR | 2014 | 94 | 71 | 24% |
| Burundi | MR | 2013 | 86 | 80 | 7% |
| Cabo Verde | MMR | 2010 | 95 | 86 | 9% |
| Cameroon | MR | 2019 | 71 | 45 | 37% |
| Central African Republic | M | N/A | 41 | 0 | N/A |
| Chad | M | 2022 | 63 | 35 | 44% |
| Comoros | MR | 2021 | 70 | 79 | −13% |
| Congo | MR | 2019 | 65 | 34 | 48% |
| Côte d'Ivoire | MR | 2021 | 70 | 43 | 39% |

**Table 1.** *Cont.*

| Country | Type of Vaccine Used | Year MCV2 Introduced | MCV1 Coverage (WUENIC 2023) | MCV2 Coverage (WUENIC 2023) | Drop-Out Rate [1] |
|---|---|---|---|---|---|
| DR Congo | M | 2022 | 52 | 18 | 65% |
| Equatorial Guinea | M | 2021 | 61 | 28 | 54% |
| Eritrea | MR | 2012 | 93 | 85 | 9% |
| Eswatini | MR | Pre-2000 | 85 | 82 | 4% |
| Ethiopia | M | 2019 | 61 | 53 | 13% |
| Gabon | M | N/A | 66 | 0 | N/A |
| Gambia | MR | 2012 | 80 | 73 | 9% |
| Ghana | MR | 2012 | 90 | 78 | 13% |
| Guinea | M | 2022 | 47 | 26 | 45% |
| Guinea-Bissau | M | 2022 | 72 | 36 | 50% |
| Kenya | MR | 2013 | 91 | 76 | 16% |
| Lesotho | MR | Pre-2000 | 90 | 82 | 9% |
| Liberia | M | 2019 | 82 | 60 | 27% |
| Madagascar | M | 2020 | 51 | 47 | 8% |
| Malawi | MR | 2015 | 87 | 65 | 25% |
| Mali | MR | 2019 | 73 | 59 | 19% |
| Mauritania | MR | 2023 | 92 | 24 | 74% |
| Mauritius | MMR | 2003 | 96 | 94 | 2% |
| Mozambique | MR | 2015 | 65 | 44 | 32% |
| Namibia | MR | 2017 | 86 | 62 | 28% |
| Niger | M | 2014 | 80 | 68 | 15% |
| Nigeria | M | 2019–2020 | 60 | 38 | 37% |
| Rwanda | MR | 2014 | 96 | 88 | 8% |
| Sao Tome and Principe | MR | 2013 | 86 | 90 | −5% |
| Senegal | MR | 2014 | 76 | 64 | 16% |
| Seychelles | MMR | Pre-2000 | 93 | 89 | 4% |
| Sierra Leone | MR | 2015 | 90 | 73 | 19% |
| South Africa | M | Pre-2000 | 80 | 84 | −5% |
| South Sudan | M | N/A | 72 | 0 | N/A |
| Togo | MR | 2019 | 72 | 58 | 19% |
| Uganda | MR | 2022 | 93 | 21 | 77% |
| United Republic of Tanzania | MR | 2014 | 91 | 78 | 14% |
| Zambia | MR | 2013 | 90 | 75 | 17% |
| Zimbabwe | MR | 2015 | 90 | 77 | 14% |

Abbreviations: M = measles vaccine; MCV1 = first dose of measles-containing vaccine; MCV2 = second dose of measles-containing vaccine; MR = measles and rubella vaccine; MMR = measles, mumps, and rubella vaccine; N/A = not applicable; WUENIC = WHO and UNICEF estimates of national immunization coverage. [1] MCV1 − MCV2 drop-out rate = (MCV1 − MCV2)/MCV1 coverage.

Among the 15 countries that have had MCV2 in their routine program for at least ten years, the mean MCV1 and MCV2 coverage levels were 90% and 83%, and the mean and median drop-out rates between MCV1 and MCV2 coverage were both 8%. In 17 countries with MCV2 in their program for between 5 and 9 years, the mean drop-out rate was 16%, with a median of 15.5%. In seven countries where MCV2 was introduced only 3–5 years ago, the average and median drop-out rate was 26% and 23% (Table 1).

As of 2022, a total of 19 countries have reported providing antigens other than MCV2 in the 2YL platform in their routine immunization programs (Table 2). Of the 19, ten provide either pentavalent, diphtheria, tetanus, and pertussis (DTP), or tetanus toxoid and diphtheria (DT) vaccine; nine provide oral polio (OPV) or inactivated polio (IPV), five meningococcal A conjugate vaccine, and two provide malaria vaccine. Higher MCV2 coverage was associated with more vaccines provided during 2YL; countries with 0, 1, or 2 additional vaccines showed an increasing MCV2 coverage (39%, 61%, and 92%, respectively) and a decreasing drop-out rate of 34%, 26%, and 11%, respectively.

**Table 2.** Vaccines other than MCV2 offered after 12 months of age to pre-school children. World Health Organization African Region, 2022. Official country reports through the WHO-UNICEF Joint Reporting Form (JRF).

| Country | Other Vaccines Provided in the 2nd Year of Life | Other Vaccines Provided by Age of School Entry |
|---|---|---|
| Algeria | None | OPV, DT and MR2 at 6 years |
| Angola | None | None |
| Benin | None | None |
| Botswana | OPV and DT at 18 months | DT at 7 years |
| Burkina Faso | Meningitis Conjugate Vaccine-4, MenA | None |
| Burundi | DTP4 | None |
| Cabo Verde | Penta4, OPV | None |
| Cameroon | None | None |
| Central African Republic | None | None |
| Chad | None | None |
| Comoros | None | None |
| Congo | None | None |
| Côte d'Ivoire | None | None |
| DR Congo | None | None |
| Equatorial Guinea | Penta4 at 18 months | None |
| Eritrea | Men-A | None |
| Eswatini | OPV at 18 months | OPV and DT at 5 years |
| Ethiopia | None | None |
| Gabon | None | None |
| Gambia | DTP4 and OPV4 at 18 months | None |
| Ghana | RTS,S and Men A at 18 months | None |
| Guinea | Men A at 15 months | None |
| Guinea-Bissau | None | None |
| Kenya | None | None |
| Lesotho | DT at 18 months | Td at 6 years |
| Liberia | None | None |

**Table 2.** *Cont.*

| Country | Other Vaccines Provided in the 2nd Year of Life | Other Vaccines Provided by Age of School Entry |
|---|---|---|
| Madagascar | None | None |
| Malawi | RTS,S4 at 22 months | None |
| Mali | None | None |
| Mauritania | None | None |
| Mauritius | Penta4 and IPV at 18 months | Tdap and IPV at 5 years |
| Mozambique | None | Td at 6 years |
| Namibia | None | OPV and DT at 5 years |
| Niger | None | None |
| Nigeria | None | None |
| Rwanda | None | None |
| Sao Tome and Principe | OPV4 at 15 months | None |
| Senegal | None | None |
| Seychelles | DPT4 and OPV4 at 18 months | DT and OPV at 6 years |
| Sierra Leone | None | None |
| South Africa | Penta4 and IPV at 18 months | Td at 6 years |
| South Sudan | None | None |
| Togo | Men A at 15 months | None |
| Uganda | None | None |
| United Republic of Tanzania | None | None |
| Zambia | OCV at 13 months | None |
| Zimbabwe | DTP4 and OPV at 18 months | None |

Abbreviations: DT = tetanus toxoid and diphtheria vaccine, children's dose; DTP4 = fourth dose of diphtheria, tetanus, and pertussis vaccine; IPV = inactivated polio vaccine; MenA = meningococcal A conjugate vaccine; MCV2 = second dose of measles-containing vaccine; MR2 = second dose of measles and rubella vaccine; OCV = oral cholera vaccine; OPV = oral polio vaccine; OPV4 = fourth dose of oral polio vaccine; Penta4 = fourth dose of pentavalent vaccine; RTS,S = RTS,S/AS01 malaria vaccine; RTS,S4 = fourth dose of malaria vaccine; Td = tetanus toxoid and diphtheria vaccine, older children and adult dose; Tdap = tetanus, diphtheria, and acellular pertussis vaccine.

The correlation between MCV2 coverage levels and health system indicators demonstrated a positive relationship, with a moderate association of 0.52 with General Governmental Health Expenditures per capita (GGHE) and 0.59 for Universal Health Coverage Service Index (UHC) (see Supplementary Figure S1).

## 4. Discussion

Following the change in the WHO policy recommendations in 2017 to include a second dose in all countries independent of first dose coverage and the availability of funding support from Gavi for introduction, there has been significant progress in MCV2 introduction from 2013 to 2022 in AFR. However, in 2023, the regional MCV2 coverage remains low at 49% compared with global MCV2 coverage of 74% [5,6], both of which are inadequate for achieving and sustaining the elimination of measles. Most countries have failed to raise their MCV2 coverage levels near MCV1 coverage levels, indicating that a large proportion of children drop out between the first and second doses. The declines in vaccination coverage during the COVID-19 pandemic have left more children unprotected against measles in 2022, risking large and disruptive outbreaks in some countries. In this study, we note that despite the trend showing an overall increase in regional-level MCV2 coverage in the past few years, the number of countries meeting the 95% target for MCV2 coverage declined in 2022, an impact of the COVID-19 pandemic [6,10]. The milestones to reaching measles elimination in AFR include the attainment of 90% coverage with MCV2 in 40% of countries by 2025 and in all countries by 2030; these will not be met unless progress is accelerated [1].

The fact that many countries continue to have low MCV2 coverage and high drop-out rates more than three years post-introduction is evidence that challenges remain with the 2YL platform. Despite the availability of initial one-time Gavi funding to support the operational costs related to introducing MCV2 in eligible countries, the preparation for MCV2 introduction in many countries has been sub-standard. Post-introduction evaluation (PIE) exercises have documented that MCV2 introductions in some countries were not implemented with meticulous logistics, social mobilization and communications, micro-planning, health worker training, revision of monitoring tools, conducting caretaker awareness for the new point of health service contact, or putting in place means of monitoring [11]. At least seven of the countries (Chad, Congo, Equatorial Guinea, Guinea, Guinea Bissau, Madagascar, and Mauritania) that introduced MCV2 since 2019 have not yet implemented comprehensive PIE exercises, which limit their ability to identify and address structural barriers in a timely manner and develop plans to increase MCV2 coverage.

A global research prioritization exercise in 2016 identified that there is a need to determine the effectiveness of strategies to increase coverage with MCV1 and MCV2, such as strategies to (1) reduce missed opportunities for vaccination (MOV), (2) improve defaulter tracing, (3) improve coverage through use of a five-dose measles vial, and (4) improve coverage using school-based platforms for the checking of vaccination status and the delivery of catch-up doses [12].

To date, evidence has been generated surrounding the effectiveness of some of these strategies. One documented barrier to increasing measles vaccination coverage has been the concern about vaccine wastage in countries using 10-dose vials, where health workers open vials only when they are certain they can utilize the majority of the doses within six hours once reconstituted. A study in Nigeria showed that vaccinators expect a minimum of six children to be present prior to opening a 10-dose MCV vial [13]. Similarly, many health facilities do not provide daily measles vaccination services, resulting in missed opportunities to deliver MVC2 [14].

As of the end of 2023, a total of 12 countries (Botswana, Cape Verde, Comoros, DR Congo, Equatorial Guinea, Eritrea, Eswatini, Lesotho, Niger, Mauritius, Seychelles, and Zimbabwe) are using five-dose or lesser-dose vials instead of the 10-dose measles-containing vaccine vials. Studies have shown that the introduction of MCV in five-dose vials leads to better health worker readiness to open vials, even with fewer eligible children at service delivery sites, and have demonstrated a statistically significant increase in both MCV1 and MCV2 coverage compared with districts using 10-dose vials [15,16].

Missed opportunities for vaccination (MOV) persist in many countries, and in one study, among children who were due for at least one vaccination dose, 76% had at least one MOV [14,17]. Many studies have documented healthcare workers' reluctance or refusal to open a multi-dose vial unless a critical number of children is gathered, especially for lyophilized vaccines such as BCG, MCV, measles-rubella (MR), and Yellow Fever (YF) vaccines [13–15,18]. Many countries have adopted school-based vaccination to reach older children with missed doses [19]. On the caregiver side, a study in Ghana found that the caregivers' awareness of the routine immunization schedule was an important determinant of childhood vaccination uptake of MCV2 and meningitis A (MenA) conjugate vaccine [20]. Other factors like maternal age, rural residency, and birth order also affected the uptake of the vaccines in the 2YL [11,20,21]. Vaccine hesitancy may also be a factor in stagnating coverage, but the impact specifically on MCV2 and other 2YL antigens has not been well described [22].

There is a moderate correlation between health system strength indicators and MCV2 coverage; both coverage and government spending on the healthcare, but are not sufficient to determine coverage, but do continue to emphasize that the degree of health care financing and universal health coverage contributes to high MCV2 coverage levels. As a caveat, these indicators do not measure the quality of services provided, nor do they reflect demand-side factors (e.g., desire for a second measles vaccination dose).

A robust 2YL platform is essential to ensure that young children are fully protected against measles and against other pathogens targeted by vaccines such as meningococcal A conjugate vaccine (Men A), a booster dose of diphtheria-tetanus-pertussis (DTP)-containing vaccine, and additional doses of pentavalent and polio vaccines. Only 19 (40%) of 47 AFR countries include DPT4 or other vaccines in the second year of life in addition to MCV2. The strengthening of the 2YL platform can be a critical point of entry for catch-up vaccination to reach children who may have missed primary doses in infancy. One analysis in South Africa found that the 2YL visit increased MCV coverage by 3%, but only 20% of children missing a pentavalent dose received a dose during this visit [23]. In addition to the 2YL platform, nine (19%) countries have scheduled vaccination appointments at the age of 5 or 6 years, coinciding with school entry. Advancing school health programs and policies requiring proof of vaccination upon school entry would help to advocate for and ensure complete measles vaccination.

The recent WHO prequalification of malaria vaccines with high national demand creates an opportunity to leverage and strengthen the 2YL platform, as many countries opt to give the fourth dose of malaria vaccine in the second year of life using established vaccination contact points [24]. Assessing the impact of malaria vaccination on increasing MCV2 and other antigens provided during the 2YL will be important to guide programs to refine vaccination schedules and service delivery approaches.

Countries are encouraged to implement detailed subnational level analysis of immunization program performance, including the 2YL platform, and as needed, conduct program reviews (either desk reviews or extensive field level reviews) and implement post-introduction evaluation to monitor the health of the 2YL and address policy and program gaps. In addition, it is important to remove any policy barriers to vaccinating eligible unvaccinated children at any age, including putting in place robust screening of vaccination status at school entry [25].

This study has several limitations. The national coverage estimates do not reflect the significant coverage diversity at the subnational level, e.g., among provinces and districts, especially in large countries [26]. In addition, data quality limitations may result in inaccurate estimates of coverage in some countries. A thorough understanding of all challenges to MCV2 service delivery, including the role of vaccine demand and quality of vaccine introduction activities, was beyond the scope of this analysis, though it likely contributes to the current challenges with improving coverage.

## 5. Conclusions

Increasing coverage of MCV2 and other vaccines in the second year of life is essential to achieving the African Regional Immunization Strategic Plan 2021–2030 and the Immunization Agenda 2030 objectives to eliminate measles and protect children from illness, disability, and death. Significant progress has been made in the African region to increase both coverage, and the number of countries offering MCV2, but no country has achieved the goal of ≥95% coverage, and only three (7%) countries have a coverage of ≥90%. Global commitment to immunization and other essential health interventions across the life course underscores the importance of strengthening the 2YL platform, increasing the utilization of five-dose vials and developing locally tailored strategies to reach children after 12 months of age, which are essential to achieving these objectives.

**Supplementary Materials:** The following supporting information can be downloaded at https://www.mdpi.com/article/10.3390/vaccines12091069/s1, Figure S1. Association of a second dose of measles-containing vaccine (MCV2) and Universal Health Coverage Service Index (UHC) and General Governmental Health Expenditures per capita (in US dollars) for countries in the African Region that had been introduced prior to 2022.

**Author Contributions:** Conceptualization: B.G.M. and M.E.S.; methodology, B.G.M. and C.H. validation, G.B.G.; formal analysis, B.G.M. and G.B.G. investigation: B.G.M. and M.E.S.; writing—original draft, B.G.M., M.E.S. and G.B.G.; writing—review and editing, C.H. and C.S.W.; supervision—C.S.W. All authors have read and agreed to the published version of the manuscript.

**Funding:** This research received no external funding.

**Institutional Review Board Statement:** Not applicable.

**Informed Consent Statement:** Not applicable.

**Data Availability Statement:** Sources for vaccination coverage data presented in this analysis were cited.

**Conflicts of Interest:** The authors declare no conflicts of interest.

## References

1. Regional Office for Africa. *Framework for the Implementation of the Immunization Agenda 2030 in the WHO African Region: Report of the Secretariat*; World Health Organization, Regional Office for Africa: Brazzaville, Congo, 2021.
2. World Health Organization. Measles vaccines: WHO position paper—April 2017. *Wkly. Epidemiol. Rec.* **2017**, *92*, 205–227.
3. World Health Organization. *Establishing and Strengthening Immunization in the Second Year of Life: Practices for Vaccination beyond Infancy*; World Health Organization: Geneva, Switzerland, 2018.
4. World Health Organization. *Working Together: An Integration Resource Guide for Immunization Services throughout the Life Course*; World Health Organization: Geneva, Switzerland, 2018.
5. World Health Organization. *Immunization Data Portal*; World Health Organization: Geneva, Switzerland, 2024; Available online: https://immunizationdata.who.int/ (accessed on 10 September 2024).
6. Minta, A.A.; Ferrari, M.; Antoni, S.; Portnoy, A.; Sbarra, A.; Lambert, B.; Hatcher, C.; Hsu, C.H.; Ho, L.L.; Steulet, C.; et al. Progress toward Measles Elimination—Worldwide, 2000–2022. *MMWR Morb. Mortal Wkly. Rep.* **2023**, *72*, 1262–1268. [CrossRef]
7. World Health Organization. *A Guide to Introducing a Second Dose of Measles Vaccine into Routine Immunization Schedules*; World Health Organization: Geneva, Switzerland, 2013.
8. Burton, A.; Monasch, R.; Lautenbach, B.; Gacic-Dobo, M.; Neill, M.; Karimov, R.; Wolfson, L.; Jones, G.; Birmingham, M. WHO and UNICEF estimates of national infant immunization coverage: Methods and processes. *Bull. World Health Organ.* **2009**, *87*, 535–541. [CrossRef]
9. World Bank. *World Development Indicator*; World Bank Group: Washington, DC, USA, 2024; Available online: https://databank.worldbank.org/source/world-development-indicators (accessed on 10 September 2024).
10. Packham, A.; Taylor, A.E.; Karangwa, M.P.; Sherry, E.; Muvunyi, C.; Green, C.A. Measles Vaccine Coverage and Disease Outbreaks: A Systematic Review of the Early Impact of COVID-19 in Low and Lower-Middle Income Countries. *Int. J. Public Health* **2024**, *69*, 1606997. [CrossRef] [PubMed]
11. Masresha, B.G.; Luce, R.; Okeibunor, J.; Shibeshi, M.E.; Kamadjeu, R.; Fall, A. Introduction of the Second Dose of Measles Containing Vaccine in the Childhood Vaccination Programs within the WHO Africa Region—Lessons Learnt. *J. Immunol. Sci.* **2018**, *17*, 113–121. [CrossRef]
12. Grant, G.B.; Masresha, B.G.; Moss, W.J.; Mulders, M.N.; Rota, P.A.; Omer, S.B.; Shefer, A.; Kriss, J.L.; Hanson, M.; Durrheim, D.N.; et al. Accelerating measles and rubella elimination through research and innovation—Findings from the Measles & Rubella Initiative research prioritization process, 2016. *Vaccine* **2019**, *37*, 5754–5761. [CrossRef] [PubMed]
13. Wallace, A.S.; Willis, F.; Nwaze, E.; Dieng, B.; Sipilanyambe, N.; Daniels, D.; Abanida, E.; Gasasira, A.; Mahmud, M.; Ryman, T.K. Vaccine wastage in Nigeria: An assessment of wastage rates and related vaccinator knowledge, attitudes and practices. *Vaccine* **2017**, *35*, 6751–6758. [CrossRef] [PubMed]
14. Olorunsaiye, C.Z.; Langhamer, M.S.; Wallace, A.S.; Watkins, M.L. Missed opportunities and barriers for vaccination: A descriptive analysis of private and public health facilities in four African countries. *Pan Afr. Med. J.* **2017**, *27* (Suppl. 3), 6. [CrossRef] [PubMed]
15. Kanagat, N.; Krudwig, K.; Wilkins, K.A.; Kaweme, S.; Phiri, G.; Mwansa, F.D.; Mvundura, M.; Robertson, J.; Kristensen, D.; Gueye, A.; et al. Health Care Worker Preferences and Perspectives on Doses per Container for 2 Lyophilized Vaccines in Senegal, Vietnam, and Zambia. *Glob. Health Sci. Pract.* **2020**, *8*, 680–688. [CrossRef] [PubMed]
16. Krudwig, K.; Knittel, B.; Karim, A.; Kanagat, N.; Prosser, W.; Phiri, G.; Mwansa, F.; Steinglass, R. The effects of switching from 10 to 5-dose vials of MR vaccine on vaccination coverage and wastage: A mixed-method study in Zambia. *Vaccine* **2020**, *38*, 5905–5913. [CrossRef] [PubMed]
17. Kabore, L.; Meda, B.; Medah, I.; Shendale, S.; Nic Lochlainn, L.; Sanderson, C.; Ouattara, M.; Kabore, W.M.F.; Betsem, E.; Ogbuanu, I.U. Assessment of missed opportunities for vaccination (MOV) in Burkina Faso using the World Health Organization's revised MOV strategy: Findings and strategic considerations to improve routine childhood immunization coverage. *Vaccine* **2020**, *38*, 7603–7611. [CrossRef] [PubMed]

18. Chirwa, G.; Wilkins, K.A.; Mercer, D.J. Descriptive study of measles vaccination second dose reporting and barriers to improving coverage in six districts in Malawi. *Pan Afr. Med. J.* **2020**, *35* (Suppl. 1), 5. [CrossRef] [PubMed]
19. Feldstein, L.R.; Fox, G.; Shefer, A.; Conklin, L.M.; Ward, K. School-based delivery of routinely recommended vaccines and opportunities to check vaccination status at school, a global summary, 2008–2017. *Vaccine* **2020**, *38*, 680–689. [CrossRef] [PubMed]
20. Muhoza, P.; Shah, M.P.; Gao, H.; Amponsa-Achiano, K.; Quaye, P.; Opare, W.; Okae, C.; Aboyinga, P.N.; Opare, K.L.; Wardle, M.T.; et al. Predictors for Uptake of Vaccines Offered during the Second Year of Life: Second Dose of Measles-Containing Vaccine and Meningococcal Serogroup A-Containing Vaccine, Ghana, 2020. *Vaccines* **2023**, *11*, 1515. [CrossRef] [PubMed]
21. Chilot, D.; Belay, D.G.; Shitu, K.; Gela, Y.Y.; Getnet, M.; Mulat, B.; Muluneh, A.G.; Merid, M.W.; Bitew, D.A.; Alem, A.Z. Measles second dose vaccine utilization and associated factors among children aged 24–35 months in Sub-Saharan Africa, a multi-level analysis from recent DHS surveys. *BMC Public Health* **2022**, *22*, 2070. [CrossRef] [PubMed]
22. Abenova, M.; Shaltynov, A.; Jamedinova, U.; Semenova, Y. Worldwide Child Routine Vaccination Hesitancy Rate among Parents of Children Aged 0–6 Years: A Systematic Review and Meta-Analysis of Cross-Sectional Studies. *Vaccines* **2023**, *12*, 31. [CrossRef] [PubMed]
23. Manandhar, P.; Wannemuehler, K.; Danovaro-Holliday, M.C.; Nic Lochlainn, L.; Shendale, S.; Sodha, S.V. Use of catch-up vaccinations in the second year of life (2YL) platform to close immunity gaps: A secondary DHS analysis in Pakistan, Philippines, and South Africa. *Vaccine* **2023**, *41*, 61–67. [CrossRef] [PubMed]
24. World Health Organization. Malaria vaccine: WHO position paper—March 2022. *Wkly. Epidemiol. Rec.* **2022**, *97*, 60–78.
25. Wiysonge, C.S.; Uthman, O.A.; Ndumbe, P.M.; Hussey, G.D. Individual and Contextual Factors Associated with Low Childhood Immunisation Coverage in Sub-Saharan Africa: A Multilevel Analysis. *PLoS ONE* **2012**, *7*, e37905. [CrossRef] [PubMed]
26. Kundrick, A.; Huang, Z.; Carran, S.; Kagoli, M.; Grais, R.F.; Hurtado, N.; Ferrari, M. Sub-national variation in measles vaccine coverage and outbreak risk: A case study from a 2010 outbreak in Malawi. *BMC Public Health* **2018**, *18*, 741. [CrossRef] [PubMed]

vaccines

MDPI

*Review*

# Serosurveillance for Measles and Rubella

**Allison M. Brady, Elina El-Badry, Eriko Padron-Regalado, Nicole A. Escudero González, Daniel L. Joo, Paul A. Rota and Stephen N. Crooke ***

Division of Viral Diseases, National Center for Immunization and Respiratory Diseases, Centers for Disease Control and Prevention, Atlanta, GA 30333, USA; par1@cdc.gov (P.A.R.)
* Correspondence: scrooke@cdc.gov

**Abstract:** Measles and rubella remain global health threats, despite the availability of safe and effective vaccines. Estimates of population immunity are crucial for achieving elimination goals and assessing the impact of vaccination programs, yet conducting well-designed serosurveys can be challenging, especially in resource-limited settings. In this review, we provide a comprehensive assessment of 130 measles and rubella studies published from January 2014 to January 2024. Methodologies and design aspects of serosurveys varied greatly, including sample size, assay type, and population demographics. Most studies utilized enzyme immunoassays for IgG detection. Sample sizes showed diverse sampling methods but favored convenience sampling despite its limitations. Studies spanned 59 countries, predominantly including adults, and revealed disparities in seroprevalence across demographics, regions, and notably among migrants and women. Age-related declines in antibodies were observed, particularly among infants, and correlations between vaccination status and seropositivity varied. We conclude with an outlook on measles and rubella serosurveillance, emphasizing the need for proper survey design and the advantages of standardized, multiplex serology assays.

**Keywords:** immune surveillance; serosurvey; seroprevalence; measles; rubella; multiplex assay; IgG antibody

## 1. Introduction

### *1.1. Measles and Rubella: Epidemiology, Disease Burden, and Elimination Efforts*

Measles and rubella continue to pose significant public health challenges despite the availability of effective vaccines and global efforts towards their elimination. Measles, caused by the measles virus, is a highly contagious disease characterized by fever, cough, coryza, conjunctivitis, and a distinctive rash, which can lead to severe health complications, particularly in unvaccinated people [1]. Rubella, often milder in children and adults, can have devastating consequences if contracted during early pregnancy, leading to congenital rubella syndrome (CRS) in the developing fetus. This syndrome can include a range of severe birth defects or fetal deaths [2]. Two doses of the measles-containing vaccine (MCV) and a single dose of the rubella-containing vaccine (RCV) can provide lifelong protection [3–5]. Moreover, high levels of measles and rubella antibodies within a population contribute to herd immunity, which helps protect individuals who are unable to be vaccinated (e.g., infants, pregnant women, and immunocompromised individuals) by reducing the overall transmission of the viruses. Despite the availability of effective vaccines for measles, the incidence of measles doubled between 2017 and 2018, a trend that continued into 2019, leading several countries to lose their measles elimination status [6]. In 2022, measles incidence trended upwards, with an estimated 136,200 deaths and 9.2 million cases, marking a 43% increase in mortality and an 18% increase in cases compared with 2021 [7]. Rubella cases dropped by 48% between 2012 and 2019 and continued to decline into 2020. However, CRS cases increased between 2012 and 2022, which can be attributed to the initiation of CRS surveillance in several large countries [8]. It is estimated that 32,000–100,000 cases of CRS occur annually, depending on the estimate model used, underscoring the persistent public health challenge posed by rubella infection [5,9–11].

To facilitate concerted efforts towards elimination, the Measles and Rubella Initiative devised the Global Measles and Rubella Strategic Plan 2012–2020, aligning with the WHO's Global Vaccine Action Plan 2011–2020 [12]. As part of this strategic plan, measles and rubella elimination was targeted in at least five WHO regions by the end of 2020 through the implementation of five core strategies [8,13]. Ultimately, complete elimination goals were not met by 2020 [14], though some progress was made. Between 2000 and 2019, global measles-containing vaccine first dose (MCV1) coverage increased from 72% to 86% [7]. Global routine measles-containing vaccine second dose (MCV2) coverage has increased steadily, from 42% in 2010 to 69% in 2018. By the end of 2019, 178 WHO member states had taken the critical step of introducing MCV2, underscoring the collective commitment towards advancing immunization initiatives and progress towards measles elimination [15]. Between 2012 and 2022, the number of countries providing rubella-containing vaccine (RCV) increased from 132 to 175, and verification of rubella elimination was documented in 98 (51%) of 194 WHO member states [8]. Unfortunately, the disruption of routine vaccination programs and supplemental immunization activities (SIAs) during the COVID-19 pandemic led to a decline in MCV1 coverage to 81% in 2021, the lowest since 2008 [7,16,17]. MCV1 coverage has begun to recover but remains alarmingly low (83% in 2022) [7]. Despite the fact that immunization averted approximately 23 million deaths between 2010 and 2018, the continued transmission of measles remains a potent reminder of the importance of sustaining robust immunization programs and surveillance systems to prevent outbreaks.

To continue efforts towards elimination, the Measles and Rubella Strategic Framework (MRSF) 2021–2030 was developed to provide a comprehensive guide on supporting global, regional, and national efforts. MRSF emphasizes strategic priorities such as integrating efforts into primary health care and universal health coverage, enhancing surveillance systems, ensuring vaccine supply, and promoting research and innovation. This framework aligns with the Immunization Agenda 2030 (IA2030) [18]. IA2030 outlines a global strategy to enhance health through immunization, in which measles and rubella elimination play a critical role, positioning measles as a "tracer" for the effectiveness of immunization programs. Measles outbreaks may indicate gaps in routine childhood immunization coverage [19]. Regardless, achieving high uniform vaccination coverage for measles and rubella remains a challenge, particularly in resource-constrained regions, and continues to impede progress towards elimination. Even for countries that have good overall coverage rates, immunization coverage in-country can vary greatly due to regional healthcare disparities, inadequate vaccine supply chain, political or social instability, or inadequate monitoring and surveillance [20]. Collectively, these challenges underscore the critical importance of enhancing surveillance systems and leveraging serosurveillance tools to monitor and address gaps in immunity. This approach can help guide the design of effective vaccination strategies aimed at preventing outbreaks and advancing toward the goal of measles and rubella elimination.

### *1.2. Antibody Response and Immune Memory to Measles and Rubella*

The WHO currently recognizes eight clades of measles (A-H); however, there is only one serotype [21]. For rubella, there are thirteen different genotypes divided into two clades (1a, 1B, 1C, 1D, 1E, 1F, 1G, 1h, 1i, 1j, 2A, 2B, and 2C); however, like measles, there is only one serotype [22]. Upon initial exposure to a virus, either through disease or vaccination, the immune system initiates a primary immune response, leading to the production of various classes of antibodies. Immunoglobulin M (IgM) antibodies are prevalent early during infection. During measles infection, IgM levels peak a few days after the onset of the rash and decrease in the subsequent weeks. Similarly, during a rubella infection, IgM is typically detectable within two to five days after rash onset and remains such for one to three months post-infection. IgM levels decline as B cells undergo class switching to produce immunoglobulin G (IgG) antibodies. Measles IgG levels peak one to two weeks after the rash onset, although low levels are detectable within a few days after the rash appears [23,24]. Anti-rubella IgG becomes detectable shortly after IgM, peaking around one to two weeks after the rash appears [25]. IgG antibodies serve as unique biomarkers of prior exposure (either by vaccination or infection) to measles and rubella, and they typically persist for life [23]. The differentiation of B cells into memory B cells is crucial for producing high-affinity IgG antibodies and establishing a sustained antibody-mediated immune response post-exposure. Additionally, memory B cells can terminally differentiate into long-lived, antibody-producing plasma cells, usually conferring protection during subsequent re-exposure to a pathogen [26]. Measles and rubella vaccines are live, attenuated viruses that cause a similar infection to wild-type viruses, although usually without symptoms. In general, the antibody response is less robust to immunization than to disease and results in lower antibody titers. However, antibody tests cannot distinguish between disease-induced and vaccination-induced antibodies.

In addition to antibody production following infection with a wild-type or vaccine virus, pathogen-specific antibodies can be transferred from one person to another in two ways. The first is prophylactic administration of pooled human immune globulin with sufficient pathogen-specific antibodies by intramuscular, intravenous, or subcutaneous injection [27]. This is a rare procedure, and the antibody duration is only a few months, so this seroprevalence is irrelevant on a population scale. The second method of antibody transfer occurs during pregnancy, when a mother transfers her own antibodies through the placenta to her baby. The titer achieved in the infant is dependent on the mother's titer and is typically roughly two-fold higher. On average, infants whose mothers have natural infection-induced immunity have higher titers than infants whose mothers have vaccine-induced immunity [28,29]. Infants of mothers who have no measles antibodies do not receive this transplacental protection. The duration of antibody protection among infants is directly related to the titer at birth and is decreasing across infant populations because of increasing proportions of mothers who have vaccine-induced or no measles immunity [29–31]. Because of the low levels of maternally derived measles antibodies and the severity of measles in infants, seroprevalence studies in infants represent a special case of serosurveys and need to be analyzed separately, typically by months of age.

In general, the measles seroprevalence in a population is highly age-dependent. Almost all infants are born with measles antibodies (provided their mother was previously vaccinated or infected), so the seroprevalence in newborns is close to 100%. However, titers in infants decrease rapidly, and, in many settings, infant titers are near zero by 4 to 6 months of age [32–35]. This is not a major risk in countries with elimination status because the likelihood of exposure to measles is very low. However, in measles-endemic countries, early infant susceptibility has led to increases in measles incidence among infants [36]. After maternal antibodies are depleted, measles seroprevalence in infants begins to increase as they are either vaccinated or infected with measles. Unfortunately, it is not possible to distinguish between maternally transferred, disease-induced, or vaccine-induced antibodies using serological testing.

The detection of IgG in serum does not necessarily indicate the presence of protective, neutralizing antibodies [37]. Functional, or neutralizing, antibodies can bind specific epitopes required for viral entry into host cells, thus preventing subsequent infections. Therefore, neutralizing antibodies are reliable indicators of protective immunity [38]. For measles, a neutralizing antibody titer of 120 milli-International Units (mIU)/mL is well established to protect against disease, although there has been some debate surrounding this in recent years [39]. The accepted correlate of protection for rubella is 10 IU/mL [40]. IgG antibodies that lack neutralizing activity (e.g., binding antibodies) are also produced during an immune response. While binding antibodies are pathogen-specific and may have other effector functions, they lack the ability to neutralize an infectious virus. Serological surveys typically assess the overall prevalence of IgG antibodies against specific pathogens in the population, irrespective of antibody activity [26].

In addition to humoral immunity, exposure to a pathogen triggers a cellular immune response. Broadly, CD4+ T cells provide essential help for several immune functions, such as affinity maturation of B cells and antibody isotype switching, while CD8+ T cells commonly exert antiviral effects by producing cytokines that suppress virus replication and eliminate infected cells. In the response to measles virus infection, T cells are considered essential for viral clearance [41]. Individuals with low or undetectable measles antibody levels have been shown to be somewhat protected against clinical measles, suggesting a significant role for cellular immunity [42]. However, the correlation between measles-specific antibody levels and the T cell immune response is poor [43]. Attempts to establish a cellular correlate of protection for rubella have failed to date [40], and no association between markers of humoral and cellular immunity has been identified [44]. Although seroprotective antibody titers for measles and rubella have been established, these correlates of protection should not be used to assess or infer the protection conferred by the cellular immune response. Additional studies are needed to establish correlates of protection specific to the cellular immune response.

### 1.3. Serosurveillance

Serosurveys are critical for understanding population-level immunity and disease burden estimates for infectious diseases. Typically, serosurveys do this by monitoring the presence of pathogen-specific IgG antibodies. For vaccine-preventable diseases (VPDs), well-designed serological surveillance studies can aid in assessing the effectiveness of vaccination programs and help identify gaps in immunity. For non-VPDs or for VPDs in countries where vaccination is not established, serosurveillance data can estimate disease burden or changes in disease exposure [45]. Unfortunately, serosurveys for estimating the disease burden of VPD can be complicated in areas with vaccination, as disease- and vaccine-induced antibodies are measured jointly and cannot be distinguished. These data can collectively guide public health decisions on vaccination policies and strategies to achieve and maintain elimination. For measles and rubella, serological surveys have been instrumental in global efforts towards elimination by evaluating immunity to identify susceptible populations or age groups, estimating disease burden in areas without vaccination, and assessing the impact of public health policies and campaigns [46]. Rubella serosurveys have also provided insights into true estimates of CRS disease burden [47].

Serosurveys often utilize enzyme immunoassays (EIAs) to assess the presence of IgG antibodies. Some EIAs and other IgG binding assays measure the total IgG antibody concentration, while others only provide a qualitative result, indicating the presence or absence of pathogen-specific IgG. EIAs can vary greatly in their sensitivity and specificity, depending on the antigen used (e.g., purified protein or whole virus lysate) as well as the assay format (e.g., direct, indirect, sandwich, or competitive EIA). These differences in assay performance can impact the ability to detect antibodies, particularly at low concentrations. One drawback of EIAs is the inability to distinguish neutralizing antibodies since these assays measure IgG binding to specific epitopes, regardless of their neutralization capacity [48]. For measles, the most abundantly produced antibodies target measles nucleoprotein, making it a common target in commercially available assays; however, nucleoprotein-specific antibodies are generally non-neutralizing; thus, total IgG titers do not correlate well with neutralization titers [48]. For rubella, the E1 glycoprotein is commonly used as the target for commercial test kits and is a target of neutralizing antibodies. EIA tests that provide a qualitative titer for rubella are designed to correspond with a protective level of antibodies; however, many studies have shown a lack of standardization [49–53]. Over time, antibody levels induced by measles and rubella vaccination may decrease [54,55]. As antibody levels wane, they may fall below the detection threshold for EIA assays that have poor sensitivity.

While EIAs are considered the standard methods for serosurveys, several studies have shown that EIAs and other immunostaining assays are less sensitive than plaque reduction neutralization tests (PRNTs), especially in the context of low antibody levels [56–58]. For measles, the plaque reduction neutralization test (PRNT) is considered the gold standard for assessing neutralizing immunity [59], while the immunocolorimetric neutralization assay is used for rubella [60]. A study by Tischer et al. demonstrated disparate positivity rates for measles between EIA, indirect immunofluorescence tests (IFT), and PRNT when serum samples were tested by each method [58]. The samples were collected from patients with known measles vaccination status but showed equivocal or negative results when initially tested with EIA several years after vaccination. Subsequent re-testing of these samples with IFT and PRNT showed positive rates of 81% for IFT and 94% for PRNT [58]. This discrepancy suggests that some EIAs may lack sufficient sensitivity to detect vaccine-induced antibodies several years post-immunization, posing potential challenges for serosurveys. However, applying neutralization assays in large-scale serosurveys is impractical due to technical difficulty, high cost, and labor-intensive processes.

Bead-based immunoassays have been around for more than two decades [61] and utilize antigen-bound beads to detect pathogen-specific IgG. Moreover, bead-based assays are often multiplexed, allowing for the simultaneous detection of antibodies to multiple pathogens in a single test. Bead-based immunoassays have been utilized for serological surveys for a variety of pathogens, including measles and rubella, and generally have robust performance characteristics, are cost-effective, and are resource-efficient [62]. A study by the National Institute of Public Health and the Environment in the Netherlands indicated a multiplexed bead-based assay (MBA) had higher sensitivity for measles and rubella IgG than individual ELISA [63]. MBA data exhibited strong correlations with ELISA data for both measles and rubella, with no cross-interference among antigens observed. Notably, MBA also demonstrated a higher correlation with PRNT than EIA [56,64]. In conclusion, MBAs present a compelling alternative to conventional EIA for detecting multiple target antibodies simultaneously in large-scale immunosurveillance studies.

## 2. Literature Review of Measles and Rubella Serosurveys (January 2014–January 2024)

### *2.1. Measles and Rubella Serosurvey Study Selection and Characteristics*

To understand the scope of measles and rubella seroprevalence surveys over the last decade, we conducted an online search using OVID (Medline, Embase, and Global Health), Cochrane Library, CINAHL, and Scopus. The search was constrained to the last 10 years (January 2014 through January 2024) and included the following keywords: 'rubella' and 'measles' combined with 'serosurvey', 'seroprevalence', 'immunity', and 'population immunity'. All search sources were last consulted on 9 January 2024. Any duplicate articles returned by the search were removed, leaving 492 results. We further excluded references that were not in English or where a full-length, peer-reviewed primary research paper or relevant seroprevalence information were not found. Additionally, any studies that focused specifically on individuals with HIV or other chronic health conditions were also excluded. This resulted in a total of 130 published studies, of which 30 described serosurveys for measles, 25 for rubella, and 75 for both. We focused our analysis on distinct populations (e.g., age, sex, occupation, or pregnancy status) and reported seroprevalence for each population individually within the paper. We also grouped studies by year of publication, country, WHO region, and vaccination status. When appropriate, medians were used to calculate the central tendency of a research outcome. Records not showing these data items were considered missing or unavailable. We did not discriminate between studies using residual samples and studies using a priori study design for estimating some outcomes in our review (e.g., overall seroprevalence). Therefore, we acknowledge that this might influence these estimations, although the extent of such influence is unknown. Supplementary Tables S1 and S2 list each population described for each published study. A 2016 review of measles and rubella seroprevalence studies published between 1998 and June 2014 found a total of 68 studies for measles and 58 for rubella [65]. In comparison, there seems to be a notable increase in the publication rate of such studies (Figure 1A).

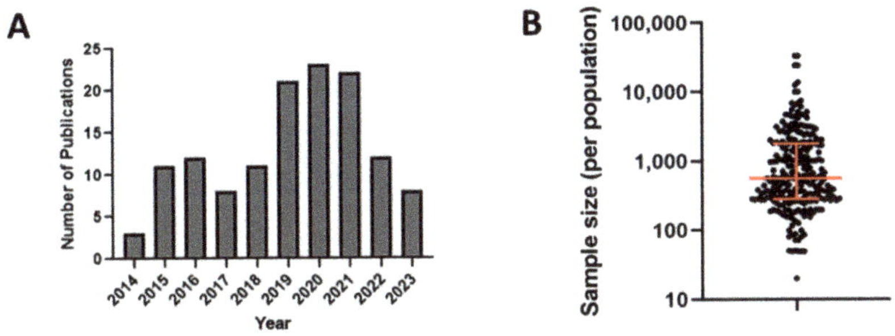


**Figure 1.** (**A**) Distribution of the number of publications by year included in the review. (**B**) Plot of serosurvey sample sizes for all included studies for measles and rubella. Red lines represent the median and interquartile range

*2.2. Serosurvey Methodology*

Of the 130 studies, 93 (71%) used EIAs to estimate IgG seroprevalence, with the most commonly used kits being Enzygnost (Siemens, Marburg, Germany, $n$ = 28) and EUROIMMUN (EUROIMMUN, Lubeck, Germany, $n$ = 20). In 25 (19%) studies, automated chemiluminescent immunoassay (CLIA), chemiluminescent microparticle immunoassay (CMIA), or enzyme-linked fluorescent assay (ELFA) technologies were utilized, with DiaSorin Liaison or Liaison XL (DiaSorin, Saluggia, Italy, $n$ = 15) being the most common. Additionally, Luminex-based MBAs were used in seven of the studies (5%). The remaining studies utilized other methods such as the hemagglutination inhibition test, rapid immunochromatographic test, particle agglutination assay, or the specific method was not indicated. Notably, one study compared the performance of the Enzygnost and EUROIMMUN IgG EIAs in a serosurvey of rubella antibodies in pregnant women [66]. In that study, the authors observed a strong qualitative (96.3%) and quantitative (mean titer difference: 0.8 IU/mL) agreement between the two tests, indicating that results between certain EIA tests may be comparable. However, the sensitivity of certain EIA kits may still cause underestimates of seroprevalence. A study in Singapore using the Enzygnost EIA as the primary test method performed further testing on all samples that were negative for measles-specific IgG and a random sampling of equivocal specimens for additional testing. Subsequent testing by PRNT revealed that approximately 75% of the samples initially categorized as measles IgG negative, along with all randomly selected samples categorized as measles IgG-equivocal, were actually seropositive. This had a significant impact on the estimated measles seroprevalence [67].

Sample sizes varied greatly across the 130 studies, ranging from sample sizes as small as 20 persons to as large as 32,502 individuals. In some instances, the seroprevalence was only reported for specific subgroups and not for the entire study population. As a result, some studies reported seroprevalence estimates for a very small number of people, with 24 (18%) studies reporting seroprevalence for groups of <200 individuals. Overall, the median sample population size for all studies was 561, and 63 (48%) studies surveyed populations of at least 1000 individuals (Figure 1B). Only 37 (28%) studies described the use of a priori sample size analysis to determine the appropriate sample size, as recommended by the WHO Guidelines for the assessment of measles and rubella seroprevalence. Other studies ($n$ = 39) described the use of sampling methods, such as multistage random cluster sampling. Most studies ($n$ = 92) did not specify a specific statistical method for participant selection. Instead, samples in those studies were obtained from residual blood donor or patient serum specimens, as well as from pre-employment or prenatal samples. Alternatively, many studies that actively recruited participants used targeted enrollment strategies, such as all students enrolled in a particular university program. The use of such opportunistic sampling is common due to its convenience and can provide local data on seroprevalence but cannot be generalized to an entire population.

## 2.3. Serosurvey Demographics

The serosurveys included a total of 59 countries; countries in the European WHO region (EUR) were most represented ($n$ = 48), followed by the Western Pacific region (WPR, $n$ = 34). In contrast, only eight studies reported data from the African region (AFR) (Figure 2A). Among the WHO regions represented in the included studies, the median measles seropositivity ranged from 88% to 93.5% (Table 1, Figure 3A). However, these estimates are certainly influenced by limited sampling in certain regions and differences among the populations studied. In particular, studies including infants at birth or early in life might have skewed the data because of waning maternal antibodies or a lack of exposure in the infants. When studies including infants were not considered, the median measles seropositivity ranged from 86.8% to 93.5% (Table 2, Figure 3B). For rubella, the median seropositivity ranged from 78.9% to 94% (Table 1, Figure 3C). When excluding studies with infants, the range is 82.6% to 94% (Table 2, Figure 3D).

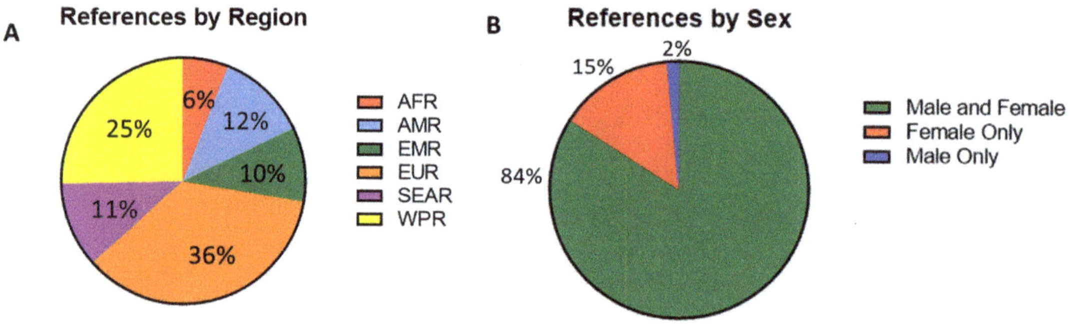


**Figure 2.** (**A**) Percent of serosurvey studies by region, percentages indicating the proportion of all included studies. African region (AFR, $n$ = 8), American region (AMR, $n$ = 16), Eastern Mediterranean region (EMR, $n$ = 13), European region (EUR, $n$ = 48), Southeast Asian region (SEAR, $n$ = 15), and Western Pacific region (WPR, $n$ = 34). (**B**) A breakdown of gender distribution among participants with percentages indicating the proportion of all included studies. Male and female ($n$ = 110), female only ($n$ = 19) and male only ($n$ = 2).

**Table 1.** Overall median seropositivity by WHO region for measles or rubella based on studies included in this review.

| Region | Measles | Rubella |
|---|---|---|
| AFR | 92.5% | 78.9% |
| AMR | 89.3% | 94% |
| EMR | 93.5% | 89.7% |
| EUR | 88% | 92.9% |
| SEAR | 91% | 86.2% |
| WPR | 91.5% | 86% |

**Table 2.** Median seropositivity by WHO region for measles or rubella based on studies included in this review, excluding studies with data from infants.

| Region | Measles | Rubella |
|---|---|---|
| AFR | 92.5% | 82.6% |
| AMR | 86.8% | 94% |
| EMR | 93.5% | 89.7% |
| EUR | 88.3% | 92.8% |
| SEAR | 91% | 87.1% |
| WPR | 91.1% | 84% |

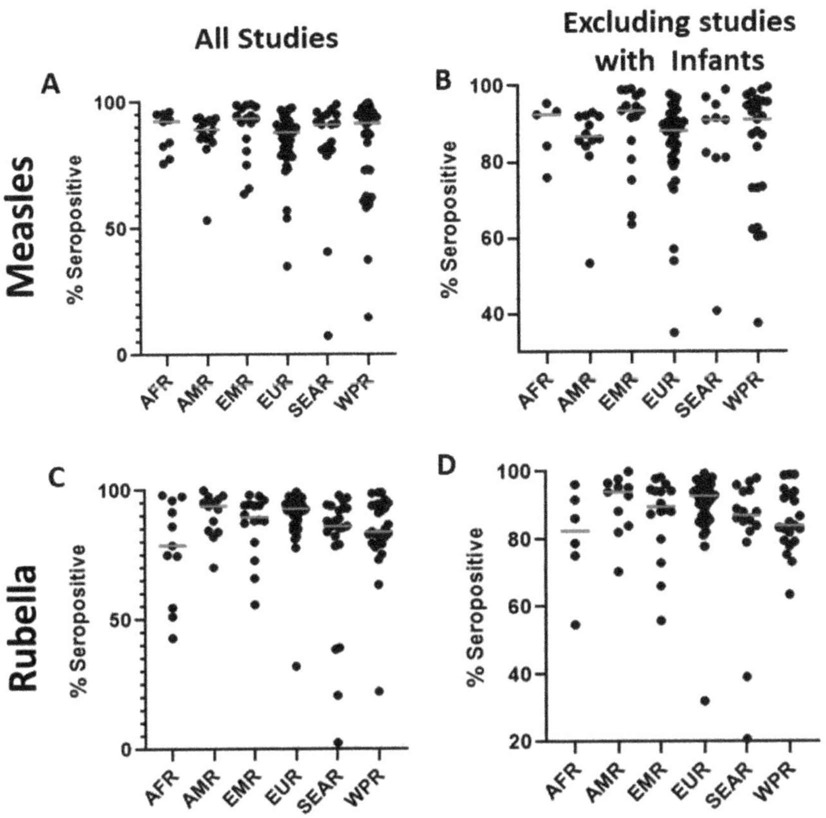


**Figure 3.** Distribution of seroprevalence for measles (**A**) and rubella (**C**) for all studies included in the literature review and the distribution of seroprevalence for measles (**B**) and rubella (**D**) excluding studies that included infants. Red line represents the median.

Twelve studies described seroprevalence in asylum seekers, refugees, international adoptees, or other immigrants or displaced peoples, and eleven of those studies examined the migration of persons into European countries from Africa, Asia, or elsewhere in Europe. Within those studies, the median seroprevalence reported in migrants into Europe (79.4% for measles and 85.1% for rubella) was lower than the median seroprevalence reported in other studies of non-migrants in the region (88.5% for measles and 93.5% for rubella). Only 13 surveys were conducted in countries listed by the UN as Least Developed Countries (LDC), and four of those studies were conducted in Zambia. Eighty-three (63%) studies were conducted in developed countries (UN Human Development index >0.8, 2021)—a significant percent increase compared to what was reported by Dimech and Mulders in 2016 [65]. Developed countries have a need to identify immunization gaps and document sufficient levels of population immunity as countries move towards elimination status.

Among the studies, 114 (87%) included adults (aged ≥18 years), 62 (47%) included adolescents (aged 15–17 years), 49 (37%) included children (aged 1–14 years), and 24 (18%) included infants (aged <1 year). Additionally, 110 (84%) of the studies included both male and female subjects. Only two studies (1%) exclusively included men, as these were cohorts of military recruits and professional sports players. Nineteen studies (15%) included only women. These studies focused on either pregnant women, women of childbearing age (WCBA), or women in universities or other workplaces (Figure 2B).

### 2.4. Overall Seroprevalence and Antibody Titers

The median measles seroprevalence reported in all studies was 89.87%, with a wide range of 7.5–99.6%. Only 16 (15%) of measles studies reported quantitative test results. Among those, the median average titer reported was 1153 mIU/mL (range = 77–25,300 mIU/mL). The median rubella seroprevalence reported was 90.5% (range = 2.5–100%). Only 17 rubella studies (17%) reported quantitative test results. Of those, the median average titer reported was 51 IU/mL (range = 4–240 IU/mL). The wide range of reported seroprevalence and antibody titers are significantly influenced by studies in older infants, which is discussed in further detail below. For this reason, the median seroprevalence (as opposed to the mean) likely gives a more accurate estimation of average seroprevalence and antibody titers globally and by region.

### 2.5. Age and Seroprevalence

Because the measles antibody is long lasting, seroprevalence in a particular birth cohort typically continues to increase as the cohort ages and experiences accumulated disease or vaccine-induced immunity. However, different birth cohorts experience different disease and immunization rates, and relative troughs in seroprevalence may be seen in some older cohorts. To assist in identifying immunity gaps, analysis of these patterns of seroprevalence is a major reason for serosurveys. In studies that analyzed age as a variable among adults, adolescents, and children younger than one year ($n$ = 78), researchers found that measles and rubella seroprevalence varied by age. Specifically, 41 studies reported an increase in measles seroprevalence among older adults compared to younger participants, as expected, whereas 22 studies observed no age-related differences. Similarly, 30 studies noted a lower rubella antibody prevalence among younger participants than older ones, but 27 studies reported no clear relationship between age and rubella antibody seroprevalence.

The median measles seroprevalence reported for studies that surveyed only infants was 90%. Among the eight studies that reported measles seroprevalence for infants only, there was a wide range of seropositivity (7.5–98%). This is due to differences in the exact age of infants in the study, and the fact that maternally acquired antibody titers wane between birth and the receipt of the measles-containing vaccine. In the four studies that further divided measles seroprevalence in infants by month of age, they all reported declining seroprevalence over the first year of life, as expected [68–71]. Differences in the exact age group studied make comparisons between studies difficult. However, there are some notable similarities. Cho et al. found that while measles seroprevalence was 94.4% in Korean infants <1 month old, seroprevalence dropped to 27.3% in 4-month-olds. Almost no infants $\geq$5 months old tested positive for the measles antibody [68]. Similarly, Muthiah et al. reported seropositivity for measles of 95% in Sri Lankan newborns, 23.1% in 7–8-month-olds, and 0% in 11–12-month-olds [69].

Only two studies examined rubella seroprevalence in infants by months of age, but the same pattern was observed as with measles. Muthiah et al. reported rubella seropositivity of 95% in Sri Lankan newborns, 9.6% in 7–8-month-olds, and 0% in 11–12-month-olds [69]. Similarly, Bassal et al. reported 80.4% rubella seropositivity in Israeli infants aged 0–6 months, compared with only 13% in infants aged 6–11 months [72]. In these studies, although each age group contained relatively few individuals, these data on measles and rubella seroprevalence in infants may cumulatively indicate a large window of susceptibility, which is most concerning for infants living in endemic settings. Whether infants should be vaccinated against measles and rubella earlier than current WHO recommendations (9 months of age in countries where transmission is ongoing) is an area of active debate. However, there is currently insufficient evidence on the long-term efficacy of early vaccination [73]. Given the increases in infant seronegativity seen in many studies, it is critical that infants be protected from exposure to measles by decreasing incidence in older populations, while research is being conducted on the immunogenicity of vaccinating infants at ages earlier than 9 months.

### 2.6. Seroprevalence and Vaccination

Sixty-eight studies had vaccination records for participants or surveyed them as to their recollection of previous vaccinations. In 24 of these, seropositivity for measles and/or rubella was reported to be positively associated with vaccination status or an increasing number of doses. Five studies found no statistically significant relationship or, interestingly, that vaccination status was negatively associated with seropositivity [74–78]. Three studies found higher titers of measles and rubella IgG in non-vaccinated individuals compared to those that had been vaccinated, as has been previously reported for individuals following infection [65,69,79–81]. This phenomenon was observed in countries that have had circulating measles or rubella viruses during the lifetime of the study participants.

Several studies reported higher seropositivity estimates for measles or rubella among the population than the percentage of participants reporting vaccination. This can be easily attributed to a prior infection with measles or the rubella virus. However, 10 studies reported lower seropositivity than the percentage of individuals either with vaccination records or those that recalled vaccination or infection [82–91]. These were typically studies of students or employees with available vaccination records. While such single-site studies can only give information on local conditions, this pattern of lower seroprevalence was observed in multiple countries spanning four WHO regions (AMR, EMR, EUR, and WPR) and may suggest instances of vaccine failure or waning immunity in the populations surveyed.

Ten studies described changes in national vaccination programs over time [80,92–100]. The results were mixed as to whether programmatic changes resulted in increased or decreased seropositivity for measles and/or rubella. For example, Gorun et al. surveyed 6914 WCBA who had undergone TORCH screening. When dividing the cohort by year of birth and vaccination program eligibility, they found the lowest rubella seroprevalence rates among the youngest cohort—82.4% of those born from 1997 to 2004 who were eligible for the measles–mumps–rubella (MMR) vaccine through the family practice system. In comparison, the seroprevalence was 95.8% in those born in 1989–1994 who were eligible for the monovalent rubella vaccine distributed in schools [92]. Coppeta et al. found no change in measles seropositivity in students following the implementation of a National Plan of Vaccine Prevention (NPVP) in Italy [100].

The effectiveness of supplementary immunization activities (SIAs) on a national or regional level was assessed in seven studies [101–107]. Of those studies, six described overall higher measles and/or rubella seroprevalence in eligible populations following a campaign, while one showed inconsistent results. Ichimura et al. evaluated the effectiveness of 2015 and 2019 SIAs in East Sepik, Papua New Guinea, and concluded that the 2019 SIA resulted in a higher measles and rubella seroprevalence in the target age group than the 2015 SIA. However, the authors note that the small number of participants ($n$ = 278) was a significant limitation. Studies assessing seroprevalence following changes in the national immunization program or the implementation of SIAs should ideally be significantly powered, have sufficient documentation of vaccination, and be conducted over an appropriate timescale in order to reliably draw definitive conclusions on the impact of these initiatives.

## 3. Discussion

### Future Considerations for Measles and Rubella Serosurveillance

Serosurveillance studies provide useful estimates of population immunity and the impact of vaccination programs, which can subsequently inform country-specific priorities and public health initiatives. Countries that have verified elimination status for measles and/or rubella, as well as countries that are approaching elimination, must document that adequate levels of population immunity are maintained or achieved. Furthermore, it is important for countries to understand the presence of gaps in population immunity, such as specific age groups or vulnerable communities that may be susceptible to measles or rubella outbreaks upon the introduction of disease. However, for accurate population-level estimates to be obtained from serosurveys, studies must have been designed and conducted appropriately.

Studies can benefit from a priori study design, including sample size calculations and a delimitation of the study population to ensure it is representative. Although it is recognized that using residual samples from other studies is a practical means to conduct serosurveillance, the results from these studies have inherent limitations. Residual samples may not be wholly representative of the overall population, preventing the generalization of immunity estimates. Also, the number of residual specimens available for testing may be limited, thereby limiting statistical power and potentially undermining confidence in the resulting immunity estimates. Even studies that incorporate active sampling into their design should carefully balance population demographics and the geographical distribution of clinical sites as best as possible to ensure a representative sample is collected. Only with a robust study design that accounts for these aspects can we confidently extrapolate results to the population of interest.

Globally standardizing testing methods and interpreting results across laboratories pose challenges for both measles and rubella [25,57,108]. As noted in our literature search, only 16 (12%) measles studies and 17 (17%) rubella studies reported a titer enabling quantitative analysis of data between studies. Most of the reviewed studies reported only qualitative data, determining the seropositive/seronegative status of samples. Comparison of qualitative data is further complicated by use of multiple different EIA platforms, which may be calibrated differently. Most commercial EIAs are designed for single patient testing, not population-level analyses, and thus have relatively high assay cutoffs, which can impact test sensitivity. Antibody titers following vaccination against measles and rubella are generally lower than following infection [109,110], which may lead to an underestimation of seroprevalence in a vaccinated population if a test with insufficient sensitivity is used. This may lead to the unnecessary implementation of vaccination campaigns or other costly public health measures, highlighting the need for sufficiently sensitive, standardized testing methods for use in serosurveillance.

In a systematic review, MBA was found to have robust sensitivity [56]. In this study, MBA for measles-specific IgG was shown to have a median sensitivity of 95% (compared to PRNT; IQR, 89.8–95.0). This sensitivity was similar to the reported median sensitivity of the Enzygnost EIA (92.1%, IQR 82.3–95.7), a commercial EIA kit that was highly employed in serosurveillance studies but has since been discontinued. Furthermore, MBA has shown a strong correlation to "gold standard" assays for evaluating immunity to measles and rubella. Measles-specific MBA has exhibited a strong correlation with PRNT, which is notable considering that most measles-specific EIAs have a poor correlation with PRNT [64]. In the case of rubella, MBA data were found to have a strong correlation with quantitative ELISA, which is commonly used for the evaluation of humoral immunity against rubella [63].

Multiplex assays, like the MBA, can also be more cost-effective than some commonly used immunoassays as they allow for the simultaneous measurement of antibody concentrations for multiple pathogens using a low sample volume [64]. This is due to the increased sample throughput and the sparing of samples and antigens, in addition to the decrease in human labor [111]. For example, 100 samples can be easily tested simultaneously for measles and rubella IgG on MBA using ~75% fewer resources (e.g., assay plates, reagents) than would be needed to test with single-plex ELISA for both pathogens. MBA also requires significantly less (~10 fold) viral antigen than is needed for conventional ELISA to test an equivalent number of specimens for measles and rubella, further highlighting the cost-savings that can be realized with multiplex testing platforms.

The capability of MBA to measure antibody levels against multiple pathogens simultaneously has additional advantages for informing public health decisions beyond monitoring existing vaccination programs. Serological MBAs can be used to quantify the burden of endemic diseases for which a vaccine has yet to be introduced into the immunization program, enabling public health programs to make informed decisions on the need and strategies for the introduction of new vaccines. Multiplex serology assays also enable programs to better leverage limited resources and strategize coordinated surveys for multiple pathogens [112]. For example, blood samples are routinely collected for different programs such as demographic and health surveys, transmission assessment surveys, and indicator surveys for HIV [23]. Serosurveillance for measles, rubella, or other pathogens could be readily integrated with these programs using MBA to maximize the use of the collected samples and related resources.

MBA has been successfully employed by the Centers for Disease Control and Prevention (CDC) for measles and rubella serosurveillance in collaboration with numerous countries and international non-profit organizations. Recently, we assessed over 2500 dried blood spots (DBS) samples from the Democratic Republic of Congo to quantify measles and rubella seroprevalence in parallel with screening of diphtheria and tetanus antibodies [113]. As the Democratic Republic of Congo has not yet implemented rubella vaccination, this illustrates the utility of MBA to simultaneously enable monitoring of vaccination programs (measles, tetanus, diphtheria), while assessing endemic disease burden (rubella) in the same survey.

MBA is amenable to technology transfer between laboratories, enabling multiplex-based serosurveillance to be conducted in multiple countries. As part of a partnership initiative for strengthening integrated serosurveillance, the CDC and the Pan-American Health Organization (PAHO) established a collaborative effort with delegates from Brazil, Mexico, and Paraguay to pilot the introduction of the MBA in their respective countries as a means of monitoring population immunity and disease transmission for multiple diseases, including measles and rubella [114]. This initiative is intended to showcase the utility of integrated serosurveillance using the MBA, combining surveillance programs that are usually addressed separately but overlap within the same populations and geographic areas. As with any serosurvey, linking the results to vaccination records and historical reports of cases and outbreaks will be critical.

## 4. Conclusions

Serosurveys remain useful tools for supporting elimination efforts for measles and rubella, but only if implemented with the appropriate design considerations and utilizing sufficiently sensitive assays to generate meaningful estimates of population immunity. Complementing overall seroprevalence data with seroprevalence estimates stratified across relevant demographic groups, such as age cohorts and geographic areas, is key for targeting interventions and assessments of program impacts. Unfortunately, this granular approach can be challenging and costly to ensure that there is sufficient statistical power across different strata. The number of published serosurveillance studies detailing measles and rubella immunity estimates has steadily increased over the past decade, yet studies largely continue to implement sub-optimal survey designs using a variety of serological assays. These limitations were previously noted by Dimech and Mulders nearly a decade ago [65,115], and we reiterate the need here for updated, standardized guidelines for conducting seroprevalence studies in support of measles and rubella elimination. Moreover, a standardized serological assay with high sensitivity—such as the MBA—will be critical for accurately assessing population immunity for measles and rubella as more countries achieve elimination.

**Supplementary Materials:** The following supporting information can be downloaded at https://www.mdpi.com/article/10.3390/vaccines12070816/s1, Supplementary Table S1: List of study populations of measles serosurveys included in literature review and Supplementary Table S2: List of study populations of rubella serosurveys included in literature review.

**Author Contributions:** Conceptualization—P.A.R. and S.N.C. developed the concept and scope of the review; Methodology—A.M.B., E.E.-B. and E.P.-R. developed methodology and criteria for the literature review; Formal analysis—A.M.B., E.E.-B., E.P.-R., N.A.E.G. and D.L.J. conducted formal analyses of the literature; Writing—Original Draft Preparation—A.M.B., E.E.-B., E.P.-R., N.A.E.G. and D.L.J. wrote the initial manuscript draft; Writing—Review and Editing—A.M.B., E.E.-B., P.A.R. and

S.N.C. reviewed and edited the manuscript; Supervision—P.A.R. and S.N.C. supervised all aspects of the work. The views are those of the authors and do not necessarily represent those of the Centers of Disease Control and Prevention or the United States Government. All authors have read and agreed to the published version of the manuscript.

**Funding:** This research received no external funding.

**Institutional Review Board Statement:** Not applicable.

**Informed Consent Statement:** Not applicable.

**Data Availability Statement:** No new data were created or analyzed in this study. Data sharing is not applicable to this article.

**Acknowledgments:** The authors would like to acknowledge the editors of this special issue of Vaccines for extending the invitation to contribute. The authors would also like to express our sincere gratitude to Mark Papania and Jim Alexander for their insightful comments and critical reading of this manuscript.

**Conflicts of Interest:** The authors declare no conflicts of interest.

## References

1. Hubschen, J.M.; Gouandjika-Vasilache, I.; Dina, J. Measles. *Lancet* **2022**, *399*, 678–690. [CrossRef] [PubMed]
2. Winter, A.K.; Moss, W.J. Rubella. *Lancet* **2022**, *399*, 1336–1346. [CrossRef] [PubMed]
3. Griffin, D.E. Measles Vaccine. *Viral Immunol.* **2018**, *31*, 86–95. [CrossRef]
4. Lambert, N.; Strebel, P.; Orenstein, W.; Icenogle, J.; Poland, G.A. Rubella. *Lancet* **2015**, *385*, 2297–2307. [CrossRef]
5. WHO. Rubella vaccines: WHO position paper—July 2020. *Wkly. Epidemiol. Rec.* **2020**, *95*, 306–324.
6. Gastanaduy, P.A.; Goodson, J.L.; Panagiotakopoulos, L.; Rota, P.A.; Orenstein, W.A.; Patel, M. Measles in the 21st Century: Progress Toward Achieving and Sustaining Elimination. *J. Infect. Dis.* **2021**, *224* (Suppl. 2), S420–S428. [CrossRef] [PubMed]
7. Minta, A.A.; Ferrari, M.; Antoni, S.; Portnoy, A.; Sbarra, A.; Lambert, B.; Hatcher, C.; Hsu, C.H.; Ho, L.L.; Steulet, C.; et al. Progress Toward Measles Elimination—Worldwide, 2000–2022. *MMWR Morb. Mortal. Wkly. Rep.* **2023**, *72*, 1262–1268. [CrossRef] [PubMed]
8. Ou, A.C.; Zimmerman, L.A.; Alexander, J.P., Jr.; Crowcroft, N.S.; O'Connor, P.M.; Knapp, J.K. Progress Toward Rubella and Congenital Rubella Syndrome Elimination—Worldwide, 2012–2022. *MMWR Morb. Mortal. Wkly. Rep.* **2024**, *73*, 162–167. [CrossRef]
9. Vynnycky, E.; Knapp, J.K.; Papadopoulos, T.; Cutts, F.T.; Hachiya, M.; Miyano, S.; Reef, S.E. Estimates of the global burden of Congenital Rubella Syndrome, 1996–2019. *Int. J. Infect. Dis.* **2023**, *137*, 149–156. [CrossRef]
10. Reef, S.E.; Icenogle, J.P.; Plotkin, S.A. The path to eradication of rubella. *Vaccine* **2023**, *41*, 7525–7531. [CrossRef]
11. Otani, N.; Shima, M.; Ueda, T.; Nakajima, K.; Takesue, Y.; Yamamoto, T.; Okuno, T. Changes in the Epidemiology of Rubella: The Influence of Vaccine-Introducing Methods and COVID-19. *Vaccines* **2023**, *11*, 1358. [CrossRef]
12. WHO. Global Measles and Rubella Strategic Plan: 2012–2020. Available online: http://apps.who.int/iris/bitstream/10665/44855/1/9789241503396_eng.pdf (accessed on 5 January 2024).
13. Orenstein, W.A.; Cairns, L.; Hinman, A.; Nkowane, B.; Olive, J.M.; Reingold, A.L. Measles and Rubella Global Strategic Plan 2012-2020 midterm review report: Background and summary. *Vaccine* **2018**, *36* (Suppl. 1), A35–A42. [CrossRef]
14. MacDonald, N.; Mohsni, E.; Al-Mazrou, Y.; Kim Andrus, J.; Arora, N.; Elden, S.; Madrid, M.Y.; Martin, R.; Mahmoud Mustafa, A.; Rees, H.; et al. Global vaccine action plan lessons learned I: Recommendations for the next decade. *Vaccine* **2020**, *38*, 5364–5371. [CrossRef]
15. WHO. National Immunization Coverage Scorecards Estimates for 2019. Available online: https://iris.who.int/bitstream/handle/10665/337665/9789240014398-eng.pdf (accessed on 5 January 2024).
16. Guglielmi, G. Pandemic drives largest drop in childhood vaccinations in 30 years. *Nature* **2022**, *608*, 253. [CrossRef]
17. WHO. Global Progress against Measles Threatened Amidst COVID-19 Pandemic. 2021. Available online: https://www.who.int/news/item/10-11-2021-global-progress-against-measles-threatened-amidst-covid-19-pandemic (accessed on 5 January 2024).
18. WHO. Measles and Rubella Strategic Framework: 2021–2030. Available online: https://iris.who.int/bitstream/handle/10665/339801/9789240015616-eng.pdf?sequence=1 (accessed on 5 January 2024).
19. WHO. *Immunization Agenda 2030 (IA2030)*; WHO: Geneva, Switzerland, 2020.
20. Lindstrand, A.; Cherian, T.; Chang-Blanc, D.; Feikin, D.; O'Brien, K.L. The World of Immunization: Achievements, Challenges, and Strategic Vision for the Next Decade. *J. Infect. Dis.* **2021**, *224* (Suppl. 2), S452–S467. [CrossRef] [PubMed]
21. World Health Organization. Genetic diversity of wild-type measles viruses and the global measles nucleotide surveillance database (MeaNS). *Wkly. Epidemiol. Rec.* **2015**, *90*, 373–380.
22. World Health Organization. Standardization of the nomenclature for genetic characteristics of wild-type rubella viruses. *Wkly. Epidemiol. Rec.* **2005**, *80*, 126–132.

23. Arnold, B.F.; Scobie, H.M.; Priest, J.W.; Lammie, P.J. Integrated serologic surveillance of population immunity and disease transmission. *Emerg. Infect. Dis.* **2018**, *24*, 1188–1194. [CrossRef]
24. El Mubarak, H.S.; Ibrahim, S.A.; Vos, H.W.; Mukhtar, M.M.; Mustafa, O.A.; Wild, T.F.; Osterhaus, A.D.; de Swart, R.L. Measles virus protein-specific IgM, IgA, and IgG subclass responses during the acute and convalescent phase of infection. *J. Med. Virol.* **2004**, *72*, 290–298. [CrossRef]
25. Dimech, W.; Grangeot-Keros, L.; Vauloup-Fellous, C. Standardization of Assays That Detect Anti-Rubella Virus IgG Antibodies. *Clin. Microbiol. Rev.* **2016**, *29*, 163–174. [CrossRef]
26. den Hartog, G.; van Binnendijk, R.; Buisman, A.M.; Berbers, G.A.M.; van der Klis, F.R.M. Immune surveillance for vaccine-preventable diseases. *Expert. Rev. Vaccines* **2020**, *19*, 327–339. [CrossRef] [PubMed]
27. Young, M.K. The indications and safety of polyvalent immunoglobulin for post-exposure prophylaxis of hepatitis A, rubella and measles. *Hum. Vaccin. Immunother.* **2019**, *15*, 2060–2065. [CrossRef]
28. Maldonado, Y.A.; Lawrence, E.C.; DeHovitz, R.; Hartzell, H.; Albrecht, P. Early loss of passive measles antibody in infants of mothers with vaccine-induced immunity. *Pediatrics* **1995**, *96*, 447–450. [PubMed]
29. Leuridan, E.; Van Damme, P. Passive transmission and persistence of naturally acquired or vaccine-induced maternal antibodies against measles in newborns. *Vaccine* **2007**, *25*, 6296–6304. [CrossRef] [PubMed]
30. Waaijenborg, S.; Hahne, S.J.; Mollema, L.; Smits, G.P., Berbers, G.A.; van der Klis, F.R.; de Melker, H.E.; Wallinga, J. Waning of maternal antibodies against measles, mumps, rubella, and varicella in communities with contrasting vaccination coverage. *J. Infect. Dis.* **2013**, *208*, 10–16. [CrossRef]
31. Caceres, V.M.; Strebel, P.M.; Sutter, R.W. Factors determining prevalence of maternal antibody to measles virus throughout infancy: A review. *Clin. Infect. Dis.* **2000**, *31*, 110–119. [CrossRef] [PubMed]
32. Kilic, A.; Altinkaynak, S.; Ertekin, V.; Inandi, T. The duration of maternal measles antibodies in children. *J. Trop. Pediatr.* **2003**, *49*, 302–305. [CrossRef]
33. Oyedele, O.O.; Odemuyiwa, S.O.; Ammerlaan, W.; Muller, C.P.; Adu, F.D. Passive immunity to measles in the breastmilk and cord blood of some nigerian subjects. *J. Trop. Pediatr.* **2005**, *51*, 45–48. [CrossRef]
34. Shilpi, T.; Sattar, H.; Miah, M.R. Determining infants' age for measles vaccination based on persistence of protective level of maternal measles antibody. *Bangladesh Med. Res. Counc. Bull.* **2009**, *35*, 101–104. [CrossRef]
35. Devecioglu, E.; Gokcay, G.; Boran, P.; Eren, T.; Yilmaz, G.; Badur, S. Prevalence of maternal measles, rubella, mumps and varicella antibodies in the first six months of life. *Mikrobiyoloji Bul.* **2018**, *52*, 324–327. [CrossRef]
36. Leuridan, E.; Sabbe, M.; Van Damme, P. Measles outbreak in Europe: Susceptibility of infants too young to be immunized. *Vaccine* **2012**, *30*, 5905–5913. [CrossRef] [PubMed]
37. Galipeau, Y.; Greig, M.; Liu, G.; Driedger, M.; Langlois, M.A. Humoral Responses and Serological Assays in SARS-CoV-2 Infections. *Front. Immunol.* **2020**, *11*, 610688. [CrossRef] [PubMed]
38. Cheedarla, N.; Hanna, L.E. Chapter 7—Functional and Protective Role of Neutralizing Antibodies (NAbs) against Viral Infections. In *Recent Developments in Applied Microbiology and Biochemistry*; Buddolla, V., Ed.; Academic Press: San Diego, CA, USA, 2019; pp. 83–93. [CrossRef]
39. Bolotin, S.; Hughes, S.L.; Gul, N.; Khan, S.; Rota, P.A.; Severini, A.; Hahne, S.; Tricco, A.; Moss, W.J.; Orenstein, W.; et al. What Is the Evidence to Support a Correlate of Protection for Measles? A Systematic Review. *J. Infect. Dis.* **2020**, *221*, 1576–1583. [CrossRef] [PubMed]
40. Plotkin, S.A. Correlates of protection induced by vaccination. *Clin. Vaccine Immunol.* **2010**, *17*, 1055–1065. [CrossRef] [PubMed]
41. Griffin, D.E. The Immune Response in Measles: Virus Control, Clearance and Protective Immunity. *Viruses* **2016**, *8*, 282. [CrossRef]
42. Haralambieva, I.H.; Kennedy, R.B.; Ovsyannikova, I.G.; Schaid, D.J.; Poland, G.A. Current perspectives in assessing humoral immunity after measles vaccination. *Expert. Rev. Vaccines* **2019**, *18*, 75–87. [CrossRef] [PubMed]
43. de Vries, R.D.; de Swart, R.L. Evaluating measles vaccines: Can we assess cellular immunity? *Expert Rev. Vaccines* **2012**, *11*, 779–782. [CrossRef] [PubMed]
44. Tosh, P.K.; Kennedy, R.B.; Vierkant, R.A.; Jacobson, R.M.; Poland, G.A. Correlation between rubella antibody levels and cytokine measures of cell-mediated immunity. *Viral Immunol.* **2009**, *22*, 451–456. [CrossRef]
45. Cutts, F.T.; Hanson, M. Seroepidemiology: An underused tool for designing and monitoring vaccination programmes in low- and middle-income countries. *Trop. Med. Int. Health* **2016**, *21*, 1086–1098. [CrossRef]
46. Patel, M.K.; Goodson, J.L.; Alexander, J.P., Jr.; Kretsinger, K.; Sodha, S.V.; Steulet, C.; Gacic-Dobo, M.; Rota, P.A.; McFarland, J.; Menning, L.; et al. Progress Toward Regional Measles Elimination—Worldwide, 2000–2019. *MMWR Morb. Mortal. Wkly. Rep.* **2020**, *69*, 1700–1705. [CrossRef]
47. Shanmugasundaram, D.; Awasthi, S.; Dwibedi, B.; Geetha, S.; Jain, M.; Malik, S.; Patel, B.; Singh, H.; Tripathi, S.; Viswanathan, R.; et al. Burden of congenital rubella syndrome (CRS) in India based on data from cross-sectional serosurveys, 2017 and 2019-20. *PLoS Negl. Trop. Dis.* **2021**, *15*, e0009608. [CrossRef] [PubMed]
48. WHO. WHO Immunological Basis for Immunization Series, Module 7: Measles Update 2020. Available online: https://iris.who.int/bitstream/handle/10665/331533/9789241516655-eng.pdf?sequence=1 (accessed on 5 January 2024).
49. Bouthry, E.; Furione, M.; Huzly, D.; Ogee-Nwankwo, A.; Hao, L.; Adebayo, A.; Icenogle, J.; Sarasini, A.; Revello, M.G.; Grangeot-Keros, L.; et al. Assessing Immunity to Rubella Virus: A Plea for Standardization of IgG (Immuno)assays. *J. Clin. Microbiol.* **2016**, *54*, 1720–1725. [CrossRef] [PubMed]

50. Dimech, W.; Panagiotopoulos, L.; Francis, B.; Laven, N.; Marler, J.; Dickeson, D.; Panayotou, T.; Wilson, K.; Wootten, R.; Dax, E.M. Evaluation of eight anti-rubella virus immunoglobulin g immunoassays that report results in international units per milliliter. *J. Clin. Microbiol.* **2008**, *46*, 1955–1960. [CrossRef] [PubMed]
51. Dimech, W.; Arachchi, N.; Cai, J.; Sahin, T.; Wilson, K. Investigation into low-level anti-rubella virus IgG results reported by commercial immunoassays. *Clin. Vaccine Immunol.* **2013**, *20*, 255–261. [CrossRef] [PubMed]
52. Enders, M.; Bartelt, U.; Knotek, F.; Bunn, K.; Strobel, S.; Dietz, K.; Enders, G. Performance of the Elecsys Rubella IgG assay in the diagnostic laboratory setting for assessment of immune status. *Clin. Vaccine Immunol.* **2013**, *20*, 420–426. [CrossRef] [PubMed]
53. WHO. Chapter 9: Manual for the Laboratory-Based Surveillance of Measles, Rubella, and Congenital Rubella Syndrome. 9 June 2018. Available online: https://www.who.int/publications/m/item/chapter-9-manual-for-the-laboratory-based-surveillance-of-measles-rubella-and-congenital-rubella-syndrome (accessed on 5 January 2024).
54. Castineiras, A.C.P.; Sales, A.C.; Picone, C.M.; Diogo, C.L.; Rossi, A.D.; Galliez, R.M.; Ferreira, O.D.C., Jr.; Castineiras, T.; Lopes, M.H.; Sartori, A.M.C. The decline of measles antibody titers in previously vaccinated adults: A cross-sectional analysis. *Rev. Inst. Med. Trop. Sao Paulo* **2024**, *66*, e4. [CrossRef] [PubMed]
55. Wang, X.; Xu, Y.; Zhang, X.; Zhang, X.; Du, J.; Che, X.; Gu, W.; Wang, J.; Jiang, W.; Liu, Y. Do adolescents need a rubella vaccination campaign? Rubella serosurvey among healthy children in Hangzhou, China. *Hum. Vaccines Immunother.* **2023**, *19*, 2254536. [CrossRef] [PubMed]
56. Lutz, C.S.; Hasan, A.Z.; Bolotin, S.; Crowcroft, N.S.; Cutts, F.T.; Joh, E.; Loisate, S.; Moss, W.J.; Osman, S.; Hayford, K. Comparison of measles IgG enzyme immunoassays (EIA) versus plaque reduction neutralization test (PRNT) for measuring measles serostatus: A systematic review of head-to-head analyses of measles IgG EIA and PRNT. *BMC Infect. Dis.* **2023**, *23*, 367. [CrossRef] [PubMed]
57. Cohen, B.J.; Doblas, D.; Andrews, N. Comparison of plaque reduction neutralisation test (PRNT) and measles virus-specific IgG ELISA for assessing immunogenicity of measles vaccination. *Vaccine* **2008**, *26*, 6392–6397. [CrossRef]
58. Tischer, A.; Gassner, M.; Richard, J.L.; Suter-Riniker, F.; Mankertz, A.; Heininger, U. Vaccinated students with negative enzyme immunoassay results show positive measles virus-specific antibody levels by immunofluorescence and plaque neutralisation tests. *J. Clin. Virol.* **2007**, *38*, 204–209. [CrossRef]
59. Ratnam, S.; Gadag, V.; West, R.; Burris, J.; Oates, E.; Stead, F.; Bouilianne, N. Comparison of commercial enzyme immunoassay kits with plaque reduction neutralization test for detection of measles virus antibody. *J. Clin. Microbiol.* **1995**, *33*, 811–815. [CrossRef] [PubMed]
60. Lambert, N.D.; Pankratz, V.S.; Larrabee, B.R.; Ogee-Nwankwo, A.; Chen, M.H.; Icenogle, J.P.; Poland, G.A. High-throughput assay optimization and statistical interpolation of rubella-specific neutralizing antibody titers. *Clin. Vaccine Immunol.* **2014**, *21*, 340–346. [CrossRef] [PubMed]
61. Reslova, N.; Michna, V.; Kasny, M.; Mikel, P.; Kralik, P. xMAP Technology: Applications in Detection of Pathogens. *Front. Microbiol.* **2017**, *8*, 55. [CrossRef]
62. Chan, Y.; Fornace, K.; Wu, L.; Arnold, B.F.; Priest, J.W.; Martin, D.L.; Chang, M.A.; Cook, J.; Stresman, G.; Drakeley, C. Determining seropositivity-A review of approaches to define population seroprevalence when using multiplex bead assays to assess burden of tropical diseases. *PLoS Negl. Trop. Dis.* **2021**, *15*, e0009457. [CrossRef]
63. Smits, G.P.; van Gageldonk, P.G.; Schouls, L.M.; van der Klis, F.R.; Berbers, G.A. Development of a bead-based multiplex immunoassay for simultaneous quantitative detection of IgG serum antibodies against measles, mumps, rubella, and varicella-zoster virus. *Clin. Vaccine Immunol.* **2012**, *19*, 396–400. [CrossRef]
64. Coughlin, M.M.; Matson, Z.; Sowers, S.B.; Priest, J.W.; Smits, G.P.; van der Klis, F.R.M.; Mitchell, A.; Hickman, C.J.; Scobie, H.M.; Goodson, J.L.; et al. Development of a Measles and Rubella Multiplex Bead Serological Assay for Assessing Population Immunity. *J. Clin. Microbiol.* **2021**, *59*, e02716-20. [CrossRef] [PubMed]
65. Dimech, W.; Mulders, M.N. A 16-year review of seroprevalence studies on measles and rubella. *Vaccine* **2016**, *34*, 4110–4118. [CrossRef]
66. Viswanathan, R.; George, S.; Murhekar, M.V.; Abraham, A.M.; Singh, M.P.; Jadhav, S.M.; Nag, V.; Naik, S.; Raut, C.; Munivenkatappa, A.; et al. Comparison of two commercial ELISA kits for detection of rubella specific IgM in suspected congenital rubella syndrome cases and rubella IgG antibodies in a serosurvey of pregnant women. *Diagn. Microbiol. Infect. Dis.* **2019**, *94*, 243–247. [CrossRef]
67. Ng, Y.; Chua, L.A.V.; Cui, L.; Ang, L.W.; Tee, N.W.S.; Lin, R.T.P.; Ma, S.; Lee, V.J.M. Seroprevalence of vaccine-preventable diseases among children and adolescents in Singapore: Results from the National Paediatric Seroprevalence Survey 2018. *Int. J. Infect. Dis.* **2020**, *92*, 234–240. [CrossRef]
68. Cho, H.K.; Lee, H.; Kim, H.W.; Kim, S.S.; Kang, H.J.; Kim, I.T.; Kim, K.H. Seroprevalences of Specific IgG Antibodies to Measles, Mumps, and Rubella in Korean Infants. *J. Korean Med. Sci.* **2016**, *31*, 1957–1962. [CrossRef]
69. Muthiah, N.; Galagoda, G.; Handunnetti, S.; Peiris, S.; Pathirana, S. Dynamics of maternally transferred antibodies against measles, mumps, and rubella in infants in Sri Lanka. *Int. J. Infect. Dis.* **2021**, *107*, 129–134. [CrossRef] [PubMed]
70. Khampanisong, P.; Pauly, M.; Nouanthong, P.; Vickers, M.A.; Virachith, S.; Xaydalasouk, K.; Black, A.P.; Muller, C.P.; Hubschen, J.M. Waning of maternal antibodies against measles suggests a large window of susceptibility in infants in lao people's Democratic republic. *Pathogens* **2021**, *10*, 1316. [CrossRef] [PubMed]
71. Gioula, G.; Exindari, M.; Melidou, A.; Minti, F.; Sidiropoulou, E.; Dionisopoulou, S.; Kiriazi, M.; Tsintarakis, E.; Malisiovas, N. Seroprevalence of measles in Northern Greece. *Acta Microbiol. Hell.* **2017**, *62*, 145–150.

72. Bassal, R.; Shohat, T.; Levin, T.; Pando, R.; Shinar, E.; Amichay, D.; Barak, M.; Ben-Dor, A.; Bar-Haim, A.; Mendelson, E.; et al. The Concordance between Mumps and Rubella Sero-Positivity among the Israeli Population in 2015. *Vaccines* **2022**, *10*, 996. [CrossRef] [PubMed]
73. Carazo, S.; Billard, M.N.; Boutin, A.; De Serres, G. Effect of age at vaccination on the measles vaccine effectiveness and immunogenicity: Systematic review and meta-analysis. *BMC Infect. Dis.* **2020**, *20*, 251. [CrossRef] [PubMed]
74. Kader, C.; Kara, M.; Gocmen, A.Y.; Erbay, A.; Polat, M.F. Antibodies against vaccine preventable diseases in pregnant women measles, mumps, rubella, varicella and tetanus in Yozgat, Turkey. *Konuralp Tip. Derg.* **2017**, *9*, 29–34. [CrossRef]
75. Rasheed, M.A.U.; Hickman, C.J.; McGrew, M.; Sowers, S.B.; Mercader, S.; Hopkins, A.; Grimes, V.; Yu, T.; Wrammert, J.; Mulligan, M.J.; et al. Decreased humoral immunity to mumps in young adults immunized with MMR vaccine in childhood. *Proc. Natl. Acad. Sci. USA* **2019**, *116*, 19071–19076. [CrossRef]
76. Yang, X.; Tang, T.; Yang, Z.; Liu, L.; Yuan, S.; Zhang, T. Evaluation of measles vaccination coverage in Lincang City, Yunnan Province, China. *Hum. Vaccines Immunother.* **2021**, *17*, 3145–3152. [CrossRef] [PubMed]
77. Freidl, G.S.; Tostmann, A.; Curvers, M.; Ruijs, W.L.M.; Smits, G.; Schepp, R.; Duizer, E.; Boland, G.; de Melker, H.; van der Klis, F.R.M.; et al. Immunity against measles, mumps, rubella, varicella, diphtheria, tetanus, polio, hepatitis A and hepatitis B among adult asylum seekers in the Netherlands, 2016. *Vaccine* **2018**, *36*, 1664–1672. [CrossRef]
78. Adam, O.; Musa, A.; Kamer, A.; Sausy, A.; Tisserand, E.; Hubschen, J.M. Seroprevalence of measles, mumps, and rubella and genetic characterization of mumps virus in Khartoum, Sudan. *Int. J. Infect. Dis.* **2020**, *91*, 87–93. [CrossRef]
79. Takemoto, K.; Nishimura, N.; Kozawa, K.; Hibino, H.; Kawaguchi, M.; Takeuchi, S.; Fujishiro, N.; Arai, S.; Gotoh, K.; Hosono, H.; et al. Time-Series Analysis Comparing the Prevalence of Antibodies against Nine Viral Species Found in Umbilical Cord Blood in Japan. *Jpn. J. Infect. Dis.* **2016**, *69*, 314–318. [CrossRef] [PubMed]
80. Vos, R.A.; Mollema, L.; van Binnendijk, R.; Veldhuijzen, I.K.; Smits, G.; Janga-Jansen, A.V.A.; Baboe-Kalpoe, S.; Hulshof, K.; van der Klis, F.R.M.; Melker, H.E. Seroepidemiology of Measles, Mumps and Rubella on Bonaire, St. Eustatius and Saba: The First Population-Based Serosurveillance Study in Caribbean Netherlands. *Vaccines* **2019**, *7*, 137. [CrossRef] [PubMed]
81. Okada, H.; Sato, T.A.; Katayama, A.; Higuchi, K.; Shichijo, K.; Tsuchiya, T.; Takayama, N.; Takeuchi, Y.; Abe, T.; Okabe, N.; et al. Comparative analysis of host responses related to immunosuppression between measles patients and vaccine recipients with live attenuated measles vaccines. *Arch. Virol.* **2001**, *146*, 859–874. [CrossRef] [PubMed]
82. Gadallah, M.; El Sayed, N.; Kandeel, A.; Moussa, I.; Mohsen, A.; Dewedar, S. Seroprevalence of rubella antibodies among adult Egyptian females aged 20–30 years. Is there a need for rubella vaccination? *Cent. Eur. J. Public Health* **2014**, *22*, 282–286. [CrossRef] [PubMed]
83. Kader, C.; Erbay, A.; Akca, N.K.; Polat, M.F.; Polat, S. Immunity of nursing students to measles, mumps, rubella, and varicella in Yozgat, Turkey. *Am. J. Infect. Control* **2016**, *44*, e5–e7. [CrossRef] [PubMed]
84. Zanella, B.; Boccalini, S.; Bonito, B.; Del Riccio, M.; Tiscione, E.; Bonanni, P.; Working Group DHS; Working Group AOUMeyer; Working Group AUSLTC; Bechini, A. Increasing Measles Seroprevalence in a Sample of Pediatric and Adolescent Population of Tuscany (Italy): A Vaccination Campaign Success. *Vaccines* **2020**, *8*, 512. [CrossRef] [PubMed]
85. Izadi, S.; Mokhtari-Azad, T.; Zahraei, S.M. Measles vaccination coverage and seroprevalence of anti-measles antibody in south-east Islamic Republic of Iran. *East. Mediterr. Health J.* **2015**, *21*, 396–402. [CrossRef]
86. Estofolete, C.F.; Milhim, B.H.G.d.A.; Franca, C.C.G.d.; Silva, G.C.D.d.; Augusto, M.T.; Terzian, A.C.B.; Zini, N.; Durigon, E.L.; Oliveira, D.B.L.; Massad, E.; et al. Prevalence of measles antibodies in Sao Jose do Rio Preto, Sao Paulo, Brazil: A serological survey model. *Sci. Rep.* **2020**, *10*, 5179. [CrossRef] [PubMed]
87. Karadeniz, A.; Akduman Alasehir, E. Seroepidemiology of hepatitis viruses, measles, mumps, rubella and varicella among healthcare workers and students: Should we screen before vaccination? *J. Infect. Public Health* **2020**, *13*, 480–484. [CrossRef]
88. Odemis, I.; Kose, S.; Akbulut, I.; Albayrak, H. Seroprevalence of measles, mumps, rubella, and varicella zoster virus antibodies among healthcare students: Analysis of vaccine efficacy and cost-effectiveness. *Rev. Esp. Quimioter.* **2019**, *32*, 525–531.
89. Chung, H.; Cho, S.K.; Joo, J.; Kim, S.K.; Kim, E.O.; Kim, M.J.; Chong, Y.P.; Choi, S.H.; Lee, S.O.; Kim, Y.S.; et al. Causes of a Low Measles Seroprevalence among Young Healthcare Workers in Korea. *Infect. Chemother.* **2023**, *55*, 388–393. [CrossRef] [PubMed]
90. Maltezou, H.C.; Karantoni, H.; Petrikkos, P.; Georgota, P.; Katerelos, P.; Liona, A.; Tsagarakis, S.; Theodoridou, M.; Hatzigeorgiou, D. Vaccination coverage and immunity levels against vaccine-preventable diseases in male Air Force recruits in Greece. *Vaccine* **2020**, *38*, 1181–1185. [CrossRef] [PubMed]
91. Jung, J.; Kim, S.K.; Kwak, S.H.; Hong, M.J.; Kim, S.H. Seroprevalence of Measles in Healthcare Workers in South Korea. *Infect. Chemother.* **2019**, *51*, 58–61. [CrossRef] [PubMed]
92. Gorun, F.; Malita, D.; Ciohat, I.; Vilibic-Cavlek, T.; Feier, H.; Tabain, I.; Craina, M.; Cretu, O.; Navolan, D. Prevalence of Rubella Antibodies among Fertile Women in the West of Romania, 18 Years after the Implementation of Immunization. *Vaccines* **2021**, *9*, 104. [CrossRef] [PubMed]
93. Holka, J.; Pawlak, K.; Ciepiela, O. Seroprevalence of IgG antibodies against measles in a selected Polish population—Do we need to be re-vaccinated? *Cent. Eur. J. Immunol.* **2019**, *44*, 380–383. [CrossRef] [PubMed]
94. Wanlapakorn, N.; Wasitthankasem, R.; Vichaiwattana, P.; Auphimai, C.; Yoocharoen, P.; Vongpunsawad, S.; Poovorawan, Y. Antibodies against measles and rubella virus among different age groups in Thailand: A population-based serological survey. *PLoS ONE* **2019**, *14*, e0225606. [CrossRef] [PubMed]

95. Plans, P.; de Ory, F.; Campins, M.; Alvarez, E.; Paya, T.; Guisasola, E.; Compte, C.; Vellbe, K.; Sanchez, C.; Lozano, M.J.; et al. Prevalence of anti-rubella, anti-measles and anti-mumps IgG antibodies in neonates and pregnant women in Catalonia (Spain) in 2013: Susceptibility to measles increased from 2003 to 2013. *Eur. J. Clin. Microbiol. Infect. Dis.* **2015**, *34*, 1161–1171. [CrossRef] [PubMed]
96. Ibrahim, N.A.; Mahallawi, W.H. Rubella Humoral Immunity Among the Saudi Population of Madinah in the Western Region of Saudi Arabia. *Viral Immunol.* **2022**, *35*, 375–380. [CrossRef] [PubMed]
97. Borocz, K.; Csizmadia, Z.; Markovics, A.; Farkas, N.; Najbauer, J.; Berki, T.; Nemeth, P. Application of a fast and cost-effective 'three-in-one' MMR ELISA as a tool for surveying anti-MMR humoral immunity: The Hungarian experience. *Epidemiol. Infect.* **2020**, *148*, e17. [CrossRef]
98. Chua, Y.X.; Ang, L.W.; Low, C.; James, L.; Cutter, J.L.; Goh, K.T. An epidemiological assessment towards elimination of rubella and congenital rubella syndrome in Singapore. *Vaccine* **2015**, *33*, 3150–3157. [CrossRef]
99. Nogareda, F.; Gunregjav, N.; Sarankhuu, A.; Munkhbat, E.; Ichinnorov, E.; Nymadawa, P.; Wannemuehler, K.; Mulders, M.N.; Hagan, J.; Patel, M.K. Measles and rubella IgG seroprevalence in persons 6 month-35 years of age, Mongolia, 2016. *Vaccine* **2020**, *38*, 4200–4208. [CrossRef] [PubMed]
100. Coppeta, L.; Biondi, G.; Lieto, P.; Pietroiusti, A. Evaluation of immunity to measles in a cohort of Medical Students in Rome, Italy. *Vaccines* **2019**, *7*, 214. [CrossRef] [PubMed]
101. Zahraei, S.M.; Mokhtari-Azad, T.; Izadi, S.; Mohammadi, M.; Sabouri, A. Seroprevalence of anti-rubella and anti-measles antibodies in women at the verge of marriage in Iran. *Vaccine* **2020**, *38*, 235–241. [CrossRef] [PubMed]
102. Murhekar, M.V.; Gupta, N.; Hasan, A.Z.; Kumar, M.S.; Kumar, V.S.; Prosperi, C.; Sapkal, G.N.; Thangaraj, J.W.V.; Kaduskar, O.; Bhatt, V.; et al. Evaluating the effect of measles and rubella mass vaccination campaigns on seroprevalence in India: A before-and-after cross-sectional household serosurvey in four districts, 2018–2020. *Lancet Glob. Health* **2022**, *10*, e1655–e1664. [CrossRef] [PubMed]
103. Hachiya, M.; Miyano, S.; Mori, Y.; Vynnycky, E.; Keungsaneth, P.; Vongphrachanh, P.; Xeuatvongsa, A.; Sisouk, T.; Som-Oulay, V.; Khamphaphongphane, B.; et al. Evaluation of nationwide supplementary immunization in Lao People's Democratic Republic: Population-based seroprevalence survey of anti-measles and anti-rubella IgG in children and adults, mathematical modelling and a stability testing of the vaccine. *PLoS ONE* **2018**, *13*, e0194931. [CrossRef]
104. Carcelen, A.C.; Mutembo, S.; Matakala, K.H.; Chilumba, I.; Mulundu, G.; Monze, M.; Mwansa, F.D.; Moss, W.J.; Hayford, K. Impact of a Measles and Rubella Vaccination Campaign on Seroprevalence in Southern Province, Zambia. *Am. J. Trop. Med. Hyg.* **2021**, *104*, 2229–2232. [CrossRef]
105. Miyano, S.; Vynnycky, E.; Pattamavone, C.; Ichimura, Y.; Mori, Y.; Nouanthong, P.; Phounphenghack, K.; Tengbriacheu, C.; Khamphaphongphane, B.; Franzel, L.; et al. Comparison of population-based measles-rubella immunoglobulin G antibody prevalence between 2014 and 2019 in Lao People's Democratic Republic: Impacts of the national immunization program. *Int. J. Infect. Dis.* **2023**, *129*, 70–77. [CrossRef]
106. Ichimura, Y.; Yamauchi, M.; Yoshida, N.; Miyano, S.; Komada, K.; Thandar, M.M.; Tiwara, S.; Mita, T.; Hombhanje, F.W.; Mori, Y.; et al. Effectiveness of immunization activities on measles and rubella immunity among individuals in East Sepik, Papua New Guinea: A cross-sectional study. *IJID Reg.* **2022**, *3*, 84–88. [CrossRef]
107. Hayford, K.; Mutembo, S.; Carcelen, A.; Matakala, H.K.; Munachoonga, P.; Winter, A.; Wanyiri, J.W.; Searle, K.; Mwansa, F.D.; Mwiche, A.; et al. Measles and rubella serosurvey identifies rubella immunity gap in young adults of childbearing age in Zambia: The added value of nesting a serological survey within a post-campaign coverage evaluation survey. *Vaccine* **2019**, *37*, 2387–2393. [CrossRef]
108. Cohen, B.J.; Audet, S.; Andrews, N.; Beeler, J.; on behalf of the WHO Working Group on Measles Plaque Reduction Neutralization Test. Plaque reduction neutralization test for measles antibodies: Description of a standardised laboratory method for use in immunogenicity studies of aerosol vaccination. *Vaccine* **2007**, *26*, 59–66. [CrossRef]
109. Anichini, G.; Gandolfo, C.; Fabrizi, S.; Miceli, G.B.; Terrosi, C.; Gori Savellini, G.; Prathyumnan, S.; Orsi, D.; Battista, G.; Cusi, M.G. Seroprevalence to Measles Virus after Vaccination or Natural Infection in an Adult Population, in Italy. *Vaccines* **2020**, *8*, 66. [CrossRef] [PubMed]
110. Bolotin, S.; Osman, S.; Hughes, S.L.; Ariyarajah, A.; Tricco, A.C.; Khan, S.; Li, L.; Johnson, C.; Friedman, L.; Gul, N.; et al. In Elimination Settings, Measles Antibodies Wane After Vaccination but Not After Infection: A Systematic Review and Meta-Analysis. *J. Infect. Dis.* **2022**, *226*, 1127–1139. [CrossRef] [PubMed]
111. van Gageldonk, P.G.; van Schaijk, F.G.; van der Klis, F.R.; Berbers, G.A. Development and validation of a multiplex immunoassay for the simultaneous determination of serum antibodies to Bordetella pertussis, diphtheria and tetanus. *J. Immunol. Methods* **2008**, *335*, 79–89. [CrossRef]
112. Arnold, B.F.; Martin, D.L.; Juma, J.; Mkocha, H.; Ochieng, J.B.; Cooley, G.M.; Omore, R.; Goodhew, E.B.; Morris, J.F.; Costantini, V.; et al. Enteropathogen antibody dynamics and force of infection among children in low-resource settings. *eLife* **2019**, *8*, e45594. [CrossRef] [PubMed]
113. Crooke, S.N.; (Centers for Disease Control and Prevention, Atlanta, GA, USA). Personal communication, 2024.

114. Pan American Health Organization. *Multiplex Bead Assay for Integrated Serological Surveillance of Communicable Diseases in the Region of the Americas. Report of the Third Regional Meeting (Cuernavaca, 4–5 March 2020)*; Pan American Health Organization: Washington, DC, USA, 2020.
115. Dimech, W.; Mulders, M.N. A review of testing used in seroprevalence studies on measles and rubella. *Vaccine* **2016**, *34*, 4119–4122. [CrossRef]

*vaccines*

MDPI

*Commentary*

# The Case for Assessing the Drivers of Measles Vaccine Uptake

**Jessica Kaufman [1,2,*], Ashleigh Rak [1], Sophia Vasiliadis [1], Navrit Brar [3], Eeman Atif [3], Jennifer White [4,5], Margie Danchin [1,2,6] and David N. Durrheim [4,5]**

[1] Vaccine Uptake Group, Murdoch Children's Research Institute, Melbourne, VIC 3052, Australia; ashleigh.rak@mcri.edu.au (A.R.); sophia.vasiliadis@mcri.edu.au (S.V.); margie.danchin@rch.org.au (M.D.)
[2] Department of Paediatrics, The University of Melbourne, Melbourne, VIC 3052, Australia
[3] Melbourne Medical School, The University of Melbourne, Melbourne, CIV 3052, Australia; nbrar@student.unimelb.edu.au (N.B.); eatif@student.unimelb.edu.au (E.A.)
[4] Health Protection, Hunter New England Local Health District, Booth Building, Wallsend Health Services Longworth Avenue, Newcastle, NSW 2287, Australia; jennifer.white3@health.nsw.gov.au (J.W.); david.durrheim@health.nsw.gov.au (D.N.D.)
[5] School of Medicine and Public Health, University of Newcastle, Newcastle, NSW 2308, Australia
[6] Department of General Medicine, The Royal Children's Hospital, Melbourne, VIC 3052, Australia
* Correspondence: jess.kaufman@mcri.edu.au

**Abstract:** Global measles cases are on the rise following disruptions to routine immunisation programs during the COVID-19 pandemic, with devastating consequences. According to the World Health Organization, the behavioural and social drivers of vaccination include what people think and feel about vaccines, social processes, motivation to vaccinate and practical barriers to vaccination. However, the drivers of measles vaccine uptake are not necessarily the same as those for other childhood vaccines, and we lack data on how these drivers specifically have changed during and since the COVID-19 pandemic. Without accurately measuring the behavioural and social drivers for measles vaccination, and ideally measuring them serially over time, countries cannot design, target and implement interventions that effectively increase and sustain measles vaccine coverage. This paper outlines what is and is not known about the behavioural and social drivers of measles vaccination and provides recommendations for improving their post-pandemic assessment.

**Keywords:** vaccination; vaccine uptake; measles; MMR; social science; barriers; vaccine hesitancy

## 1. Background

The current worldwide resurgence in measles cases is a critical global health issue. From 2021 to 2022, the estimated number of measles cases worldwide increased by 18% to 9,232,300, and the number of World Health Organization (WHO) countries experiencing large or disruptive outbreaks increased from 22 to 37 out of 194 [1]. In the same period, estimated measles deaths increased by 43% to 136,200, and the first months of 2024 demonstrate the perpetuation of these disturbing trends [1].

While measles is among the most infectious communicable diseases in the world, it is also preventable [2]. The measles vaccine has saved more lives than any other vaccine [1,3]. However, very high coverage—over 95% of the population—is required to prevent devastating outbreaks [4]. Since the start of the COVID-19 pandemic in 2020, routine childhood vaccination rates have dropped 3% worldwide [5]. The detrimental impact was particularly pronounced for measles: global first dose measles-containing vaccine (MCV) coverage declined from 86% pre-pandemic to 81% in 2021, the lowest coverage since 2008 [1]. Despite some early recovery in 2022, 40 million children missed a measles vaccine dose [1]. The greatest declines have been seen in low- and middle-income countries [6], but high-income countries have also been impacted [7–9].

The reasons for this decline are multifactorial. Deployment of immunisers away from childhood vaccination to delivering COVID-19 vaccines to older age groups had an immediate impact. However, while childhood immunisation services have now been restored, coverage has not bounced back to pre-pandemic levels. Vaccine confidence and trust have also been impacted by the pandemic; in 2021, confidence in vaccines declined in almost all countries, according to data from the Vaccine Confidence Project [5]. As the World Health Organization Regional Verification Commission Chairs warn, the global drop in routine childhood vaccination threatens progress towards measles elimination and puts millions of children at risk of measles and other life-threatening vaccine-preventable diseases like polio and pertussis [6,10].

## 2. The Behavioural and Social Drivers of Measles Vaccination

Measles is one of many serious vaccine-preventable diseases, but the factors affecting measles vaccine uptake are not necessarily the same as those for other childhood vaccines. Coverage data can only tell us which locations or demographic groups have low uptake, but not why. It is now imperative that we understand the social and behavioural drivers of measles vaccination—separate from other childhood vaccines—so countries can develop tailored, cost-effective solutions for increasing coverage.

A number of frameworks have been proposed to explain the drivers of vaccine uptake. For example, the 3Cs (highlighting Convenience, Complacency and Confidence) is one of the foundational models of vaccine hesitancy [11], while the 5As (Access, Affordability, Awareness, Acceptance and Activation) was designed specifically for application by diverse stakeholders to plan and target interventions [12]. The WHO Behavioural and Social Drivers (BeSD) of Vaccination framework includes many of the same social and behavioural drivers as these other models, organised into four categories: what people think and feel about vaccines, social processes, motivation to vaccinate and practical barriers to vaccination [13,14]. Uniquely, however, the BeSD framework is accompanied by both qualitative and quantitative data collection instruments and comprehensive supporting guidance for measuring these drivers. Without accurate measurement and, ideally, measuring serially over time, it is easy to assume that the main barriers are hesitancy or misinformation, when the actual issue may be access or availability or a complex mix of multiple factors. Below, we outline what is and is not known about the behavioural and social drivers of measles vaccination.

### 2.1. Thinking and Feeling

The way people think and feel about measles vaccination continues to be influenced by the discredited 1998 Lancet study reporting fraudulent data linking the measles, mumps and rubella (MMR) vaccine to autism. Although this study was formally retracted by the Lancet more than a decade ago, its pervasive impact remains. For example, studies from Australia and Saudi Arabia have found that up to 10% of parents are still concerned about a potential link between autism and the MMR vaccine [15,16]. A review of studies from the United States found that fear of autism was the most frequently cited reason for hesitancy about the MMR vaccine [17]. This was also the primary concern cited by over 70% of surveyed Somali parents in Minnesota, where a significant measles outbreak occurred in 2019 [18]. While a recent Australian study found that the belief that vaccines cause autism increased from 8.7% in 2017 to 14.4% in 2023 [19], very few other studies have compared evidence of pre- and post-pandemic beliefs, highlighting the need for repeated assessment of drivers of under- and non-vaccination.

Vaccine safety concerns are a significant factor in parents' decision-making about measles vaccines. Some parents seek alternative vaccination schedules that delay measles vaccination or separate the components of the MMR vaccine [20], despite the risks and lack of supportive evidence for this practice [21]. Measles coverage can also be affected by vaccine safety signals about other vaccines that impact confidence in all childhood vaccines [22]. In the Philippines, the Dengvaxia vaccine for dengue fever caused the death of 14 vaccinated children out of 800,000 vaccinated in 2016–2017, after which the vaccine campaign was stopped [23]. Vaccine confidence plummeted: while 93% strongly agreed that vaccines were important in 2015, this figure dropped to just 32% in 2018 [24], and

MCV1 coverage declined to 77% [25]. The resulting measles outbreak resulted in over 47,000 cases with more than 630 measles deaths in 2019 [26]. While coverage of DTP1 had recovered to 75% in the Philippines by 2022, MCV1 coverage remained worryingly low at 69% [25].

### 2.2. Social Processes

Measles vaccine decision-making is influenced by external social processes. For example, the origins of the modern anti-vaccine movement can be largely traced to the media coverage of the MMR controversy of the 1990s [27,28]. The MMR vaccine itself has been singled out by anti-vaccine activists and influencers [29], whose goal is to shape social norms. Religious leaders have also exerted significant influence on measles vaccination. In 2018, a fatwa was issued by Islamic clerics in Indonesia stating that the measles-containing vaccine was haram, or made using forbidden processes or ingredients. This caused vaccination rates to drop significantly across the country and especially in Aceh, a province ruled by sharia law [30]. Similarly, a study from Thailand found that religious opposition was the primary barrier to measles vaccination [31].

One of the most significant measles outbreaks of recent years, in Samoa, was caused by a policy decision. Following two fatal vaccine reconstitution errors, where a muscle relaxant was accidentally used, the country temporarily suspended the entire measles vaccination program. This decision dramatically undermined confidence in vaccination, and the country's ongoing measles outbreak worsened, with 83 deaths in children due to a drop in measles coverage [32]. Understanding the specific social processes that affect measles vaccination decisions is critical, as these may differ between vaccines.

### 2.3. Practical Issues

The practical issues affecting vaccine uptake are multifactorial and can be unique in relation to measles vaccination. For example, stock-outs of measles vaccines specifically have been a major challenge in countries like Romania [33]. The vaccine is heat-sensitive, requiring meticulous cold chain management and reconstitution that complicates storage and delivery and increases the risk of secondary vaccine failure [34]. As a live attenuated vaccine, it can be more reactogenic than inactivated vaccines. The side effects are usually delayed 5 to 10 days, with fever and a measles-like rash occurring in 10–25% of recipients [35]. Even though these side effects are generally mild, parents frequently cite the challenge of taking time off work to care for a child after vaccination as a barrier to uptake [36].

## 3. What Do We Know about How the Pandemic Has Changed the Drivers of Measles Uptake?

For the reasons outlined above, it is conceivable that measles vaccination has been differentially impacted by the pandemic in many unique and important ways. However, despite the urgent global concern about measles resurgence and inadequate measles vaccine coverage, there is a gap in our understanding of how the social and behavioural drivers of measles vaccination have changed during and since the COVID-19 pandemic. While many studies assessing factors that influence measles vaccine uptake have been published since 2020, most report pre-pandemic data [37–39]. Of the few that did report data collected since the start of the pandemic, lack of knowledge about MMR was a commonly cited issue [31,40]. These studies highlight the need for ongoing parental education on the measles vaccine and the protection it can provide to children and their communities. However, educational interventions alone may not be sufficient to improve uptake if there are more complex barriers, such as low levels of vaccine literacy [41], or if other barriers like access issues remain in place [42,43]. This is why it is critical to repeatedly and systematically assess a range of systemic factors and social and behavioural drivers over time to identify growing problems and lingering barriers.

We need serial data on drivers of measles vaccination—and granular data on MCV uptake—if we are to design, target and implement interventions that effectively increase and sustain measles vaccine coverage. It may be that these drivers are the same as for other childhood vaccines, but, given the importance and threat measles poses, we cannot assume this to be the case. We must make concerted efforts to understand the drop-off in measles coverage in different demographic groups and settings.

Validated tools focused on social or behavioural factors associated with measles vaccine uptake are very limited. Some studies have adapted the Parent Attitudes towards Childhood Vaccination (PACV) scale [37] or the WHO Vaccine Hesitancy Scale (VHS) [44], and one MMR attitudinal scale has been validated in the UK [45]. However, all of these instruments focus on acceptance issues alone and do not capture data on practical access issues. The WHO Tailoring Immunization Programmes approach employs the COM-B behaviour change wheel to qualitatively assess barriers to uptake, including practical issues [46], but this approach is complex, resource intensive, and can be difficult to deploy rapidly and repeatedly. The WHO BeSD tools address both access and acceptance issues and have been designed for use globally, particularly in low- and middle-income countries, but they are not customised for individual vaccines.

Using validated tools to understand and address the drivers of vaccination is a global priority [13]. There is now an urgent need to adapt these or other instruments to capture measles-specific data on a routine basis or when there are precipitous drops in coverage. While academic researchers may be best suited to conduct full psychometric validation of new or adapted tools, governments and public health organisations should at least look to existing validated tools rather than creating them from scratch. Ideally, existing tools should be subject to both forward and back translation to the required language and pilot tested with the target population to ensure clarity and relevance [47]. Serial surveillance of social and behavioural drivers of vaccination should be conducted alongside vaccine uptake monitoring. Coverage data from national immunisation registers, integrated with data from multiple agencies, show gaps in specific demographic and socioeconomic groups and locations but provide no data on why the gaps exist. The Immunization Agenda 2030 includes the concrete indicator of achieving 90% global coverage for MCV2 and achieving measles elimination in every WHO region [48]. The WHO Joint External Evaluation tool also has a first dose MCV indicator, but we strongly recommend countries consider indicators for vaccine drivers, with a focus on measles.

With these data, countries can apply qualitative approaches to tailor interventions to address country and sub-national specific measles concerns.

We make the following recommendations:

- At a macro level, health departments should invest in and encourage a learning health systems approach to systematically collect data and apply it to inform evidence-based care and decision-making [49–51]. Some academic institutions offer online short courses and fellowship programs for low- and middle-income country leaders [52,53].
- Countries should ideally establish serial surveillance of the social and behavioural drivers of measles vaccine uptake (e.g., vaccine confidence, concerns and social influences) over time. Short-form instruments, such as the five-item BeSD key indicators, may be suitable for embedding in existing population surveys. Partnerships with academic institutions should be considered for local validation of measurement instruments.
- Interventions should be evidence-based and targeted to address specific barriers identified through surveillance. A recent systematic review and meta-analysis maps behavioural interventions against the BeSD domains, identifying provider recommendations (social processes domain) and on-site vaccination (practical issues domain) as the most effective strategies to improve uptake [54].
- In addition to aligning with identified barriers, interventions should be locally tailored through community co-design. Measles vaccine uptake may be particularly susceptible to concerns about vaccine safety. Community-led and -owned approaches to encourage and sustain vaccine demand are critical, such as building the capacity

of health workers, community leaders and faith leaders to advocate for vaccination [54,55]. These groups are often highly trusted and influential but benefit from specific vaccine education and vaccine communication skills training.
- Assessing perceived vaccine accessibility, affordability and availability is critical, even in settings where vaccinations are provided free of charge [56]. Governments should prioritise guaranteeing availability and optimal supply of vaccines. Officials should employ evidence-based risk communication and response approaches to address vaccine safety signals while maintaining public trust.

**Author Contributions:** Conceptualisation, J.K., M.D. and D.N.D.; Writing—original draft preparation, J.K., M.D., A.R. and D.N.D.; Writing—review and editing, J.K., M.D., A.R., S.V., E.A., N.B., J.W. and D.N.D. All authors have read and agreed to the published version of the manuscript.

**Funding:** This research received no external funding.

**Conflicts of Interest:** The authors state that they have no conflicting interests.

## References


1. Minta, A.A.; Ferrari, M.; Antoni, S.; Portnoy, A.; Sbarra, A.; Lambert, B.; Hatcher, C.; Hsu, C.H.; Ho, L.L.; Steulet, C.; et al. Progress Toward Measles Elimination—Worldwide, 2000–2022. *MMWR Morb. Mortal. Wkly. Rep.* **2023**, *72*, 1262–1268. [CrossRef] [PubMed]
2. Paterson, B.J.; Kirk, M.D.; Cameron, A.S.; D'Este, C.; Durrheim, D.N. Historical data and modern methods reveal insights in measles epidemiology: A retrospective closed cohort study. *BMJ Open* **2013**, *3*, e002033. [CrossRef]
3. Global Immunization Efforts Have Saved at Least 154 Million Lives over the Past 50 Years. Geneva/New York/Seattle: World Health Organization, UNICEF, Gavi, The Bill and Melinda Gates Foundation. 24 April 2024. Available online: https://www.who.int/news/item/24-04-2024-global-immunization-efforts-have-saved-at-least-154-million-lives-over-the-past-50-years (accessed on 17 June 2024).
4. De Serres, G.; Gay, N.J.; Farrington, C.P. Epidemiology of transmissible diseases after elimination. *Am. J. Epidemiol.* **2000**, *151*, 1039–1048, discussion 1049–1052. [CrossRef]
5. United Nations Children's Fund. *The State of the World's Children 2023: For Every Child, Vaccination*; United Nations Research Institute for Social Development: Florence, Italy, 2023.
6. COVID-19 Pandemic Leads to Major Backsliding on Childhood Vaccinations, New WHO, UNICEF Data Shows. Geneva/New York: UNICEF. 15 July 2021. Available online: https://www.unicef.org/press-releases/covid-19-pandemic-leads-major-backsliding-childhood-vaccinations-new-who-unicef-data (accessed on 17 June 2024).
7. Harker, R. *Childhood Immunisation Statistics. Commons Library Research Briefing*; House of Commons Library: London, UK, 1 March 2024. Available online: https://commonslibrary.parliament.uk/research-briefings/cbp-8556/ (accessed on 17 June 2024).
8. Te Whatu Ora Health New Zealand. Immunisation Coverage 2023. Available online: https://www.tewhatuora.govt.nz/for-the-health-sector/vaccine-information/immunisation-coverage/ (accessed on 17 June 2024).
9. Australian Government Department of Health and Aged Care. Childhood Immunisation Coverage 2023. Available online: https://www.health.gov.au/topics/immunisation/immunisation-data/childhood-immunisation-coverage (accessed on 17 June 2024).
10. Durrheim, D.N.; Andrus, J.K.; Tabassum, S.; Bashour, H.; Githanga, D.; Pfaff, G. A dangerous measles future looms beyond the COVID-19 pandemic. *Nat. Med.* **2021**, *27*, 360–361. [CrossRef]
11. MacDonald, N.E.; Hesitancy, S.W.G.o.V. Vaccine hesitancy: Definition, scope and determinants. *Vaccine* **2015**, *33*, 4161–4164. [CrossRef]
12. Thomson, A.; Robinson, K.; Vallee-Tourangeau, G. The 5As: A practical taxonomy for the determinants of vaccine uptake. *Vaccine* **2016**, *34*, 1018–1024. [CrossRef] [PubMed]
13. World Health Organization. Understanding the behavioural and social drivers of vaccine uptake WHO Position Paper—May 2022. *Wkly. Epidemiol. Rec.* **2022**, *97*, 209–224.
14. World Health Organization. *Behavioural and Social Drivers of Vaccination: Tools and Practical Guidance for Achieving High Uptake*; World Health Organization: Geneva, Switzerland, 2022.
15. Alshammari, S.Z.; AlFayyad, I.; Altannir, Y.; Al-Tannir, M. Parental Awareness and Attitude about Childhood Immunization in Riyadh, Saudi Arabia: A Cross-Sectional Study. *Int. J. Environ. Res. Public Health* **2021**, *18*, 8455. [CrossRef] [PubMed]
16. Danchin, M.H.; Costa-Pinto, J.; Attwell, K.; Willaby, H.; Wiley, K.; Hoq, M.; Leask, J.; Perrett, K.P.; O'Keefe, J.; Giles, M.L.; et al. Vaccine decision-making begins in pregnancy: Correlation between vaccine concerns, intentions and maternal vaccination with subsequent childhood vaccine uptake. *Vaccine* **2018**, *36*, 6473–6479. [CrossRef]
17. Novilla, M.L.B.; Goates, M.C.; Redelfs, A.H.; Quenzer, M.; Novilla, L.K.B.; Leffler, T.; Holt, C.A.; Doria, R.B.; Dang, M.T.; Hewitt, M.; et al. Why Parents Say No to Having Their Children Vaccinated against Measles: A Systematic Review of the Social Determinants of Parental Perceptions on MMR Vaccine Hesitancy. *Vaccines* **2023**, *11*, 926. [CrossRef]

18. Christianson, B.; Sharif-Mohamed, F.; Heath, J.; Roddy, M.; Bahta, L.; Omar, H.; Rockwood, T.; Kenyon, C. Parental attitudes and decisions regarding MMR vaccination during an outbreak of measles among an undervaccinated Somali community in Minnesota. *Vaccine* **2020**, *38*, 6979–6984. [CrossRef] [PubMed]
19. Kaufman, J.; Hoq, M.; Rhodes, A.; Measey, M.; Danchin, M. Post-pandemic increase in parent misperceptions about routine childhood vaccines in Australia. *Med. J. Aust.* 2024, in press.
20. Dempsey, A.F.; Schaffer, S.; Singer, D.; Butchart, A.; Davis, M.; Freed, G.L. Alternative vaccination schedule preferences among parents of young children. *Pediatrics* **2011**, *128*, 848–856. [CrossRef] [PubMed]
21. Offit, P.A.; Moser, C.A. The problem with Dr Bob's alternative vaccine schedule. *Pediatrics* **2009**, *123*, e164–e169. [CrossRef] [PubMed]
22. Mabale, M.A.A.; Tejero, L.M.S.; Montes, L.A.; Collante, M.T.M.; Tempongko, M.S.B.; Tolabing, M.C.C. Implications of information heard about Dengvaxia on Filipinos' perception on vaccination. *Vaccine* **2024**, *42*, 1673–1681. [CrossRef] [PubMed]
23. The Lancet Infectious Diseases. Infectious disease crisis in the Philippines. *Lancet Infect. Dis.* **2019**, *19*, 1265. [CrossRef] [PubMed]
24. Larson, H.J.; Hartigan-Go, K.; de Figueiredo, A. Vaccine confidence plummets in the Philippines following dengue vaccine scare: Why it matters to pandemic preparedness. *Hum. Vaccin. Immunother.* **2019**, *15*, 625–627. [CrossRef] [PubMed]
25. World Health Organization; UNICEF. Philippines: WHO and UNICEF Estimates of Immunization Coverage: 2022 Revision. 2023. Available online: https://cdn.who.int/media/docs/default-source/country-profiles/immunization/2023-country-profiles/immunization_phl_2023.pdf?sfvrsn=6f71b3f3_3&download=true (accessed on 29 April 2024).
26. International Federation of Red Cross and Red Crescent Societies. Philippines: Measles Outbreak—Operation Update—Re-Emergence of Vaccine Preventable Diseases—Measles Outbreak—DREF n° MDRPH032 (12 March 2020). 2020. Available online: https://reliefweb.int/report/philippines/philippines-measles-outbreak-operation-update-re-emergence-vaccine-preventable (accessed on 17 June 2024).
27. Holton, A.; Weberling, B.; Clarke, C.E.; Smith, M.J. The Blame Frame: Media Attribution of Culpability About the MMR–Autism Vaccination Scare. *Health Commun.* **2012**, *27*, 690–701. [CrossRef] [PubMed]
28. Walsh, S.; Thomas, D.R.; Mason, B.W.; Evans, M.R. The impact of the media on the decision of parents in South Wales to accept measles-mumps-rubella (MMR) immunization. *Epidemiol. Infect.* **2015**, *143*, 550–560. [CrossRef]
29. Gottlieb, S.D. Vaccine resistances reconsidered: Vaccine skeptics and the Jenny McCarthy effect. *BioSocieties* **2016**, *11*, 152–174. [CrossRef]
30. Rochmyaningsih, D. Indonesian fatwa causes immunization rates to drop. *Science* **2018**, *362*, 628–629. [CrossRef] [PubMed]
31. Sirithammaphan, U.; Chaisang, U.; Pongrattanamarn, K. Barriers to measles mumps rubella vaccine acceptance in the three southern border provinces of Thailand. *Clin. Exp. Vaccine Res.* **2023**, *12*, 298–303. [CrossRef] [PubMed]
32. Thornton, J. In the aftermath: The legacy of measles in Samoa. *Lancet* **2020**, *395*, 1535–1536. [CrossRef] [PubMed]
33. Habersaat, K.B.; Pistol, A.; Stanescu, A.; Hewitt, C.; Grbic, M.; Butu, C.; Jackson, C. Measles outbreak in Romania: Understanding factors related to suboptimal vaccination uptake. *Eur. J. Public Health* **2020**, *30*, 986–992. [CrossRef] [PubMed]
34. Breakwell, L.; Moturi, E.; Helgenberger, L.; Gopalani, S.V.; Hales, C.; Lam, E.; Sharapov, U.; Larzelere, M.; Johnson, E.; Masao, C.; et al. Measles Outbreak Associated with Vaccine Failure in Adults--Federated States of Micronesia, February–August 2014. *MMWR Morb. Mortal. Wkly. Rep.* **2015**, *64*, 1088–1092. [CrossRef]
35. Jeong, S.Y.; Choe, Y.J.; Lee, D.H.; Kim, E.Y.; Kim, M.N.; Kim, S.J.; Lee, G.H.; Kang, H.J.; Han, M.G. Measles vaccine-associated rash illness amidst measles elimination: National surveillance data, South Korea. *J. Med. Virol.* **2022**, *94*, 4539–4541. [CrossRef]
36. Kaufman, J.; Tuckerman, J.; Bonner, C.; Durrheim, D.N.; Costa, D.; Trevena, L.; Thomas, S.; Danchin, M. Parent-level barriers to uptake of childhood vaccination: A global overview of systematic reviews. *BMJ Glob. Health* **2021**, *6*, e006860. [CrossRef] [PubMed]
37. Nwangwu, C.C.; Chike, A.E.; Ijeoma, I.O.E. Cross-sectional Survey on Parental Perception and Attitude on Measles Vaccine: Low Hospital Measles Case Presentation in Rural Area in Enugu Nigeria. *J. Clin. Diagn. Res.* **2021**, *15*, 14–19. [CrossRef]
38. Sabahelzain, M.M.; Moukhyer, M.; Bosma, H.; van den Borne, B. Determinants of Measles Vaccine Hesitancy among Sudanese Parents in Khartoum State, Sudan: A Cross-Sectional Study. *Vaccines* **2022**, *10*, 6. [CrossRef]
39. Toll, M.; Li, A. Vaccine sentiments and under-vaccination: Attitudes and behaviour around Measles, Mumps, and Rubella vaccine (MMR) in an Australian cohort. *Vaccine* **2021**, *39*, 751–759. [CrossRef]
40. Hussein, S.Z.; Mardia, N.; Amirah, M.; Hashim, R.; Abu Bakar, S.H. Knowledge and Practice of Parents Towards Measles, Mumps and Rubella Vaccination. *Malays. J. Med. Sci. MJMS* **2022**, *29*, 90–98. [CrossRef] [PubMed]
41. Badua, A.R.; Caraquel, K.J.; Cruz, M.; Narvaez, R.A. Vaccine literacy: A concept analysis. *Int. J. Ment. Health Nurs.* **2022**, *31*, 857–867. [CrossRef] [PubMed]
42. Lu, Y.; Wang, Q.; Zhu, S.; Xu, S.; Kadirhaz, M.; Zhang, Y.; Zhao, N.; Fang, Y.; Chang, J. Lessons learned from COVID-19 vaccination implementation: How psychological antecedents of vaccinations mediate the relationship between vaccine literacy and vaccine hesitancy. *Soc. Sci. Med.* **2023**, *336*, 116270. [CrossRef] [PubMed]
43. Isonne, C.; Iera, J.; Sciurti, A.; Renzi, E.; De Blasiis, M.R.; Marzuillo, C.; Villari, P.; Baccolini, V. How well does vaccine literacy predict intention to vaccinate and vaccination status? A systematic review and meta-analysis. *Hum. Vaccin. Immunother.* **2024**, *20*, 2300848. [CrossRef] [PubMed]
44. Sabahelzain, M.M.; Dubé, E.; Moukhyer, M.; Larson, H.J.; Borne, B.v.d.; Bosma, H. Psychometric properties of the adapted measles vaccine hesitancy scale in Sudan. *PLoS ONE* **2020**, *15*, e0237171. [CrossRef] [PubMed]

45. Brown, K.; Fraser, G.; Ramsay, M.; Shanley, R.; Cowley, N.; van Wijgerden, J.; Toff, P.; Falconer, M.; Hudson, M.; Green, J.; et al. Attitudinal and Demographic Predictors of Measles-Mumps-Rubella Vaccine (MMR) Uptake during the UK Catch-Up Campaign 2008–2009: Cross-Sectional Survey. *PLoS ONE* **2011**, *6*, e19381. [CrossRef] [PubMed]
46. World Health Organization Regional Office for Europe. TIP: Tailoring Immunization Programmes. 2019. Available online: https://www.who.int/europe/publications/i/item/9789289054492 (accessed on 17 June 2024).
47. Cruchinho, P.; Lopez-Franco, M.D.; Capelas, M.L.; Almeida, S.; Bennett, P.M.; Miranda da Silva, M.; Teixeira, G.; Nunes, E.; Lucas, P.; Gaspar, F.; et al. Translation, Cross-Cultural Adaptation, and Validation of Measurement Instruments: A Practical Guideline for Novice Researchers. *J. Multidiscip. Healthc.* **2024**, *17*, 2701–2728. [CrossRef] [PubMed]
48. Immunization Agenda 2030: Progress towards global immunization goals and implementation of the Immunization Agenda 2030. In Proceedings of the Executive Board 154th Session, Geneva, Switzerland, 4 December 2023.
49. Sheikh, K.; Abimbola, S. (Eds.) *Learning Health Systems: Pathways to Progress*; Flagship report of the Alliance for Health Policy and Systems Research; World Health Organization: Geneva, Switzerland, 2021.
50. Witter, S.; Sheikh, K.; Schleiff, M. Learning health systems in low-income and middle-income countries: Exploring evidence and expert insights. *BMJ Glob. Health* **2022**, *7*, e008115. [CrossRef] [PubMed]
51. Lozano, P.M.; Lane-Fall, M.; Franklin, P.D.; Rothman, R.L.; Gonzales, R.; Ong, M.K.; Gould, M.K.; Beebe, T.J.; Roumie, C.L.; Guise, J.M.; et al. Training the next generation of learning health system scientists. *Learn. Health Syst.* **2022**, *6*, e10342. [CrossRef] [PubMed]
52. The University of Melbourne. The Applied Learning Health Systems Short Course. 2024. Available online: https://mdhs.unimelb.edu.au/digitalhealth/learn/applied-learning-healthcare-system-short-course (accessed on 17 June 2024).
53. Murdoch Children's Research Institute. Asia-Pacific Vaccine Research Seminar Series. 2024. Available online: https://www.mcri.edu.au/news/events/asia-pacific-vaccine-research-seminar-series (accessed on 17 June 2024).
54. Malik, A.A.; Ahmed, N.; Shafiq, M.; Elharake, J.A.; James, E.; Nyhan, K.; Paintsil, E.; Melchinger, H.C.; Team, Y.B.I.; Malik, F.A.; et al. Behavioral interventions for vaccination uptake: A systematic review and meta-analysis. *Health Policy* **2023**, *137*, 104894. [CrossRef]
55. Kaufman, J.; Overmars, I.; Leask, J.; Seale, H.; Chisholm, M.; Hart, J.; Jenkins, K.; Danchin, M. Vaccine Champions Training Program: Empowering Community Leaders to Advocate for COVID-19 Vaccines. *Vaccines* **2022**, *10*, 1893. [CrossRef] [PubMed]
56. Attwell, K.; Hannah, A.; Leask, J. COVID-19: Talk of 'vaccine hesitancy' lets governments off the hook. *Nature* **2022**, *602*, 574–577. [CrossRef] [PubMed]

*vaccines*

MDPI

*Review*

# The Problem with Delaying Measles Elimination

**Natasha S. Crowcroft [1,2,3,*], Anna A. Minta [1], Shelly Bolotin [2,3,4,5], Tania Cernuschi [1], Archchun Ariyarajah [2,3,6], Sébastien Antoni [1], Mick N. Mulders [1], Anindya S. Bose [1] and Patrick M. O'Connor [1]**

1 Immunization, Vaccines and Biologicals, World Health Organization, 1211 Geneva, Switzerland; muldersm@who.int (M.N.M.); bosea@who.int (A.S.B.)
2 Dalla Lana School of Public Health, University of Toronto, Toronto, ON M5S 3H2, Canada
3 Centre for Vaccine Preventable Diseases, University of Toronto, Toronto, ON M5S 3H2, Canada
4 Department of Laboratory Medicine and Pathobiology, University of Toronto, Toronto, ON M5S 3H2, Canada
5 Public Health Ontario, Toronto, ON M5G 1V2, Canada
6 ICES, Toronto, ON M4N 3M5, Canada
* Correspondence: crowcroftn@who.int

**Abstract:** Measles is a highly infectious disease leading to high morbidity and mortality impacting people's lives and economies across the globe. The measles vaccine saves more lives than any other vaccine in the Essential Programme of Immunization and is also the most cost-effective vaccine, with an extremely high return on investment. This makes achieving measles elimination through vaccination a key child health intervention, particularly in low-income countries, where the overwhelming majority of measles deaths continue to occur. All countries and regions of the world have committed to achieving measles elimination, yet many have faced challenges securing political commitment at national and global levels and predictable, timely, and flexible support from global donors, and experienced setbacks during the COVID-19 pandemic. This has happened against a backdrop of stagnant measles vaccination coverage and declining enthusiasm for vertical programmes, culminating in a World Health Organization Strategic Advisory Group of Experts (WHO SAGE) review of the feasibility of measles eradication in 2019. Sustaining the elimination of measles long term is extremely difficult, and some countries have lost or nearly lost their measles elimination status in the face of ongoing importation of cases from neighbouring or closely connected countries in which elimination had been delayed. Thus, a widening equity gap in measles immunisation coverage creates challenges for all countries, not just those facing the greatest burden of measles morbidity and mortality. Delaying elimination of measles in some countries makes it cumulatively harder for all countries to succeed for three principal reasons: increased inequity in measles immunisation coverage makes outbreaks more likely to happen and to be larger; political will is very difficult to sustain; and immunity may wane to a point that transmission is re-established. New strategies are needed to support countries and regions in their vision for a world without measles, including ways to galvanise domestic, regional and global resources and ignite the political will that is essential to make the vision a reality.

**Keywords:** Measles; elimination; vaccination programmes; waning immunity; vaccine equity

## 1. Introduction

Measles elimination is an example of a truly country-led initiative. All countries have committed to measles elimination. All six World Health Organization (WHO) regions have established measles elimination goals, following the lead of the Pan American Health Organization (PAHO). However, degrees of progress, definitions and processes for verification, as well as target dates vary [1–8].

Measles elimination is defined as the absence of endemic measles virus transmission in a country, region or other defined geographic area for ≥12 months in the presence of a high-quality surveillance system that meets the targets of key performance indicators [9].

Following the model developed for polio eradication, regions have established mechanisms for verifying that countries have achieved measles elimination based on careful work by National Verification Committees (NVCs) for Measles and Rubella elimination that is reviewed by Regional Verification Commissions (RVCs). The RVCs verify measles elimination for individual countries when sufficient evidence is presented by the NVC that endemic measles transmission has been interrupted for at least three years. The key prerequisites to achieving measles elimination are high vaccination coverage with two doses of a measles vaccine, a well-performing surveillance system that can detect measles cases quickly, and a health system that can detect and respond quickly and effectively to potential outbreaks. A country with at least 95% coverage of two doses of a measles vaccine, accredited laboratories, high-quality surveillance and monitoring, and a rapid effective outbreak response mechanism will both eliminate measles and achieve vaccine equity. Gaps in the implementation of any parts of these systems can lead to children, adolescents and adults remaining unprotected and measles outbreaks occurring.

This article looks beyond the short- to medium-term implications of delays to measles elimination to examine long-term factors and risks to consider strategically. Measles elimination is primarily the task of governments supported in the country by various key institutions and civil society organizations and within regions by various partners including UNICEF and WHO, but the global level is an important component of the measles and rubella ecosystem that is driving progress towards elimination, and this article takes a global perspective. The objective of this review is to assess what impact delays will have on the likelihood of achieving and sustaining elimination in all regions. We consider this from three key perspectives in turn: the societal impact of increasing inequity, the implications of biological aspects, such as waning measles immunity; and the importance of solidarity between nations and regions.

## 2. Context

One of the seven impact goal indicators of the current global immunisation strategy (the Immunization Agenda 2030, IA2030) is that all countries achieve the endorsed disease control, elimination and eradication targets which include measles along with maternal and neonatal tetanus, rubella and polio [10]. Despite widespread support for IA2030, there is a lack of appetite among countries, donors and partners for another disease-specific eradication programme in light of the challenges and experiences in the polio eradication efforts over the past two decades. Regardless, countries and regions have progressed their elimination ambitions by establishing region-specific target dates for the elimination of measles in all regions and in four of six regions for rubella. Based on RVC reports, by the end of 2023, 43% of countries had eliminated measles and 51% had eliminated rubella [11]. Strong routine immunisation programmes have helped countries achieve elimination, with 32% of measles eliminated or verified countries reaching the target routine first dose measles vaccine coverage of at least 95% compared with 19% of endemic countries. In addition, good surveillance is a critical determinant of success, supported by the Global Measles and Rubella Laboratory Network which provides high-quality laboratory surveillance of measles and rubella in nearly every country. However, data also show that strong routine immunisation is neither necessary nor sufficient for achieving or sustaining measles elimination since 68% of the eliminated or verified countries did not achieve the 95% routine immunisation coverage target (Table 1). Nearly all countries that have eliminated measles have done so by a combination of campaigns and various levels of routine immunisation coverage, and some have relied mainly on campaigns.

**Table 1.** The strength of routine immunisation, measured by whether the first dose of measles vaccination (MCV1) coverage reaches the recommended target of at least 95% and the country's measles elimination status.

| Category | Number of Countries | MCV1 >95% | MCV1 <95% |
|---|---|---|---|
| Verified | 82 | 28 (34%) | 54 (66%) |
| Eliminated | 21 | 5 (24%) | 16 (76%) |
| Endemic | 85 | 16 (19%) | 69 (81%) |
| Re-established endemic transmission post-verification | 5 | 2 (40%) | 3 (60%) |
| No report | 1 | 1 (100%) | 0 (0%) |

Data source: Regional Verification Reports shared in confidence with WHO HQ by WHO regions.

Only one entire WHO region, the Americas, has so far succeeded in eliminating measles, in 2016, but unfortunately lost that status in 2019 and is now working to regain it [12]. Three regions—Europe, Southeast Asia, and the Western Pacific—have also faced challenges in some countries but made tremendous progress in others, even during the pandemic of COVID-19. The African (AFR) and Eastern Mediterranean (EMR) WHO Regions are further behind the others, but recently EMR has verified four countries as having eliminated measles, and AFR has started the process of verifying its first countries. A coordinated and concerted global and regional approach is essential to achieve regional elimination given the very high transmission rate for measles and high population mobility between neighbouring countries and to almost anywhere for some highly connected countries and communities [13,14]. Hence, lack of progress in one country or region has an impact on other countries and regions in an increasingly interconnected world. In response, regions are working closely with countries on cross-border surveillance and collaboration. Furthermore, a coordinated effort brings economies of scale, such as opportunities to direct global funding and vaccine supply where most needed in the interest of global health security and opportunities for peer learning between countries and regions.

Measles has re-emerged in several countries following verification of elimination, for reasons related to weak health systems, vaccine access or hesitancy in the face of the reintroduction of the virus from outside the borders [15,16]. Such outbreaks cause several issues. Firstly, measles outbreaks are extremely disruptive in any setting, with severe impact on the health of those infected, contributing to poverty through health care costs and the corollaries of reduced child survival and subsequent negative impact on economic development, as well as disrupting and overburdening the health care system. Secondly, measles outbreaks in countries that had previously been verified as measles eliminated may undermine relatively fragile confidence in the whole immunisation programme of a country, and thirdly, as mentioned above, such outbreaks often spread to other countries depending on how connected the country's population is to other parts of the world and how rapidly the outbreak transmission is interrupted. On the positive side, outbreaks often garner media attention, particularly in previously verified countries, offering an important advocacy opportunity for strengthening immunisation services and outbreak response capacity as well as increasing political attention and will to safeguard previous gains. Measles cases are also an important reminder for parents and health workers of the importance of immunisation in general.

Conversely, as time passes post-verification of measles elimination, the perceived risk of measles decreases because people no longer see measles cases, and they consequently do not see a need for vaccination—a great example of the prevention paradox [17]. As a consequence, it becomes increasingly difficult to sustain high vaccine demand and coverage, and harder to sustain measles elimination.

The theme of 'no one is safe until everyone is safe' perfectly describes the solidarity required between nations in making progress together in achieving measles elimination, since measles is a threat everywhere. In that context, it is important to consider the implications of delays to achieving elimination from regional and global perspectives as an important motive for bringing nations together around their common goals. A lesson from polio eradication efforts has been not to leave the most challenging countries to last. The reasons are not just because of the explicit inequity but also because this means all countries must sustain elimination for even longer periods, with ongoing risk of measles importations and outbreaks—a lesson that the measles field is trying to leverage through prioritising resources to a small group of large countries that are anticipated to have the greatest difficulty achieving and sustaining measles elimination.

The Global Immunization Strategy, IA2030, includes the concept of measles as a tracer of immunisation system strengths and weaknesses. The phrase "measles as a tracer" is used to refer to the way in which measles outbreaks shine a light on immunity gaps which reflect failures of health systems to identify and reach missed children with vaccination [18]. Tackling measles immunity gaps can generate enormous gains for the whole of a country's immunisation programme and, if leveraged intelligently, can also generate important gains for other health and social programmes. Within IA2030, the Measles Rubella Strategic Framework 2021–2030 (MRSF) was launched in 2021 with the goal of supporting all regions in achieving their measles elimination goals [19]. MRSF is supported first and foremost by regional resolutions on measles and rubella elimination [20, 21]. Global leadership and coordination for implementation of the MRSF are delivered by the Measles & Rubella Partnership which comprises the American Red Cross, the Bill and Melinda Gates Foundation (BMGF), the Global Alliance for Vaccines and Immunization (Gavi), the U.S. Centers for Disease Control and Prevention (CDC), UNICEF, the UN Foundation and WHO.

Important context for the MRSF is a WHO SAGE feasibility assessment from 2019, which indicates that measles eradication was set to be very hard to achieve within proximate timescales. Given large differences between the starting points of the six WHO regions, the fact that global coverage of both the first dose of measles- vaccine had stalled for a decade, and considerable uncertainty about when or how quickly coverage might increase, predictions of when measles transmission might be interrupted were pessimistic. The report concluded that it was premature to set a global eradication target [22], even if that is the end goal. This has set the tone for the global measles ecosystem ever since, with the reluctance of donors to support elimination activities. The report recommended the elaboration of a set of pre-conditions to meet that would signal when the world could and should go big and go fast towards the goal of measles eradication. The authors emphasised the risks of delaying elimination and recommended that all countries and regions accelerate progress towards achieving and maintaining measles and rubella elimination goals. At that time measles vaccine coverage had stagnated for a decade finishing with the largest epidemic year since 1996. Since then, global coverage has fallen further due to the COVID-19 pandemic, especially in low-income countries that are also furthest away from achieving measles elimination.

### *2.1. Implications of Delays to Measles Elimination for Health Inequity, and Equity for Elimination*

Inequities in measles immunisation cause delays in achieving measles elimination and delays to elimination increase inequity. Delays create a vicious cycle whereby, for multiple reasons, the longer it takes a country to achieve elimination the harder it may be for that country and for other countries to succeed (Figure 1). It is therefore apt that the concept of "measles as a tracer" articulated in the Immunization Agenda 2030 incorporates the role of measles in revealing inequity in protection from vaccine-preventable diseases. The Sustainable Development Goals (SDGs) also reflect this concept in using coverage of the second dose of measles vaccine, administered during the second year of life, as an indicator of the fully vaccinated child [23].

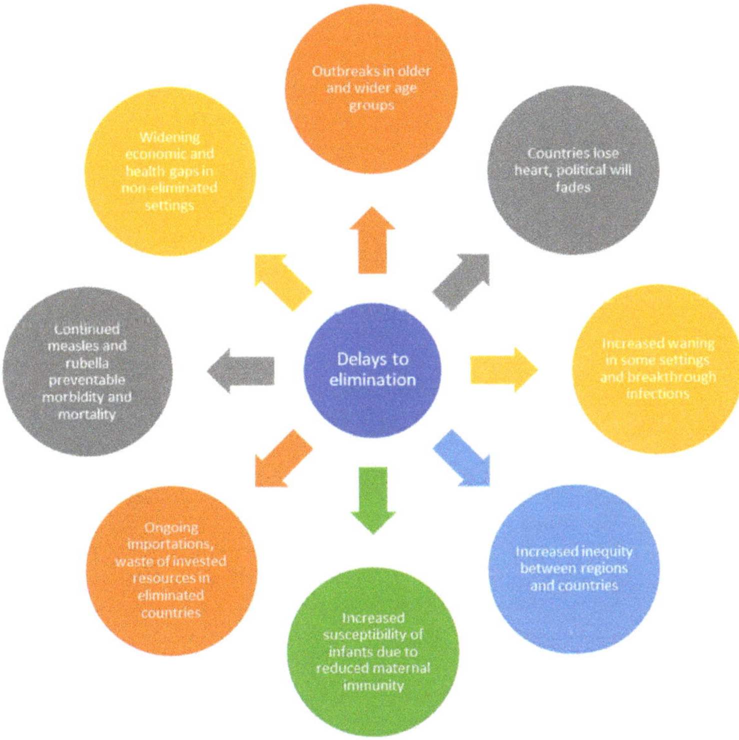


**Figure 1.** The implications of delays to achieving measles elimination.

Inequities in outcomes from measles can be conceptualised as operating at three different levels: within countries, between countries, and at the regional-global nexus. The first level gets the most focus, which is inequity within countries, for example, individuals living in rural areas have more barriers to accessing immunisation services due to weakness in primary health care, lack of government political will, lack of resources, conflict or other reasons [24]. The second level is the inequity between countries, usually assessed by some group proxy characteristic, such as gross national income. The third level is a combined regional/global nexus that relates to the will and capacity of regional and global communities to mobilise resources, catalyse progress and generate solidarity between nations.

*2.2. Inequity within Countries*

At the within-country level, inequity in protection from measles makes elimination more difficult to achieve. This is because the more unprotected individuals cluster together, the higher the coverage that is needed to interrupt transmission [25]. This occurs whatever the cause of the inequity—whether due to economic or geographical barriers, religious, racial or any other type of discrimination, or political reasons. Greater clustering of unprotected individuals also increases the likelihood and size of outbreaks. This effect has been demonstrated through mathematical modelling but is also easy to understand by imagining a thousand unvaccinated children living in one community and comparing the risk of measles with the same number of unvaccinated children spread evenly through a population of several million, in which measles transmission would be far less likely. Because measles is so infectious, any clusters of unprotected children are at risk of getting measles, and higher degrees of clustering of unprotected children increase the risk of outbreaks occurring sooner and being larger.

From an equity perspective, the children who remain unprotected from measles also tend to be disadvantaged in multiple other ways, including being at greater risk of already being malnourished as well as of becoming malnourished because of measles, and of dying from measles. Countries within the WHO African and Eastern Mediterranean Regions account for only 24% of the world's population, yet 92% of measles deaths in 2022 occurred in these regions [9]. Measles is, therefore, not only a tracer of immunisation programme performance, but also a tracer of the outcome of that performance measured in cases and deaths, and also reflects multiple inequities in such settings (Figure 1) [26].

Within countries, excellent immunisation systems are required to achieve both equity and measles elimination since these are interdependent. We have sufficient evidence, including from increasingly diverse settings, about what it takes to succeed in achieving measles elimination. The technical tools needed to eliminate measles, which include a highly effective vaccine, systems for supply, immunisation delivery, surveillance, and data monitoring, and rapid outbreak response, are effective if fully implemented. Hence the most frequent challenges facing countries in sustaining elimination have largely been political and programmatic, including suboptimal financial and human resources investments, lack of services in hard-to-reach geographical areas [27], cold chain failures, turning children away to avoid opening a vaccine vial for one or two children (even though using one dose from a 10-dose vial is cost-effective [28]). Barriers to protection are related to failure to vaccinate rather than vaccine failure [29]. For various reasons, countries are not yet sufficiently prioritising access to primary health care. If inequities in access to measles vaccines are similar to those tracked for the third dose of diphtheria, tetanus and pertussis vaccine (DTP3) then these have been increasing since 2015 and, along with TB, account for an increasing trend in between-country inequality [30].

The reasons for low coverage and the characteristics of communities most at risk vary tremendously from place to place. In order to take appropriate action, local knowledge and high-quality local and subnational data are needed. Indeed, national data may be quite misleading. This is well-illustrated by the mismatch with measles incidence found in one country where the local incidence varied 100-fold within the country, in part due to movements of high-risk refugees due to conflict; once again, infection is shown to be concentrated in a vulnerable group [31].

In countries that have sub-optimal measles vaccination coverage, delays in achieving elimination allow the average age at infection to increase which creates multiple challenges (Figure 1). Vaccine coverage that is too low to interrupt transmission will decrease rates of infection compared to no vaccination, leaving susceptibility gaps as children age. This effect can increase the risk of measles to infants through transmission from older children and adults who had remained susceptible. Furthermore, given that nearly all countries use combined measles and rubella vaccine, this also has implications for achieving rubella elimination goals because increasing the age for rubella infection may increase congenital rubella syndrome (CRS) if susceptible children are not protected before they become adults. Measles is a tracer of rubella immunity gaps for countries using measles and rubella-containing vaccines since rubella is less infectious and may be epidemiologically silent, in contrast to measles.

Examples of measles outbreaks among older children and adults are becoming more widespread, most recently shown by outbreaks in Europe [32]. These include breakthrough infections that in general are milder and less infectious than typical measles [33,34]. Efforts to reach healthy young adults with vaccines can be more expensive and less effective than reaching children through routine immunisation system, and outbreaks in older persons are challenging to control because healthy young adults do not regularly interact with the health system and many countries lack an immunisation system for older children and adults. The increased age at time of infection can be mitigated in countries that rely on regular campaigns by widening the age range that is targeted, but funders often default to a 9–59-month age range to avoid the additional costs.

### 2.3. Inequity between Countries

With regards to inequity between countries and regions, delays and uneven progress towards achieving measles elimination have increased inequity because measles cases have become concentrated in the countries and communities facing multiple crises, including fragile economies, mass population migration, weak health systems, climate change-related disasters and conflict. These countries are more likely to have measles outbreaks and are also most likely to be disrupted by outbreaks. They are the last to benefit from measles elimination whilst having the most to benefit from elimination. Such countries are most likely to be found in the African and Eastern Mediterranean regions. Countries represented in the Americas, Europe and Western Pacific WHO regions have moved more quickly and further than other regions, leveraging political will and access to resources, and in so doing the global equity gap has widened. The Southeast Asia region has made amazing progress over the past decade, most notably in India [35].

The COVID-19 pandemic set many countries back in terms of immunisation coverage generally and measles vaccine coverage specifically, particularly in Low-Income Countries (LICs). Currently, 54% (105/194) of the world's countries are assessed to be at high risk of experiencing measles outbreaks by the end of 2024 based on immunity profiles derived from reported routine and campaign immunisation coverage (Personal Communication Dr. Patrick O'Connor). The risk of measles outbreaks is highest in countries where coverage is lowest and where inequity within the country is very high, with LICs disproportionately experiencing both of these characteristics (Table 2). The lack of timeliness of measles vaccination campaigns in such settings is a major cause of inequity; this can and has led to thousands of preventable deaths.

**Table 2.** Average WHO/UNICEF Estimates of National Immunization Coverage (WUENIC) of Measles-containing vaccine, 1st dose (MCV1) and Measles-containing vaccine, 2nd dose (MCV2) in 2022 and annual measles incidence per million in 2022 by Low-, Middle- and High-Income Country status (LIC, MIC and HIC).

| Country Status | Dose | Coverage (%) | Incidence, Cases per Million |
|---|---|---|---|
| Low income | MCV1 | 66 | 98 |
| Low income | MCV2 | 40 | |
| Middle income | MCV1 | 86 | 18 |
| Middle income | MCV2 | 79 | |
| High income | MCV1 | 93 | 0.4 |
| High income | MCV2 | 91 | |
| Global | MCV1 | 83 | 24 |
| Global | MCV2 | 74 | |

Source: the WHO Immunization Data Portal for coverage and cases by World Bank Income category. Available at https://immunizationdata.who.int/, accessed on 11 July 2024.

### 2.4. The Global and Regional Nexus

At global, regional and country levels, the attention and commitment to measles and rubella is not commensurate with the public health burden or impact of prevention. Measles is the most cost-effective vaccine and saves more lives than any other vaccine, accounting for an estimated 60% of lives saved since the launch of EPI in 1974 [36]. Measles is one of the most cost-effective interventions a country can make, with a return on investment of more than $50 for every dollar spent [37]. Measles is also one of the diseases that display the greatest level of "negative externalities" across countries. For example, an infant in one country who is too young to be vaccinated can be infected because of a failure to control measles in another country—making it, a perfect target for multilateral engagement and resolution. Added to this, rubella is globally the most common preventable cause of congenital birth defects. Nevertheless, more energy, advocacy, and funding are dedicated to other immunisation priorities, often influenced by external interests in the use of funds within LICs. This does little to enable the establishment of strong and sustainable country-level institutions that drive equitable primary health systems, universal health care access and improved health status of populations. Such changes will not be easy to achieve and require a rebalance of power in global health which encompasses measures to enact decolonisation and raise countries' voices [38,39].

## 3. Delays to Measles Elimination and Waning Immunity

Countries in which a large proportion of the population has become immune through measles rather than vaccination can generally rely on the life-long immunity conferred by wild measles virus infection [40]. In contrast, in eliminated settings evidence is growing that vaccine-derived immunity is not lifelong, which raises the spectre of elimination being a time-limited state in some settings and with some schedules.

Most of the available data on the waning of immunity following vaccination comes from countries that vaccinate at 12 months of age or later [41]. Even in these countries, data are somewhat limited but seem to indicate that protection wanes relatively slowly and does not fall below the threshold of protection over a timescale of many decades [42]. These estimates align well with the sustained elimination that has been achieved in many countries where routine immunisation coverage has been high enough using schedules that start earliest at 12 months of age. Emerging data on vaccination within the schedule most commonly in use in countries with endemic transmission, where the first dose of measles vaccination is usually given at 9 months, seem to indicate that waning occurs more quickly than in countries where the first dose is given at 12 months. Modelling seroprevalence data from China, where the first dose is given at 8 months of age, indicates that IgG antibody concentrations would drop below the protective threshold of 200 mIU/mL around 5 years after the first dose and 13 years after the second dose of a measles vaccine, or at 14.3 years of age [43]. These modelling findings need to be followed closely to see if they translate into reduced programmatic effectiveness. A study of the impact of an early first dose of measles vaccine in the Netherlands given at 6 months of age found much more rapid waning compared with the standard schedule starting at 14 months, resulting in more than 10% of children becoming susceptible to measles by as early as 4 years of age [44]. These data are alarming and seem to indicate the need for countries that give the first dose early to consider moving their first dose of MCV1 later to 9–12 months or potentially to introduce an additional (third) routine MCV dose. These findings also raise concern about the sustainability of measles elimination in countries that start the first dose early in a routine program.

As countries spend increasing time in a state of elimination, the likelihood increases of breakthrough infections in fully vaccinated individuals. The critical question is how transmissible breakthrough infections are. Infections in previously immune individuals are generally mild and transmit rarely to other people, and if this situation persists then they may not present a significant risk to maintaining measles elimination. Conversely, if early immunisation increases the risk of breakthrough infections and their infectiousness, then the risk arises that these may start to contribute to the epidemiology of measles transmission [45].

Based on accumulating evidence of waning immunity, delays to eliminating measles could make elimination ultimately harder to achieve as older cohorts protected by infection age out, and the immunity of younger cohorts starts waning, especially if breakthrough cases are infectious enough to jeopardise elimination [46].

A different waning immunity issue to consider affects young infants. Infants are protected during their first few months of life by maternal antibodies. Here the evidence is very clear, that mothers whose immunity is vaccine-derived pass on much lower levels of antibodies to infants compared to mothers who are immune due to previous measles infection [47,48]. This immunity is not just lower but wanes more quickly. Hence in highly vaccinated communities, infants are susceptible to measles at a much younger age than in endemic settings, and this can increase their risk should measles elimination be delayed or not sustained (Figure 1). Whether this represents a risk to infants, in general, depends largely on whether countries sustain measles elimination. In elimination settings, infants are protected by herd immunity generated by the vaccination programme until they are old enough to be protected directly by vaccination. However, they risk infection due to the importation of measles from an endemic country or through travel to such a setting.

## 4. Discussion

### 4.1. Sustainability of Elimination Is a Major Challenge and Requires Solidarity between Countries and Regions

In an ideal world, countries and regions would move forward towards elimination in coordinated lockstep because together they are stronger. As long as some regions and countries remain in a state of endemicity, all other countries have greater risk and require larger investments to maintain their elimination state. The achievement of measles elimination in the Americas illustrates this perfectly; it benefited all countries of the region by greatly reducing importations of measles due to travel within the region.

Countries that have large populations, remote communities, are federalised, have decentralised health systems, experience other health emergencies including COVID-19, climate-change-related disasters, economic crisis or conflict, waning vaccine demand and high levels of inequity, will have problems achieving and sustaining measles elimination. Several countries in these categories have achieved but then lost their elimination status; some have subsequently been reverified as having eliminated measles. The loss of measles elimination status has happened for multiple interrelated reasons including failures to address the accumulation of susceptible children, delayed campaigns, late outbreak response, mass migration, financial crisis, conflict, and vaccine hesitancy. The ideal setting for sustaining elimination is a small peaceful island state with a highly equitable society, strong universally available and accessible health care, a population that trusts in its institutions and health care providers, and with few visitors or mass movements of people. Nevertheless, the majority of the 78 countries that have achieved and sustained measles elimination have succeeded without the benefit of this idyllic setting, including countries, such as Haiti and Venezuela which have faced many challenges [49]. Such achievements are a tribute both to the countries themselves and to the community of countries and the region that have together supported each country in achieving its goal.

### 4.2. Delaying Elimination Is a Major Risk for Sustainability

Sustainability is possibly the most important determinant of success for most countries and also the hardest to achieve. It is a key attribute that has been relatively neglected in measles elimination strategies. The longer we wait, the harder it will be to sustain elimination and the more likely that measles mortality and disability will resurge. In facing challenges as enormous as measles and, in the face of constrained resources, rigorous focus is needed on what is essential.

### 4.3. Diverse Tools and Strategies Are Available to Push Forward Measles Elimination

Measles could be described as an ancient pandemic. Combat against it is ongoing. The world could learn from the COVID-19 pandemic during which equitable access to vaccines was not achieved despite attempts to coordinate globally. For measles, we have it all, with a visible disease, cheap, cost-effective and abundant vaccine and opportunities to innovate in diverse ways, such as by implementing 5-dose vials and new campaign strategies or accelerating new technology, such as MR microarray patch vaccines (MAPs) and rapid diagnostic tests (RDTs) [50–52]. We have the technological ability to deliver reliable accurate and timely surveillance and coverage data down to subnational levels, particularly important for understanding where action needs to be taken to raise coverage in large, decentralised and heterogeneous countries. As coverage increases in a country, the requirements for investment in high-quality information systems for surveillance and coverage increase, including home-based records, electronic immunisation registries and school entry checks to identify missed children. Where trust in vaccines has been shaken, tools and methods exist for social listening to understand vaccine confidence and how to raise it. We could build evidence on waning immunity by tracking breakthrough infections, especially in countries that start routine measles immunisation at 6, 8 or 9 months. The high-performing Global Measles Rubella Laboratory Network (GMRLN) is also a key resource for global health security and pandemic response. Recent pandemics have been respiratory diseases, as are measles and rubella. Vaccines have been key to the response and should be integral to the global health security agenda.

Such diverse tools and strategies, if implemented for measles and rubella, would not just help countries achieve and sustain measles and rubella elimination but also enhance a life course approach to immunisation and health. This is where the measles and rubella teams can work with other health initiatives to strengthen routine immunisation together, including the "second year of life platform". School entry requirements may also help generate sustainable progress.

### 4.4. The Gap in Political Will for Measles Elimination Requires Strong Global Advocacy

We have nearly all the elements to achieve elimination but miss a key essential ingredient, which is sufficient political will to seize this opportunity. The 78 countries that have eliminated measles show us that it is possible even in very difficult settings. If momentum can be generated, many more countries are set to follow suit, but focused action is needed to ensure accelerated progress in the African and Eastern Mediterranean regions to address the regional equity gap. Lessons we can take from the Global Polio Eradication Initiative (GPEI) include the need for intensified resources in countries where the greatest impact can be made in order to raise up all countries together, relentless advocacy at all levels, strong collaboration with other initiatives, and clearly defined benchmarks and milestones towards elimination. Building momentum towards measles elimination requires not just concerted advocacy efforts but also support from global leaders in immunisation.

### 4.5. Country Voices Need to Be Elevated and Economic Benefits of Elimination Emphasised

Successful countries and regions have demonstrated that pursuing measles and rubella elimination goals relies on financing for countries as well as high-level political championing, yet resources are currently shrinking. When routine measles vaccine coverage is below 90%, countries must implement regular catch-up strategies or campaigns as a rescue strategy to reach unimmunised children and prevent outbreaks. Immunization campaigns are expensive and unpopular with country ministries of health and finance, and with donors, despite the costs of the outbreaks that occur without campaigns, but there is no escaping the need for them until routine immunisation systems are stronger. Countries with coverage below 80% face a vicious cycle of needing such frequent campaigns, often every two years, that it becomes very challenging for them to strengthen their routine immunisation systems. This campaign trap can be broken through assistance in building the strong routine immunisation systems needed to stop this rapid cycle of campaigns, but this takes time and in the interim needs to be strongly supported through a proactive and evolutionary multi-year campaign strategy. Combined with more effective and integrated health campaign planning, as is underway through the work of the Measles & Rubella Partnership (M&RP), other disease-specific initiatives and partners, more impact can be achieved with limited resources [53,54]. Helping the few countries yet to use the rubella vaccine to meet the requirements for its introduction could also be a stepping stone towards measles elimination.

We have taken a global perspective in this piece and should reflect on the implications of this viewpoint in the context of the call to decolonise global health and raise country voices [55]. Truly country-led sustainable approaches to development could force a more sustainable approach to materialise, maybe through further engagement of emerging Global South voices and leadership by large middle-income countries. In discussing inequity and measles, we should reframe the discussion from some countries being behind on progress to all countries being behind for as long as children everywhere are not being reached equally. Measles does not respect institutional boundaries, so neither should we in trying to stop its spread. There are not just health or economic benefits to be considered, there are real risks and measurable costs to failing to sustain elimination (Figure 1). For example, the question should be asked: would measles be a worthwhile investment for Development Banks established by high-burden countries? For every $1 spent, we estimate a return on investment of more than $58 [56]. There is much to be gained from investing in measles elimination.

## 5. Conclusions

We cannot expect to bring about change by repeating past strategies. New and creative solutions are desperately needed to create and drive momentum towards the agreed measles and rubella goals. At the same time, we should not delay using the strategies we know to be effective while we wait for new ones that are, as yet, untested. We already have the technical tools to finish this unfinished pandemic of measles. What is missing is political leaders and global, regional and country-level actors to join forces around a common goal and make major progress in combatting one of the world's most burdensome diseases. Essential to these efforts is a higher ambition to address increasing inequity and strengthen health systems to reach unreached communities. The ultimate end game is to eradicate measles, but that effort cannot start until countries are ready and at the starting line for a final push, and the starting line is still far away. The resources and commitment to get there are out of step with the magnitude of the problem. It is time to correct that disparity and find the will and tenacity to act.

**Funding:** A.A. received funding from the Canadian Institutes of Health Research (CIHR) and the Canadian Immunization Research Network (CIRN).

**Acknowledgments:** With thanks to helpful editorial comments from Katrina Kretsinger, Kate O'Brien and Ann Lindstrand.

**Conflicts of Interest:** SB is director of The Centre for Vaccine Preventable Diseases at the University of Toronto, which operates using a mix of funding sources, including university funds, grant funding, and donations from vaccine manufacturers. The Centre has a robust set of governance processes at the school to ensure independent operation of the Centre and its Faculty and Staff. The authors alone are responsible for the views expressed in this article and they do not necessarily represent the views, decisions or policies of the institutions with which they are affiliated. Some of the content has been changed during institutional approval processes.

## References

1. Teleb, N.; Atta, H.; Hajjeh, R. Measles and rubella elimination in the Eastern Mediterranean Region: Successes and challenges. *East. Mediterr. Health J.* **2019**, *25*, 667–668. [CrossRef] [PubMed]
2. Lemos, D.R.Q.; Franco, A.R.; Garcia, M.H.d.O.; Pastor, D.; Bravo-Alcantara, P.; de Moraes, J.C.; Domingues, C.; Cavalcanti, L.P.d.G. Risk analysis for the reintroduction and transmission of measles in the post-elimination period in the Americas. *Rev. Panam. Salud Publica* **2017**, *41*, e157. [CrossRef] [PubMed] [PubMed Central]
3. Lewis-Bell, K.N.; Irons, B.; Ferdinand, E.; Jackson, L.L.; Figueroa, J.P. The Expanded Program on Immunization in the English- and Dutch-speaking Caribbean (1977–2016): Reasons for its success. *Rev. Panam. Salud Publica* **2017**, *41*, e127. [CrossRef] [PubMed] [PubMed Central]
4. Muscat, M.; Ben Mamou, M.; Shefer, A.; Jankovic, D.; Deshevoy, S.; Butler, R. The State of Measles and Rubella in the WHO European region. *Rev. Esp. Salud Publica* **2015**, *89*, 345–351, (In English, Spanish). [CrossRef] [PubMed]
5. Musa, N.; Ghoniem, A.; Hsu, C.H.; Mubarak, S.; Sume, G.; Sharifuzzaman, M.; Bak, J.; Hutin, Y.; Teleb, N.; Crowcroft, N.; et al. Progress toward Measles Elimination—World Health Organization Eastern Mediterranean Region, 2019–2022. *Mmwr. Morb. Mortal. Wkly. Rep.* **2024**, *73*, 139–144. [CrossRef] [PubMed] [PubMed Central]

6. Durrheim, D.N.; Baker, M.G.; Capeding, M.R.; Goh, K.T.; Lee, D.; Papania, M.; Rota, P.A.; Soo, T.L.; Tsang, T.H.; Xu, A. Accelerating measles elimination in the Western Pacific Region during the calm between the storms. *Lancet Reg. Health West. Pac.* **2022**, *23*, 100495. [CrossRef] [PubMed] [PubMed Central]
7. Masresha, B.G.; Hatcher, C.; Lebo, E.; Tanifum, P.; Bwaka, A.M.; Minta, A.A.; Antoni, S.; Grant, G.B.; Perry, R.T.; O'Connor, P. Progress toward Measles Elimination—African Region, 2017–2021. *Mmwr. Morb. Mortal. Wkly. Rep.* **2023**, *72*, 985–991. [CrossRef] [PubMed] [PubMed Central]
8. Bahl, S.; Khanal, S.; Sangal, L.; Tabassum, S.; Ungchusak, K.; Andrus, J. Measles and rubella elimination: Protecting children through immunization in South-East Asia Region (SEAR). *Lancet Reg. Health Southeast Asia* **2023**, *18*, 100303. [CrossRef] [PubMed] [PubMed Central]
9. Minta, A.A.; Ferrari, M.; Antoni, S.; Portnoy, A.; Sbarra, S.; Lambert, B.; Hatcher, C.; Hsu, C.H.; Ho, L.; Steulet, C.; et al. Progress Toward Measles Elimination—Worldwide, 2000–2022. *Mmwr. Morb. Mortal. Wkly. Rep.* **2023**, *72*, 1262–1268. [CrossRef]
10. Immunization Agenda 2030 Scorecard. Available online: https://scorecard.immunizationagenda2030.org/ (accessed on 14 May 2024).
11. O'Connor, Patrick personal communication, based on confidential Regional Verification Reports of the World Health Organization Regional Offices. 2023.
12. PAHO Regional Framework for the Monitoring and Re-Verification of Measles, Rubella, and Congenital Rubella Syndrome Elimination in the Americas. Available online: https://iris.paho.org/bitstream/handle/10665.2/55074/9789275124062_eng.pdf?sequence=5&isAllowed=y (accessed on 5 June 2024).
13. McDonald, R.; Ruppert, P.S.; Souto, M.; Johns, D.E.; McKay, K.; Bessette, N.; McNulty, L.X.; Crawford, J.E.; Bryant, P.; Mosquera, M.C.; et al. Notes from the Field: Measles Outbreaks from Imported Cases in Orthodox Jewish Communities—New York and New Jersey, 2018–2019. *Mmwr. Morb. Mortal. Wkly. Rep.* **2019**, *68*, 444–445. [CrossRef]
14. De Serres, G.; Markowski, F.; Toth, E.; Landry, M.; Auger, D.; Mercier, M.; Bélanger, P.; Turmel, B.; Arruda, H.; Boulianne, N.; et al. Largest Measles Epidemic in North America in a Decade—Quebec, Canada, 2011: Contribution of Susceptibility, Serendipity, and Superspreading Events. *J. Infect. Dis.* **2013**, *207*, 990–998. [CrossRef] [PubMed]
15. Parums, D.V. A Review of the Resurgence of Measles, a Vaccine-Preventable Disease, as Current Concerns Contrast with Past Hopes for Measles Elimination. *Med. Sci. Monit.* **2024**, *30*, e944436. [CrossRef] [PubMed] [PubMed Central]
16. Paniz-Mondolfi, A.E.; Tami, A.; Grillet, M.E.; Márquez, M.; Hernández-Villena, J.; Escalona-Rodríguez, M.A.; Blohm, G.M.; Mejías, I.; Urbina-Medina, H.; Rísquez, A.; et al. Resurgence of Vaccine-Preventable Diseases in Venezuela as a Regional Public Health Threat in the Americas. *Emerg. Infect. Dis.* **2019**, *25*, 625–632. [CrossRef] [PubMed] [PubMed Central]
17. Rose, G. Strategy of prevention: Lessons from cardiovascular disease. *Br. Med. J.* **1981**, *282*, 1847–1851. [CrossRef] [PubMed]
18. World Health Organization Geneva. Immunization Agenda 2030: A Global Strategy to Leave No One Behind. 1 April 2020. Available online: https://www.who.int/teams/immunization-vaccines-and-biologicals/strategies/ia2030 (accessed on 21 January 2024).
19. World Health Organization Geneva. The Measles Rubella Strategic Framework 2021–2030. Available online: https://www.who.int/publications/i/item/measles-and-rubella-strategic-framework-2021-2030 (accessed on 21 January 2024).
20. Pan American Health Organization Elimination of Measles, Rubella, and Congenital Rubella Syndrome in the Region of the Americas. Available online: https://www3.paho.org/hq/dmdocuments/2012/CE150-INF-6-C-e.pdf (accessed on 25 April 2024).
21. O'Connor, P.; Jankovic, D.; Muscat, M.; Ben-Mamou, M.; Reef, S.; Papania, M.; Singh, S.; Kaloumenos, T.; Butler, R.; Datta, S. Measles and rubella elimination in the WHO Region for Europe: Progress and challenges. *Clin. Microbiol. Infect.* **2017**, *23*, 504–510. [CrossRef] [PubMed]
22. WHO SAGE Feasibility Assessment of Measles and Rubella Eradication October 8, 2019. Available online: https://terrance.who.int/mediacentre/data/sage/SAGE_Docs_Ppt_Oct2019/4_session_measles_and_rubella_vaccines/Oct2019_session4_feasibility_assessment_Measles-Rubella_eradication.pdf (accessed on 8 April 2024).
23. Sustainable Development Goals. Available online: https://sdgs.un.org/goals (accessed on 14 March 2024).
24. Local Burden of Disease Vaccine Coverage Collaborators. Mapping routine measles vaccination in low- and middle-income countries. *Nature* **2021**, *589*, 415–419. [CrossRef] [PubMed]
25. Truelove, S.A.; Graham, M.; Moss, W.J.; Metcalf, C.J.E.; Ferrari, M.J.; Lessler, J. Characterizing the impact of spatial clustering of susceptibility for measles elimination. *Vaccine.* **2019**, *37*, 732–741. [CrossRef] [PubMed]
26. Durrheim, D.N.; Crowcroft, N.S. The price of delaying measles eradication. *Lancet Public Health* **2017**, *2*, E130–E131. [CrossRef] [PubMed]
27. Goodson, J.L.; Rota, P.A. Innovations in vaccine delivery: Increasing access, coverage, and equity and lessons learnt from measles and rubella elimination. *Drug Deliv. Transl. Res.* **2022**, *12*, 959–967. [CrossRef]
28. Byberg, S.; Fisker, A.B.; Thysen, S.M.; Rodrigues, A.; Enemark, U.; Aaby, P.; Benn, C.S.; Griffiths, U.K. Cost-effectiveness of providing measles vaccination to all children in Guinea-Bissau. *Glob. Health Action* **2017**, *10*, 1329968. [CrossRef]
29. Hinman, A.R.; Orenstein, W.A.; Mortimer, E.A., Jr. When, where, and how do immunizations fail? *Ann. Epidemiol.* **1992**, *2*, 805–812. [CrossRef] [PubMed]
30. World Health Organization and World Bank. Tracking Universal Health Coverage 2023 Global Monitoring Report. Available online: https://iris.who.int/bitstream/handle/10665/374059/9789240080379-eng.pdf?sequence=1 (accessed on 16 May 2024).

31. Comfort, H.; Lafta, R.K.; Flaxman, A.D.; Hagopian, A.; Duber, H.C. Association between Subnational Vaccine Coverage, Migration, and Incident Cases of Measles, Mumps, and Rubella in Iraq, 2001–2016. *Front. Public Health* **2022**, *9*, 689458. [CrossRef] [PubMed]
32. ECDC Measles on the Rise in the EU/EEA: Considerations for Public Health Response. Available online: https://www.ecdc.europa.eu/sites/default/files/documents/measles-eu-threat-assessment-brief-february-2024.pdf (accessed on 27 April 2024).
33. Kurata, T.; Kaida, Y.; Kanbayashi, D.; Motomura, K. Achieving measles elimination and emerging modified measles: Longitudinal measles epidemiology from 1982 to 2021 in Osaka Prefecture, Japan. *Vaccine* **2024**, *42*, 271–286. [CrossRef] [PubMed]
34. Cherry, J.D.; Zahn, M. Clinical Characteristics of Measles in Previously Vaccinated and Unvaccinated Patients in California. *Clin. Infect. Dis.* **2018**, *67*, 1315–1319. [CrossRef] [PubMed]
35. Khanal, S.; Kassem, A.M.; Bahl, S.; Jayantha, L.; Sangal, L.; Sharfuzzaman, M.; Bose, A.S.; Antoni, S.; Datta, D.; Alexander, J.P., Jr. Progress toward Measles Elimination—South-East Asia Region, 2003–2020. *Mmwr. Morb. Mortal. Wkly. Rep.* **2022**, *71*, 1042–1046. [CrossRef] [PubMed]
36. Shattock, A.J.; Johnson, H.C.; Sim, S.Y.; Carter, A.; Lambach, P.; Hutubessy, R.C.W.; Thompson, K.M.; Badizadegan, K.; Lambert, B.; Ferrari, M.J.; et al. Contribution of vaccination to improved survival and health: Modelling 50 years of the Expanded Programme on Immunization. *Lancet* **2024**. *ahead of print*. [CrossRef] [PubMed]
37. Sim, S.Y.; Watts, E.; Constenia, D.; Brenzel, L.; Patenaude, B.N. Return on Investment from Immunization against 10 Pathogens in 94 Low- and Middle-income countries, 2011–2030. *Health Aff.* **2020**, *39*, 1343–1353. [CrossRef] [PubMed]
38. Mogaka, O.F.; Stewart, J.; Bukusi, E. Why and for whom are we decolonising global health? *Lancet Glob. Health* **2021**, *9*, e1359–e1360. [CrossRef] [PubMed]
39. Kunnuji, M.; Shawar, Y.R.; Neill, R.; Manoj, M.; Shiffman, J. Why 'elevating country voice' is not decolonizing global health: A frame analysis of in-depth interviews. *PLoS Glob. Public Health* **2023**, *3*, e0001365. [CrossRef] [PubMed] [PubMed Central]
40. Hughes, S.L.; Bolotin, S.; Khan, S.; Li, Y.; Johnson, C.; Friedman, L.; Tricco, A.C.; Hahné, S.J.M.; Heffernan, J.M.; Dabbagh, A.; et al. The effect of time since measles vaccination and age at first dose on measles vaccine effectiveness—A systematic review. *Vaccine* **2020**, *38*, 460–469. [CrossRef]
41. Guerra, F.M.; Crowcroft, N.S.; Friedman, L.; Deeks, S.L.; Halperin, S.A.; Severini, A.; Hatchette, T.F.; Bolotin, S. Immunity of Canadians and Risk of Epidemics (iCARE) Network. Waning of measles maternal antibody in infants in measles elimination settings—A systematic literature review. *Vaccine* **2018**, *6*, 1248–1255. [CrossRef] [PubMed]
42. Bolotin, S.; Osman, S.; Hughes, S.L.; Ariyarajah, A.; Tricco, A.C.; Khan, S.; Li, L.; Johnson, C.; Friedman, L.; Gul, N.; et al. In Elimination Settings, Measles Antibodies Wane After Vaccination but Not After Infection: A Systematic Review and Meta-Analysis. *J. Infect. Dis.* **2022**, *226*, 1127–1139. [CrossRef] [PubMed]
43. Wang, Q.; Wang, W.; Winter, A.K.; Zhan, Z.; Ajelli, M.; Trentini, F.; Wang, L.; Li, F.; Yang, J.; Xiang, X.; et al. Long-term measles antibody profiles following different vaccine schedules in China, a longitudinal study. *Nat. Commun.* **2023**, *14*, 1746. [CrossRef] [PubMed]
44. Brinkman, I.D.; de Wit, J.; Smits, G.P.; Ten Hulscher, H.I.; Jongerius, M.C.; Abreu, T.C.; van der Klis, F.R.M.; Hahné, S.J.M.; Koopmans, M.P.G.; Rots, N.Y.; et al. Early Measles Vaccination During an Outbreak in the Netherlands: Short-Term and Long-Term Decreases in Antibody Responses Among Children Vaccinated before 12 Months of Age. *J. Infect. Dis.* **2019**, *220*, 594–602. [CrossRef] [PubMed] [PubMed Central]
45. Fappani, C.; Gori, M.; Canuti, M.; Terraneo, M.; Colzani, D.; Tanzi, E.; Amendola, A.; Bianchi, S. Breakthrough Infections: A Challenge towards Measles Elimination? *Microorganisms* **2022**, *10*, 1567. [CrossRef] [PubMed] [PubMed Central]
46. Bolotin, S.; Crowcroft, N.S.; Hughes, S.L.; De Serres, G. Letter to the editor: Measles outbreak in Gothenburg urban area, Sweden, 2017 to 2018: Low viral load in breakthrough infections. *Eurosurveillance* **2019**, *24*, 1900465. [CrossRef] [PubMed] [PubMed Central]
47. Leuridan, E.; Hens, N.; Hutse, V.; Ieven, M.; Aerts, M.; Van Damme, P. Early waning of maternal measles antibodies in era of measles elimination: Longitudinal study. *BMJ* **2010**, *340*, c1626. [CrossRef]
48. Science, M.; Savage, R.; Severini, A.; McLachlan, E.; Hughes, S.L.; Arnold, C.; Richardson, S.; Crowcroft, N.; Deeks, S.; Halperin, S.; et al. Measles Antibody Levels in Young Infants. *Pediatrics* **2019**, *144*, e20190630. [CrossRef] [PubMed]
49. Tohme, R.A.; Francois, J.; Cavallaro, K.F.; Paluku, G.; Yalcouye, I.; Jackson, E.; Wright, T.; Adrien, P.; Katz, M.A.; Hyde, T.B.; et al. Expansion of Vaccination Services and Strengthening Vaccine-Preventable Diseases Surveillance in Haiti, 2010–2016. *Am. J. Trop. Med. Hyg.* **2017**, *97* (Suppl. 4), 28–36. [CrossRef] [PubMed] [PubMed Central]
50. Krudwig, K.; Knittel, B.; Karim, A.; Kanagat, N.; Prosser, W.; Phiri, G.; Mwansa, F.; Steinglass, R. The effects of switching from 10 to 5-dose vials of MR vaccine on vaccination coverage and wastage: A mixed-method study in Zambia. *Vaccine* **2020**, *38*, 5905–5913. [CrossRef]
51. Hasso-Agopsowicz, M.; Crowcroft, N.; Biellik, R.; Gregory, C.J.; Menozzi-Arnaud, M.; Amorij, J.P.; Gilbert, P.A.; Earle, K.; Frivold, C.; Jarrahian, C.; et al. Accelerating the Development of Measles and Rubella Microarray Patches to Eliminate Measles and Rubella: Recent Progress, Remaining Challenges. *Front. Public Health* **2022**, *10*, 809675. [CrossRef] [PubMed] [PubMed Central]
52. Brown, D.W.; Warrener, L.; Scobie, H.M.; Donadel, M.; Waku-Kouomou, D.; Mulders, M.N.; Rota, P.A. Rapid diagnostic tests to address challenges for global measles surveillance. *Curr. Opin. Virol.* **2020**, *41*, 77–84. [CrossRef] [PubMed]
53. Measles & Rubella Partnership. Available online: https://measlesrubellapartnership.org/ (accessed on 17 May 2024).
54. Health Campaign Effectiveness Coalition. Available online: https://campaigneffectiveness.org/ (accessed on 17 May 2024).

55. McCoy, D.; Kapilashrami, A.; Kumar, R.; Rhule, E.; Khosla, R. Developing an agenda for the decolonization of global health. *Bull. World Health Organ.* **2024**, *102*, 130–136. [CrossRef] [PubMed] [PubMed Central]
56. Ozawa, S.; Clark, S.; Portnoy, A.; Grewal, S.; Brenzel, L.; Walker, D. Return on investment from childhood immunization in low- and middle-income countries, 2011–2020. *Health Aff.* **2016**, *35*, 199–207. [CrossRef] [PubMed]

vaccines

MDPI

*Review*

# Using Regular High-Quality Serosurveys to Identify and Close National Immunity Gaps—Measles and Rubella Elimination in Japan

**Tomimasa Sunagawa [1,*], Yusuke Kobayashi [1,*], Yoshihiro Takashima [2], Hajime Kamiya [3], Tomoe Shimada [1], Kazutoshi Nakashima [4], Satoru Arai [1], Kiyosu Taniguchi [5], Keiko Tanaka-Taya [6] and Nobuhiko Okabe [7]**

1 National Institute of Infectious Diseases, Tokyo 162-8640, Japan
2 Osaka University Center for Infectious Disease Education and Research, Osaka 565-0871, Japan
3 Graduate School of Medicine, Mie University, Tsu 514-8507, Japan
4 Department of Health Science, Faculty of Sports and Health Science, Daito Bunka University, Tokyo 175-8571, Japan
5 Department of Pediatrics, Mie National Hospital, National Hospital Organization, Tsu 514-0125, Japan
6 Kanagawa Prefectural Institute of Public Health, Kanagawa 253-0087, Japan
7 Kawasaki City Institute for Public Health, Kanagawa 210-0821, Japan
* Correspondence: sunatomi@niid.go.jp (T.S.); yusuke-k@niid.go.jp (Y.K.); Tel.: +81-3-5285-1111 (T.S. & Y.K.)

**Abstract:** In Japan, periodic measles outbreaks occurred mainly among young children under the routine immunization program with one dose of the measles-containing vaccine (MCV). A second dose of MCV was introduced in 2006. During a nationwide measles resurgence in 2007–2008, the most affected age group was teenagers. The national serological surveillance for vaccine-preventable diseases made it clear that there was a measles immunity gap among teenagers who had not received a second dose of MCV. To fill this immunity gap, nationwide non-selective supplementary immunization activities (SIAs) were carried out as a five-year program from April 2008 to March 2013 by providing an opportunity to be vaccinated with the measles and rubella vaccine during the first year of junior high school (12–13 years old) and the last year of high school (17–18 years old). The SIA was conducted with the strong involvement of local governments in charge of vaccination delivery and collaboration between the health and education sectors. Japan was verified as achieving measles elimination in 2015 and this has been sustained to date. The challenge of rubella elimination following a similar strategy of a serological diagnosis of an immunity gap and targeted vaccination is also discussed.

**Keywords:** measles; rubella; elimination; immunity gaps; serological surveillance; SIAs

## 1. Introduction

### 1.1. Objectives of This Review

Measles and rubella are viral and representative vaccine-preventable diseases [1]. Measles can lead to serious complications such as pneumonia, encephalitis, and death is airborne and spread by respiratory droplets. Rubella is generally a milder illness than measles but it poses a significant risk to pregnant women and can cause congenital rubella syndrome (CRS), leading to serious birth defects such as heart abnormalities, cataracts, and deafness. There are highly effective vaccines for both measles and rubella, and they are generally used as a combination vaccine [2,3].

The world has had the shared goal of eliminating the endemic transmission of measles and rubella viruses, which will also result in the elimination of CRS. For example, the Region of the Americas (PAHO), consisting of 35 member states, declared measles elimination in 2016 (two of these countries lost their elimination certification in 2018, but only one is currently pending reverification), and rubella elimination in 2015, with remaining to date.

This has been achieved through the implementation of PAHO-recommended surveillance and immunization strategies [4]. In the Western Pacific Region consisting of 27 member states including Japan, as of May 2024, 8 countries and regions had been verified as having achieved and sustained measles elimination, with 7 verified for rubella elimination [5].

We describe and discuss how Japan, as a country using national serological surveillance to routinely identify measles immunity gaps, planned strategies to fill them and then monitored the impact of these strategies. We consider the impact on achieving and sustaining measles elimination. We also analyze and discuss the application of the same approach to achieving rubella elimination.

### *1.2. Immunization Program in Japan*

In Japan, while the Ministry of Health, Labor, and Welfare has overall responsibility for the national immunization program [1], implementation of the program is principally carried out by municipalities (local governments) ($n$ = 1718) based on the Immunization Act [6]. Currently, the majority of vaccines are administered at local medical facilities where physicians contracted by municipalities provide vaccination services. The physician records the date, dose, and lot number of vaccines administered in the Maternal and Child Health Handbook and sends the filled vaccine screening questionnaire to the local government so that the medical facility can be reimbursed. The local government retains the form and calculates the local vaccination coverage.

### *1.3. Serological Surveillance Programme in Japan*

Serological surveillance in Japan was launched in 1962 and it has been called the National Epidemiological Surveillance of Vaccine-Preventable Diseases (NESVPD) since the enforcement of the Infectious Diseases Control Law in 1999. Local public health institutes participate each fiscal year (hereafter FY; from April to March in Japan), collaborating with health facilities to collect blood samples according to the numbers of targeted areas and subjects, with serological analysis for VPDs such as measles and rubella. The results are to be shared with NIID and feedback is provided to the public [7]. For example, in FY 2023, the survey was conducted in 23 prefectures and 23 areas with 4554 people targeted for measles serology, with a total of 18 prefectures, 24 areas, and 5982 people targeted for rubella serology [7].

### *1.4. Measles and Rubella Control with Vaccination in Japan, 1979–2005*

Under the routine immunization program, from October 1978 to March 1995, the measles vaccine (MV) was given to both boys and girls aged 12–72 months. From August 1977 to March 1995, the rubella vaccine (RV) was given to only girls aged 12–15 years. From April 1995 to March 2006, the measles and rubella vaccine (MRV) was given to children (both boys and girls) aged 12 to 90 months [8,9]. Accurate coverage was estimated from 1995 and, since that time, MRV coverage has been maintained above 90%. While the targeted age range for MRV vaccination in Japan was wide, local clinicians were encouraged to administer the measles-containing vaccine (MCV) as soon as possible after the child's first birthday, and MCV coverage at the first year of age has increased since the early 2000s.

In 1947, measles became a reportable disease for surveillance in Japan. From 1983 to 2007, the occurrence of both measles and rubella was monitored by the pediatric sentinel surveillance system involving around 3000 pediatric hospitals and clinics [8,9]. From 1999 to 2007, sentinel surveillance for adult measles was also operational [8]. There were several measles resurgences recorded, with cases from sentinel sites exceeding 50,000 cases in a number of years (e.g., 1983, 1984, 1987, and 1991) (Figure 1A) [10,11].

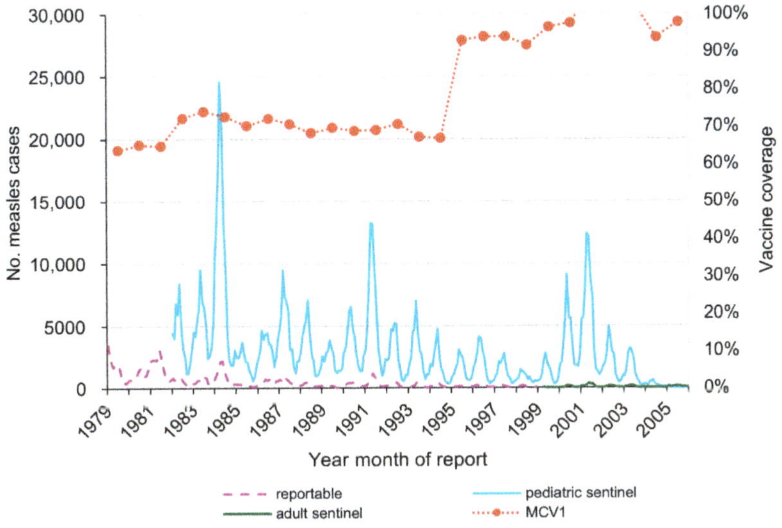


**(A)**

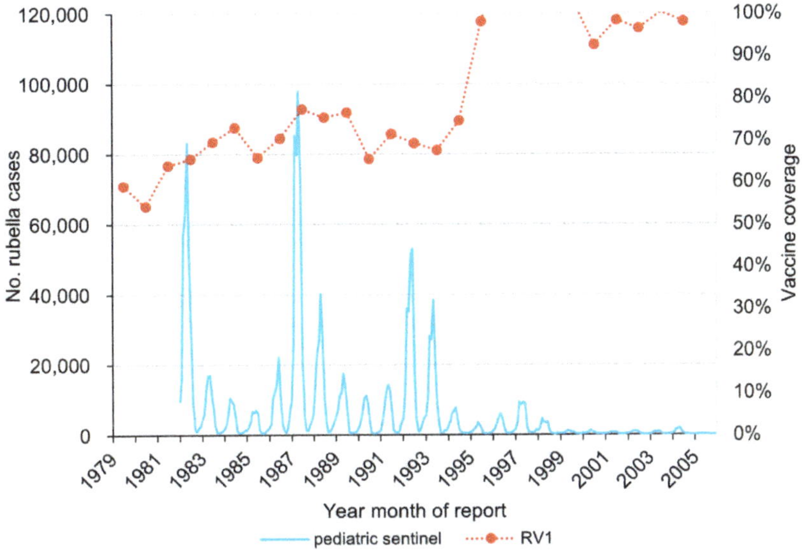


**(B)**

**Figure 1.** Measles and rubella vaccination * and aggregated numbers from sentinel sites † in Japan, 1979–2005. (**A**) Measles. (**B**) Rubella. MV, measles vaccine; RV, rubella vaccine. * Vaccine coverage = number of people immunized (the Report on Regional Public Health Services)/total population of standard immunization age period (as of October 1). The numerator is the number of people who received vaccinations out of the total number of people eligible for vaccinations, while the denominator is the population newly eligible for vaccinations each year, so the coverage rate may exceed 100%. † Since 1947, measles has been a reportable disease for surveillance. Since 1983, measles has been reported as pediatric sentinel surveillance. Under the current law (Infectious Diseases Control Law), measles and rubella have been reported as sentinel surveillance from 1999 to 2007. During 1999–2008, measles in adults was reported from hospitalized sentinel sites.

### 1.5. Measles Outbreak in 2007–2008

In Japan, the second dose of MRV (MRV-2) was introduced into the routine vaccination program in 2006 for children aged 5–7 years with the first dose of MRV (MRV-1) given to children aged 12–24 months. While MRV-1 had been given with high coverage since 1995 (>90%) and MRV-2 was introduced with high coverage (80%) in 2006, the country experienced a nationwide measles resurgence in 2007–2008 [1,8], which triggered the development and implementation of a national strategy and plan of action for measles elimination in Japan ("Guidelines for the Prevention of Specific Infectious Diseases Related to Measles", hereinafter "Guidelines") [12].

### 1.6. Measles Elimination Program

The Guidelines were prepared to address and overcome several critical challenges in measles elimination in Japan, which included (1) the existence of large immunity gaps among adolescents; (2) the limited production capacity of domestic MCV, where around 1.2 million doses were produced by three domestic vaccine manufactures annually in 2005 for the routine MCV-1 and 2.3 million doses of MCV-1 and MCV-2 in 2006 [13]; (3) insufficient information on how to implement elimination-focused vaccination programs among municipalities; (4) limited experiences and technical capacity of local government to conduct nationwide case-based measles and rubella surveillance including active case investigation started in 2008; and (5) insufficient awareness of the importance of preventing measles in schools and immunization for high-school-aged students.

To overcome those challenges, the Guidelines includes strategies and activities to (1) strengthen routine vaccination with MRV-1 (for children aged 12–24 months) and MRV-2 (for children aged 5–6 years), with cohorts born after 2000 specifically targeted; (2) identify birth cohorts with higher susceptibility to measles virus infection and transmission using the national serological surveillance system; (3) develop and conduct a nationwide non-selective catch-up measles and rubella supplemental immunization activity (MR-SIA) to fill large immunity gaps with full consideration of the national capacity for vaccine supply; (4) achieve and maintaine high vaccination coverage in all municipalities; (5) enhance case-based surveillance with aggressive case and outbreak investigations to detect and report all measles cases with laboratory confirmation and virus genotyping; (6) clearly determine the roles and responsibilities of national and local governments in planning and implementing elimination activities; (7) fully involve the education sector for the vaccination of adolescents; (8) strengthen the outbreak response by local government in collaboration with the NIID; and (9) sensitize the public.

### 1.7. Progress and Achievements

From 2008 to 2012, strategies in the Guidelines were intensively and rigorously implemented across the country, resulting in the last detection of endemic measles virus (genotype D5) in 2010 [14] and the confirmation of the interruption of endemic virus transmission in 2012. In 2015, the WHO's Western Pacific Regional Verification Commission for Measles and Rubella Elimination (RVC) verified Japan to have achieved measles elimination [15]. Since then, measles elimination has been successfully sustained even under the pressure of multiple measles virus importation from endemic countries, particularly during the regional measles resurgence in the Western Pacific in 2013–2016 and the global measles resurgence in 2018–2019 (Figure 2) [10,11,16,17].

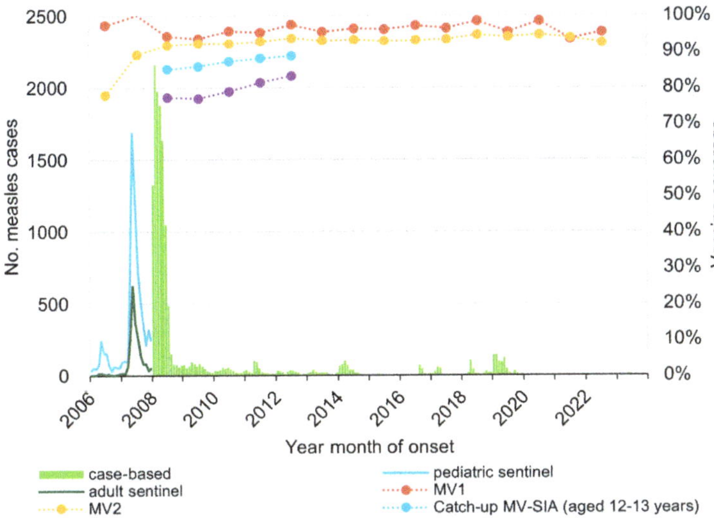


(A)

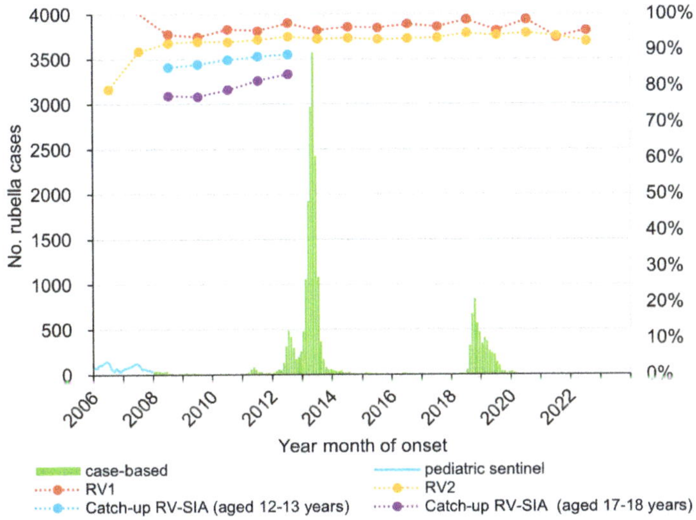


(B)

**Figure 2.** Measles and rubella vaccination * and occurrence † in Japan, 2006–2022. (**A**) Measles. (**B**) Rubella. MV, measles vaccine; RV, rubella vaccine. * Vaccine coverage = number of people immunized (the Report on Regional Public Health Services)/total population of standard immunization age period (as of October 1). The numerator is the number of people who received vaccinations out of the total number of people eligible for vaccinations, while the denominator is the population newly eligible for vaccinations each year, so the coverage rate may exceed 100%. † Since 2008, all measles cases have been reported.

## 2. Materials and Methods

This study is a narrative review. We have used measles and rubella surveillance data, which are publicly available, from the National Epidemiological Surveillance of Infectious Diseases (NESID), serological data from the National Epidemiological Surveillance of Vaccine-Preventable Diseases (NESVPD), and technical guidelines prepared by the National

Institute of Infectious Diseases (NIID) and issued by the Ministry of Health, Labor, and Welfare (MHLW).

NESID mainly consists of (1) pathogen reporting (laboratory-based surveillance) and (2) patient reporting [18]. For NESVPD [7], local public health institutes collaborate and share results with NIID.

We analyzed and characterized a measles resurgence in 2008, the transmission of measles virus in 2013–2022, and rubella resurgences in 2013–2014 and 2018–2019 and reviewed the impact of strategies and activities carried out from 2008 described in the National Strategy and Plan of Action for Measles Elimination on measles elimination and rubella elimination in Japan.

As this study utilized publicly available surveillance data with only aggregated information, ethical approval was not required.

## 3. Results

### 3.1. Measles Outbreak in 2007–2008

Before 2007, measles surveillance was carried out at sentinel sites for children and adults (rubella only for children), and a major measles outbreak starting in 2007 was obvious from both sentinel surveillance systems. With the transition to nationwide case-based surveillance for both measles and rubella in 2008, we focus our description on 2008. There were 11,013 measles cases reported from January to December 2008. Among them, 2363 (21.5%), 1580 (14.3%), and 2866 (27.2%) were reported from the cohorts born in FY 2000–2008, FY 1995–1999, and FY 1990–1994, respectively, with 63.0% of reported cases aged younger than 15 years (Figures 2A and 3A) [10,19].

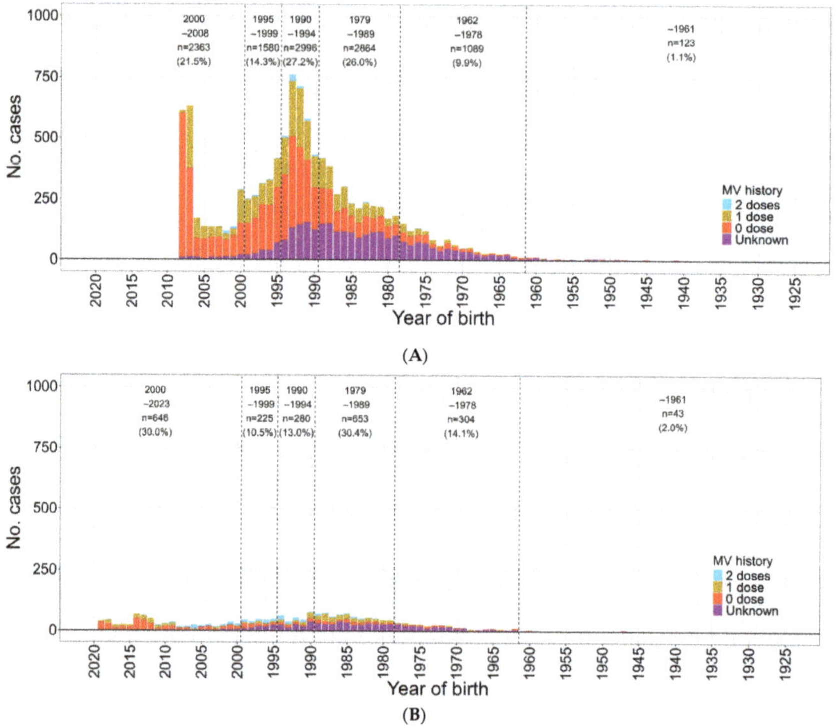


**Figure 3.** Measles cases (confirmed) by year of birth and vaccination history during measles outbreak (January–December 2008 and January 2013–December 2023); (**A**) January–December 2008 ($n$ = 11,015). (**B**) January 2013–December 2023 ($n$ = 2151). MV, measles vaccine.

*3.2. Determination of Immunity Gaps to Be Filled*

NESVPD revealed and confirmed that there was a significant measles immunity gap among the cohorts born in FY 1995–1999 and FY 1990–1994 compared with other birth cohorts (Figure 4) [7].

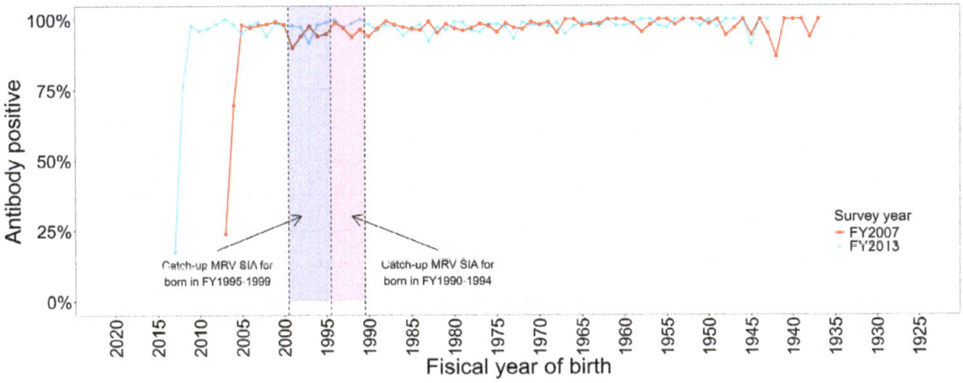


**Figure 4.** Measles antibody positive rate (PA $\geq$ 1:16) by year of birth in 2007 and 2013. MRV, measles and rubella vaccine; SIA, supplementary immunization activity; FY, fiscal year.

*3.3. Immunization Strategy 2008–2012 and 2013 to Date*

To fill the immunity gap among the cohorts born in FY 1990–1999 and establish high population immunity among all birth cohorts born after FY 2000, the immunization strategy developed was to (1) double the production of domestic MRV from 2.3 million in 2006 to 4.7 million per year from 2008 to 2012 to cover 20 birth cohorts with either routine childhood vaccination or the catch-up MR-SIA over five years; and (2) provide MRV to four birth cohorts from 2008 to 2012 through (i) routine MRV-1 at the age of 12–24 months (the cohorts born in 2008–2012), (ii) routine MRV-2 at the age of 5–6 years (the cohorts born in 2000–2007), (iii) the catch-up MR-SIA at the age of 12–13 years (the first year at junior high school) (the cohorts born between 1995 and 1999), and (iv) the catch-up MR-SIA at the age of 17–18 years (the last year at the senior high school) (the cohorts born between 1990 and 1994).

Routine MRV-1 and MRV-2 coverage was achieved and sustained at >90% (Figure 2A,B). The proportion of prefectures ($n$ = 47) with catch-up coverage at the age of 12–13 years and 17–18 years >85% continued to increase from 76.6% to 87.2% and 23.4% to 68.1%, respectively, from 2008 to 2012. More than 90% of prefectures have maintained the coverage of routine MRV-1 and MRV-2 >90% from 2010 to date (Table 1) [20].

Vaccination coverage of the 12–13-year-old and 17–18-year-old SIAs increased every year, starting at 85.1% and 77.3% in 2008, respectively, and ending at 88.8% and 83.2% in 2012, respectively, through the enhanced engagement of local governments and local medical associations and the support of schools, teachers, and parents (Table 2) [13,20].

*3.4. Impact of the Immunization Strategy on Measles*

The last chain of endemic measles transmission due to the genotype D5 virus was confirmed to have been interrupted in May 2010. Since then and up to the end of 2023, Japan has experienced multiple importations of genotypes D9, H1, D8, and B3 measles viruses, particularly between 2016 and 2019. Some of these resulted in small clusters of import-related measles cases among inadequately vaccinated young adults, but rigorous case and outbreak investigation confirmed that each was controlled within a relatively short period with four or fewer generations of virus transmission in limited geographical areas (e.g., within a prefecture) without large-scale outbreaks developing (Figure 5) [17,21].

**Table 1.** Number and percentage of prefectures in Japan ($n$ = 47) by the coverage of measles and rubella vaccination, 2008–2022.

| Vaccination | Coverage % | FY2008 *n* | FY2008 % | FY2009 *n* | FY2009 % | FY2010 *n* | FY2010 % | FY2011 *n* | FY2011 % | FY2012 *n* | FY2012 % | FY2013 *n* | FY2013 % | FY2014 *n* | FY2014 % | FY2015 *n* | FY2015 % | FY2016 *n* | FY2016 % | FY2017 *n* | FY2017 % | FY2018 *n* | FY2018 % | FY2019 *n* | FY2019 % | FY2020 *n* | FY2020 % | FY2021 *n* | FY2021 % | FY2022 *n* | FY2022 % |
|---|---|---|---|---|---|---|---|---|---|---|---|---|---|---|---|---|---|---|---|---|---|---|---|---|---|---|---|---|---|---|---|
| Routine MRV-1 (the aged 1 year) | >90 | 45 | 95.7 | 44 | 93.6 | 47 | 100 | 46 | 97.9 | 47 | 100 | 47 | 100 | 47 | 100 | 47 | 100 | 47 | 100 | 47 | 100 | 47 | 100 | 47 | 100 | 47 | 100 | 46 | 97.9 | 46 | 97.9 |
| | 85–90 | 2 | 4.3 | 3 | 6.4 | 0 | 0.0 | 1 | 2.1 | 0 | 0.0 | 0 | 0.0 | 0 | 0.0 | 0 | 0.0 | 0 | 0.0 | 0 | 0.0 | 0 | 0.0 | 0 | 0.0 | 0 | 0.0 | 1 | 2.1 | 1 | 2.1 |
| | <85 | 0 | 0.0 | 0 | 0.0 | 0 | 0.0 | 0 | 0.0 | 0 | 0.0 | 0 | 0.0 | 0 | 0.0 | 0 | 0.0 | 0 | 0.0 | 0 | 0.0 | 0 | 0.0 | 0 | 0.0 | 0 | 0.0 | 0 | 0.0 | 0 | 0.0 |
| Routine MRV-2 (the aged 6 years) | >90 | 42 | 89.4 | 41 | 87.2 | 46 | 97.9 | 44 | 93.6 | 46 | 97.9 | 44 | 93.6 | 45 | 95.7 | 45 | 95.7 | 46 | 97.9 | 46 | 97.9 | 47 | 100 | 47 | 100 | 47 | 100 | 45 | 95.7 | 44 | 93.6 |
| | 85–90 | 5 | 10.6 | 6 | 12.8 | 1 | 2.1 | 3 | 6.4 | 1 | 2.1 | 3 | 6.4 | 2 | 4.3 | 2 | 4.3 | 1 | 2.1 | 1 | 2.1 | 0 | 0.0 | 0 | 0.0 | 0 | 0.0 | 2 | 4.3 | 3 | 6.4 |
| | <85 | 0 | 0.0 | 0 | 0.0 | 0 | 0.0 | 0 | 0.0 | 0 | 0.0 | 0 | 0.0 | 0 | 0.0 | 0 | 0.0 | 0 | 0.0 | 0 | 0.0 | 0 | 0.0 | 0 | 0.0 | 0 | 0.0 | 0 | 0.0 | 0 | 0.0 |
| Catch-up MRV SIA (the aged 13 years) | >90 | 19 | 40.4 | 19 | 40.4 | 19 | 40.4 | 25 | 53.2 | 25 | 53.2 | | | | | | | | | | | | | | | | | | | | |
| | 85–90 | 17 | 36.2 | 16 | 34.0 | 18 | 38.3 | 15 | 31.9 | 16 | 34.0 | | | | | | | | | | | | | | | | | | | | |
| | <85 | 11 | 23.4 | 12 | 25.5 | 10 | 21.3 | 7 | 14.9 | 6 | 12.8 | | | | | | | | | | | | | | | | | | | | |
| Catch-up MRV SIA (the aged 17 years) | >90 | 2 | 4.3 | 3 | 6.4 | 4 | 8.5 | 7 | 14.9 | 10 | 21.3 | | | | | | | | | | | | | | | | | | | | |
| | 85–90 | 9 | 19.1 | 10 | 21.3 | 15 | 31.9 | 19 | 40.4 | 22 | 46.8 | | | | | | | | | | | | | | | | | | | | |
| | <85 | 36 | 76.6 | 34 | 72.3 | 28 | 59.6 | 21 | 44.7 | 15 | 31.9 | | | | | | | | | | | | | | | | | | | | |

MRV, measles and rubella vaccine; SIA, supplementary immunization activity; FY, fiscal year.

**Table 2.** Comparison of vaccination coverage by catch-up SIA.

**A. Catch-Up SIA for Measles Elimination**

| Vaccination | Year of Birth | | FY 2008 | FY 2009 | FY 2010 | FY 2011 | FY 2012 | Total |
|---|---|---|---|---|---|---|---|---|
| Catch-up MRV SIA (the aged 12–13 years) | FY 1995–1999 | No. targeted | 1,192,612 | 1,194,878 | 1,200,301 | 1,207,874 | 1,190,773 | 5,986,438 |
| | | No. vaccinated | 1,015,341 | 1,026,892 | 1,047,356 | 1,064,727 | 1,057,237 | 5,211,553 |
| | | Coverage | 85.1% | 85.9% | 87.3% | 88.1% | 88.8% | 87.0% |
| Catch-up MRV SIA (the aged 17–18 years) | FY 1990–1994 | No. targeted | 1,224,084 | 1,213,204 | 1,214,161 | 1,201,664 | 1,235,125 | 6,088,238 |
| | | No. vaccinated | 946,593 | 933,891 | 957,506 | 978,440 | 1,027,607 | 4,844,037 |
| | | Coverage | 77.3% | 77.0% | 78.9% | 81.4% | 83.2% | 79.6% |

**B. Catch-Up SIA for Rubella Elimination**

| Vaccination | Year of Birth | | | FY 2019 | FY 2020 | FY 2021 | FY 2022 | FY 2023 * | Other | Total |
|---|---|---|---|---|---|---|---|---|---|---|
| Catch-up RV SIA | Male FY 1962–1978 | Antibody test | No. targeted | - | - | - | - | - | - | 15,374,162 † |
| | | | No. tested | 1,245,330 | 1,769,990 | 847,962 | 531,596 | 253,175 | 66,307 | 4,714,360 |
| | | | Coverage | - | - | - | - | - | - | 30.7% |
| | | RV | No. vaccinated | 270,113 | 359,312 | 200,419 | 121,390 | 55,154 | 13,097 | 1,019,485 |
| | | | Coverage | - | - | - | - | - | - | 6.6% |

MRV, measles and rubella vaccine; RV, rubella vaccine; SIA, supplementary immunization activity; FY, fiscal year. * As of November 2023; † As of April 2019.

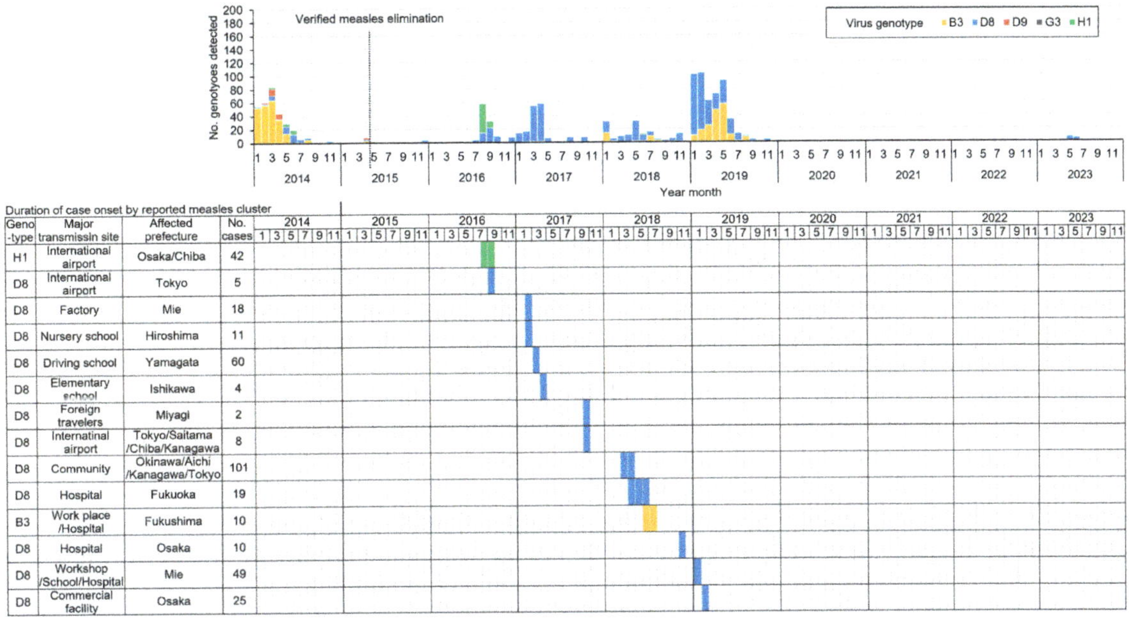


**Figure 5.** Detected measles virus genotypes and reported measles clusters, 2014–2023.

The Catch-up MR SIA at the age of 12–13 years and 17–18 years conducted in 2008–2012 with enhanced routine MRV-1 and MRV-2 coverage from 2006 established high population immunity among the cohorts born after 1990 and enabled Japan to achieve and sustain measles elimination and prevent the re-establishment of endemic transmission due to imported measles virus.

### 3.5. Impact of the Immunization Strategy on Rubella

The story of progress regarding rubella elimination is different. There were two nationwide rubella outbreaks in 2012–2013 and 2018–2019 (Figures 2B and 6).

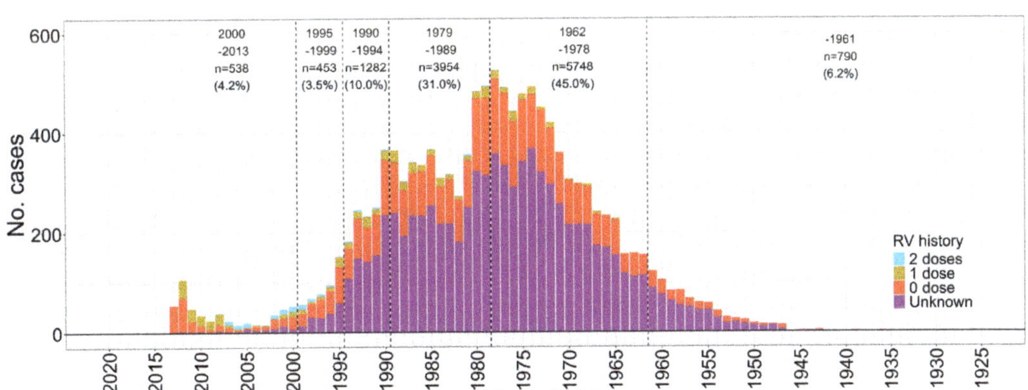


**(A-1)**

**Figure 6.** *Cont.*

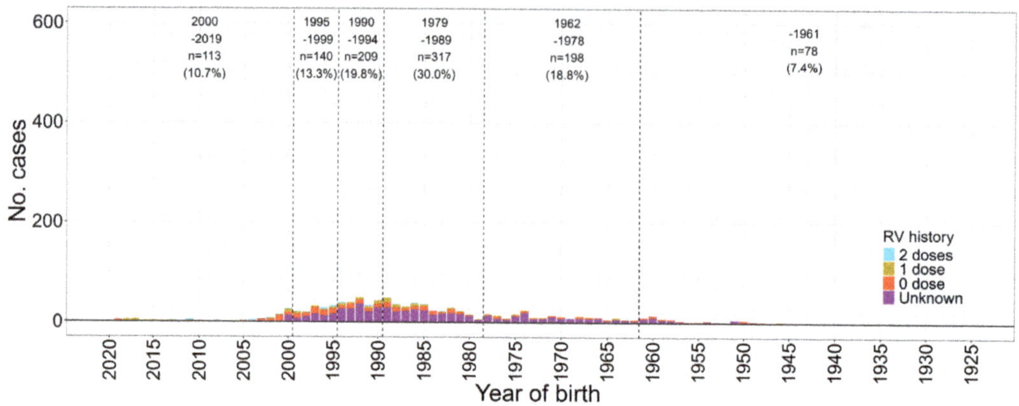


(A-2)

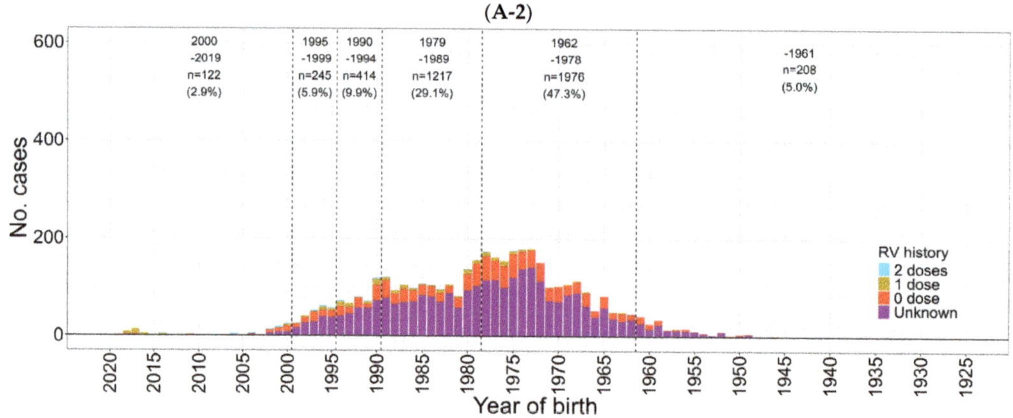


(B-1)

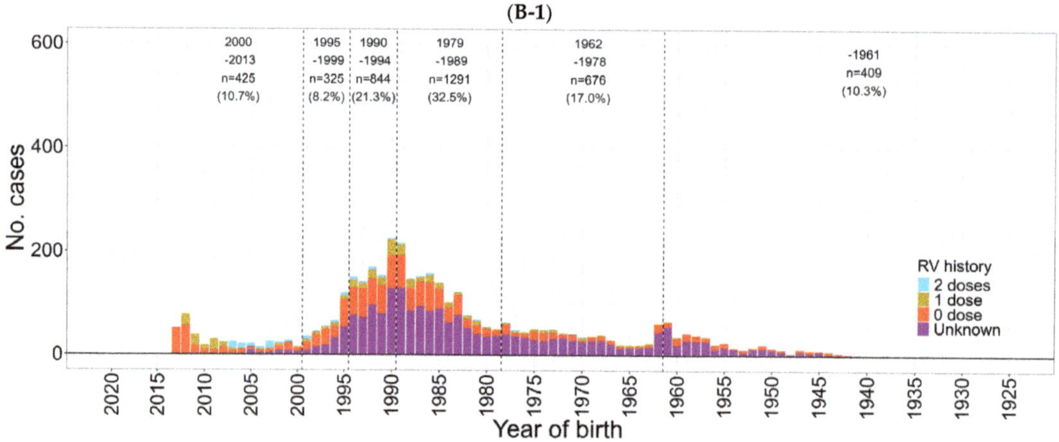


(B-2)

**Figure 6.** Rubella cases (confirmed) by sex, year of birth, and vaccination history during rubella outbreaks in January 2012–December 2013 and in January 2018–December 2019. (**A-1**) Male, January 2012–December 2013 ($n$ = 12,765). (**A-2**) Female, January 2012–December 2013 ($n$ = 3970). (**B-1**) Male, January 2018–December 2019 ($n$ = 4182). (**B-2**) Female, January 2018–December 2019 ($n$ = 1055). RV, rubella vaccine.

During the 2012–2013 outbreak, 16,730 cases of rubella were reported. Among them, 12,763 (76.1%) were male and, among these male rubella cases, 3951 (31.0%), 5749 (45.0%), and 792 (6.2%) were from cohorts born in FY 1979–1989, FY 1962–1978, and FY 1961 and before, respectively. The male and female cohorts born after 1990 accounted for 17.7% and 40.1%, respectively (Figure 6A-1,A-2). Following this outbreak, 45 infants with CRS were identified, 12 of whom died within the first year of life [22].

During the 2018–2019 outbreak, 5237 cases of rubella were reported. Among them, 4182 (79.9%) were male and, among male cases of rubella, 1216 (29.1%), 1978 (47.3%), and 208 (5.0%) were reported from the cohorts born in FY 1979–1989, FY 1962–1978, and FY 1961 and before, respectively. The male and female cohorts born after 1990 accounted for 18.7% and 43.6% of cases, respectively (Figure 6B-1,B-2) [10,23]. Following the outbreak during 2018–2019, six infants with CRS were identified (no deaths at the time of report) [24].

### 3.6. Rubella Outbreaks in 2012–2013 and 2018–2019

The outbreaks pointed to large population rubella immunity gaps among male cohorts born in FY 1962–1989, from which 78.0% and 79.9% of male rubella cases were reported during both rubella outbreaks in 2012–2013 and 2018–2019, respectively. Male rubella cases born in FY 1962–1978 and 1979–1989 accounted for 34.3% and 23.6%, respectively, of the total rubella cases reported during the 2012–2013 outbreak and for 37.8% and 23.2%, respectively, of the total rubella cases reported during the 2018–2019 outbreak (Figure 6). NESVPD confirmed a large immunity gap among male cohorts born in 1979–1989, as well as in FY 1962–1978 (Figure 7) [7]. This assisted in identifying the group of adult males that were offered screening for rubella immunity and rubella vaccination as required on the basis of their individual serological laboratory results.

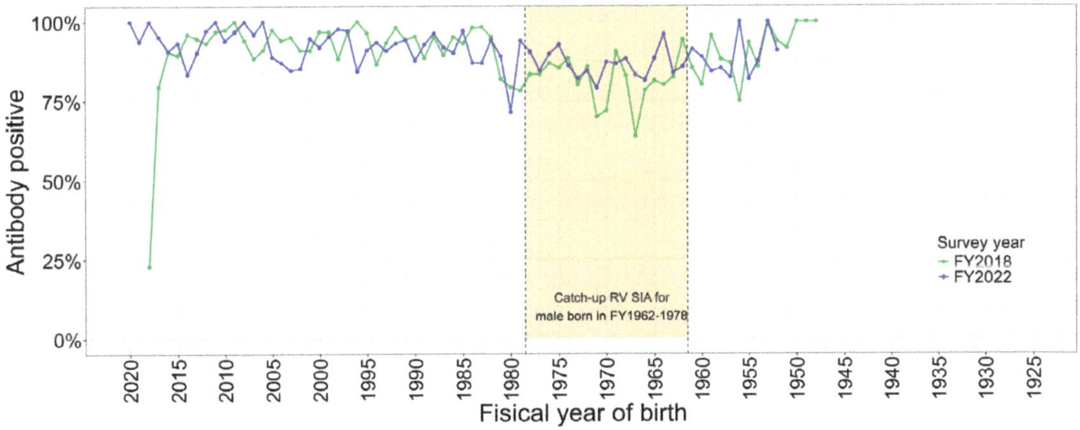


**Figure 7.** Rubella antibody positive rate (PA $\geq$ 1:8) among male population by year of birth in 2018 and 2022. RV, rubella-containing vaccine; SIA, supplementary immunization activity; FY, fiscal year.

## 4. Discussion

An in-depth epidemiologic analysis of the 2007–2008 nationwide resurgence of endemic measles virus transmission supported by the case-based measles and rubella surveillance system established during the resurgence together with the national serological surveillance system revealed birth cohorts with large immunity gaps causing the nationwide measles resurgence and helped to determine susceptible age groups (i.e., children and adolescents). They were targeted through a special vaccination program for achieving measles elimination with a time-limited surge of domestic vaccine production capacity, multifaceted engagement and coordination among different levels of governments across the country, enhanced collaboration between the health and education sectors, and the strengthened outbreak response capacity of national and local government public health sectors.

Implementation of this 5-year special vaccination program, which conducted a nationwide non-selective catch-up MRV-SIAs providing school students with a one-year opportunity for two age cohorts simultaneously, successfully established high-enough population immunity among the 20 cohorts born between 1990 and 2012 to interrupt endemic transmission, enabling the country to achieve and be verified for achieving measles elimination in 2015. This nationwide program also established strong momentum for preventing measles throughout the country, which enabled Japan to achieve and sustain very high routine MRV-1 and MRV-2 coverage ongoing in all prefectures, thus preventing the reestablishment of endemic measles virus transmission following importations even during the regional measles resurgence in the Western Pacific Region in 2013–2016 and the worldwide measles resurgence in 2018–2019.

Despite this successful achievement and maintenance of measles elimination in Japan in the last 15 years, the goal announced for rubella elimination in 2014 [25] has not yet been achieved. The main difference is clearly demonstrated through the epidemiology of recent rubella outbreaks and confirmed through population serology, with the high-risk population group for rubella virus infection and transmission being adult males aged above 40 years.

The catch-up MRV-SIA launched in 2019 to achieve rubella elimination in Japan after the nationwide rubella outbreak in 2018–2019 provided an opportunity for men who were born between FYs 1962 and 1978 to receive RCV after the confirmation of insufficient immunity against rubella by low antibody titer (≦1:8) of hemagglutination inhibition (HI) (selective MRV-SIA following antibody test). The national goal for this catch-up program was to increase population immunity based on NESVPD among men born in FY 1962 to 1978 from 80% (in 2018) to 90% by the end of March 2022. However, between 2019 and November 2023, only 4.71 million men had presented for an antibody test among a total of 15.4 million men born in FY 1962–1978 (30.7%), and 1.02 million men had received RCV (6.6% of this population) [26]. With the majority of people having weekday work, a vaccination program depending on the results of antibody titer measurements would involve at least two absences from work, and thus, this population is difficult to reach.

The use of serological surveillance for measles and rubella elimination is a strategy that has been used in multiple countries. For example, the United Kingdom has used serological studies to monitor immunity levels, guide vaccination strategies, and play an important role in maintaining elimination [27]. Germany also regularly conducts serological surveys to inform public health interventions and ensure high immunity levels [28]. Japan's approach is consistent with these international practices and demonstrates the value of continuous surveillance and adapted strategies using serological surveillance to achieve and sustain measles and rubella elimination.

A unique strategy in Japan was the implementation of a time-phased, intensified routine vaccination program based on incidence trends, historical vaccination schedules, and serological surveillance. From the experience in Japan, to obtain effective results with the multi-year SIA method for target populations determined by the results of serological surveillance, etc., it was important that the department(s) to which the target population belonged was clear and that the active administrative approach over a long period was possible. When the expected intervention was passive and left to the voluntary efforts of individuals or groups, progress was slow. It was also considered important that the operational procedures be as flexible and simple as possible, but further research is needed.

The trends in serological surveillance for measles may suggest that a certain level of herd immunity has been formed in Japan. However, serological surveillance cannot identify individuals with insufficient or weakened immunity due to the vaccine, nor can it detect populations with low levels of immunity. From this perspective, it is important for Japan to detect and respond to individuals and groups with gaps in measles immunity, and further indicates the need for a strategy to continue maintaining a high level of herd immunity against measles through two doses of measles vaccine [29].

## 5. Limitations

This study has several limitations that need to be acknowledged. Our findings are based on the interpretation of existing data and literature, which may be subject to publication bias and the availability of studies. This means that it could involve potential underreporting and misclassification of cases. Additionally, variations in laboratory testing and reporting practices over the years may affect data consistency.

## 6. Conclusions

The target population with immunity gaps to be filled should be carefully determined before launching nationwide large-scale catch-up SIAs. Detailed epidemiological analysis of outbreaks using case-based surveillance and field investigation supported by strong laboratory networks are essential for determining this target population. National serological surveillance has been a powerful asset for planning nationwide large-scale catch-up SIAs. In countries with limited vaccine supplies but gaps in immunity, pre-screening strategies to detect people for a nationwide SIA may be an option.

Serological surveillance can also play a pivotal role in monitoring the impact of these targeted SIAs and how successful they have been in closing the detected immunity gaps.

**Author Contributions:** Conceptualization, T.S. (Tomimasa Sunagawa) and Y.T.; methodology, T.S. (Tomimasa Sunagawa), Y.K. and Y.T.; software, Y.K.; validation, H.K., K.N., K.T.-T., K.T. and N.O.; formal analysis, Y.K. and Y.T.; investigation, T.S. (Tomimasa Sunagawa), Y.K., H.K., T.S. (Tomoe Shimada), K.N., S.A., K.T.-T. and K.T.; resources, T.S. (Tomimasa Sunagawa); data curation, T.S. (Tomimasa Sunagawa), Y.K., H.K. and S.A.; writing—original draft preparation, T.S. (Tomimasa Sunagawa), Y.K. and Y.T.; writing—review and editing, H.K., K.N., S.A., K.T., K.T. and N.O.; visualization, Y.K.; supervision, T.S. (Tomimasa Sunagawa); project administration, N.O. All authors have read and agreed to the published version of the manuscript.

**Funding:** This research received no external funding.

**Acknowledgments:** This research is based on publicly available information that was reported to the NESID or NESVPD systems from local governments, including prefectural and municipal HCs and Public Health Institutes (PHIs). The authors gratefully appreciate staff members from HCs, PHIs, and local government headquarters, along with the reporting physicians and relevant practitioners for serological surveillance. The authors thank MHLW for leading the measles and rubella elimination as a risk management organization. This article is provided solely for informational purposes by volunteers and does not represent the views of any affiliated organization.

**Conflicts of Interest:** The authors declare no conflicts of interest.

## References

1. Kamiya, H.; Kamidani, S.; Saitoh, A. An Introduction to the Japanese Immunization Program: Past, Present, and Future Perspectives. *Pediatr. Infect. Dis. J.* **2023**, *42*, e154–e157. [CrossRef] [PubMed]
2. Centers for Disease Control and Prevention. Measles Symptoms and Complications. Available online: https://www.cdc.gov/measles/signs-symptoms/index.html (accessed on 30 June 2024).
3. Reef, S.E. Rubella and congenital rubella syndrome. *Bull. World Health Organ.* **1998**, *76*, 156. [PubMed]
4. Rey-Benito, G.; Pastor, D.; Whittembury, A.; Durón, R.; Pacis-Tirso, C.; Bravo-Alcántara, P.; Ortiz, C.; Andrus, J. Sustaining the Elimination of Measles, Rubella and Congenital Rubella Syndrome in the Americas, 2019–2023: From Challenges to Opportunities. *Vaccines* **2024**, *12*, 690. [CrossRef] [PubMed]
5. World Health Organization. Regional Office for the Western Pacific. Measles-Rubella Bulletin. 2024. Available online: https://iris.who.int/handle/10665/375987 (accessed on 21 July 2024).
6. Immunization Act (Act No. 68 of 1948), Last Version: Act No. 103 of 2013. Available online: https://www.japaneselawtranslation.go.jp/ja/laws/view/2964/en#je_ch1at1 (accessed on 30 April 2024).
7. National Institute of Infectious Diseases. National Epidemiological Surveillance of Vaccine-Preventable Diseases. Available online: https://www.niid.go.jp/niid/ja/yosoku-index.html (accessed on 30 April 2024).

8. Sunagawa, T.; Shimada, T.; Ueno-Yamamoto, K.; Yamashita, K.; Tanaka-Taya, K.; Tada, Y.; Yasui, Y.; Matsui, T.; Taniguchi, K.; Kobayashi, J.; et al. Progress toward measles elimination—Japan, 1999–2008. *MMWR Morb. Mortal. Wkly. Rep.* **2008**, *57*, 1049–1052.
9. Tanaka-Taya, K.; Satoh, H.; Arai, S.; Yamagishi, T.; Yahata, Y.; Nakashima, K.; Sugawara, T.; Ohkusa, Y.; Matsui, T.; Saito, T.; et al. Nationwide rubella epidemic—Japan, 2013. *MMWR Morb. Mortal. Wkly. Rep.* **2013**, *62*, 457–462.
10. National Institute of Infectious Diseases. Annual Report of National Epidemiological Surveillance of Infectious Diseases. Available online: https://www.niid.go.jp/niid/ja/idsc2/8217-nenpou-archive.html (accessed on 30 April 2024). (In Japanese)
11. Ministry of Health, Labour and Welfare. Number of Routine Immunizations Administered. Available online: https://www.mhlw.go.jp/topics/bcg/other/5.html (accessed on 30 April 2024). (In Japanese)
12. Ministry of Health, Labour and Welfare. Guidelines for the Prevention of Specific Infectious Diseases Related to Measles (Version on 28 December 2017). Available online: https://data.e-gov.go.jp/data/dataset/mhlw_20140917_0627/resource/de775472-d9f2-497f-a42d-241079670011 (accessed on 30 April 2024). (In Japanese)
13. Japan Association of Vaccine Industries. Q&A for Vaccine Practitioners and Basic of Vaccine. Available online: http://www.wakutin.or.jp/medical/index.html (accessed on 30 April 2024). (In Japanese)
14. National Institute of Infectious Diseases. Monthly Reports of Measles Virus Isolation/Detection, July 2008–December 2011 as Part of Infectious Agents Surveillance Report. Available online: https://idsc.niid.go.jp/iasr/prompt/graph/masin111e.gif (accessed on 30 April 2024).
15. World Health Organization. Brunei Darussalam, Cambodia, Japan Verified as Achieving Measles Elimination (27 March 2015). Available online: https://www.who.int/westernpacific/news/item/27-03-2015-brunei-darussalam-cambodia-japan-verified-as-achieving-measles-elimination (accessed on 30 April 2024).
16. National Institute of Infectious Diseases. Infectious Diseases Weekly Report. Available online: https://www.niid.go.jp/niid/ja/idwr.html (accessed on 30 April 2024). (In Japanese)
17. Regional Office for the Western Pacific, World Health Organization. Measles-Rubella Bulletin. Available online: https://iris.who.int/handle/10665/197909 (accessed on 30 April 2024).
18. National Institute of Infectious Diseases. Infectious Diseases Weekly Report. New Articles, Surveillance Data, Trend Graph. Available online: https://www.niid.go.jp/niid/en/idwr-e.html (accessed on 30 April 2024).
19. National Institute of Infectious Diseases. Notified Measles Cases in Japan (Preliminary Figures, Weekly). Available online: https://www.niid.go.jp/niid/en/measles-e/655-idsc/2180-measles-e.html (accessed on 30 April 2024).
20. Ministry of Health, Labour and Welfare. Measles and Rubella Vaccination Coverage. Available online: https://www.mhlw.go.jp/bunya/kenkou/kekkaku-kansenshou21/hashika.html (accessed on 30 April 2024). (In Japanese)
21. National Institute of Infectious Diseases. Infectious Agents Surveillance Report. Available online: https://www.niid.go.jp/niid/ja/iasr.html (accessed on 30 April 2024). (In Japanese)
22. Kanai, M.; Kamiya, H.; Okuno, H.; Sunagawa, T.; Tanaka-Taya, K.; Matsui, T.; Oishi, K.; Kitajima, H.; Takeda, M.; Mori, Y. Epidemiology of Congenital Rubella Syndrome Related to the 2012–2013 Rubella Epidemic in Japan. *J. Pediatr. Infect. Dis. Soc.* **2022**, *11*, 400–403. [CrossRef] [PubMed]
23. National Institute of Infectious Diseases. Notified Rubella Cases in Japan (Preliminary Figures, Weekly). Available online: https://www.niid.go.jp/niid/ja/rubella-m-111/700-idsc/2131-rubella-doko.html (accessed on 30 April 2024).
24. National Institute of Infectious Diseases. Regarding congenital rubella syndrome reported from 2019 to 2021. *Infect. Agents Surveill. Rep.* **2022**, *43*, 3–4. (In Japanese)
25. Ministry of Health, Labour and Welfare. Guidelines for the Prevention of Specific Infectious Diseases Related to Rubella (Revised on 21 December 2017 from the Original Version on 28 March 2014). Available online: https://www.mhlw.go.jp/file/06-Seisakujouhou-10900000-Kenkoukyoku/0000186690.pdf (accessed on 30 April 2024). (In Japanese)
26. Hori, A.; Yoshii, S.; Isaka, Y.; Wada, K. Factors associated with participation in an ongoing national catch-up campaign against rubella: A cross-sectional internet survey among 1680 adult men in Japan. *BMC Public Health* **2021**, *21*, 292. [CrossRef] [PubMed]
27. Public Health England. UK Measles and Rubella Elimination Strategy 2019. Available online: https://assets.publishing.service.gov.uk/media/5c35e849ed915d732cade0a5/UK_measles_and_rubella_elimination_strategy.pdf (accessed on 30 June 2024).
28. Robert Koch Institute. Annual Status Update on Measles and Rubella Elimination in Germany 2022. Available online: https://www.rki.de/DE/Content/Kommissionen/NAVKO/Berichte/Bericht_2022_en.pdf?__blob=publicationFile (accessed on 30 June 2024).
29. Plans-Rubió, P. Vaccination coverage for routine vaccines and herd immunity levels against measles and pertussis in the world in 2019. *Vaccines* **2021**, *9*, 256. [CrossRef] [PubMed]

*vaccines*

MDPI

*Article*

# Strengthening of Vaccine-Preventable Disease (VPD) Surveillance to Enhance National Health Capacity and Security: Perspective from India

**Arun Kumar [1,*], Ratnesh Murugan [1], Satishchandra Donkatti [1], Deepa Sharma [1], Nirmal Kaundal [1], Tigran Avagyan [1], Pawan Kumar [2], Sunil Bahl [3], Sudhir Khanal [4] and Vinod Bura [4]**

1 World Health Organization, National Public Health Support Network, Country Office, New Delhi 110029, India; muruganr@who.int (R.M.); donkattis@who.int (S.D.); sharmade@who.int (D.S.); kaundaln@who.int (N.K.); avagyant@who.int (T.A.)

2 Ministry of Health and Family Welfare, Government of India, New Delhi 110011, India; drpawan.kumar@gov.in

3 Public Health Expert, Formerly with World Health Organization, South-East Asia Region, New Delhi 110001, India; bahlsk@gmail.com

4 World Health Organization, South-East Asia Region, New Delhi 110001, India; khanals@who.int (S.K.); burav@who.int (V.B.)

* Correspondence: akumar@who.int; Tel.: +91-11-66564800; Fax: +91-11-26162996

**Abstract:** The Government of India, in collaboration with the World Health Organization (WHO), established the National Polio Surveillance Project (NPSP) in 1997 and initiated acute flaccid paralysis (AFP) surveillance to achieve the goal of polio eradication. The WHO South-East Asia Region, comprising of 11 countries, including India, was certified as polio-free in March 2014. India was also validated to have eliminated maternal and neonatal tetanus in May 2015. Over the years, the surveillance of other vaccine-preventable diseases (VPDs) was integrated with AFP surveillance in the country. Outbreak-based measles–rubella (MR) surveillance was initiated in 2005 using AFP surveillance as a platform, case-based fever–rash (FR) surveillance started in 2021 as one of the strategies to achieve measles and rubella elimination in the country. The surveillance of diphtheria, pertussis, and neonatal tetanus was integrated with AFP surveillance in a phased manner during 2015–2022. The surveillance system for VPDs in India, supported by a laboratory network of 10 polio laboratories, 28 measles–rubella laboratories, and 20 diphtheria–pertussis laboratories, has enhanced the national health capacity and security. The setting up and expansion of the surveillance system in the country involved the important component of capacity building of personnel on various components of surveillance, including case identification, case investigation, sample collection and shipment, data analysis and public health response. These capacities have been used effectively during other emergencies, such as the recent COVID-19 pandemic, as well as during outbreaks of other diseases and natural calamities.

**Keywords:** surveillance; vaccine-preventable disease; acute flaccid paralysis; fever–rash; laboratory

## 1. Introduction

Vaccine-preventable disease (VPD) surveillance is defined as the routine ongoing collection, analysis, and dissemination of health data of vaccine-preventable diseases which includes the following functions: the detection and notification of health events, collection and consolidation of pertinent data, investigation and confirmation of VPDs, routine analysis and creation of reports, and feedback of information to persons providing data [1]. VPD surveillance is critical for monitoring the overall immunization program performance. The evidence generated through surveillance helps to identify outbreaks and take appropriate public health measures, guide the introduction of new vaccines, detect changes in disease epidemiology, and monitor the status of disease elimination or eradication.

The universal immunization program (UIP) of India is one of the largest routine immunization programs in the world. The annual birth cohort of the country is nearly 26 million. The diseases for which vaccines are provided under UIP are tuberculosis, polio, diphtheria, pertussis, tetanus, hepatitis B, *H. influenzae*, rotavirus, pneumococcus, measles, rubella, and Japanese Encephalitis (Table 1) [2].

**Table 1.** National immunization schedule—India [3].

| Age | Vaccines Given |
|---|---|
| Birth | BCG, OPV 0, Hepatitis B birth dose |
| 6 weeks | OPV 1, Pentavalent 1 *, Rotavirus 1, fractional IPV 1, PCV 1 |
| 10 weeks | OPV 2, Pentavalent 2, Rotavirus 2 |
| 14 weeks | OPV 3, Pentavalent 3, Rotavirus 3, fractional IPV 2, PCV 2 |
| 9–12 months | MR 1, JE 1 **, PCV booster, fIPV 3 |
| 16–24 months | MR 2, JE 2 **, DPT booster 1, OPV booster |
| 5–6 years | DPT booster 2 |
| 10 years | Td |
| 16 years | Td |
| Pregnant mother | Td 1, Td 2, Td booster *** |

OPV: oral poliovirus vaccine; IPV: inactivated poliovirus vaccine; PCV: pneumococcal conjugate vaccine; MR: measles–rubella vaccine; JE: Japanese Encephalitis vaccine; DPT: diphtheria, pertussis, and tetanus vaccine; Td: tetanus and adult diphtheria. * Pentavalent: diphtheria, pertussis, tetanus, hepatitis B, and *Hemophilus influenzae* type b. ** JE in endemic districts only. *** One dose if previously vaccinated within three years.

In India, the Immunization Division of the Ministry of Health and Family Welfare is responsible for the management of the immunization program and, with the technical support of the World Health Organization's National Public Health Support Network (WHO-NPSN), is also responsible for the quality and breadth of VPD surveillance in the country.

The Government of India, in collaboration with the World Health Organization, established the National Polio Surveillance Project (NPSP) in 1997 to support the case-based, laboratory-supported acute flaccid paralysis (AFP) surveillance system as one of the strategies to achieve polio eradication [4]. A polio laboratory network was also established in the same year. The environmental surveillance for poliovirus detection was initiated in 2001 at three sites in Mumbai as a supplement to the AFP surveillance system. The number of sites for environmental surveillance was expanded over the years, and currently, there exist 63 sites in 32 cities of 14 states.

The expansion of the AFP surveillance system to cover a broader range of infectious diseases was a critical part of the founding vision back in 1996. Building upon the existing AFP surveillance system of the polio eradication initiative, India initiated an outbreak-based measles–rubella (MR) surveillance system in a few states in 2005 and expanded this to all states by 2015. The country transitioned from an outbreak-based to case-based MR surveillance between 2016 and 2019. Beginning in 2018, fever–rash (FR) surveillance was piloted in three states of the country (Karnataka, Madhya Pradesh, and Odisha), and based on the findings from this pilot study, FR surveillance expanded to the entire country in 2021 wherein the suspected case definition was broadened to include all cases of fevers with maculopapular rashes (Figure 1). These efforts helped in increasing the sensitivity of measles–rubella surveillance in the country [5].

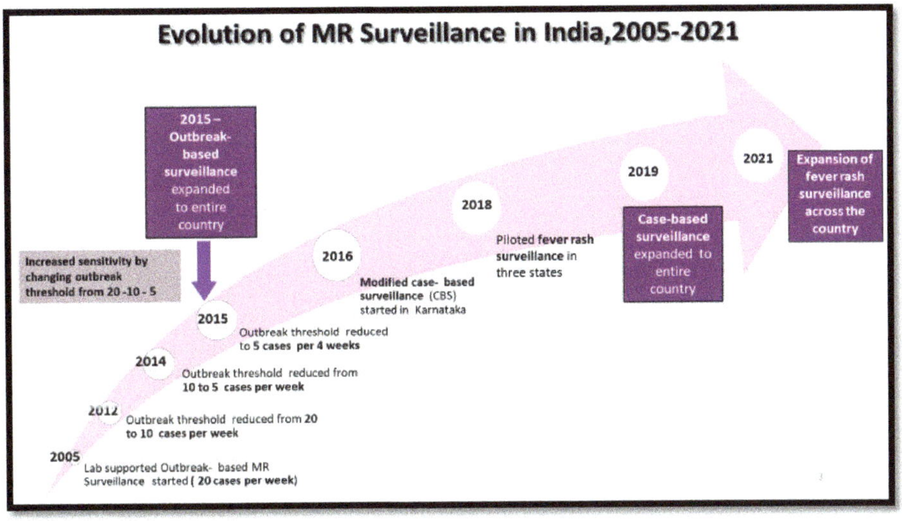


**Figure 1.** Evolution of MR surveillance system in India.

In 2015, the government mandated the WHO-NPSP to support laboratory-supported case-based diphtheria–pertussis–neonatal tetanus (DPT) surveillance in the country. The objective of this surveillance was to generate evidence to guide the immunization program of the country. This surveillance was added to the existing AFP-MR surveillance system in 2015 and was gradually expanded to all states of the country by August 2022 [5,6].

It is important to note that in 2004, the Government of India initiated an 'Integrated Disease Surveillance Project—IDSP' and included several VPDs, such as cholera, diphtheria, hepatitis A, influenza, JE, measles, meningococcal meningitis, mumps, pertussis, pneumococcal disease, polio, rubella, typhoid, and varicella, under this project. The main purpose of this surveillance system is to detect early warning signals of impending outbreaks and to help initiate an effective response in a timely manner. IDSP is a passive surveillance system that collects limited epidemiological data, does not collect data on immunization status of cases, and has limited involvement of the private sector and informal sectors [7].

The Indian Council of Medical Research—National Institute of Epidemiology (ICMR-NIE) has conducted sentinel surveillance for congenital rubella syndrome (CRS) since 2016. As of January 2024, there are 13 sentinel sites for CRS surveillance in the country.

Public health capacity is the ability to achieve stated public health objectives at the national, regional, and global levels with respect to both ongoing and emerging health problems [8]. Building the public health capacity is the process of improving the ability of the public health workforce to meet its objectives and to perform better. The public health workforce is the central component of the national public health capacity, which also includes infrastructural components such as resources, facilities, and appropriate technology [9].

Public health security is defined as the activities required, both proactive and reactive, to minimize the danger and impact of acute public health events that endanger people's health [10]. The International Health Regulation (IHR) 2005 calls for a strengthened national capacity for surveillance and control; prevention, alert, and response to international public health emergencies beyond the traditional short list of required reporting; global partnership and collaboration; and rights, obligations, accountability, and procedures of monitoring [11].

India's VPD surveillance program has enhanced both the public health capacity as well as the public health security. The aim of this article is to share insights into how the work towards strengthening and implementing comprehensive VPD surveillance has provided guidance for strengthening the national health capacity and national health security.

## 2. Methods

This article explains the processes related to the laboratory-supported VPD surveillance system in India conducted by the immunization division with the technical support of the WHO-NPSN.

### 2.1. VPD Surveillance Structure

A geographically well-distributed reporting network in the form of reporting units (RU) and informer units (IU) exists in the country.

1. Reporting units send regular weekly reports, including nil reports. As of January 2024, there are 12,022 reporting units in the country.
2. Informer units (IU) inform cases but do not send any weekly reports [3–5]. As of January 2024, there are 39,217 informer units in the country.

Taken together, more than 51,000 reporting sites have been established across the country. The reporting network involves both the public (~40%) and private (~60%) sectors, including Indian System of Medicine, i.e., AYUSH (Ayurveda, Yoga, Unani, Siddha, and Homeopathy), and other practitioners, based on the health-seeking behaviour of the community. Based on the potential of seeing suspected VPD cases, the reporting sites are classified into three priority categories—very high, high, and low. The VPD surveillance network stood the test of time during the COVID-19 pandemic as the reporting of AFP and FR cases continued during the pandemic.

### 2.2. Capacity Building of the Reporting Network

The reporting network is regularly sensitized for the identification and timely notification of suspected VPD cases. In 2023, approximately 5500 district and sub-district level workshops and >125,000 active case searches (ACSs) were conducted at these reporting sites. These ACS visits are important to assess the knowledge gaps existing among the health staff involved with VPD surveillance as well as to provide an opportunity to sensitize them. Surveillance posters and audio-visuals have been used to sensitize the health staff on the importance of VPD surveillance and overall surveillance processes.

### 2.3. Response to Reported VPD Cases

More than 90% of the suspected VPD cases get investigated within 48 h of notification by trained medical officers. The epidemiological data are collected through a case investigation form (CIF). Samples are collected as per the surveillance protocol and are shipped to the designated WHO-accredited laboratories in a timely manner under the required cold chain conditions.

### 2.4. Laboratory Network for VPD Surveillance

There are 58 VPD laboratories in the country for polio, MR, and diphtheria–pertussis (DP). These laboratories ensure the timely testing of samples to guide the surveillance and immunization program of the country. The WHO-NPSN with support from the government provides technical guidance and capacity building support for sample testing and quality assurance in these laboratories.

#### 2.4.1. Polio Laboratory Network

To maintain the achievement of the polio-free status, the country continues to have eight WHO-accredited polio laboratories since 1997 and two sewage sample concentration laboratories since 2016 (Figure 2). These polio laboratories are part of Global Polio Laboratory Network (GPLN).

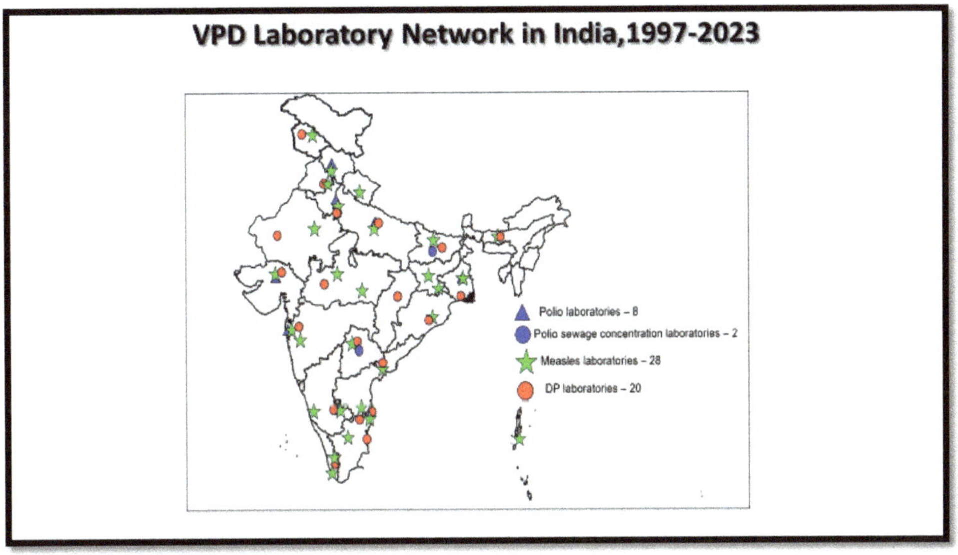


**Figure 2.** VPD laboratory network (polio, MR, and DP).

2.4.2. MR Laboratory Network

The MR laboratory network was established in 2005 based on the framework of polio laboratories and expanded to 28 laboratories to support the elimination program (Figure 2). Two of them are regional reference laboratories, seven are national laboratories, and nineteen are sub-national laboratories. The National Institute of Virology (NIV), Mumbai (for sequencing), and King Institute of Preventive Medicine (KIPM), Chennai (for serology), are designated as regional reference laboratories [12].

2.4.3. DP Laboratory Network

The DP laboratory network was established in 2015 to support the surveillance program for the control of diseases and timely public health interventions. The gradual expansion of DP laboratories has been carried out with the expansion of DPT surveillance all over the country. As of 2023, there are 20 DP laboratories in the country, and the Christian Medical College (CMC) at Vellore has been designated to serve as the reference laboratory (Figure 2). These laboratories perform bacterial culture and molecular and serologic testing.

## 3. Results

Continuous efforts have been made to strengthen the VPD surveillance system in India, including the following:

- Identification and sensitization of potential informers (faith healers, temple sites, Indian System of Medicine [ISM] practitioners, and others): There has been an expansion of the reporting network to increase VPD surveillance reporting. From 41,800 reporting sites in 2015, the network has expanded to more than 51,000 reporting sites in the country.
- · Capacity building of health functionaries: Between January 2020 and December 2023, more than 22,000 workshops on surveillance have been conducted, with more than 400,000 health personnel trained and oriented on VPDs through these cascaded training sessions across India. In 2023, approximately 5500 workshops were conducted at health facilities.

- Active case searches (ACSs) at the reporting sites: Between January 2020 and December 2023, more than 500,000 ACS visits have been made by government officers (District Immunization Officers/District Surveillance Officers/Surveillance Nodal Medical Officers) and WHO-NPSN Surveillance Medical Officers. In 2023 alone, more than 125,000 of these ACS visits were conducted at health facilities.
- Expansion of VPD laboratory network across the country: The expansion of surveillance has resulted in the expansion of both virology and bacteriology laboratories in the country. There is a strong component of quality assurance and quality control in these laboratories.
- Program review: Annually, two to three state-level VPD surveillance reviews are conducted in the country. These reviews have integrated the UIP reviews as well. Further, there is a close tracking of the progress of the immunization and surveillance program in the country through task force meetings, which are conducted periodically, usually monthly.
- Efficient data analysis and feedback mechanism: At the time of the initiation of AFP surveillance in 1997, data collation and analysis were mainly conducted using an Excel-based system. From 2005 to June 2023, the data management had been conducted through an offline epi-info based system called the Surveillance Information Management system (SIMS). From July 2023, the VPD surveillance data are being managed through a real time web-based tool called the 'vaccine-preventable disease surveillance information management system (VSIMS)'.

As a result of the continuous efforts listed above, the VPD surveillance system has improved, as evident in the improvement of cardinal indicators of VPD surveillance mentioned below.

### *3.1. AFP Surveillance*

The country continues to maintain and sustain the quality of AFP surveillance with indicators above the global recommended levels. The non-polio AFP rate for the country is well above the global recommended target (≥1 per 100,000 populations of less than 15 years of age). In 2023, the non-polio AFP rate was 5.8. Similarly, stool adequacy at the national level in 2023 was 89%—again above the global recommended target (≥80% of AFP cases, where two adequate stool specimens were collected within 14 days of paralysis onset) [13].

### *3.2. Measles and Rubella Surveillance*

Over the years, MR surveillance has been strengthened in the country, especially as evidenced by the recent trend in non-measles–non-rubella (NMNR) discard rate, which is the globally accepted cardinal indicator for measuring MR surveillance sensitivity. The NMNR discard rate has shown tremendous progress, as a result of various surveillance strengthening efforts, and has improved from 0.53 in 2018 to 5.61 in 2023 (as of 10 January 2024) (Figure 3). This is two and half times greater than the global recommended standards of ≥2 per 100,000 population [14].

Additionally, the percentage of cases with adequate serum specimen collected within 28 days of rash onset was found to be above the global recommended target in 2023 (95% in 2023).

Measles–rubella outbreaks: The country's sensitive surveillance has detected measles/ rubella outbreaks in areas of immunity gaps. In 2023, of the 2225 suspected outbreaks investigated, 1215 were lab-confirmed measles outbreaks, and 13 were lab-confirmed rubella outbreaks [14]. Appropriate public health response measures were initiated, and more than 30 million children were vaccinated through MR campaigns and special immunization drives, including the outbreak response immunization in 2023.

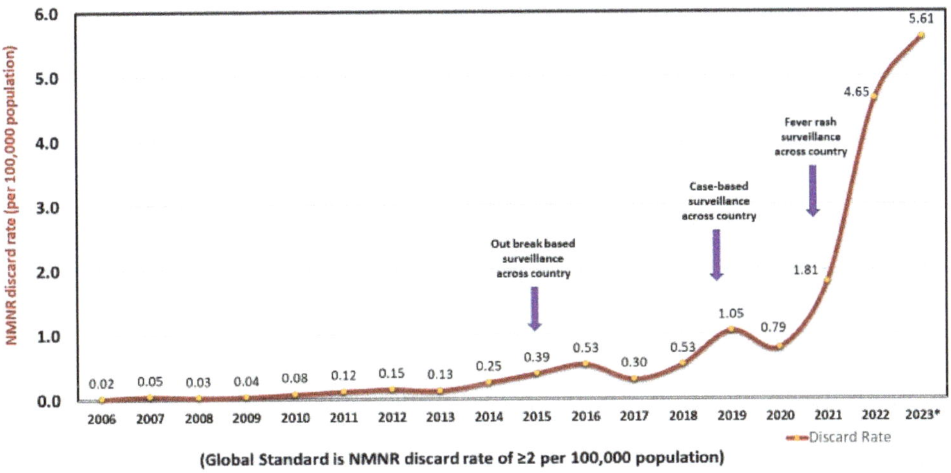


**Figure 3.** Non-measles–non-rubella discard rate (per 100,000 population), India, 2006–2023 *. * data as on 10 January 2024.

With the enhancement of surveillance sensitivity, the number of fever-rash cases reported to the surveillance program increased from 33,379 in 2021 to 154,372 in 2023. Few of the case characteristics have been detailed in Table 2.

**Table 2.** Distribution of fever–rash cases by age, sex, and setting, 2021–2023.

| | | 2021 | 2022 | 2023 |
|---|---|---|---|---|
| Fever–rash cases | | 33,379 | 112,226 | 154,372 |
| Age group | <5 years | 50% | 53% | 48% |
| | 5–10 years | 20% | 24% | 26% |
| | >10 years | 30% | 23% | 26% |
| Sex | Male | 56% | 55% | 55% |
| | Female | 44% | 45% | 45% |
| Setting | Rural | 71% | 64% | 69% |
| | Urban | 29% | 36% | 31% |

*3.3. Diphtheria, Pertussis, and Neonatal Tetanus Surveillance*

DPT surveillance guides the immunization program of the country.

Diphtheria: A total of 3724 suspected diphtheria cases have been reported in the country in 2023, compared to 3318 cases in 2022. Approximately 75% cases in 2022 and 80% cases in 2023 were in persons above five years of age. The overall incidence of suspected diphtheria cases at the national level was 2.3 and 2.7 per million population in 2022 and 2023, respectively.

Pertussis: A total of 4876 suspected pertussis cases have been reported in the country in 2023, compared to 4412 cases in 2022. Approximately 54% cases in 2022 and 63% cases in 2023 were in children below five years of age. The overall incidence of suspected pertussis cases at the national level was 2.3 and 2.7 per million population in 2022 and 2023, respectively.

Neonatal tetanus: Sixty-two cases of neonatal tetanus have been reported in the country in 2023, compared to the sixty-five cases reported in 2022. None of the districts in the country had neonatal tetanus cases above the elimination level, i.e., ≥1 NT case per 1000 live births during 2022 and 2023. Based on the surveillance data, the Standing

Working Group on VPD surveillance under the National Technical Advisory Group on Immunization (NTAGI) has recommended that 'a post-validation MNTE assessment should be considered in select districts which have reported several neonatal tetanus cases, even though the rate of disease is below the rate used to define MNTE' [15].

### 3.4. VPD Laboratory Network

The laboratory network has immensely supported the VPD surveillance in the country. The timely provision of results by the laboratories has led to a timely response in the community. The number of samples processed by these laboratories over the years is shown below in Table 3.

**Table 3.** Sample testing load at VPD surveillance laboratories.

| Year | 1997–2023 | 2005–2023 | 2006–2023 | 2014–2023 | 2019–2023 |
|---|---|---|---|---|---|
| Polio (AFP) | 1,721,408 | | | | |
| Polio (ES) | | 17,100 | | | |
| MR (Serology) | | | 309,200 | | |
| MR (Molecular) | | | | 161,364 | |
| Diphtheria (TS) | | | | | 16,985 |
| Pertussis (NPS and Serology) | | | | | 23,256 |

AFP, acute flaccid paralysis; ES, environmental surveillance; TS, throat swab; NPS, nasopharyngeal swab.

## 4. Discussion

Continuous efforts have been made to strengthen the VPD surveillance system in India, which has resulted in enhancing the national health capacity and security. The best practices adopted are listed below.

### 4.1. Best Practices towards Health Capacity Enhancement

#### 4.1.1. Capacity Building of Health Personnel

High-quality cascaded training workshops with simulation exercises on the VPD outbreak investigation and response has helped in strengthening the outbreak response. The sensitization of frontline health workers, potential informers, and community leaders and the engagement of private health sector have strengthened the surveillance system, thereby improving the outbreak detection and response capacity. In 2023, 85% of the suspected diphtheria cases were notified within 7 days of onset of sore throat, and 95% of the notified cases were investigated within 48 h of notification. Approximately 95% of the notified suspected FR cases were investigated within 48 h, and adequate serological samples were collected in 97% of cases. In 2023, 1215 measles outbreaks were identified, and in 98% of these outbreaks, public health response activities were conducted, including outbreak response immunization.

#### 4.1.2. Ensuring Quality of Surveillance System at Par with the Global Standards

The verification and desk review of the case investigation forms of suspected VPDs by Surveillance Medical Officers of the WHO-NPSN, District Immunization Officers/Nodal Medical officers has ensured the reliable and quality data of VPDs to assess the disease burden. Such independent reviews of the investigation forms provide an extra layer of quality control for effective surveillance. These data are being used to provide guidance for policy decisions and to formulate evidence-based recommendations.

#### 4.1.3. Surveillance-Guided Program Planning and Implementation

Reliable and timely information is being provided through an effective and sensitive VPD surveillance for immediate public health response- and evidence-based policy decisions for program planning and implementation.

The surveillance data of AFP system helped in the identification of areas at high risk of polio transmission, which further helped in targeted mop-up campaigns, served as the final blow to interrupt the wild poliovirus (WPV) transmission. This has guided India to achieve and sustain their polio-free status since 13 January 2011. The best example is the development of the Kosi River operational plan to overcome the challenges in the access-compromised area (ACA) of Kosi River basin, which was the hub of WPV transmission in the state of Bihar. The plan was implemented successfully for several mop-up campaigns for polio, which resulted in a sharp decline in missed children during polio supplementary immunization activity (SIA) by the end of 2011 (1.4% missed children) as compared to 2008 (13.0% missed children) before the implementation of the plan. As a result, Bihar significantly reduced the transmission of WPV type 1 in the high transmission season and interrupted polio transmission in the main polio reservoir. With the help of this plan, the capacity was built to respond to exceptional circumstances like floods in the Kosi riverine area [16].

The AFP surveillance system has been leveraged to also support case-based, laboratory-supported measles–rubella surveillance. Based on the surveillance data, outbreak-based MR surveillance transitioned from the aggregate reporting of disease to case-based disease surveillance. MR surveillance has provided data for action in the form of policy decisions to introduce rubella-containing vaccines in the immunization program and to plan wide age-range MR SIAs across the country. As one of the key strategy, MR surveillance is guiding the progress towards the achievement of MR elimination in India [17].

The learned findings of the AFP and MR surveillance systems have been utilized to expand surveillance of other VPDs—diphtheria, pertussis and neonatal tetanus. The laboratory-supported surveillance data of diphtheria in 2017 and 2018 indicated a higher diphtheria burden in the age group of 5 years and above. The National Technical Advisory Group on Immunization (NTAGI) reviewed the surveillance data and recommended the introduction of the Td vaccine in UIP, replacing the TT vaccine in line with global recommendations, which was substantiated by the evidence of the age shift that was observed in diphtheria surveillance data. This resulted in the change from the TT vaccine to the Td vaccine in the adolescent age group of 10 years and 16 years as well as to pregnant women, a critical milestone in India's effort to enhance the overall capacity of primary care and public health services [18].

#### 4.1.4. Strengthening of VPD Surveillance and Routine Immunization (RI) Program [19]

- High-risk areas identified through VPD surveillance were linked to RI session sites to improve immunization coverage;
- Advocacy and accountability framework through state, district/city, and block task forces for the polio program were utilized for other VPD surveillance and RI program reviews;
- VPD surveillance field reviews integrated the UIP field review to identify the gaps in the surveillance and routine immunization program, thereby strengthening VPD surveillance and RI;
- The identification and enlistment of areas vulnerable to MR outbreaks and carrying out the risk reprioritization of outbreak areas into high-risk areas for risk mitigation measures are crucial to prevent the outbreaks. This has resulted in the strengthening of the immunization and health system [20].

#### 4.1.5. Epidemic Response Team (ERT) at State/District/Block Levels

ERTs have been constituted at the state and district levels as a preparedness measure to rapidly respond to VPD outbreaks. At the state level, the State Immunization Officer, State

Surveillance Officer from IDSP, and Sub-regional Team Leader and, at the district level, the District Immunization Officer (DIO), District Surveillance Officer (DSO), and Surveillance Medical Officer of NPSN are providing direct oversight to the state and district ERTs, respectively. The constitution and effective coordination of all the key players of the ERT at all levels for immediate public health responses have been found to be critical towards initiating early investigations and implementing public health response measures. During the COVID-19 pandemic, the WHO-NPSN SMOs coordinated at the district and block levels to mobilize the ERT to support contact tracing, home quarantine, and home isolation.

#### 4.1.6. VPD Surveillance System Backed by an Effective Network of Diagnostic Laboratories

Laboratory networks play a pivotal role in the accurate and timely confirmation of infections supporting public health response to the disease and thus become an essential component of the disease surveillance system. These laboratory networks guide programs for disease control, elimination, and eradication [21].

An efficient AFP and environmental surveillance system for poliovirus detection has continuously been supported by the WHO-accredited laboratory network for the virological diagnosis of polioviruses. Considering the sensitivity of environmental surveillance in detecting the silent transmission of WPV/vaccine-derived poliovirus (VDPV), ES has been expanded further in Rajasthan, Punjab, Jammu, and Kashmir in 2022–2023, all near the international border with Pakistan, which is still endemic for WPV1. ES was successfully used to demonstrate the end of WPV transmission in the country as well as to judge the effectiveness of polio immunization campaigns, and post polio-free certification, it is used as supplementary surveillance to screen presence of any WPV/VDPV in the country [22–25].

Twenty-eight MR laboratory networks are supporting laboratory-based surveillance to reach MR elimination goal in the country, while 20 bacteriology laboratories are supporting the control of diphtheria–pertussis. The diagnosis and case classification through the results obtained from these laboratory support programs take quick actions for mass immunization or develop additional strategies to control the infection/outbreaks.

Nearly all the VPD laboratories belong to the public sector and have the capacity to detect the viral and bacteriological pathogens, as necessitated.

#### 4.1.7. Leveraging VPD Surveillance System for COVID-19 Response and Other Public Health Priorities

The efforts towards nurturing VPD surveillance in the country that included the expansion of the reporting network, capacity building, case notification, sample collection, and shipment proved immensely useful during the COVID-19 pandemic. The existing VPD surveillance and IDSP platforms were utilized effectively to operationalize the collection of case data during the recent COVID-19 pandemic. The medical officers involved with the investigation of VPD cases were trained to investigate the COVID-19 cases and collect information on a case investigation form that was developed for influenza-like illness (ILI) and severe acute respiratory infection (SARI) [26].

In 11 cities of the country, the environmental surveillance sites for poliovirus detection were leveraged for the detection of SARS CoV-2 RNA. Eight polio labs were involved with testing sewage samples for SARS CoV-2, in addition to testing for polioviruses. The evidence generated through this surveillance demonstrated a linear relation between the increase in the load of COVID-19 cases detected through case-based surveillance and positivity in the sewage sample, thereby demonstrating the utility of the system.

As a part of the COVID-19 surveillance strengthening efforts, laboratories played a pivotal role in surveillance while maintaining good quality within the laboratory network, which helped in identifying control measures for the disease. The WHO supported the quality of laboratory network operating under the Ministry of Health and Family Welfare, the Indian Council of Medical Research, and the National Centre for Disease Control by providing an external quality assurance panel (EQAP) [27]. Out of 1312 laboratories which participated, 91% qualified by achieving ≥80% scores, thus assuring the quality of testing under these laboratories for COVID-19 detection.

These measures led to a timely detection of COVID-19 cases and guided the implementation of rapid public health response measures.

The task forces established earlier for polio elimination at the district and state levels were utilized for the COVID-19 pandemic and ensured good intersectoral coordination for effective public health response measures, including for COVID-19 vaccination coverage.

Taking the learned findings of VPD surveillance and routine immunization, training modules were developed for capacity building of the stakeholders for the COVID-19 vaccination program at all levels. Cascaded training was conducted across the country to build the capacity of health staff. India has extended support to other countries through capacity building and the sharing of their experience on the rollout of the COVID-19 vaccine.

Other public health priorities: During 2016–2022, under the EIS and FETP, the WHO-NPSN network provided support in detailed epidemiologic investigations of the select outbreaks of cholera, acute diarrheal disease, dengue, chicken pox, typhoid, malaria, hepatitis A, H1N1, and Kyasanur Forest Disease (KFD). VPD surveillance tools were used to strengthen KFD surveillance in the vulnerable districts of Karnataka. The capacity of the local government was built for surveillance and outbreak responses, including conducting vaccination campaigns for KFD control [28].

The NPSN personnel have also been involved in flood/cyclone responses in the states of Kerala, Odisha, and Tamil Nadu in recent years. The staff supported the public health response to communicable diseases during the floods and also strengthened surveillance for communicable diseases in these areas.

### *4.2. Best Practices towards Health Security Enhancement*

#### 4.2.1. Governance Mechanism and Intersectoral Coordination

With strong governance in the form of task forces at various levels and good intersectoral coordination, the strategies of polio eradication were effectively implemented that led to the polio-free status in India. The findings were carried forward to track and review the MR elimination progress and to strengthen outbreak preparedness and response measures for other VPDs like MR, diphtheria, and pertussis.

#### 4.2.2. Cross-Border Cooperation

Infectious diseases do not respect international borders. Cross-border coordination for vaccination strategies and surveillance proved essential for the eradication of polio. The best example is the expansion of environmental surveillance sites for poliovirus detection in select cities along the Indo-Pakistan border and the vaccination sites along the borders of the country with neighboring countries, notably Bangladesh, Nepal, and Pakistan.

#### 4.2.3. Data Management System

An efficient and robust data management system is in place with the capacity to detect impending outbreaks through early warning signals for immediate public health responses. The triangulation of vaccination coverage and VPD surveillance data helps to better understand the immunity gaps in the population and support policy decisions targeted towards strengthening the immunization system.

#### 4.2.4. Support in Public Health Emergencies of National and International Concern

The capacity built over the years among the VPD surveillance staff in India has been used during public health emergencies outside the country such as during the Ebola outbreak in Western Africa, polio outbreak in Nigeria, and diphtheria outbreak in Cox's Bazar. The same has been replicated in India, most recently with regard to the COVID-19 pandemic. An adequate VPD surveillance system backed by an effective network of WHO-accredited diagnostic laboratories enhance the country's capacity to detect and manage other communicable diseases of public health concern.

## 5. Strengths and Limitations of the Surveillance System

Strengths: The surveillance system for VPDs in India extends across the length and breadth of the country, covering every district of every state and union territory of the country. The reporting network for VPDs includes health facilities both from the public and private sectors and can be adjusted based on the health-seeking behavior of the community to individual diseases. The system is a case-based, laboratory-supported system that is able to generate detailed information on cases and outbreaks of individual diseases that contributes to the control/elimination of such diseases. The surveillance system has a built-in component of active surveillance that improves the reporting of the VPDs that are under the surveillance. The data management and analysis component of the system not only ensures collation of the large data base but also ensures the availability of real-time information that can be put to programmatic action at the state and district levels, in addition to policy decision making at the national level. Indicators to measure the sensitivity of the system are well defined and used to assess the same at the national and subnational levels, based on which gaps in quality can be identified and appropriate changes made to enhance quality. The system has ensured building national capacity for surveillance and public health response to several diseases, even those outside of the scope of the current system.

Limitations: The surveillance system is resource intensive and needs dedicated staff and finances to support the field implementation and laboratory testing of samples. Integration with IDSP will require a revision in the protocols of IDSP so that the system can serve the needs for VPDs, especially those that are targeted for elimination.

## 6. Conclusions

India initiated VPD surveillance with AFP surveillance in 1997, and over the years, AFP surveillance has been strengthened and environmental, MR surveillance, other VPDs like diphtheria, pertussis, and neonatal tetanus have been integrated into this surveillance system. The geographically well-distributed WHO-accredited/proficient VPD surveillance laboratories are an integral component of the surveillance system.

India's experience with VPD surveillance strengthening efforts has guided the immunization program. It has enhanced the national health capacity and security in terms of detection and response to VPDs, thereby contributing to the eradication of polio, the elimination of maternal and neonatal tetanus, efforts towards the elimination of measles and rubella, and the control of diphtheria, pertussis, and other VPDs. The efforts made to maintain the VPD surveillance system have the potential to contribute to support the surveillance of other diseases, thereby enhancing national health capacity and security.

**Author Contributions:** Conceptualization, A.K., R.M. and S.K.; Methodology, A.K., R.M., S.D. and D.S; Validation, A.K. and R.M.; Formal analysis, A.K., R.M., S.D. and D.S.; Data curation, A.K., R.M., S.D. and D.S.; Writing—original draft, A.K., R.M., S.D., D.S. and N.K.; Writing—review and editing, A.K., R.M., T.A., P.K., S.B. and S.K.; Supervision, T.A., P.K., S.B., V.B. and S.K.; Project administration, T.A. and V.B. All authors have read and agreed to the published version of the manuscript.

**Funding:** This research received no external funding.

**Institutional Review Board Statement:** Not applicable.

**Informed Consent Statement:** Not applicable.

**Data Availability Statement:** The raw data supporting this article will be made available by the authors without undue reservation.

**Acknowledgments:** We thank the VPD surveillance field team and data team of National Public Health Support Network (NPSN).

Conflicts of Interest: The authors declare no conflicts of interest.

## References

1. World Health Organization. Vaccine Preventable Diseases Surveillance Standards. Available online: https://www.who.int/teams/immunization-vaccines-and-biologicals/immunization-analysis-and-insights/surveillance/surveillance-for-vpds/vpd-surveillance-standards (accessed on 8 April 2024).
2. Ministry of Health and Family Welfare; Government of India. *A Big Leap Towards Measles & Rubella Elimination. Intensified Mission Indradhanush 5.0, Operational Guidelines*; Government of India: New Delhi, India, 2023.
3. Ministry of Health and Family Welfare; Government of India. National Immunization Schedule. Available online: https://nhm.gov.in/New_Updates_2018/NHM_Components/Immunization/report/National_%20Immunization_Schedule.pdf (accessed on 8 April 2024).
4. Child Health Division; Department of Family Welfare Ministry of Health & Family Welfare New Delhi. *Field Guide. Surveillance of Acute Flaccid Paralysis*, 3rd ed.; Ministry of Health & Family Welfare: New Delhi, India, 2005.
5. Ministry of Health and Family Welfare; Government of India. *Measles and Rubella Surveillance Field Guide 2020*; Government of India: New Delhi, India, 2020.
6. Ministry of Health and Family Welfare; Government of India. *Surveillance of Diphtheria, Pertussis and Neonatal Tetanus, Field Guide, India*, 1st ed.; Government of India: New Delhi, India, 2020.
7. Blanchard, J.; Washington, R.; Becker, M.; Vasanthakumar, N.; Madangopal, K.; Sarwal, R.; Becker, M. *Vision 2035: Public Health Surveillance in India. A White Paper*; NITI Aayog/Government of India: New Delhi, India, 2020.
8. Brown, L.; LaFond, A.; Macintyre, K. *Measuring Capacity Building*; Carolina Population Center/University of North Carolina: Chapel Hill, NC, USA, 2001.
9. Beaglehole, R.; Dal Poz, M.R. Public health workforce: Challenges and policy issues. *Hum. Resour. Health* **2003**, *1*, 4. [CrossRef]
10. World Health Organization. Health Security. Available online: https://www.who.int/health-topics/health-security#tab=tab_1 (accessed on 8 April 2024).
11. World Health Organization. International Health Regulations. 2005. Available online: https://www.who.int/publications/i/item/9789241580410 (accessed on 8 April 2024).
12. Sharma, D.; Sangal, L.; Vijay, N.; Nalavade, U.; Krishnasamy, K.; Pawar, S.; Kaur, H.; Narayan, J.; Rane, S.; Narkar, M. Expansion of the measles and rubella laboratory network, India. *Bull. World Health Organ.* **2022**, *100*, 247–255. [CrossRef]
13. World Health Organization. *Health. Acute Flaccid Paralysis Surveillance Bulletin*; World Health Organization: Geneva, Switzerland, 2024.
14. World Health Organization. *Health. Measles Rubella Surveillance Bulletin*; World Health Organization: Geneva, Switzerland, 2024.
15. World Health Organization. *Health. Diphtheria, Pertussis and Neonatal Tetanus Surveillance Bulletin*; World Health Organization: Geneva, Switzerland, 2024.
16. Ministry of Health and Family Welfare; Government of India. *Polio Eradication Initiative, Bihar. Kosi Operational Plan Bihar. Standard Operating Procedures*; Government of India: New Delhi, India, 2009.
17. Ministry of Health and Family Welfare; Government of India. *Introduction of Measles Rubella Vaccine (Campaign and Routine Immunization. National Operational Guidelines*; Government of India: New Delhi, India, 2017.
18. Ministry of Health and Family Welfare; Government of India. *Strengthening Td 10 and Td 16 Vaccine Implementation. Operational Guidelines and Strategic Plan*; Government of India: New Delhi, India, 2019.
19. Ministry of Health and Family Welfare; Government of India. *Immunization Handbook for Medical Officers*, 2nd ed.; Government of India: New Delhi, India, 2017.
20. Ministry of Health and Family Welfare; Government of India. *Roadmap to Measles & Rubella Elimination in India by 2023*; Government of India: New Delhi, India, 2022.
21. Mulders, M.N.; Serhan, F.; Goodson, J.L.; Icenogle, J.; Johnson, B.W.; Rota, P.A. Expansion of Surveillance for Vaccine-preventable Diseases: Building on the Global Polio Laboratory Network and the Global Measles and Rubella Laboratory Network Platforms. *J. Infect. Dis.* **2017**, *216* (Suppl. 1), S324–S330. [CrossRef] [PubMed]
22. Manor, Y.; Handsher, R.; Halmut, T.; Neuman, M.; Bobrov, A.; Rudich, H.; Vansover, A.; Shulman, L.; Kew, O.; Mendelson, E. Detection of poliovirus circulation by environmental surveillance in the absence of clinical cases in Israel and the Palestinian authority. *J. Clin. Microbiol.* **1999**, *37*, 1670–1675. [CrossRef]
23. Pöyry, T.; Stenvik, M.; Hovi, T. Viruses in sewage waters during and after a poliomyelitis outbreak and subsequent nationwide oral poliovirus vaccination campaign in Finland. *Appl. Environ. Microbiol.* **1998**, *30*, 212–222. [CrossRef] [PubMed]
24. Avoort, H.G.V.D.; Reimerink, J.H.; Ras, A.; Mulders, M.N.; Van Loon, A.M. Isolation of epidemic poliovirus from sewage during the 1992–3 type 3 outbreak in The Netherlands. *Epidemiol. Infect.* **1995**, *114*, 481–491. [CrossRef]
25. Deshpande, J.M.; Shetty, S.J.; Siddiqui, Z.A. Environmental surveillance system to track wild poliovirus transmission. *Appl. Environ. Microbiol.* **2003**, *69*, 2919–2927. [CrossRef] [PubMed] [PubMed Central]
26. National Centre for Disease Control; Government of India. *Standard Operating Procedures (SOPs) for Investigation of a Suspected COVID-19 Case Using Case Investigation Form (CIF)*; Government of India: New Delhi, India, 2020.

27. Kaur, H.; Mukhopadhyay, L.; Gupta, N.; Aggarwal, N.; Sangal, L.; Potdar, V.; Inbanathan, F.Y.; Narayan, J.; Gupta, S.; Rana, S.; et al. External quality assessment of COVID-19 real time reverse transcription PCR laboratories in India. *PLoS ONE* **2022**, *17*, e0263736. [CrossRef]
28. Directorate of Health and Family Welfare Services; Government of Karnataka. *Operational Manual Kyasanur Forest Disease*; Government of Karnataka: Karnataka, India, 2020.

vaccines

MDPI

Article

# Lessons from Recent Measles Post-Campaign Coverage Surveys Worldwide

M. Carolina Danovaro-Holliday [1,*], Mitsuki Koh [1], Claudia Steulet [1], Dale A. Rhoda [2] and Mary Kay Trimner [2]

1 World Health Organization, 1211 Geneva, Switzerland
2 Biostat Global Consulting, Worthington, OH 43085, USA; dale.rhoda@biostatglobal.com (D.A.R.)
* Correspondence: danovaroc@who.int

**Abstract:** Background: Measles elimination strategies include supplementary immunization activities (SIAs) to rapidly fill immunity gaps. Post-campaign coverage surveys (PCCSs) are recommended to assess SIA coverage. We characterized selected PCCSs performed following recent SIAs, highlighting specific challenges and strengths, and provide recommendations for improvement. Methods: We extracted national SIA data from the global measles/MR SIA database for the period of 2020–2023 and reviewed PCCS reports available at the World Health Organization headquarters. We extracted selected information on PCCS implementation, including information about the implementer, sampling, and main results. Results: Only 15 of 66 countries (23%) with a national-level SIA performed since 2020 had a PCCS report available. We reviewed those reports, plus six more, following three 2019 SIAs with a delayed PCCS and two PCCSs following large subnational SIAs (Kenya 2021 and Yemen 2023). All 24 PCCS reports available were from Gavi-eligible countries, with 15 from South Saharan Africa (Cameroon, the Democratic Republic of the Congo, and Ethiopia had two PCCSs). Eleven (45.8%) PCCSs were conducted within three months of the end of the SIA. All included sampling information and most had percentage of participation. Description of the interviewers' profiles varied but was limited. PCCS coverage was lower than administrative data in all but two instances. All PCCSs collected data on previous measles vaccination status that would allow exploring indicators on the SIA reaching previously measles zero-dose children. Of the 12 PCCSs reporting coverage among previously measles zero-dose children, nine reported coverage among this group of more than 50% (range: 12% and 91.6%). Conclusion: Even though a PCCS following an SIA is recommended and a requirement in Gavi-supported countries, most SIAs are not followed by a PCCS and, when performed, the timeliness of survey implementation needs improvement. Recent PCCSs were independently conducted and reports included basic survey information, but analysis and presentation of survey results vary particularly for measles zero-dose-related indicators. More guidance and technical support on how to implement PCCSs, including standardization of reports and more in-depth PCCS analyses, may help improve reporting and use of available PCCS data.

**Keywords:** measles; post-campaign coverage surveys; supplementary immunization activities; coverage

## 1. Background

Since the launch of the Expanded Program on Immunization (EPI) 50 years ago, over 154 million vaccine-preventable deaths have been averted, with measles vaccination contributing in a great extent to this achievement [1]. The World Health Organization (WHO) recommends two doses of a measles-containing vaccine (MCV) to be given in routine immunization (RI) [2]. In addition, supplementary immunization activities (SIAs) are a common strategy used to fill immunity gaps resulting from incomplete vaccination through RI services [3,4]. SIAs have been part of measles elimination strategies since their development in the 1990s [4,5]. During an SIA, age- and place-eligible persons, most often children, are vaccinated regardless of their previous vaccination status. In most low- and middle-income countries, SIAs occur every 2–5 years, as the number of measles-susceptible persons accumulate from incomplete vaccination coverage with one or two doses [3,6–8]. SIAs have been found to be more equitable in reaching children than routine immunization in several countries [9], and their timeliness and performance have been under much scrutiny recently [10,11]. Most countries have now also introduced rubella vaccination and use measles-rubella-containing (MR) vaccines, with SIAs effectively contributing to rubella control and elimination [12,13]. During the COVID-19 pandemic, not only did MCV1 and MCV2 coverage decline globally [14–16], but also many SIAs were cancelled or postponed [17]. MCV coverage is yet to reach pre-pandemic levels globally. As a result, several outbreaks are now occurring across the globe [18–20].

To be effective, SIAs need to reach high and homogenous coverage; reaching communities and children previously missed by RI is particularly important. To evaluate the coverage reached by an SIA, the Measles and Rubella Partnership (former Measles Rubella Initiative) recommends implementing an independent post-campaign coverage survey (PCCS) within three months of SIA implementation. For measles and MR SIAs implemented with support from Gavi, the Vaccine Alliance, a PCCS following WHO guidance is required [21–23]. A PCCS does not replace intra-campaign monitoring using real-time monitoring of the process, administrative data, and rapid convenience monitoring [3,24–26]. However, a PCCS is considered an important tool to estimate the coverage reached by the SIA, to evaluate coverage among children who were previously zero-dose measles vs. those who had been previously vaccinated, and to better understand enablers and barriers to vaccination [22,27].

Concerns have been raised about the quality of vaccination coverage surveys in general and for those following measles campaigns in particular [25,28]. In 2015, the WHO released new survey guidance, first as a working draft and in 2018 as a final product, and accompanying analytical software to overcome some of the challenges [22,28]. Countries have since moved toward conducting independent, probability sampling, vaccination coverage surveys that use probability sampling. This manuscript explores the implementation of PCCSs following measles and MR SIAs since 2020, in addition to selected PCCSs not included in a related publication manuscript published in 2021 [21]. It also characterizes the PCCSs conducted, highlighting specific challenges and strengths, and provides recommendations for improvement.

## 2. Methods

We extracted SIA data from the measles/MR SIA database and reviewed the PCCS reports available at the World Health Organization headquarters as of 11 July 2024. We restricted the analysis to PCCSs conducted since 2020, as a summary of PCCSs conducted between 2017 and 2019 was published by Cutts et al. [21]. However, PCCS reports for 2019 SIAs that were not included in that publication were also included here.

We extracted data on country, vaccine type, SIA date, target age group, estimated target population, administrative coverage, and conduct of the PCCS. For the available PCCS reports, we extracted information on whether it was a national-level survey, dates of field work, sample size, SIA cards or finger marking seen, profile of the implementing partner, sampling approach, length of training, the composition of teams and the supervision provided, and whether the PCCS included questions related to barriers and enablers to vaccination or on reasons for no vaccination. Regarding the results, we extracted information on whether a description of the sample, including the exclusion of certain areas and clusters, was presented. We also extracted MCV RI coverage, SIA overall coverage, and information related to measles zero-dose children, including the proportion receiving their first MCV dose in the SIA, SIA coverage among previously measles zero-dose children, and proportion who remained measles zero-dose after the SIA. Two of the authors (MCD-H and MK) extracted the data in an Excel file, and when one was unsure, both authors reviewed at the report together.

## 3. Results

Review of the WHO SIA database identified 66 countries that had conducted non-outbreak response, national-level, or rolling SIAs between 2020 and 21 June 2024 (Supplemental Table S1). Of them, 15 (23%) had a PCCS with a report available; Ethiopia had two. We also included six additional PCCS reports following 2019 SIAs that were not included by Cutts et al. [21], as well as one PCCS report from Kenya, for a subnational SIA in 2021 and one from Yemen, for a subnational SIA in 2023, but both covered a large proportion of the country. Cameroon and DRC had PCCSs that evaluated 2019 SIAs. In total, our analysis included 24 PCCS reports (Tables 1 and 2). All PCCSs were implemented at the national level, except for Kenya, which included only the 22 counties where the SIA took place, and Yemen, where the SIA and PCCS were conducted only in the southern governorates. The Somalia PCCS excluded one large northern region, although the SIA was also conducted there. For the Central African Republic, only 57% of enumeration areas available in the list of enumeration areas were deemed accessible and kept in the sampling frame. Eleven PCCSs (45.8%) were implemented within three months of the SIA; four PCCSs (16.7%) were implemented at about one year or more after the SIA. In terms of implementers, four were conducted by the National Bureau of Statistics (NBS) and all but two at least mentioned collaborating or using a sampling frame from the NBS. Twenty-three PCCSs reported having performed a weighted analysis, although in one it was unclear if weighting was performed according to the sampling strategy or only to aggregate the country-level estimates. For Syria, weighting was not performed as per NBS guidance due to the current situation of moving populations and unavailability of accurate population data at any administrative level. Ten (43%) were led by independent consultants or organizations and four (20.8%) were led by an academic institution or a research organization.

Twenty-one (87.5%) reports indicated having referred to the 2018 WHO Vaccination Coverage Cluster Survey Reference Manual, with one referring to an outdated version (2005), and most described the key sampling elements. All but two reports described exclusions or furnished the response rate. Sample sizes varied, but most PCCSs were large, with all having >1000 children. Regarding field implementation, dates were explicitly stated in all but one report. The description of the composition of the teams varied broadly, with the profile and gender of interviewers rarely described (data not displayed in the table, as the reports varied widely). Seventeen PCCS reports mentioned ethical clearance being obtained and two (Chad and Kenya) indicated that the survey was considered a programmatic evaluation and thus ethical clearance not required. The other five reports had no mention of ethical review, although explicit information on informed consent was available for three (the two PCCSs from Cameron and the one in Nigeria) of these five. Copies of the questionnaires were included in 19 reports (79.2%). Of relevance, all but one of the PCCSs were performed using computer-assisted personal interviewing (CAPI) and at least seventeen (70.8%) collected GPS coordinates. We did not explicitly extract information on whether geospatial analyses were conducted, but from reading the reports, we noted that maps were not frequently included. Finally, all PCCSs included a section on reasons for no vaccination, with two mentioning the Behavioral and Social Drivers of Vaccination (BeSD) framework.

**Table 1.** Summary of basic characteristics of post-campaign coverage surveys (PCCSs) following measles supplementary immunization activities.

| Measles Supplementary Immunization Activities (SIAs) | | | | | | | | Post-Campaign Coverage Surveys (PCCSs) | | | | | | | | | | | | | | | |
|---|---|---|---|---|---|---|---|---|---|---|---|---|---|---|---|---|---|---|---|---|---|---|---|
| Basics | | | | | | | | Basics | | | | | Sampling | | | | | | | | | | |
| # | Year of PCCS | Country | WHO Region | Target Age Group in Months | Estimated Target Population | Admin Coverage % | SIA Month/Year | Month/Year of Field Work | Delay Between SIA & PCCS (in Months) | Lead Implementer | Ethical Clearance Mentioned | Questionnaire/Data Collection Form Included in Report | # of Clusters Selected/Included | # of Households Interviewed | # of Children Included | Description of Response Rates of Clusters | Description of Response Rates of Households | Primary Sampling Units | Household Enumeration Done | Involvement of NBS/CSO | Data Collection Tools | GPS Coordinates Collected | Software Used for Analysis |
| 1 | 2019 | Democratic People's Republic of Korea | SEAR | 9 months-15 years old | 5,873,914 | 99.7 | Oct-19 | Winter | NA | Country-led | Yes | Yes | 41 | 1312 (31 HH in each cluster) | 1180 | Yes | Yes | Census enumeration blocks | Yes | Yes | CSPro | No | SPSS |
| 2 | 2019 | Zimbabwe | AFR | 9–59 months | 1,776,546 | 91 | Sep-19 | Nov-19 | 2 months | Not specified | Yes | Yes | 470 | 8110 planned *actual number included missing | 3796 planned *actual number included missing | No | No | Enumeration areas | Yes | Yes | ODK | NR | Stata |
| 3 | 2020 | Burkina Faso | AFR | 9–59 months | 3,078,334 | 106 | Nov-19 | Aug–Sept 2020 | 9–10 months | Independent consultant | Yes | No | 548 | 17,650 | 8457 | Yes | Yes | Enumeration areas | Not mentioned | Sampling frame from NBS | ODK | NA | SPSS and Stata |
| 4 | 2020 | Cameroon | AFR | 9–59 months | 3,339,090 | 92 | Dec-19 | June–July 2020 | 6–7 months | Research Organization | Not mentioned. Informed consent was obtained. | Yes | 396 | 4866 | 4671 | Yes | Yes | Enumeration areas | Yes | Sampling frame from NBS | ODK | Yes | SPSS |
| 5 | 2020 | Ethiopia | AFR | 9–59 months | 14,181,143 | 102.8 | June–July 2020 | Oct 2020–Jan 2021 | 4–6 months | Research Organization | Yes | Yes | 1016 Tigray was excluded | 10,143 | 12,867 | Yes | Yes | Enumeration areas | Yes | Sampling frame from NBS | CSPro | Yes | Stata, VCQI |
| 6 | 2020 | Uganda | AFR | 9 months to less than 15 years old | 18,200,970 | 107 | Oct-19 | Dec 2019–Jan 2020 | 2–3 months | Academic Institution | Yes | No | 363 | 5174 | 12,025 | Yes (written as coverage rate) | Yes | Enumeration areas | Yes | Sampling frame from NBS | ODK | NA | Stata |
| 7 | 2021 | Central African Republic † | AFR | 6–59 months 5–10 years | 1,209,256 | 102 for 6–59 m 85.5 for 5–10 yrs | Phase 1: Mar-2020 Phase 2: Aug-2020 | Dec 2020 Bangui, March–April 2021 rest | 8–11 months | Independent consultant | Yes | Yes | 240 | 3172 | 5674 | Yes | Yes | Enumeration areas | Yes | Sampling frame from NBS | ODK | Yes (difficulties noted) | SPSS |
| 8 | 2021 | Chad | AFR | 9–59 months | 1,792,830 (Phase1) 1,623,518 (Phase2) | 108.8 (Phase1) 107.5 (Phase2) | Jan- 2021 (Phase1) Mar-2021 (Phase2) | Mar–April 2022 | ~1 year | Independent consultant | The survey technical committe considered that the survey was not reasearch and thus it was not needed to present the protocol to an ethical comittee Informed consent was obtained | Yes | 695 | 15,793 | 11,601 | Yes | Yes | Enumeration areas, with segmentation | Yes | Yes | ODK | Yes, at least for clusters | SPSS and Stata |
| 9 | 2021 | Democratic Republic of the Congo | AFR | 6–59 months | 18,167,926 | 101.6 | Oct-Dec 2019 | Nov–Dec 2021 | ~2 years | Independent consultant | Yes | Yes | 728 | 81,740 | 21,575 | Yes | Yes | Enumeration areas | Yes | Yes | CSPro | Yes | SPSS, EpIInfo |
| 10 | 2021 | Kenya ‡ | AFR | 9–59 months | 3,374,464 | 111 | June–July 2021 | Jul-21 | <3 months | NBS | Considered programmatic evaluation. No ethical clearance was sought. Informed consent was obtained. | No | 477 | 4404 | 5409 | Yes, but by Region | Yes | Enumeration areas | Not for the PCCS. Sample was from available up-to-date sampling frame maintained by NBS. | Yes | Survey Solution application with digitization of the questionnaire and integration of maps. | Yes | Not mentioned |
| 11 | 2021 | Nepal | SEAR | 9–59 months | 2,548,336 | 101 | Feb–Mar 2020 (Phase 1) Mar–July 2020 (Phase 2) | Sept–Nov 2021 | >1 year | Family Welfare Division Department of Health Services MOH | Yes | Yes | 342 | 7180 | 3715 | Yes | Yes | List of wards (some were merged or segmented) | Yes | Yes | CSPro | Yes | SPSS |
| 12 | 2021 | Pakistan | EMR | 9 months-15 years old | 90,262,980 | 105 | Nov-21 | Nov 2021–Jan 2022 | <3 months | Contech International Health Consultants | Yes | Yes | 1584 | 15,840 | 31,871 | Yes | Yes | Enumeration areas | Yes | Yes. Technical and sampling frame | Proprietary android-based CAPI application from implementing partner | No | Stata, VCQI |

**Table 1.** *Cont.*

| | | | | | | | | | | | | | | | | | | | | | | | |
|---|---|---|---|---|---|---|---|---|---|---|---|---|---|---|---|---|---|---|---|---|---|---|---|
| Measles Supplementary Immunization Activities (SIAs) | | | | | | | | Post-Campaign Coverage Surveys (PCCSs) | | | | | | | | | | | | | | | |
| Basics | | | | | | | | Basics | | | | | Sampling | | | | | | | | | | |
| # | Year of PCCS | Country | WHO Region | Target Age Group in Months | Estimated Target Population | Admin Coverage % | SIA Month/Year | Month/Year of Field Work | Delay Between SIA & PCCS (in Months) | Lead Implementer | Ethical Clearance Mentioned | Questionnaire/ Data Collection Form Included in Report | # of Clusters Selected/Included | # of Households Interviewed | # of Children Included | Description of Response Rates of Clusters | Description of Response Rates of Households | Primary Sampling Units | Household Enumeration Done | Involvement of NBS/CSO | Data Collection Tools | GPS Coordinates Collected | Software Used for Analysis |
| 13 | 2021 | Zambia | AFR | 9–59 months | 3,398,230 | 91.3 | Nov-20 | Oct-21 | >1 year | Not specified | No | No | 272 | 5155 | 4590 | No | Yes | Enumeration areas | Yes | Yes | The questionnaire was programmed into a CAPI application using survey solutions, a World Bank software application | | Not mentioned? |
| 14 | 2022 | Burundi | AFR | 9–59 months | 1,683,300 | 93 | Jan-22 | Oct–Nov 2022 | 10–11 months | NBS | Not mentioned | Yes | 540 | 32,177 | 20,618 | Yes | Yes | Ennumeration areas | Yes | Yes | KoboCollect | Yes | SPSS and Stata |
| 15 | 2022 | Madagascar | AFR | 6–59 months | 4,355,433 | 95.11 | May–June 2022 | Aug–Sept 2022 | 3 months | International consultant with Directorate of Demography and Social Statistics (DDSS) of the NBS | Yes | Yes | 123 | 3055 | 1421 | Yes | Yes | Enumeration areas | Yes | Yes | CSPro | Yes | SPSS and Stata |
| 16 | 2022 | Somalia | EMR | children of 0–59 months for tOPV, 06–59 months for MCV and Vitamin A and 12–59 months for deworming | 2,566,955 | 90 | Nov-22 | Feb-23 | 3 months | Independent consultant/cabinet | Yes | Yes | 450 | 17,539 | 21,740 | No | No | Lists of accessible areas (not mentioned in detail) | Not mentioned | Not mentioned | Survey123 | Yes | SPSS, Stata, ArcGIS |
| 17 | 2022 or 2023 | Syrian Arab Republic | EMR | 6 months-5 years | 2,494,498 | 75.62 | Oct–Nov 2022 | Dates not provided. 2023? | NA | Independent consultant | Yes | No | 99 | 5982 | 3581 | Yes | Yes | Sub-districts | Yes | Yes, technical advise | Paper-based | No | EpiInfo |
| 18 | 2023 | Cameroon | AFR | 9–59 months | 5,564,940 | 94.38 | Jul-23 | Sept–Oct 2023 | <3 months | NBS | No. Informed consent was obtained. | Yes | 395 | 5711 | 3546 | Yes | Yes | Enumeration areas | Yes | Yes | CSPro | Yes | SPSS, Stata, VCQI |
| 19 | 2023 | Democratic Republic of the Congo | AFR | 6–59 months | 6,454,490 (May) 7,359,339 (August) 5,273,383 (September) | 103.6 (May) 85.7 (August) 101.1 (September) | Three phases: April, June and Aug 2023. | October–December 2023 in Block 1, Phase 2 in Block 2 and part of Block 3 from January to March 2024, then Phase 3 in the rest of the provinces in March–April 2024. | 6 to 10 months | Independent consultant | Yes | Yes | 728 | 10,920 | 9627 | Yes | Yes | Enumeration areas | Yes | Yes | CSPro | Yes | SPSS, EpIInfo |
| 20 | 2023 | Malawi | AFR | 9–59 months | 3,169,522 | 82.4 | May-23 | Jun-23 | <3 months | International consultant and NBS | Yes | Yes | 205 | 4715 | 8485 | Yes | Yes | Enumeration areas | Yes | Yes | CSPro | Yes | Stata, VCQI |

**Table 1.** *Cont.*

| | | | | Measles Supplementary Immunization Activities (SIAs) | | | | | | | | | | Post-Campaign Coverage Surveys (PCCSs) | | | | | | | | | | |
|---|---|---|---|---|---|---|---|---|---|---|---|---|---|---|---|---|---|---|---|---|---|---|
| | | | | Basics | | | | | Basics | | | | | Sampling | | | | | | | | |
| # | Year of PCCS | Country | WHO Region | Target Age Group in Months | Estimated Target Population | Admin Coverage % | SIA Month/Year | Month/Year of Field Work | Delay Between SIA & PCCS (in Months) | Lead Implementer | Ethical Clearance Mentioned | Questionnaire/ Data Collection Form Included in Report | # of Clusters Selected/Included | # of Households Interviewed | # of Children Included | Description of Response Rates of Clusters | Description of Response Rates of Households | Primary Sampling Units | Household Enumeration Done | Involvement of NBS/CSO | Data Collection Tools | GPS Coordinates Collected | Software Used for Analysis |
| 21 | 2023 | Niger | AFR | 6–59 m or 9–59 m depending on district | 5,098,682 | 105 | Dec 2022–Jan 2023 | Mar–April 2023 | 3 months | Independent consultant | Yes | Yes | 270 | 5334 | 4655 | Yes | Yes | Ennumeration areas | Yes | Yes | ODK | Yes | SPSS |
| 22 | 2023 | Nigeria | AFR | 9–59 months | 4,298,149 (October) 1,090,330 (November) 5,021,611 (December) | 96.67 (October) 103.95 (November) 4,823,266 (December) | Oct 2023–Jan 2024 | Dec 2023–Jan 2024 | <3 months | NBS | No. Informed consent was obtained. | Yes | 740 (560 in 14 states plus 180 in 6 local area governments in Borno) | 7399 | 6987 | Yes | Yes | Enumeration areas | Yes | Yes | CSPro | Yes | Stata, VCQI |
| 23 | 2023 | Yemen ‡ | EMR | 6–59 months | 1,267,083 | 91 | September–October 2023 | Oct-23 | <3 months | Research Organization | Yes | Yes | 1547 | 18,564 | 29,549 | Yes | Yes | Harahs | No | No | ODK | No | Excel |
| 24 | 2024 | Ethiopia | AFR | | | 98.7 | Dec 2022–April 2023 | Dec 2023–Jan 2024 | >1 year | Research Organization | Yes | Yes | 1272 | 12,702 | 15,763 | Yes | Yes | Enumeration areas | Yes | Sampling frame from NBS | Kobo Toolbox | Yes | Stata, VCQI |

AFR = World Health Organization African Region; EMR = World Health Organization Middle Eastern Region; SEAR = World Health Organization South-East Asian Region NBS = National Bureau of Statistics; NA = not available; NR = not reported, but potentially available; VCQI = Vaccination Coverage Quality Indicators tool; † Areas considered secure; ‡ Subnational.

**Table 2.** Summary of main results of post-campaign coverage surveys (PCCSs) following measles supplementary immunization activities (SIAs) and related coverage levels.

| | | | | | Results | | | | | | | |
|---|---|---|---|---|---|---|---|---|---|---|---|---|
| # | Year of PCCS | Country | WHO Region | MCV1 Coverage in Year of Start of SIA | Admin Coverage % | SIA Cards or Finger Marking Seen | SIA Coverage (95% CI) | % Routine Immunization (RI) Cards Seen (Age Group If Not All) | RI MCV1 Coverage % (95% CI) (Age Group If Not All) | SIA Dose Was the First MCV Dose Received by Child % (95%CI) | SIA Coverage Among Zero-Dose % (95%CI) | Child Remained Measles Zero-Dose After SIA % (95%CI) |
| 1 | 2019 | Democratic People's Republic of Korea | SEAR | 98 | 99.7 | Almost all were verified by record in Primary Health Facility. Only recall were 7 children who had records in a different health facility | 99.9% (99.09–99.87) | NA | 81% yes, 18.6% unsure, 0.4% no | NR | NA | NA |
| 2 | 2019 | Zimbabwe | AFR | 85 | 91 | NR | 78.7% (77.35–79.98) | NA | NA | NR | NR | NR |

**Table 2.** *Cont.*

| # | Year of PCCS | Country | WHO Region | MCV1 Coverage in Year of Start of SIA | Admin Coverage % | SIA Cards or Finger Marking Seen | SIA Coverage (95% CI) | % Routine Immunization (RI) Cards Seen (Age Group If Not All) | RI MCV1 Coverage % (95% CI) (Age Group If Not All) | SIA Dose Was the First MCV Dose Received by Child % (95%CI) | SIA Coverage Among Zero-Dose % (95%CI) | Child Remained Measles Zero-Dose After SIA % (95%CI) |
|---|---|---|---|---|---|---|---|---|---|---|---|---|
| | | | | | | Results | | | | | | |
| 3 | 2020 | Burkina Faso | AFR | 88 | 106 | 38.7% (87.8% received one) | 84.4% (83.6–85.2%) | 93% 12–23 months 81% 24–35 months | 87,8% 12–23 m 84.8% 24–35 m | NR | NR | 4.80% |
| 4 | 2020 | Cameroon | AFR | 61 | 92 | 8.30% | 69.7% (68.34–71.01) | NA | NR | 35.70% | NR | NR |
| 5 | 2020 | Ethiopia | AFR | 59 | 102.8 | 81.10% | 81.5% (80.0–83.0%) | NA | 80.30% | NR | 56.70% | 8.10% |
| 6 | 2020 | Uganda | AFR | 87 | 107 | 48.5 (78.4% received one) | 94.4% (93.0–95.5) | 25.30% | 85.40% | 12.00% | NR | 2.60% |
| 7 | 2021 | Central African Republic † | AFR | 41 | 102 for 6–59 m 85.5 for 5–10 yrs | 25% (83% received one) | 94.6% (92.9–96.0%) | NA | 25.2% 12–23 m 15.3% 24–35 m | NR | NR | 3.40% |
| 8 | 2021 | Chad | AFR | 53 | 108.8 (Phase1) 107.5 (Phase2) | 11% (19% reported not having received a card) | 77.4% (74.8–79.8%) | NA | Available as an analysis added later, not in main report. 41.1% 12–23 m 28.2% 24–35 m | NR | 73.5% (IC95%:70.2–76.5%) | 20% (IC95%: 17.6–22.5%) |
| 9 | 2021 | Democratic Republic of the Congo | AFR | 65 | 101.6 | 6.89%; 4.93% (correctly filled in) | 87.52% (87.50–87.53%) | NR | 80.70% | NR | 61.06%. | 7.61% |
| 10 | 2021 | Kenya ‡ | AFR | 90 | 111 | NR | 84.20% | NA | NA | NR | 80.10% | NR |
| 11 | 2021 | Nepal | SEAR | 87 | 101 | 43% | 84% (82–87) Phase 1: 87% (85–89) phase 2: 81% (77–85) | 51.40% | 95.50% | Small sample size of previously zero-dose | Small sample size of previously zero-dose | NR |
| 12 | 2021 | Pakistan | EMR | 81 | 105 | 80% | 93.6% (92.7–94.4) | 47% | 71.5% (and 10% unkown status) 79% for children under 2 years | NR | NR | NR |

**Table 2.** *Cont.*

| | | | | | | | | | Results | | | |
|---|---|---|---|---|---|---|---|---|---|---|---|---|
| **#** | **Year of PCCS** | **Country** | **WHO Region** | **MCV1 Coverage in Year of Start of SIA** | **Admin Coverage %** | **SIA Cards or Finger Marking Seen** | **SIA Coverage (95% CI)** | **% Routine Immunization (RI) Cards Seen (Age Group If Not All)** | **RI MCV1 Coverage % (95% CI) (Age Group If Not All)** | **SIA Dose Was the First MCV Dose Received by Child % (95%CI)** | **SIA Coverage Among Zero-Dose % (95%CI)** | **Child Remained Measles Zero-Dose After SIA % (95%CI)** |
| 13 | 2021 | Zambia | AFR | 96 | 91.3 | NA | 68.90% | 63% had documented evidence | 88.5 | NA | NA | NA |
| 14 | 2022 | Burundi | AFR | 89 | 93 | 15% | 88.60% | 91.8% 12–23 m<br>86.1% 24–35 m | 85.90% | NR | NR | NR |
| 15 | 2022 | Madagascar | AFR | 44 | 95.11 | 56.30% | 65.3% (56.8–72.9) | NA | 69.50% | NR | NR | 19.20% |
| 16 | 2022 | Somalia | EMR | 46 | 90 | NA | 86.0 (83.7–88.0) | 25% 12–23 | 65% | NR | 33.1%<br>14.1% 12–23 m<br>37.2% 24–35 m | NR |
| 17 | 2022 or 2023 | Syrian Arab Republic | EMR | 52 | 75.62 | 54.40% | 80.7% (79.35%–81.94%) | NA | 82.8 12–23 m<br>93.6 24–59 m | NR | 54.30% | NR |
| 18 | 2023 | Cameroon | AFR | 71 | 94.38 | 31.8% (84.9% received a card) | 69.5 (66.4–72.5) | NA | NR | 22.10% | 62.30% | 13.3% |
| 19 | 2023 | Democratic Republic of the Congo | AFR | 52 | 103.6 (May)<br>85.7 (August)<br>101.1 (September) | 12.88% | 94.60% (94.60%–94.61%) | ~3.5% (3.47% vaccinated by card seen) | 78.30% | NR | 75.01% | NA |
| 20 | 2023 | Malawi | AFR | 87 | 82.4 | 38.8% | 75.7% (72.3–79.0) | NA | NR | NR | 27.6% for 12–35 m | NR |
| 21 | 2023 | Niger | AFR | 65 | 105 | 71.8% (86.2% received one) | 92.7% (90.8–94.1) | NA | NA | NR | 91.60% | 4.60% |
| 22 | 2023 | Nigeria | AFR | 60 | 96.67 (October)<br>103.95 (November)<br>4,823,266 (December) | 47% card and 9.9% finger marking | 87% (84–90) | NR | NR | 12% | NR | NR |
| 23 | 2023 | Yemen ‡ | EMR | 45 | 91 | NA | 84.2% (95% CI: 83.8–84.6) | NA | NR | NR | 12% | NR |
| 24 | 2024 | Ethiopia | AFR | 55 | 98.7 | 16% | 87.10% | 3940 (~25%) | 73.80% | 14.00% | 72% | NR |

AFR = World Health Organization African Region; EMR = World Health Organization Middle Eastern Region; SEAR = World Health Organization South-East Asian Region; NBS = National Bureau of Statistics; NA = not available; NR = not reported, but potentially available; † Areas considered secure; ‡ Subnational.

The main PCCS results and comparisons to administrative data and routine coverage with the first dose of a measles-containing vaccine (MCV1) are included in Table 2. PCCS SIA coverage was lower than the administrative coverage included in the SIA database, apart from DPR Korea and the accessible areas of Syria. Regarding ascertainment of SIA vaccination, 19 had vaccination cards or finger marking as proof of vaccination in the SIA (range: 6.9–81.1%). One third of the PCCSs reported SIA coverage that was below the WHO/UNICEF Estimate of National Immunization Coverage (WUENIC) for one dose of a measles-containing vaccine. Twenty PCCS reports (83.3%) included at least one of the indicators related to zero-dose measles. Of the 12 PCCSs reporting coverage among previously measles zero-dose children, nine had coverage of more than 50% (range: 12% and 91.6%). DPR Korea and Nepal explored this indicator but unvaccinated children in the sample were extremely few. Only the Zambia PCCS report did not allow ascertaining whether the collected data would allow calculating at least one of the three measles zero-dose SIA coverage indicators included in our table.

Only one anonymized database was available to WHO-HQ. This PCCS had been re-analyzed, in 2023, using the tool Vaccination Coverage Quality Indicators (VCQI) [29] upon request from stakeholders. In this PCCS, which excluded one large northern region and security-compromised areas, SIA coverage among children previously vaccinated with either one or 2+ measles doses was strikingly higher than among those who had no previous MCV dose. Table 3 illustrates the VCQI output for a given age-group.

**Table 3.** Measles SIA vaccination coverage by previous vaccination status, children aged 24–35 months, Somalia (minus one large northern region) PCCS 2023.

| Number of Measles Vaccine Doses Prior to SIA | Vaccinated During SIA (%) | 95% CI (%) | Vaccinated During SIA (Weighted N) | Weighted N |
|---|---|---|---|---|
| Zero | 37.2 | (31.8, 42.8) | 81 | 217 |
| 1 Dose | 92.8 | (89.5, 95.1) | 540 | 582 |
| 2+ Doses | 90.9 | (86.6, 94.0) | 812 | 894 |
| Somalia 2023 (Total) | 84.7 | (81.6, 87.3) | 1433 | 1692 |

Secondary analyses were conducted to better understand SIA coverage heterogeneity. Table 4 describes measles SIA coverage, the number of children in the sample, and the number of clusters, by state. It then indicates the number of clusters where all surveyed children were found vaccinated, those where the proportion was >50% but <100%, and then the clusters where the proportion of vaccinated children was ≤50%. The design effect (DEFF) and intra-cluster correlation coefficient (ICC) are also included for each stratum. Both parameters were high, with the DEFF ranging from 10.8 to 28.5, which is largely above the parameters used in sample size calculations. The large value observed here is due to the high ICC and an unusually high number of respondents per cluster.

**Table 4.** Measles SIA coverage, the number of children in the sample, and the number of clusters, by state. Somalia (minus one large northern region) PCCS 2023.

| State | % Vac'd During SIA | Total # Children | Total # of Clusters | # Clusters with 100% Children vac'd' | # Clusters with >50–99.9% Children vac'd | # Clusters with ≤50% Children vac'd | DEFF | ICC |
|---|---|---|---|---|---|---|---|---|
| Banadir | 89.8 | 3604 | 74 | 13 | 57 | 4 | 11.7 | 0.2216 |
| Galmudug | 86.1 | 3338 | 76 | 10 | 61 | 5 | 10.8 | 0.1634 |
| Hirshabelle | 82.6 | 4372 | 76 | 17 | 47 | 12 | 28.5 | 0.4284 |
| Jubbaland | 83.8 | 2781 | 76 | 29 | 39 | 8 | 26.7 | 0.4465 |
| Puntland | 88.6 | 3279 | 73 | 18 | 52 | 3 | 14.0 | 0.2361 |
| Southwest | 87 | 3542 | 75 | 20 | 48 | 7 | 17.7 | 0.2791 |
| Total | 87 | 20,916 | 450 | 107 | 304 | 39 | 21.3 | 0.3116 |

DEFF: design effect; ICC: intra-cluster correlation coefficient. For PCCS, ICC values of 1/6 = 0.167 are considered conservative [21].

An organ pipe plot [21,30], as recommended by the WHO Vaccination Coverage Survey Manual, was produced for all 6 states included in the PCCS (Figure 1—illustrative). Cluster-level SIA proportion vaccinated (indicated by the individual columns) varied considerably across State X.

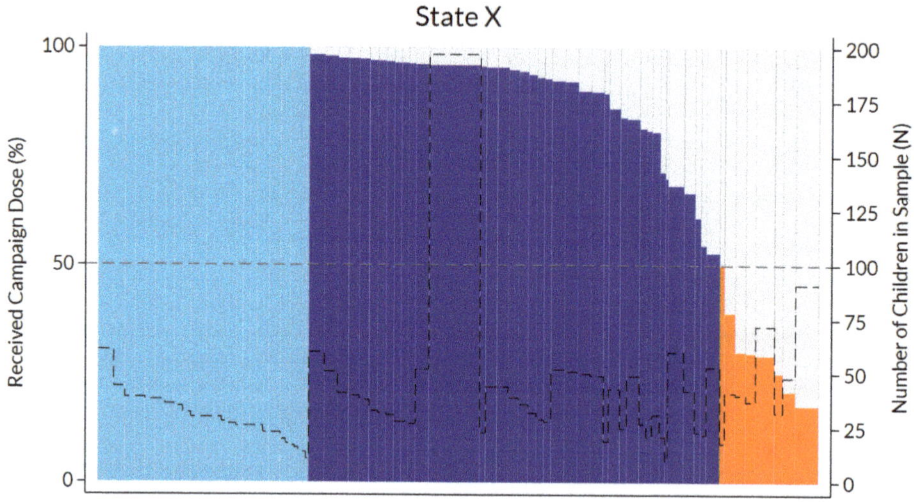


**Figure 1.** Organ pipe plot of proportion of children vaccinated per cluster in State X. Somalia (minus one large northern region one large northern region) PCCS 2023.

Figure footnote: Clusters are sorted left-to-right in descending order of coverage. In this representation, clusters with 100% sample coverage are light blue, those with 50.01–99.99% are dark blue, and those with 0–50% are shown in orange. The thin gray dashed line that varies in height from cluster to cluster indicates the number of respondents per cluster and its values are read using the right vertical axis.

Only two other PCCS reports reviewed for this work included calculation of the intra-cluster correlation coefficient (ICC) or design effect (DEFF), parameters that are useful to inform sample size calculations in future PCCS.

## 4. Discussion

Though measles SIAs are performed in many parts of the world, few countries use PCCSs to evaluate their performance. All PCCSs for which the WHO had access to reports were conducted in Gavi-eligible countries, and most in Sub Saharan Africa. If we compare our findings with previous reviews [21,25], the use of probability sampling and weighted analysis is encouraging; most PCCSs are explicit in indicating that current WHO guidance is being considered. The independence of implementers and quality of reports has also improved compared to previous studies.

Many challenges remain, however. Not all countries can implement a PCCS, and this is evident from the fact that only Gavi eligible countries had PCCS reports available. Also, the timing of PCCS implementation is of particular concern. Only about half of the PCCSs explored here were implemented within three months of the SIA, though our findings are confounded by the limitations to field activities imposed by the COVID-19 pandemic.

Administrative coverage levels tend to overestimate campaign coverage compared to coverage obtained from PCCS. This finding is not surprising. Administrative coverage can be affected by inaccurate denominators and errors in tallying and aggregating doses. For SIAs, vaccination of children outside the target age while tallying them as within the age range is not uncommon.

Only five PCCS coverage levels were above 90%, and only one >95%. We also observed that measles SIA coverage was lower than routine MCV1 coverage for a third of the PCCSs included. This was unexpected, as SIAs, by their nature, conduct intensive outreach and social mobilization. This warrants more exploration, as it may also be that as documentation of vaccine doses received improves, children who are already vaccinated may be less likely to go for an additional dose.

The next questions after seeing coverage that is insufficient to stop measles transmission are: where coverage was not reached and why. While PCCSs can provide clues, these answers would be better addressed by better intra-campaign monitoring and rapid convenience monitoring before stopping vaccination. We did not explore these aspects of SIA implementation but would argue that they need strengthening judging by the SIA coverage reached in most recent campaigns and their heterogeneity in reaching previously unvaccinated children [4,21,27,31]. Furthermore, to our knowledge, only campaign coverage is broadly accepted and recommended as an indicator of measles SIA quality and impact. The establishment of more criteria to assess SIAs was recommended by the Measles & Rubella Strategic Framework 2021–2030 published at the beginning of the decade [32].

Conducting a PCCS is not always easy. The PCCSs included here tend to be large, with over 1000 children. The more clusters in a survey, the more resources are needed to reach the different areas. In addition to the challenges linked to the normal work of reaching selected places, interviewing families takes time and effort. Four reports explicitly mentioned the violence that survey teams faced, with one survey team even being kidnapped in a country in central Africa. To this end, one should consider under what situations a PCCS may not be the best use of resources or may not warrant the risk that field work may entail. Also, complementary monitoring tools may need to be used in insecure areas and others that are not included in normal sampling frames. Decision support tools may be worth considering. Time elapsed between the SIA and the PCCS may be a consideration. Senegal implemented a selective SIA in 2021. It was an SIA of particular interest because it involved screening and listing children aged 9 to 59 months (performed in Oct 2021) and then vaccination of these children at fixed and outreach sites (in November 2021); children not on the lists but who came to a site without documentation of having previously received two doses of MR vaccine were also to be vaccinated. Unfortunately, a PCCS was not conducted until 2023, and at the time of this writing, in July 2024, the report is not available. Another example where a PCCS may not be the best option is when an SIA is known to not have reached high coverage, using administrative data and a narrative of the issues, complemented or not with rapid convenience monitoring, may be a better option. This was the case in Indonesia outside of Java in 2017–2018 and the Gambia in 2022. Another example might be that of South Sudan, where after performing an SIA in 2023 decided to prioritize campaign evaluation and rapid field assessments, and their PCCS was paired with a planned RI vaccination coverage survey that was scheduled for late 2023, after the rainy season. This survey is yet to be implemented. Recent outbreaks affecting mainly children aged 1–4 years suggest that coverage was likely insufficient [33]. More needs to be done to triangulate data from intra-campaign monitoring and administrative coverage with PCCS findings to better inform the proposed decision support algorithms [3,31].

When PCCSs are implemented, exploiting the findings and the available data should be of utmost priority. The WHO and partners make available analytical software and a detailed list of indicators [29]. However, most of the surveys described in the reports accessible to us did not use them. This may reflect limited awareness or other barriers that we need to further explore. In addition to coverage and the availability of sociodemographic variables that would allow exploring factors associated with no vaccination, most PCCSs now collect GPS coordinates. They also have information about reasons for no vaccination, and more recent PCCSs are starting to use the Behavioral and Social Drivers of Immunization (BeSD) [34] framework to explore barriers and enablers to vaccination.

Some of the countries included here used survey data to conduct exploratory analysis on factors linked to not being vaccinated. Nigeria explored geographic differences in measles vaccination in RI vs. SIAs [27]. The analysis showed that the SIA reached more homogenous coverage than the RI, but that there are areas where many children are missed by both approaches. Furthermore, geolocated campaign and RI coverage data can be extremely useful to modelers when modeling disease transmission and outbreak risk, which can help to inform disease control targeting [10,11,31,35–39]. However, unlike well-established household survey programs, there is no PCCS database repository. The example presented here allowed exploring heterogeneity in coverage. The results, which represent areas that were accessible to surveyors, warrant better exploring why coverage among measles zero-dose children was so much lower than that for those who had been previously vaccinated. Countries should be encouraged to make anonymized databases available to the WHO, the IA2030 Measles and Rubella Partnership, and other stakeholders, as is done by most household surveys. Furthermore, we support the initiative by the IA2030 Partnership to establish data analysis cooperation in countries conducting coverage surveys with additional analyses performed by local analysts, close in time to the PCCS, and engaging with EPI programs to promote data use.

Our analysis has several limitations. First, we included only national SIAs that were not for outbreak response. We may have accidentally left out SIAs that should have been included. Second, we may not have the reports of all PCCSs conducted. This is less likely for Gavi-eligible countries, as the authors reached out to Gavi and the US Centers for Disease Control and Prevention (CDC) to seek reports. However, non-Gavi eligible countries may not share PCCS reports with the WHO. Third, we selected only a few characteristics of the PCCS and the reports from a long list of recommended items in the survey checklist recommended by Cutts et al. [21] and adopted by Gavi. Also, we did not compare the reports to the elements recommended in the recently introduced "Preferred Reporting Items for Complex Sample Survey Analysis" (PRICSSA) checklist [40]. Fourth, two authors extracted data from the PCCS reports, and as they were not structured according to our list of items, we may have misrepresented some data; we did not attempt to reach PCCS teams for clarifications. Lastly, having an item in a report does not guarantee good survey implementation. There are many challenges to conducting field enumeration and sampling, identifying pre-selected clusters boundaries and pre-selected households, and to interviewing people, particularly to ascertain vaccination status when a card or other documentation is not available. Caregivers' ability to accurately recall vaccination experience for each of their children can be challenging, and more so the longer the time lag between the SIA and the survey. Analysis of data collected using complex sampling, particularly the appropriate weight calculations, and use of sample design parameters in statistical packages is challenging. We did not have access to any analytical codes, except for the VCQI code used for one PCCS performed by two co-authors (DR and MKT). Nevertheless, we believe that our main findings remain solid: not all SIAs are followed by a PCCS and, when performed, timeliness remains a concern; more PCCSs appear to be following current recommendations; survey coverage tends to be lower than administrative SIA results; and more analysis could be performed with the data that are collected by PCCS analysts and, if made available, by measles modelers and other stakeholders.

Gavi contracted out two PCCSs in 2024, one for Burkina Faso and one for Laos, in an attempt to ensure PCCS timeliness and quality survey implementation. Neither report is available for review yet. This work will present an opportunity to explore the pros and cons of a centralized contracting approach, as well as to explicitly triangulate PCCS results with other data to better inform decision making.

The WHO is coordinating a thorough update to the 2018 Vaccination Coverage Cluster Survey Reference Manual [22] and accompanying software tools [29] in 2024–2026. This presents an opportunity to further engage with countries and the IA2030 Measles and Rubella Partnership to ensure that the revised guidance includes options for areas where regular sampling is problematic, clearer standardization for reports, more guidance on analyses beyond descriptive statistics, and more hands-on capacity-building activities if a stakeholder analysis identifies this as useful.

Measles is so exceedingly contagious that very high vaccination coverage is required to prevent outbreaks from spreading through a population. High-quality, independent, probability-based assessments of campaign coverage will be useful both for refining SIA planning and execution to consistently achieve high coverage rates, especially among measles zero-dose children.

**Supplementary Materials:** The following supporting information can be downloaded at: https://www.mdpi.com/article/10.3390/vaccines12111257/s1. Table S1: List of measles campaigns, global measles supplemental immunization activity (SIA) database.

**Author Contributions:** Conceptualization, M.C.D.-H.; Data compilation: C.S.; Data extraction M.C.D.-H. and M.K.; Survey data analysis, D.A.R. and M.K.T. All authors have read and agreed to the published version of the manuscript.

**Funding:** This research received no external funding.

**Institutional Review Board Statement:** This study did not require ethical approval as it is a secondary data analysis.

**Informed Consent Statement:** Informed consent was obtained from all subjects participating in the surveys described in this study.

**Data Availability Statement:** Data is contained within the article.

**Conflicts of Interest:** M.C.D.-H., C.S., and M.K. for the World Health Organization (WHO). The authors alone are responsible for the views expressed in this publication and they do not necessarily represent the decisions, policy, or views of the WHO. D.A.R. and M.K.T. declare that the research was conducted in the absence of any commercial or financial relationships that could be construed as a potential conflict of interest. Authors Dale A. Rhoda and Mary Kay Trimner are employed by the company Biostat Global Consulting. The remaining authors declare that the research was conducted in the absence of any commercial or financial relationships that could be construed as a potential conflict of interest.

## References


1. Shattock, A.J.; Johnson, H.C.; Sim, S.Y.; Carter, A.; Lambach, P.; Hutubessy, R.C.W.; Thompson, K.M.; Badizadegan, K.; Lambert, B.; Ferrari, M.J.; et al. Contribution of vaccination to improved survival and health: Modelling 50 years of the Expanded Programme on Immunization. *Lancet* **2024**, *403*, 2307–2316. [CrossRef] [PubMed]
2. World Health Organization. Measles vaccines: WHO position paper. *Wkly. Epidemiol. Rec.* **2017**, *92*, 205–227.
3. World Health Organization. *Planning and Implementing High-Quality Supplementary Immunization Activities for Injectable Vaccines: Using an Example of Measles-Rubella Vaccines—Field Guide*; WHO: Geneva, Switzerland, 2016. Available online: https://www.who.int/publications/i/item/9789241511254 (accessed on 15 October 2024).
4. Strebel, P.; Grabowsky, M.; Hoekstra, E.; Gay, A.; Cochi, S. Evolution and Contribution of a Global Partnership against Measles and Rubella, 2001–2023. *Vaccines* **2024**, *12*, 693. [CrossRef] [PubMed]
5. De Quadros, C.A.; Hersh, B.S.; Nogueira, A.C.; A Carrasco, P.; Da Silveira, C.M. Measles eradication: Experience in the Americas. *Bull. World Health Organ.* **1998**, *76* (Suppl. 2), 47–52. [PubMed]
6. Verguet, S.; Johri, M.; Morris, S.K.; Gauvreau, C.L.; Jha, P.; Jit, M. Controlling measles using supplemental immunization activities: A mathematical model to inform optimal policy. *Vaccine* **2015**, *33*, 1291–1296. [CrossRef]
7. Prada, J.; Metcalf, C.; Takahashi, S.; Lessler, J.; Tatem, A.; Ferrari, M. Demographics, epidemiology and the impact of vaccination campaigns in a measles-free world—Can elimination be maintained? *Vaccine* **2017**, *35*, 1488–1493. [CrossRef]
8. Auzenbergs, M.; Fu, H.; Abbas, K.; Procter, S.R.; Cutts, F.T.; Jit, M. Health effects of routine measles vaccination and supplementary immunisation activities in 14 high-burden countries: A Dynamic Measles Immunization Calculation Engine (DynaMICE) modelling study. *Lancet Glob. Health* **2023**, *11*, e1194–e1204. [CrossRef]
9. Portnoy, A.; Jit, M.; Helleringer, S.; Verguet, S. Comparative Distributional Impact of Routine Immunization and Supplementary Immunization Activities in Delivery of Measles Vaccine in Low- and Middle-Income Countries. *Value Health* **2020**, *23*, 891–897. [CrossRef] [PubMed]
10. Portnoy, A.; Jit, M.; Helleringer, S.; Verguet, S. Impact of measles supplementary immunization activities on reaching children missed by routine programs. *Vaccine* **2018**, *36*, 170–178. [CrossRef] [PubMed] [PubMed Central]
11. Rosenfeld, K.A.; Frey, K.; McCarthy, K.A. Optimal Timing Regularly Outperforms Higher Coverage in Preventative Measles Supplementary Immunization Campaigns. *Vaccines* **2024**, *12*, 820. [CrossRef] [PubMed] [PubMed Central]
12. Yan, L.; Jing, M.; Dapeng, Y. Rubella vaccines: WHO position paper. *Wkly. Epidemiol. Rec.* **2020**, *95*, 27.

13. Ou, A.C.; Zimmerman, L.A.; Alexander, J.P.; Crowcroft, N.S.; O'connor, P.M.; Knapp, J.K. Progress Toward Rubella and Congenital Rubella Syndrome Elimination—Worldwide, 2012–2022. *Mmwr-Morb. Mortal. Wkly. Rep.* **2024**, *73*, 162–167. [CrossRef] [PubMed]
14. Minta, A.A.; Ferrari, M.; Antoni, S.; Portnoy, A.; Sbarra, A.; Lambert, B.; Hatcher, C.; Hsu, C.H.; Ho, L.L.; Steulet, C.; et al. Progress Toward Measles Elimination—Worldwide, 2000–2022. *Mmwr-Morbidity Mortal. Wkly. Rep.* **2023**, *72*, 1262–1268. [CrossRef] [PubMed]
15. Rachlin, A.; Danovaro-Holliday, M.C.; Murphy, P.; Sodha, S.V.; Wallace, A.S. Routine Vaccination Coverage—Worldwide, 2021. *Mmwr-Morbidity Mortal. Wkly. Rep.* **2022**, *71*, 1396–1400. [CrossRef]
16. Muhoza, P.; Danovaro-Holliday, M.C.; Diallo, M.S.; Murphy, P.; Sodha, S.V.; Requejo, J.H.; Wallace, A.S. Routine Vaccination Coverage—Worldwide, 2020. *Mmwr-Morbidity Mortal. Wkly. Rep.* **2021**, *70*, 1495–1500. [CrossRef]
17. Ho, L.L.; Gurung, S.; Mirza, I.; Nicolas, H.D.; Steulet, C.; Burman, A.L.; Danovaro-Holliday, M.C.; Sodha, S.V.; Kretsinger, K. Impact of the SARS-CoV-2 pandemic on vaccine-preventable disease campaigns. *Int. J. Infect. Dis.* **2022**, *119*, 201–209. [CrossRef]
18. CDC. Global Measles Outbreaks. Global Measles Vaccination. Published 13 May 2024. Available online: https://www.cdc.gov/global-measles-vaccination/data-research/global-measles-outbreaks/index.html (accessed on 15 October 2024).
19. e Clinical Medicine Concerning global rise in measles cases. *eClinicalMedicine* **2024**, *68*, 102502. [CrossRef]
20. Parums, D.V. A Review of the Resurgence of Measles, a Vaccine-Preventable Disease, as Current Concerns Contrast with Past Hopes for Measles Elimination. *Med. Sci. Monit.* **2024**, *30*, e944436-1–e944436-10. [CrossRef]
21. Cutts, F.T.; Danovaro-Holliday, M.C.; Rhoda, D.A. Challenges in measuring supplemental immunization activity coverage among measles zero-dose children. *Vaccine* **2021**, *39*, 1359–1363. [CrossRef]
22. World Health Organization. *Vaccination Coverage Cluster Surveys: Reference Manual*; WHO: Geneva, Switzerland, 2018.
23. Measles and Measles-Rubella Vaccine Support. Available online: https://www.gavi.org/types-support/vaccine-support/measles-and-measles-rubella (accessed on 15 October 2024).
24. Luman, E.T.; Cairns, K.L.; Perry, R.; Dietz, V.; Gittelman, D. Use and abuse of rapid mnitoring to assess coverage during mass vaccination campaigns. *Bull. World Health Organ.* **2007**, *85*, 651. [CrossRef]
25. Kaiser, R.; E Shibeshi, M.; Chakauya, J.M.; Dzeka, E.; Masresha, B.G.; Daniel, F.; Shivute, N. Surveys of measles vaccination coverage in eastern and southern Africa: A review of quality and methods used. *Bull. World Health Organ.* **2015**, *93*, 314–319. [CrossRef] [PubMed]
26. Cutts, F.T.; Izurieta, H.S.; Rhoda, D.A. Measuring Coverage in MNCH: Design, Implementation, and Interpretation Challenges Associated with Tracking Vaccination Coverage Using Household Surveys. *PLoS Med.* **2013**, *10*, e1001404. [CrossRef] [PubMed]
27. Utazi, C.E.; Wagai, J.; Pannell, O.; Cutts, F.T.; Rhoda, D.A.; Ferrari, M.J.; Dieng, B.; Oteri, J.; Danovaro-Holliday, M.C.; Adeniran, A.; et al. Geospatial variation in measles vaccine coverage through routine and campaign strategies in Nigeria: Analysis of recent household surveys. *Vaccine* **2020**, *38*, 3062–3071. [CrossRef] [PubMed]
28. Danovaro-Holliday, M.C.; Dansereau, E.; Rhoda, D.A.; Brown, D.W.; Cutts, F.T.; Gacic-Dobo, M. Collecting and using reliable vaccination coverage survey estimates: Summary and recommendations from the "Meeting to share lessons learnt from the roll-out of the updated WHO Vaccination Coverage Cluster Survey Reference Manual and to set an operational research agenda around vaccination coverage surveys", Geneva, 18–21 April 2017. *Vaccine* **2018**, *36*, 5150–5159. [CrossRef] [PubMed]
29. Biostat Global Consulting. Vaccination Coverage Quality Indicators (VCQI)—Resources [Internet]. 2024. Available online: http://www.biostatglobal.com/VCQI_RESOURCES.HTML (accessed on 23 August 2024).
30. Prier, M.L.; Rhoda, D.A. Organ Pipe Plots for Clustered Datasets—Visualize Disparities in Cluster-Level Coverage [Internet]. Stata Conference 2018; Columbus, Ohio. Available online: https://github.com/BiostatGlobalConsulting/organ-pipe-plots/blob/master/opplot_presentation.pptx (accessed on 23 August 2024).
31. Cutts, F.T.; Ferrari, M.J.; Krause, L.K.; Tatem, A.J.; Mosser, J.F. Vaccination strategies for measles control and elimination: Time to strengthen local initiatives. *BMC Med.* **2021**, *19*, 2. [CrossRef]
32. World Health Organization. *Measles and Rubella Strategic Framework 2021–2030*; World Health Organization: Geneva, Switzerland, 2020.
33. Measles Cases in the AFRO Region. South Sudan. Available online: https://www.afro.who.int/sites/default/files/2024-06/Measles%20Outbreak%20and%20Response%20Weekly%20Situation%20Update_Week%2019,%202024.pdf (accessed on 23 August 2024).
34. Behavioral and Social Drivers of Immunization. Available online: https://www.who.int/teams/immunization-vaccines-and-biologicals/essential-programme-on-immunization/demand (accessed on 15 October 2024).
35. Akpan, G.U.; Mohammed, H.F.; Touray, K.; Kipterer, J.; Bello, I.M.; Ngofa, R.; Stein, A.; Seaman, V.; Mkanda, P.; Cabore, J. Conclusions of the African Regional GIS Summit (2019): Using geographic information systems for public health decision-making. *BMC Proc.* **2022**, *16* (Suppl. 1), 3. [CrossRef]
36. Utazi, C.E.; Aheto, J.M.; Wigley, A.; Tejedor-Garavito, N.; Bonnie, A.; Nnanatu, C.C.; Wagai, J.; Williams, C.; Setayesh, H.; Tatem, A.J.; et al. Mapping the distribution of zero-dose children to assess the performance of vaccine delivery strategies and their relationships with measles incidence in Nigeria. *Vaccine* **2022**, *41*, 170–181. [CrossRef]
37. Arambepola, R.; Yang, Y.; Hutchinson, K.; Mwansa, F.D.; Doherty, J.A.; Bwalya, F.; Ndubani, P.; Musukwa, G.; Moss, W.J.; Wesolowski, A.; et al. Using geospatial models to map zero-dose children: Factors associated with zero-dose vaccination status before and after a mass measles and rubella vaccination campaign in Southern province, Zambia. *BMJ Glob. Health* **2021**, *6*, e007479. [CrossRef] [PubMed]

38. Gebreslasie, M.T. A review of spatial technologies with applications for malaria transmission modelling and control in Africa. *Geospat. Health* **2015**, *10*, 239–247. [CrossRef] [PubMed]
39. Fatima, M.; O'keefe, K.J.; Wei, W.; Arshad, S.; Gruebner, O. Geospatial Analysis of COVID-19: A Scoping Review. *Int. J. Environ. Res. Public Health* **2021**, *18*, 2336. [CrossRef] [PubMed] [PubMed Central]
40. Seidenberg, A.B.; Moser, R.P.; West, B.T. Preferred Reporting Items for Complex Sample Survey Analysis (PRICSSA). *J. Surv. Stat. Methodol.* **2023**, *11*, 743–757. [CrossRef]

vaccines

MDPI

*Article*

# On the Path to Measles and Rubella Elimination Following Rubella-Containing Vaccine Introduction, 2000–2023, Namibia

**Balcha G. Masresha [1,*], Messeret E. Shibeshi [1], Roselina de Wee [2], Nicholas Shapumba [3], Takudzwa Sayi [4], Susan E. Reef [5] and James L. Goodson [4]**

1 African Regional Office, World Health Organization, Brazzaville P.O. Box 06, Congo; eshetum@who.int
2 Country Office, World Health Organization, Windhoek P.O. Box 3444, Namibia; deweer@who.int
3 Expanded Programme on Immunization, Namibia Ministry of Health and Social Services, Windhoek 13198, Namibia
4 Global Immunization Division, US Centers for Disease Control and Prevention, Atlanta, GA 30333, USA; prp2@cdc.gov (T.S.); fez9@cdc.gov (J.L.G.)
5 Independent Consultant, Atlanta, GA 30329, USA; susanreef4@gmail.com
* Correspondence: masreshab@who.int

**Abstract:** Introduction: The WHO Measles and Rubella Strategic Framework 2021–2030 within the Immunization Agenda 2030 includes both measles and rubella elimination goals and provides guidance to countries for planning and implementing the measles and rubella elimination strategies. Namibia has been implementing measles elimination strategies since 1997. Methods: We reviewed and described the implementation of measles and rubella elimination strategies and the programmatic and epidemiological situation in Namibia during 2000–2023. Namibia introduced a rubella-containing vaccine (RCV) in 2016 as a combined measles–rubella (MR) vaccine using a MR catch-up campaign, targeting a wide age range based on detailed analysis and triangulation of multiple key data sources including MR vaccination coverage, MR case-based surveillance, detailed measles outbreak investigations, and serosurveys. Results: In 2020, estimated MCV1 coverage in Namibia reached 90% and has been sustained at 91% in 2021 and 2022. MCV2 was introduced in 2016, and the estimated MCV2 coverage has steadily increased to 79% in 2022. Following the MCV2 introduction and the implementation of the wide age range MR catch-up campaign in 2016, annual measles and rubella incidence decreased substantially. During 2017–2023, the period following the implementation of the catch-up MR vaccination SIA in 2016, average annual measles incidence per million population in Namibia decreased by 97% from the average during 2010–2016. Similarly, the average annual rubella incidence decreased by 95% from 2010–2016 to 2017–2023. Discussion: Successful implementation of the 2016 wide age range campaign and maintaining high routine immunization coverage likely led to the significant reduction in measles and rubella incidence in Namibia. To sustain the reduction in measles and rubella incidence and attain the elimination targets, Namibia needs to attain and maintain high routine immunization coverage with both doses of the MR vaccine and implement timely and high-quality periodic MR follow-up SIAs. High-quality elimination-standard measles and rubella surveillance will help guide strategies and serve as the basis for the eventual verification of measles and rubella elimination in Namibia according to the WHO-recommended framework.

**Keywords:** measles; rubella; Namibia; incidence; elimination

## 1. Introduction

Measles remains a major cause of child mortality worldwide, and rubella is the leading cause of birth defects among all infectious diseases globally [1–4], despite the availability of safe and effective measles and rubella vaccines since the 1960s. Both diseases are among a handful that have been identified for possible eradication [5,6]. The feasibility and benefits of measles and rubella elimination are well established, and global progress toward elimination continues to be made [7–12]. Elimination of both diseases is optimally achieved by implementing synergistic integrated strategies that include using an inexpensive, safe, and highly effective combined measles and rubella vaccine, case-based disease surveillance for rash-fever illness to detect and confirm both diseases, and rapid outbreak response [13]. To introduce a rubella-containing vaccine (RCV) in a national immunization program, the WHO recommends first using a combined measles–rubella (MR) vaccine in a national wide age range catch-up campaign and then using the MR vaccine for all recommended vaccination opportunities, including the two routine doses, periodic SIAs, and measles outbreak response immunizations (ORIs). During measles ORIs, using MR is critically important since measles is a tracer for identifying areas of weakness in immunization services, low vaccination coverage, and immunity gaps for both measles and rubella [14–16].

The basic reproductive number ($R_0$) ranges from 9 to 18 for measles and from 4 to 7 for rubella, depending on context-specific variables [17,18]; recent analyses suggest that rubella $R_0$ can be even lower in some settings [19]. Herd immunity thresholds for measles are higher than for rubella, and while both vaccines are highly effective, vaccine effectiveness for the rubella vaccine is slightly higher than the measles vaccine; therefore, the integrated MR elimination strategies are generally driven by measles epidemiology. Historically, national immunization programs have sequentially introduced the two vaccines, with the measles vaccine first and the rubella vaccine introduction coming some years later [18,20]. By the end of 2023, only 19 countries worldwide remained without rubella vaccine introduction, nearly all in the African Region. Rubella vaccine introduction with MR offers an important opportunity to close any remaining measles population immunity gaps while maximizing population immunity for rubella.

Global efforts to eliminate measles and rubella are ongoing. In 2012, the World Health Assembly endorsed the Global Vaccine Action Plan (GVAP), which aimed at extending the full benefits of the EPI to all and setting a target to eliminate measles and rubella in five of six WHO regions by 2020 [5,21–24]. As of 2024, all six WHO regions had established a measles elimination goal, and five a rubella elimination goal. The WHO African Region Member States established measles and rubella elimination goals in 2011 and 2021 [25,26], respectively; and the WHO provided a regional elimination strategic framework to support countries in the region [27,28].

Namibia is a WHO African Region Member State and middle-income country situated in the southwestern part of the African continent. The country shares land borders with South Africa, Botswana, Angola, and Zambia and had an estimated population of 2.5 million in 2021 [29,30]. The country is dry and sparsely inhabited with the Kalahari Desert in the east and the Namib Desert in the coastal regions; 67% of inhabitants are rural dwellers. Following the declaration of national independence in 1990, Namibia established the national Ministry of Health and Social Services (MoHSS) Expanded Programme on Immunization (EPI). Measles vaccination in the population initially began prior to independence in 1983 with the introduction of one dose of the measles vaccine given to infants at nine months of age. Starting in 2016, a routine second dose of the measles-containing vaccine (MCV2) is provided at 15 months of age through ongoing immunization services. The RCV was also introduced in 2016, following which the monovalent measles vaccine was replaced by a combined MR vaccine for all vaccination activities based on WHO recommendations [31–33].

During 1997–2009, measles SIAs started with a catch-up campaign in 1997 for children 9 months–14 years of age, and then periodic follow-up SIAs in 2000, 2003, 2006, and 2009 for children 9–59 months of age. Reported administrative coverage for those campaigns ranged from 89% to 104% (a value > 100% indicates that the number of doses administered exceeded the estimated target population); no post-campaign coverage surveys were implemented. Following the initial catch-up measles SIA in 1997, which reached 677,538 children aged 9 months–14 years, Namibia experienced a period of very low measles incidence for approximately five years [34,35]. After this period of very low incidence, periodic measles outbreaks with lower incidence than in the pre-vaccination era restarted, similar to patterns documented in other settings [35]. Measles outbreaks in Namibia during 2002–2003, 2009–2011, and 2013–2014 were well documented [36]. These outbreaks were characterized by shifting measles epidemiology over time that included increases in the age of infection of cases. In 2010, Ogbuanu et al. conducted a comprehensive detailed outbreak investigation and found that 38% of confirmed measles cases were in persons $\geq$ 15 years of age during 2009–2011 [37,38]. Additionally, an analysis of the case-based surveillance data from 2014 found that 21% of measles cases were in persons $\geq$ 25 years of age [39].

Seroprevalence surveys (serosurveys) were completed to further characterize population immunity for measles, rubella, and polio and to identify age groups with susceptibility for evidence to help guide measles and rubella elimination and polio eradication efforts in Namibia, [40–42]. These serosurveys of a randomly selectedage-stratified patient subset of previously collected and stored serum specimens from the MoHSS national HIV surveys among pregnant women aged 15–44 years and were completed in 2008 and 2010; (the results were previously published elsewhere [40–42]). In both serosurveys, the lowest measles seroprevalence was among persons 15–19 years of age, and overall measles seropositivity did not differ significantly between 2008 (87%) and 2010 (87%) despite a large measles outbreak occurring in the interim [40,41]. In 2010, measles seropositivity among those aged 15–19, 20–24, 25–29, 30–34, 34–39, and 40–44 years was 56%, 71%, 77%, 80%, 88%, and 91% respectively. In 2010, rubella seropositivity by 5-year age group among those aged 15–19, 20–24, 25–29, 30–34, 34–39, and 40–44 years was 83%, 86%, 82%, 86%, 88%, and 90% respectively. Women from urban residences had significantly higher rubella seroprevalence (87%) compared with women from rural residences (83%) ($p < 0.001$) [40,41].

The findings from surveillance data of increased age-specific measles incidence in older age groups, combined with the identified population immunity gaps in older age groups from the measles and rubella serosurveys, provided strong evidence of MR susceptibility in older age groups and helped define the target age group for the 2016 SIA. The epidemiological shift to older age groups following increasing vaccination coverage, a shift observed in other settings [43], was well described in Namibia during measles outbreak investigations during 2009–2010. Based on the evidence, a key decision was made by the Namibia MoHSS to use an expanded target age group in the next SIA to provide MR vaccinations for persons 9 months–39 years of age. The national MR SIA was implemented during 11–22 July 2016 and had reported administrative coverage of > 100%. It was the first opportunity to provide the RCV through the EPI in the country, and, therefore, to prevent rubella infection and make progress toward achieving rubella elimination. The SIA was followed by the introduction of the RCV in the national EPI schedule per the WHO guidance [31]. We reviewed and described the implementation of measles and rubella elimination strategies and the programmatic and epidemiological situation during 2000–2023 to document and share experiences from Namibia in advancing progress toward the goal of measles and rubella elimination.

## 2. Methods

**Routine Immunization Services:** The national estimated population was 2,133,188 in 2009 and included 69,067 surviving infants, 300,260 children < 5 years of age, and 839,112 children < 15 years of age. In 2009, life expectancy was 53 years for males and 62 years for females, and the under-five mortality rate was 69 per 1000 live births. The MoHSS is organized into three levels—national, regional, and district—with district health centers serving as the primary service delivery level. Namibian citizens who possess a registration card (called a health passport) receive all health services free of charge after payment of a nominal registration fee. In addition to the MoHSS, some immunization services are delivered through fee for services in the private sector. The national EPI provides ongoing daily immunization services at health facilities and outreach sites and during periodic SIAs at fixed post sites and by mobile teams. Vaccine doses are administered to eligible persons during daily immunization services and periodic SIAs are reported from the health facilities to the provinces and onward to the national level. Sub-national and national administrative coverage data are calculated by the EPI by dividing the number of children vaccinated during vaccination activities by the number of children in the vaccination target age group the program reports it intends to vaccinate based on estimated population denominators. The country reports the national-level coverage annually to the WHO and UNICEF as part of the annual Joint Reporting Form (JRF) process. The WHO and UNICEF use the reported administrative coverage data and any available survey results to generate the WHO/UNICEF estimates of national immunization coverage (WUENIC) for each antigen provided through routine immunization services [44]. Data from private sector immunization services were not available. We analyzed reported vaccination data for routine immunization services from the JRF and WUENIC during 2000–2023.

**Supplemental Immunization Activities:** The periodic measles and MR SIAs are implemented with the objective of achieving $\geq$ 95% vaccination coverage; generally, the SIAs occur every 2–5 years, depending on the rate of accumulation of measles-susceptibility, primarily based on children missed by routine immunization services [45,46]. The SIAs are designed to reach all children in the target age group and include special strategies to reach areas with large numbers of unvaccinated or "zero-dose" children [47]. The number of doses provided during SIAs is tallied at the service delivery level and compiled for reporting up to the provincial level and then the national level. The SIA administrative coverage is calculated by the EPI using the administrative method of dividing the number of children vaccinated during the SIA by the number of children in the SIA target age group for the vaccination; the denominators are based on the 2001 and 2011 census projections. SIA coverage data are reported to the WHO using official SIA technical reports. We analyzed technical reports and post-campaign surveys (PCCSs) from measles and measles–rubella SIAs implemented during 2000–2023 [48].

**Measles and Rubella Incidence and Case-based Surveillance Performance**: Nationwide measles case-based surveillance with the support of the national laboratory for serological case confirmation was established in 1998 in Namibia. Suspected measles cases were defined as illnesses characterized by a generalized maculopapular rash and fever and at least one of the following: cough, coryza, or conjunctivitis, or any case suspected to be measles by a clinician. For suspected cases, patient age, sex, address, number of measles vaccination doses received, and date of most recent measles vaccination were collected by a clinician on a standard case report form. Blood specimens were collected from persons with suspected measles cases identified within 30 days of onset and tested for measles-specific immunoglobulin M (IgM) antibodies at the national measles reference laboratory using a standard enzyme-linked immunosorbent assay. Specimens tested without a positive result were then tested for rubella-specific IgM antibodies. Confirmed measles cases were defined by either a positive result for measles IgM antibody testing, by epidemiological linkage, or clinically compatible case classification. Confirmed rubella cases were defined by a positive test result for the rubella IgM antibody. An epidemiologically linked case was defined as a case-patient with illness that met the suspected case definition and had contact ('contact' defined according to surveillance guidelines as living in same district or adjacent districts with plausibility of transmission) with a laboratory-confirmed measles case with rash onset within the preceding 30 days. The national case-based surveillance database and the serological laboratory database were shared by MoHSS with the WHO weekly. We analyzed the measles and rubella surveillance data from 2010 to 2023 to describe the measles and rubella epidemiology and the quality of surveillance performance measured using the WHO-recommended performance indicators. Two key performance indicators were analyzed: (1) the non-measles febrile rash illness (NMFRI) rate (target: $\geq$ 2 per 100,000 population) and (2) the proportion of districts that have investigated $\geq$ 1 suspected case of measles with blood specimen (target: $\geq$ 80% of districts) annually. The confirmed measles incidence per million population was calculated by dividing the total number of confirmed measles cases (confirmed by laboratory, epidemiological linkage, and clinically compatible case classification) by the total population based on the official projections from the census estimates. The incidence of confirmed rubella was calculated using the number of laboratory-confirmed rubella cases as the numerator and the same denominator as used for measles incidence [49].

*Measles Immunity Profile*

Estimating measles immunity gaps can help guide immunization programs in monitoring program performance, identifying when the next SIAs should be conducted and identifying age groups that have the largest measles immunity gaps. The WHO recommends countries monitor the risk of measles outbreaks by estimating the accumulated number of measles-susceptible preschool children, and preventing outbreaks by conducting SIAs before that number reaches the equivalent of one birth cohort. This approach has been found to be programmatically useful in preventing large outbreaks. We generated the national measles immunity profile to estimate the number of persons immune by MCV1, MCV2, and SIAs and the number of measles-susceptible persons by year of birth. The estimated percentage of measles-susceptible persons is multiplied by the number of persons by age to estimate the total number of measles-susceptible persons by age as of 31 December 2023. To estimate a profile as of 31 December 2023, MCV1 and MCV2 coverage data points in 2023 were assumed to be the same as the WUENIC for 2022, the last year available. PCCS estimates were used for SIA coverage, and if unavailable, we used administrative coverage.

## 3. Results

**Ongoing Immunization Services:** Estimated MCV1 coverage in Namibia was 75% in 2010, and it steadily increased to 85% in 2015 and then fluctuated between 75% and 82% until 2019 (Figure 1). In 2020, estimated MCV1 coverage reached 90% and was sustained at 91% in both 2021 and 2022. After MCV2 was introduced in the childhood vaccination schedule in 2016, estimated MCV2 coverage steadily increased from 32% in 2017 to 79% in 2022. Since RCV introduction in 2016, the EPI has switched from using a monovalent measles vaccine to a combined MR vaccine for all doses, and RCV coverage is represented by the measles vaccination coverage data.

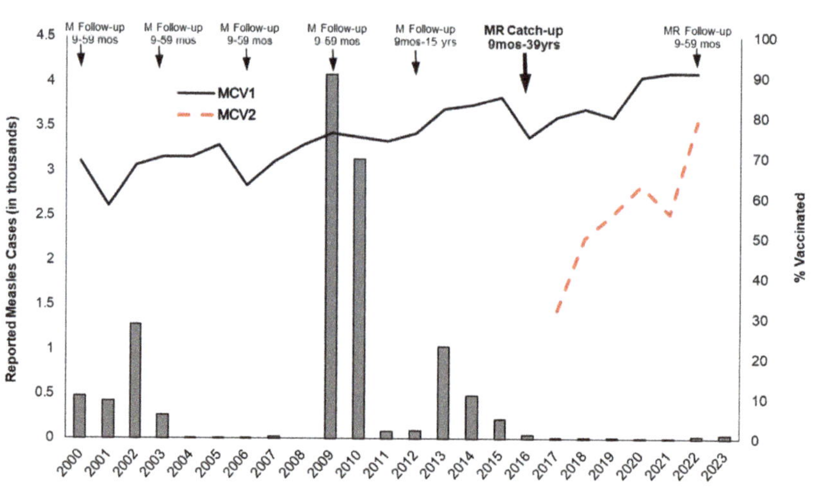


**Figure 1.** National coverage with the first dose of the measles-containing vaccine (MCV1) and second dose (MCV2), supplemental immunization activities, and reported measles cases, 2000–2023, Namibia. Notes: M = measles, MR = measles–rubella, mos = months, yrs = years; World Health Organization (WHO) and United Nations Children's Fund (UNICEF) estimates of national immunization coverage; data from the Joint Reporting Form submitted to the WHO and UNICEF by member states with the official number of measles cases in the country for the year, http://immunizationdata.who.int (accessed on 11 June 2024).

**Supplemental Immunization Activities:** In 2012, Namibia conducted a nationwide measles SIA for children aged 9 months–15 years (Table 1). The reported SIA administrative coverage for the 2012 SIA was 91%, and a PCCS that estimated nationwide SIA coverage was 97%. In 2016, Namibia conducted a wide age range catch-up MR SIA for persons aged 9 months–39 years as part of the strategy for RCV introduction. A total of 1,908,193 persons were vaccinated during the nationwide MR SIA, with 103% reported administrative coverage, and 77% of districts reported ≥95% administrative coverage. In 2022, a follow-up MR SIA for children aged 9–59 months was implemented with a reported 95% administrative coverage. A PCCS was not performed following SIAs in 2016 and 2022.

**Table 1.** National measles and measles–rubella supplementary immunization activities, 2000–2023, Namibia.

| Year | Type of SIAs | Target Age Group | Number of Persons Targeted | Number of Persons Vaccinated | Administrative Coverage | Proportion of Districts with ≥95% Coverage | SIA Coverage by Survey |
|---|---|---|---|---|---|---|---|
| 2000 | M Follow-up | 9–59 months | 285,504 | 257,590 | 80% | N/A | N/A |
| 2003 | M Follow-up | 9–59 months | 340,000 | 318,240 | 94% | N/A | N/A |
| 2006 | M Follow-up | 9–59 months | 353,270 | 318,905 | 97% | N/A | N/A |
| 2009 | M Follow-up | 9–59 months | 246,501 | 256,006 | 104% | N/A | N/A |
| 2012 | M Follow-up | 9 months–15 years | 972,163 | 885,259 | 91% | 100% | 97% |
| 2016 | MR Catch-up | 9 months–39 years | 1,859,857 | 1,908,193 | 103% | 77% | N/A |
| 2022 | MR Follow-up | 9–59 months | 309,916 | 293,705 | 95% | 53% | N/A |

Notes: M = measles, MR = measles–rubella, SIAs = supplementary immunization activities, N/A = not available.

**Measles and Rubella Incidence:** During 2010–2016, the average annual incidence per million persons was 163.9 (range: 5.0 to 656.4) for measles and 53.3 (range: 5.0 to 172.9) for rubella. The laboratory-confirmed measles incidence per million population sharply fell from 88.3 in 2015 to 5.0 in 2016 (the year of the MR catch-up SIAs) and was 7.5 in 2017. Similarly, the confirmed rubella incidence per million persons declined from 172.9 in 2015 to 15.4 in 2016 and 7.1 in 2017. During 2017–2023, the period following the implementation of the catch-up MR vaccination SIA in 2016, the average annual measles incidence per million population in Namibia was 4.9 (range: 0.7–10.5) and decreased 97% from the average during 2010–2016, with the total number of reported confirmed cases decreasing from 2698 during 2010–2016 to 113 during 2017–2023 (Table 2). Similarly, the average annual rubella incidence per million population in Namibia was 2.7, with a range from 0.4 to 7.1. The average annual rubella incidence decreased 95.4% from 2010–2016 to 2017–2023 with the total number of confirmed rubella cases decreasing from 885 during 2010–2016 to 52 during 2017–2023; a total of 4 reported rubella cases occurred among WCBA during 2017–2023 (Table 2).

**Table 2.** Laboratory-confirmed measles and rubella cases by sex, setting, and age group, Namibia, 2010–2023.

| | | | | | Setting * | | | | Age Group | | | | | | | | | | | |
|---|---|---|---|---|---|---|---|---|---|---|---|---|---|---|---|---|---|---|---|---|
| | Time Period | Cases † | Female | | Rural | | Urban | | <1 y | | 1–4 y | | 5–9 y | | 10–14 y | | ≥15 y | | Women of Reproductive Age (15–49 y) | |
| | Years | n | n | % | n | % | n | % | n | % | n | % | n | % | n | % | n | % | n | % |
| Measles | 2010–2016 | 2698 | 1328 | 49 | 1124 | 65 | 602 | 35 | 74 | 3 | 708 | 26 | 568 | 21 | 342 | 13 | 707 | 26 | 702 | 29 |
| | 2017–2023 | 113 | 49 | 43 | 31 | 27 | 82 | 73 | 0 | 0 | 44 | 39 | 47 | 42 | 8 | 7 | 3 | 3 | 3 | 3 |
| Rubella | 2010–2016 | 885 | 465 | 53 | 314 | 39 | 482 | 61 | 2 | 2 | 171 | 21 | 343 | 42 | 197 | 24 | 111 | 13 | 110 | 13 |
| | 2017–2023 | 52 | 27 | 52 | 15 | 29 | 37 | 71 | 0 | 0 | 13 | 30 | 18 | 41 | 8 | 18 | 5 | 11 | 4 | 9 |

Notes: * Setting classification was reported as either urban or rural; the percentages are of those without a missing value. † Total number of laboratory-confirmed cases detected through the national case-based surveillance system with specimens tested at the national measles reference laboratory using a standard enzyme-linked immunosorbent assay. The national measles and rubella case-based surveillance uses a case definition of rash, fever, and at least one of cough, coryza, and conjunctivitis, to rash and fever; under-reporting of measles and rubella cases is common and well documented.

*3.1. Measles and Rubella Case-Based Surveillance Performance*

Measles and rubella case-based surveillance performance in Namibia met the key indicator target for assessing the sensitivity of the system of ≥2 NMFRI annually since 2010 (Table 3). The key indicator target for nationwide case confirmation by laboratory testing of ≥80% of districts reporting cases with a blood specimen annually was met 5 (36%) times during 2010–2023. In recent years since 2020, the surveillance system performance steadily improved; the NMFRI increased from 3.7 to 12.5 and the proportion of districts reporting cases with a blood specimen increased from 18% to 74% during 2021–2023. However, since 2018, the percentage of districts that investigated at least one measles-suspected case with a blood specimen per year was <80%, indicating suboptimal surveillance performance and likely under-reporting of measles and rubella.

**Table 3.** Measles and rubella case-based surveillance performance, 2010–2023, Namibia.

| Year | % Districts that Investigated at Least One Measles-Suspected Case with a Blood Specimen per Year (Target: ≥ 80%) | Non-Measles Febrile Rash Illness Rate per 100,000 Population (Target: ≥ 2 per Million Population) |
|---|---|---|
| 2010 | 82% | 22.6 |
| 2011 | 82% | 18.9 |
| 2012 | 73% | 16.0 |
| 2013 | 59% | 6.8 |
| 2014 | 73% | 16.5 |
| 2015 | 75% | 45.6 |
| 2016 | 85% | 10.9 |
| 2017 | 100% | 16.9 |
| 2018 | 91% | 11.3 |
| 2019 | 76% | 7.3 |
| 2020 | 76% | 7.8 |
| 2021 | 18% | 3.7 |
| 2022 | 68% | 5.5 |
| 2023 | 74% | 12.5 |

*3.2. Measles Immunity Profile*

The estimated number of measles-susceptible children less than 5 years of age was 42,954 as of December 31, 2023, which was 64% of the number of children born in the most recent year, far below the size of one birth cohort, suggesting that population immunity was sufficient to prevent measles outbreaks at that time (Figure 2). Among older children, the highest measles susceptibility remained among those aged 6 years (19%), 7 years (37%), and 8 years (11%), primarily because these birth cohorts were not fully covered by the implemented SIAs. The SIA strategy protected adults born since 1980, reducing measles susceptibility to <10% in each adult birth cohort. For adults born prior to national independence in 1990, MCV1 coverage estimates were not available; therefore, population immunity for those cohorts was based on SIA coverage only and likely underestimated population immunity.

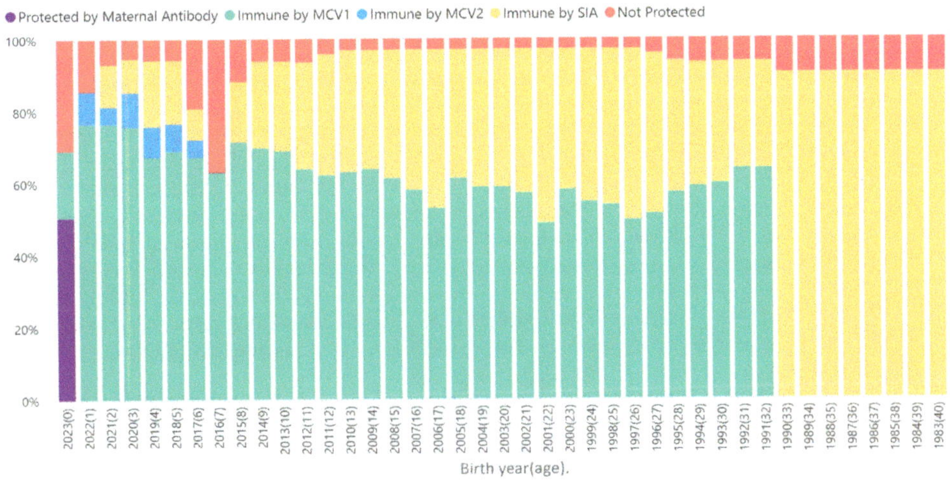


**Figure 2.** National measles immunity profile as of 31 December 2023, Namibia. Notes: MCV1 = first dose of the measles-containing vaccine; MCV2 = second dose of the measles-containing vaccine; SIAs = supplementary immunization activities. The number of measles-susceptible children under 5 years of age was projected to be 42,954 by 31 December 2023, which was 0.64 times the number of children born in the most recent year.

## 4. Discussion

Our analysis showed that Namibia achieved substantial reductions in both measles and rubella incidence following the implementation of elimination strategies, including the introduction of the RCV with the wide age range catch-up SIA in 2016. Since this pivotal SIA, along with the other ongoing elimination strategies, the annual incidence for both measles and rubella has remained <5 per million population, the elimination threshold, and, in fact, at or near zero reported cases. The country has not experienced any large and disruptive measles or rubella outbreaks as it did before 2016. The successful measles campaign in Namibia suggests that sustaining very high (≥ 95%) two-dose MR vaccination rates might not be required to substantially reduce or even interrupt measles and rubella virus transmission in an African context. Further, considering the lower reproductive number of rubella, the measles immunity profile indicated that the EPI, through the use of the MR vaccine, has maintained sufficient levels of population immunity to prevent both measles and rubella outbreaks.

A decline in reported rubella incidence to near zero after the implementation of a wide-age range MR SIA for RCV introduction is consistent with previously described findings in other settings [50–53]. Prior to the introduction of the RCV in the WHO African Region (AFR), the rubella virus circulated widely throughout the region and primarily infected young children [54]. Estimates from the three largest serosurveys of women of child-bearing age (WCBA) in the AFR prior to the use of the RCV found that rubella susceptibility was 6–16% among WCBA [54]. During 2002–2009 in the AFR, of the 25,631 confirmed rubella cases, 25,097 (98%) had information on age; 3% were infants < 1 year, 28% were 1–4 years, 47% were 5–9 years, 16% were 10–14 years, and 5% were ≥15 years of age, and the mean age of persons with rubella virus infection was 7.3 years [54]. In Namibia during 2002–2009, of the 545 laboratory-confirmed rubella cases, 481 (88.3%) were less than 15 years of age, while 58 (11%) were ≥15 years of age, all in WCBA. Sentinel surveillance for congenital rubella syndrome (CRS) has not been established in Namibia; therefore, the dearth of CRS data makes it difficult to fully estimate the impact of RCV use on disease burden. However, the implementation of high-performing case-based surveillance provided data showing that reported rubella cases decreased to ≤10 annually, and there were only four reported rubella cases among WCBA during 2017–2023.

The analysis and triangulation of multiple key data sources including MR vaccination coverage, MR case-based surveillance, detailed measles outbreak investigations, programmatic risk assessments, and serosurveys provided critical evidence to support the decision made by the country to implement the wide age range MR SIA in 2016 [36–38,40,41,43,55–57]. Before RCV introduction in Namibia, analysis of surveillance data and outbreak investigations for both measles and polio indicated an epidemiological shift in susceptibility to older age groups and outbreaks following virus importations from cross-border population movement with neighboring countries [36–38,43,55,56]. Moreover, the 2013 DHS Survey in Namibia documented wide variations in MCV1 coverage among the provinces, leading to geographically clustered measles susceptibility in the population and corresponding to the areas with increased measles incidence during outbreaks, which were identified as areas with high risk in programmatic risk assessments [58].

Some limitations of the data need to be considered when interpreting the results. First, administrative vaccination coverage for both routine immunization services and SIAs can be biased by inaccurate estimates of population denominators and incorrect reporting of doses delivered, resulting in the need for careful interpretation of the coverage data. Since a PCCS was not implemented in 2016 or 2022, the reported administrative SIA coverage could not be triangulated with survey estimates. Second, under-reporting of measles and rubella through surveillance is well documented; therefore, the surveillance data analyses were representative of reported cases and did not account for undetected and unreported cases, including those cases that may have been seen in the private sector but not included in the nationwide surveillance reporting. Third, comparisons of annual measles and rubella case totals and incidences may be inaccurate if the completeness of case reporting varies from year to year. Finally, surveillance performance around the time of the COVID-19 pandemic indicated that the country was not able to fully document measles and rubella cases as was expected, and so the data likely did not reflect the actual epidemiology of these diseases.

To sustain the reduction in measles and rubella incidence and attain the elimination targets, Namibia needs to achieve and maintain high routine immunization coverage with both doses of the MR vaccine and implement timely and high-quality periodic MR follow-up SIAs, and high-quality elimination-standard MR case-based surveillance need to be implemented [13,27]. The identified measles susceptibility remaining among children born during 2015–2017 heightens the risk for outbreaks and may need to be addressed with targeted vaccination activities to sustain elimination. If an outbreak does occur, these cohorts likely will have a higher age-specific incidence since measles epidemiology reflects susceptibility in the population. A similar scenario from susceptible cohorts that were missed by the SIA strategy was observed in a measles outbreak in Dar es Salaam, Tanzania, during 2006–2007 [59,60]; analysis of the surveillance data during the outbreak investigation revealed cohorts missed by previous SIAs likely contributed to the outbreak occurrence and needed to be covered rapidly during local outbreak response immunizations and a subsequent national follow-up SIA using a wide target age group. Like trends widely documented in other countries, vaccination coverage in Namibia was affected during the COVID-19 pandemic, with a flattening of the MCV1 coverage trend during 2020–2022 and a decline in MCV2 coverage in 2021 [61,62]. Surveillance performance was also noted to have dropped in 2021, with only 18% of districts having reported suspected measles or rubella cases. Sensitive surveillance and targeted efforts to close immunity gaps will be critical to prevent large outbreaks of measles or rubella when virus importations occur. As of early 2024, South Africa has not yet introduced the RCV nationwide in the immunization schedule, and sustained rubella virus transmission is ongoing in South Africa [63]. Angola has very low routine vaccination coverage and has been experiencing large measles and rubella outbreaks, posing ongoing risks of virus transmission across borders into Namibia and other countries. Maintaining high-performing case-based surveillance and capacity for rapid outbreak response will be essential for Namibia to quickly confirm cases and identify and address immunity gaps to stop outbreaks and sustain elimination.

Successful implementation of the 2016 wide age range campaign, along with the other ongoing elimination strategies, likely led to the interruption of endemic measles and rubella viruses in the country, with sporadic cases likely related to importations from neighboring countries that remain endemic for both diseases. However, verification of measles and rubella elimination in Namibia will be needed following the WHO-recommended verification framework [27,64]. The WHO verification framework recommends documentation of required evidence through a national verification committee (NVC) report to the regional verification commission (RVC) to define metrics and key evidence for monitoring progress toward the regional goals for measles and rubella elimination [25–27,64]. The interruption of endemic rubella or measles virus transmission is defined as at least 12 months without ongoing local transmission. When interruption of transmission is sustained for 36 months, the RVC weighs the available evidence from the NVC by applying the WHO verification framework [65]. Genotypic documentation of measles and rubella virus strains is critical as part of the process of documenting progress towards elimination and as key evidence for the verification of the elimination of measles and rubella. Given the documented progress toward measles and rubella elimination achieved in Namibia, it is recommended that the NVC compile and submit a report to the RVC for verification.

The IA2030 MRSF includes measles and rubella elimination as a goal and provides guidance to countries for planning and implementing measles and rubella elimination strategies [45]. As of the end of 2022, the elimination of endemic rubella has been verified in 93 countries [28], and measles elimination has been verified in 83 countries [66]; however, none of these countries are in the WHO African Region. Of the 19 countries globally remaining without the RCV, 15 are in the African Region and account for nearly the entire global burden of CRS, highlighting the gross inequities of access to the RVC. Efforts should be made to ensure resources are made available to support universal RCV introduction, including in the remaining 15 countries in the African Region. The implementation of the initial nationwide wide age range MR SIA and periodic follow-up MR SIAs to achieve and maintain population immunity to eliminate rubella and CRS is a golden opportunity for building population immunity and has the additional benefit of reducing any remaining measles susceptibility in older children and young adults if included in the MR SIA target age group to achieve and maintain the elimination of both rubella and measles [36,54,67].

Namibia is currently on track to be one of the first countries in the WHO African Region to be verified for achieving the elimination of both measles and rubella. Until all countries in the region introduce the RCV and make substantial progress toward measles and rubella elimination, the risk for virus importations will remain high. Therefore, it is essential the country maintains high population immunity, as well as high-performing case-based surveillance and robust capacity for rapid outbreak response, to detect and stop outbreaks. Efforts by global partners should be accelerated to ensure expedited universal access and use of the RCV to support measles and rubella elimination. Measles and rubella elimination were both achieved in the Region of the Americas (although re-certification for measles elimination is pending after the re-established endemic virus appears to have been interrupted) and the other regions, including the WHO African Region, will also achieve these goals with continued progress like that achieved in Namibia [50–53].

**Author Contributions:** Conceptualization, B.G.M. and J.L.G.; methodology, B.G.M. and J.L.G.; software, T.S. and J.L.G.; validation, B.G.M., M.E.S., R.d.W., N.S., T.S., S.E.R. and J.L.G.; formal analysis, B.G.M. and J.L.G.; investigation, B.G.M., N.S., R.d.W. and J.L.G.; resources, B.G.M., M.E.S., R.d.W., N.S. and J.L.G.; data curation, B.G.M., M.E.S., R.d.W., N.S., T.S. and J.L.G.; writing—original draft preparation, B.G.M. and J.L.G.; writing—review and editing, B.G.M., T.S., S.E.R. and J.L.G.; visualization, B.G.M.; T.S.; and J.L.G.; supervision, B.G.M. and J.L.G.; project administration, B.G.M. and J.L.G. All authors have read and agreed to the published version of the manuscript.

**Funding:** This research received no external funding.

**Institutional Review Board Statement:** Not applicable.

**Informed Consent Statement:** Not applicable.

**Data Availability Statement:** Sources for vaccination coverage and population data presented in this analysis were cited. Data for generating the national population immunity profiles were the WHO-UNICEF Estimates of National Immunization Coverage (available at https://immunizationdata.who.int/, accessed on 16 June 2024) and population data from United Nations Population Division (available at https://population.un.org/wpp/, accessed on 16 June 2024).

**Acknowledgments:** The authors would like to recognize the efforts of all staff of the Expanded Programme on Immunization, surveillance officers, and laboratory staff in Namibia. The findings and conclusions in this report are those of the authors and do not necessarily represent the official position of the Centers for Disease Control and Prevention.

**Conflicts of Interest:** The authors declare no conflict of interest.

## References

1. Vynnycky, E.; Adams, E.; Cutts, F.; Reef, S.; Navar, A.; Simons, E.; Yoshida, L.-M.; Brown, D.W.J.; Jackson, C.; Strebel, P.; et al. Using Seroprevalence and Immunisation Coverage Data to Estimate the Global Burden of Congenital Rubella Syndrome, 1996–2010: A Systematic Review. *PLoS ONE* **2016**, *11*, e0149160. [CrossRef]
2. Patel, M.; Gacic Dobo, M.; Strebel, P.; Dabbagh, A.; Mulders, M.; Okwo Bele, J.-M.; Dumolard, L.; Rota, P.; Kretsinger, K.; Goodson, J. Progress Toward Regional Measles Elimination—Worldwide, 2000–2015. *MMWR Morb. Mortal. Wkly. Rep.* **2016**, *65*, 1228–1233. [CrossRef] [PubMed]
3. United Nations General Assembly. *United Nations Millennium Declaration*; United Nations General Assembly: New York, NY, USA, 2000; Available online: http://www.un.org/millenniumgoals/ (accessed on 10 May 2017).
4. World Health Organization. *Global Vaccine Action Plan 2011–2020*; World Health Organization: Geneva, Switzerland, 2012. Available online: http://www.who.int/immunization/global_vaccine_action_plan/GVAP_doc_2011_2020/en/index.html (accessed on 15 January 2020).
5. Strebel, P.M.; Cochi, S.L.; Hoekstra, E.; Rota, P.A.; Featherstone, D.; Bellini, W.J.; Katz, S.L. A World without Measles. *J. Infect. Dis.* **2011**, *204* (Suppl. 1), S1–S3. [CrossRef] [PubMed]
6. Durrheim, D.N.; Crowcroft, N.S. The price of delaying measles eradication. *Lancet Public Health* **2017**, *2*, e130–e131. [CrossRef]
7. Robbins, F.C. Prospects for Worldwide Control of Measles: Discussion I. *Rev. Infect. Dis.* **1983**, *5*, 619–620. [CrossRef]
8. Dowdle, W.; Cochi, S. The principles and feasibility of disease eradication. *Vaccine* **2011**, *29* (Suppl. 4), D70–D73. [CrossRef]
9. Thompson, K.M.; Badizadegan, N. Modeling the transmission of measles and rubella to support global management policy analyses and eradication investment cases. *Risk Anal.* **2017**, *in press*. [CrossRef]
10. International Task Force for Disease Eradication. Recommendations of the International Task Force for Disease Eradication. *MMWR Recomm. Rep. Morb. Mortal. Wkly. Rep. Recomm. Rep.* **1993**, *42*, 1–38.
11. Strebel, P.M.; Papania, M.J.; Gastañaduy, P.A.; Goodson, J.L. Measles Vaccines. In *Vaccines*, 7th ed.; Plotkin, S., Orenstein, W., Offit, P., Edwards, K.M., Eds.; Elisevier: Philadelphia, PA, USA, 2018; pp. 579–618.
12. Shattock, A.J.; Johnson, H.C.; Sim, S.Y.; Carter, A.; Lambach, P.; Hutubessy, R.C.W.; Thompson, K.M.; Badizadegan, K.; Lambert, B.; Ferrari, M.J.; et al. Contribution of vaccination to improved survival and health: Modelling 50 years of the Expanded Programme on Immunization. *Lancet* **2024**, *403*, 2307–2316. [CrossRef]
13. WHO. Measles and Rubella Strategic Framework: 2021–2030. Available online: https://www.who.int/publications/i/item/measles-and-rubella-strategic-framework-2021-2030 (accessed on 5 October 2021).
14. Goodson, J.L.; Alexander, J.P.; Linkins, R.W.; Orenstein, W.A. Measles and rubella elimination: Learning from polio eradication and moving forward with a diagonal approach. *Expert Rev. Vaccines* **2017**, *16*, 1203–1216. [CrossRef]
15. World Health Organization. *Immunization Agenda 2030 (IA2030)*; World Health Organization: Geneva, Switzerland, 2020. Available online: http://www.immunizationagenda2030.org/ (accessed on 1 June 2024).
16. World Health Organization. *Measles Outbreak Guide*; World Health Organization: Geneva, Switzerland, 2022.
17. Guerra, F.M.; Bolotin, S.; Lim, G.; Heffernan, J.; Deeks, S.L.; Li, Y.; Crowcroft, N.S. The basic reproduction number (R0) of measles: A systematic review. *Lancet Infect. Dis.* **2017**, *17*, e420–e428. [CrossRef] [PubMed]
18. Rota, P.; Moss, W.; Takeda, M.; de Swart, R.; Thompson, K.; Goodson, J. Measles. *Nat. Rev. Dis. Primers* **2016**, *2*, 16049. [CrossRef] [PubMed]
19. Nakase, T.; Brownwright, T.; Okunromade, O.; Egwuenu, A.; Ogunbode, O.; Lawal, B.; Akanbi, K.; Grant, G.; Bassey, O.O.; Coughlin, M.M.; et al. The impact of sub-national heterogeneities in demography and epidemiology on the introduction of rubella vaccination programs in Nigeria. *Vaccine* **2024**, *42*, 125982. [CrossRef]
20. World Health Organization. Meeting of the International Task Force for Disease Eradication, November 2015. *Wkly. Epidemiol. Rec.* **2016**, *91*, 61–71.

21. Nguku, P.M.; Sharif, S.K.; Mutonga, D.; Amwayi, S.; Omolo, J.; Mohammed, O.; Farnon, E.C.; Gould, L.H.; Lederman, E.; Rao, C.; et al. An investigation of a major outbreak of Rift Valley fever in Kenya: 2006–2007. *Am. J. Trop. Med. Hyg.* **2010**, *83*, 5–13. [CrossRef]
22. Strebel, P.; Grabowsky, M.; Hoekstra, E.; Gay, A.; Cochi, S. Evolution and Contribution of a Global Partnership against Measles and Rubella, 2001–2023. *Vaccines* **2024**, *12*, 693. [CrossRef]
23. Perry, R.; Gacic Dobo, M.; Dabbagh, A.; Mulders, M.; Strebel, P.; Okwo Bele, J.-M.; Rota, P.; Goodson, J. Progress toward regional measles elimination-worldwide, 2000–2013. *MMWR Morb. Mortal. Wkly. Rep.* **2014**, *63*, 1034–1038.
24. World Health Organization. Global Measles and Rubella Strategic Plan 2012–2020. Available online: http://www.who.int/immunization/newsroom/Measles_Rubella_StrategicPlan_2012_2020.pdf (accessed on 15 January 2020).
25. Regional Committee for Africa. *Measles Elimination by 2020: A Strategy for the African Region*; World Health Organization, Regional Office for Africa: Brazzaville, Congo, 2011.
26. Regional Committee for Africa. *Framework for the Implementation of the Immunization Agenda 2030 in the WHO African Region: Report of the Secretariat*; World Health Organization, Regional Office for Africa: Brazzaville, Congo, 2021.
27. Masresha, B.G.; Hatcher, C.; Lebo, E.; Tanifum, P.; Bwaka, A.M.; Minta, A.A.; Antoni, S.; Grant, G.B.; Perry, R.T.; O'Connor, P. Progress Toward Measles Elimination—African Region, 2017–2021. *MMWR Morb. Mortal. Wkly. Rep.* **2023**, *72*, 985–991. [CrossRef]
28. Ou, A.C.; Zimmerman, L.A.; Alexander, J.P., Jr.; Crowcroft, N.S.; O'Connor, P.M.; Knapp, J.K. Progress Toward Rubella and Congenital Rubella Syndrome Elimination—Worldwide, 2012–2022. *MMWR Morb. Mortal. Wkly. Rep.* **2024**, *73*, 162–167. [CrossRef]
29. World Bank. World Bank Country Economy Classification by Income. 2023. Available online: https://datahelpdesk.worldbank.org/knowledgebase/articles/906519-world-bank-country-and-lending-groups (accessed on 18 February 2024).
30. United Nations Population Division. World Population Prospects. 2022. Available online: https://population.un.org/wpp/Download/Standard/Population/ (accessed on 28 April 2024).
31. World Health Organization Organisation Mondiale de la Santé. Rubella vaccines: WHO position paper—July 2020—Note de synthèse: Position de l'OMS concernant les vaccins antirubéoleux. *Wkly. Epidemiol. Rec. Relev. Épidémiol. Hebd.* **2020**, *95*, 306–324.
32. Namibia Ministry of Health and Social Services; Expanded Programme on Immunization. *Namibia Strategic Plan for Expanded Programme on Immunization 2018–2022*; WHO Namibia Country Office: Windhoek, Namibia, 2017.
33. World Health Organization. Namibia: WHO and UNICEF Estimates of Immunization Coverage: 2022 Revision. 2023. Available online: https://cdn.who.int/media/docs/default-source/country-profiles/immunization/2023-country-profiles/immunization_nam_2023.pdf?sfvrsn=c1e915f0_3&download=true (accessed on 28 April 2024).
34. Biellik, R.; Madema, S.; Taole, A.; Kutsulukuta, A.; Allies, E.; Eggers, R.; Ngcobo, N.; Nxumalo, M.; Shearley, A.; Mabuzane, E.; et al. First 5 years of measles elimination in southern Africa: 1996–2000. *Lancet* **2002**, *359*, 1564–1568. [CrossRef] [PubMed]
35. McLean, A. After the honeymoon in measles control. *Lancet* **1995**, *345*, 272. [CrossRef]
36. Shibeshi, M.E.; Masresha, B.G.; Smit, S.B.; Biellik, R.J.; Nicholson, J.L.; Muitherero, C.; Shivute, N.; Walker, O.; Reggis, K.; Goodson, J.L. Measles resurgence in southern Africa: Challenges to measles elimination. *Vaccine* **2014**, *32*, 1798–1807. [CrossRef]
37. Ogbuanu, I.U.; Zeko, S.; Chu, S.Y.; Muroua, C.; Gerber, S.; De Wee, R.; Kretsinger, K.; Wannemuehler, K.; Gerndt, K.; Allies, M.; et al. Maternal, fetal, and neonatal outcomes associated with measles during pregnancy: Namibia, 2009–2010. *Clin. Infect. Dis.* **2014**, *58*, 1086–1092. [CrossRef] [PubMed]
38. Ogbuanu, I.U.; Muroua, C.; Allies, M.; Chitala, K.; Gerber, S.; Shilunga, P.; Mhata, P.; Kriss, J.L.; Caparos, L.; Smit, S.B.; et al. Measles outbreak reveals measles susceptibility among adults in Namibia, 2009–2011. *S. Afr. Med. J.* **2016**, *106*, 715–720. [CrossRef] [PubMed]
39. World Health Organisation African Regional Office. *Measles and Rubella Case-Based Surveillance Data Analysis*; Presented at measles technical meeting; WHO African Regional Office: Brazzaville, Congo, 2014.
40. Jonas, A.; Cardemil, C.V.; Beukes, A.; Anderson, R.; Rota, P.A.; Bankamp, B.; Gary, H.E., Jr.; Sawadogo, S.; Patel, S.V.; Zeko, S.; et al. Rubella immunity among pregnant women aged 15–44 years, Namibia, 2010. *Int. J. Infect. Dis.* **2016**, *49*, 196–201. [CrossRef]
41. Cardemil, C.V.; Jonas, A.; Beukes, A.; Anderson, R.; Rota, P.A.; Bankamp, B.; Gary, H.E., Jr.; Sawadogo, S.; Patel, S.V.; Zeko, S.; et al. Measles immunity among pregnant women aged 15–44 years in Namibia, 2008 and 2010. *Int. J. Infect. Dis.* **2016**, *49*, 189–195. [CrossRef]
42. Cardemil, C.V.; Jonas, A.; Gerber, S.; Weldon, W.C., 3rd; Oberste, M.S.; Beukes, A.; Sawadogo, S.; Patel, S.V.; Zeko, S.; Muroua, C.; et al. Poliovirus immunity among pregnant females aged 15–44 years, Namibia, 2010. *J. Infect. Dis.* **2014**, *210* (Suppl. 1), S136–S142. [CrossRef]
43. Goodson, J.L.; Masresha, B.G.; Wannemuehler, K.; Uzicanin, A.; Cochi, S. Changing Epidemiology of Measles in Africa. *J. Infect. Dis.* **2011**, *204*, S205–S214. [CrossRef]
44. Burton, A.; Monasch, R.; Lautenbach, B.; Gacic-Dobo, M.; Neill, M.; Karimov, R.; Wolfson, L.; Jones, G.; Birmingham, M. WHO and UNICEF estimates of national infant immunization coverage: Methods and processes. *World Health Organ. Bull. World Health Organ.* **2009**, *87*, 535–541. [CrossRef]
45. Simons, E.; Mort, M.; Dabbagh, A.; Strebel, P.; Wolfson, L. Strategic planning for measles control: Using data to inform op-timal vaccination strategies. *J. Infect. Dis.* **2011**, *204* (Suppl. S1), S28–S34. [CrossRef] [PubMed]

46. World Health Organization Organisation Mondiale de la Santé. Measles vaccines: WHO position paper—April 2017—Note de synthèse de l'OMS sur les vaccins contre la rougeole—Avril 2017. *Wkly. Epidemiol. Rec. Relev. Épidémiol. Hebd.* **2017**, *92*, 205–227.
47. World Health Organization. *Planning and Implementing High-Quality Supplementary Immunization Activities for Injectable Vaccines Using an Example of Measles and Rubella Vaccines: Field Guide*; World Health Organization: Geneva, Switzerland, 2016.
48. Namibia Ministry of Health and Social Services; Expanded Programme on Immunization. *Namibia Measles and Measles-Rubella Campaign Technical Reports Reported to the World Health Organization (WHO)*. Presented at technical meeting; WHO African Regional Office: Congo, Brazzaville, 2012–2021.
49. WHO Regional Office for Africa Office. African Regional Guidelines for Measles and rubella Surveillance. 2015. Available online: https://www.afro.who.int/sites/default/files/2017-06/who-african-regional-measles-and-rubella-surveillance-guidelines_updated-draft-version-april-2015_1.pdf (accessed on 28 April 2024).
50. Luce, R.; Masresha, B.G.; Katsande, R.; Fall, A.; Shibeshi, M.E. The Impact of Recent Rubella Vaccine Introduction in 5 Countries in The African Region. *J. Immunol. Sci.* **2018**, *16*, 108–112. [CrossRef]
51. Su, Q.; Ma, C.; Wen, N.; Fan, C.; Yang, H.; Wang, H.; Yin, Z.; Feng, Z.; Hao, L.; Yang, W. Epidemiological profile and progress toward rubella elimination in China. 10 years after nationwide introduction of rubella vaccine. *Vaccine* **2018**, *36*, 2079–2085. [CrossRef]
52. Castillo-Solorzano, C.; Marsigli, C.; Bravo-Alcantara, P.; Flannery, B.; Ruiz Matus, C.; Tambini, G.; Gross-Galiano, S.; Andrus, J.K. Elimination of rubella and congenital rubella syndrome in the Americas. *J. Infect. Dis.* **2011**, *204* (Suppl 2), S571–S578. [CrossRef]
53. Centers for Disease Control and Prevention. Progress toward control of rubella and prevention of congenital rubella syndrome—Worldwide, 2009. *MMWR Morb. Mortal. Wkly. Rep.* **2010**, *59*, 1307–1310.
54. Goodson, J.L.; Masresha, B.; Dosseh, A.; Byabamazima, C.; Nshimirimana, D.; Cochi, S.; Reef, S. Rubella Epidemiology in Africa in the Prevaccine Era, 2002–2009. *J. Infect. Dis.* **2011**, *204*, S215–S225. [CrossRef]
55. Kidd, S.; Goodson, J.; Aramburu, J.; Morais, A.; Gaye, A.; Wannemuehler, K.; Buffington, J.; Gerber, S.; Wassilak, S.; Uzicanin, A. Poliomyelitis outbreaks in Angola genetically linked to India: Risk factors and implications for prevention of outbreaks due to wild poliovirus importations. *Vaccine* **2011**, *29*, 3760–3766. [CrossRef] [PubMed]
56. World Health Organization. Outbreak of polio in adults—Namibia, 2006. *MMWR Morb. Mortal. Wkly. Rep.* **2006**, *55*, 1198–1201.
57. Kriss, J.; De Wee, R.; Lam, E.; Kaiser, R.; Shibeshi, M.; Ndevaetela, E.-E.; Muroua, C.; Shapumba, N.; Masresha, B.; Goodson, J. Development of the World Health Organization Measles Programmatic Risk Assessment Tool Using Experience from the 2009 Measles Outbreak in Namibia. *Risk Anal.* **2017**, *37*, 1072–1081. [CrossRef]
58. The Nambia Ministry of Health and Social Services (MoHSS); ICF International. *Namibia Demographic and Health Survey 2013*; MoHSS/Namibia and ICF International: Windhoek, Namibia, 2014.
59. Goodson, J.L.; Perry, R.T.; Mach, O.; Manyanga, D.; Luman, E.T.; Kitambi, M.; Kibona, M.; Wiesen, E.; Cairns, K.L. Measles outbreak in Tanzania, 2006–2007. *Vaccine* **2010**, *28*, 5979–5985. [CrossRef] [PubMed]
60. Goodson, J.; Wiesen, E.; Perry, R.; Mach, O.; Kitambi, M.; Kibona, M.; Luman, E.; Cairns, K.L. Impact of measles outbreak response vaccination campaign in Dar es Salaam, Tanzania. *Vaccine* **2009**, *27*, 5870–5874. [CrossRef]
61. Harris, R.C.; Chen, Y.; Côte, P.; Ardillon, A.; Nievera, M.C.; Ong-Lim, A.; Aiyamperumal, S.; Chong, C.P.; Kandasamy, K.V.; Mahenthiran, K.; et al. Impact of COVID-19 on routine immunisation in South-East Asia and Western Pacific: Disruptions and solutions. *Lancet Reg. Health West Pac.* **2021**, *10*, 100140. [CrossRef]
62. Gaythorpe, K.A.; Abbas, K.; Huber, J.; Karachaliou, A.; Thakkar, N.; Woodruff, K.; Li, X.; Echeverria-Londono, S.; Ferrari, M.; Jackson, M.L.; et al. Impact of COVID-19-related disruptions to measles, meningococcal A, and yellow fever vaccination in 10 countries. *Elife* **2021**, *10*, 67023. [CrossRef] [PubMed]
63. Hong, H.; Malfeld, S.; Smit, S.; Makhathini, L.; Fortuin, M.; Motsamai, T.; Tselana, D.; Manamela, M.J.; Motaze, N.V.; Ntshoe, G.; et al. A retrospective 5-year review of rubella in South Africa prior to the introduction of a rubella-containing vaccine. *PLoS ONE* **2022**, *17*, e0265870. [CrossRef]
64. Masresha, B.; Luce, R., Jr.; Tanifum, P.; Lebo, E.; Dosseh, A.; Mihigo, R. The African Region early experience with structures for the verification of measles elimination—A review. *Pan Afr. Med. J.* **2020**, *35*, 2. [CrossRef] [PubMed]
65. WHO. Guidance for evaluating progress towards elimination of measles and rubella. *Wkly. Epidemiol. Rec.* **2018**, *93*, 544–552.
66. Minta, A.A.; Ferrari, M.; Antoni, S.; Portnoy, A.; Sbarra, A.; Lambert, B.; Hatcher, C.; Hsu, C.H.; Ho, L.L.; Steulet, C.; et al. Progress Toward Measles Elimination—Worldwide, 2000–2022. *MMWR Morb. Mortal. Wkly. Rep.* **2023**, *72*, 1262–1268. [CrossRef]
67. Andrus, J.K.; de Quadros, C.A.; Solórzano, C.C.; Periago, M.R.; Henderson, D.A. Measles and rubella eradication in the Americas. *Vaccine* **2011**, *29* (Suppl. 4), D91–D96. [CrossRef]

*vaccines*

MDPI

*Article*

# Optimal Timing Regularly Outperforms Higher Coverage in Preventative Measles Supplementary Immunization Campaigns

**Katherine A. Rosenfeld *, Kurt Frey and Kevin A. McCarthy**

Institute for Disease Modeling, Bill and Melinda Gates Foundation, Seattle, WA 98109, USA
* Correspondence: katherine.rosenfeld@gatesfoundation.org

**Abstract:** Measles threatens the lives and livelihoods of tens of millions of children and there are countries where routine immunization systems miss enough individuals to create the risk of large outbreaks. To help address this threat, measles supplementary immunization activities are time-limited, coordinated campaigns to immunize en masse a target population. Timing campaigns to be concurrent with building outbreak risk is an important consideration, but current programmatic standards focus on campaigns achieving a high coverage of at least 95%. We show that there is a dramatic trade-off between campaign timeliness and coverage. Optimal timing at coverages as low as 50% for areas with weak routine immunization systems is shown to outperform the current standard, which is delayed by as little as 6 months. Measured coverage alone is revealed as a potentially misleading performance metric.

**Keywords:** measles; immunization; modeling

## 1. Introduction

Since the 1900s, measles has killed tens of millions. Today, the threat of measles varies widely between low-, middle-, and high-income countries, and in the most challenged regions the disease threatens a similar order of children, mostly under the age of 5 and often the most vulnerable [1]. Measles supplementary immunization activities (SIAs) are an important programmatic tool to stop large outbreaks and interrupt transmission [2]. These are time-limited, coordinated campaigns to immunize en masse a target population that has been missed by the routine immunization (RI) system. SIAs can be run at the national or subnational scale, and fill immunity gaps by immunizing children with a dose of measles-containing vaccine (MCV) [3].

The timeliness of these campaigns has been known to be a critical component of campaign planning and execution [4–7], particularly due to the high infectivity of the measles virus and the rapidly escalating nature of outbreaks (e.g., [8]). The true impact of a measles campaign is the burden averted by preventing/precluding outbreaks. However, the burden averted cannot be directly measured and must be estimated from modeled counterfactuals. Currently, the standard proxy for measuring a campaign's quality is 95% coverage both overall and in every district [9]. While coverage is a critical measure of campaign quality, it only captures one side of the task: what proportion of children received an MCV dose through the SIA. However, it cannot capture whether the SIA reached them prior to infection by the circulating virus.

While the role of timeliness is generally appreciated, the campaign planning and financing cycle is long, and the actual date of campaign execution can be delayed from the epidemiologically optimal timing for many reasons, including civil conflict/insecurity, vaccine and device shortages, and cold-chain space [9]. This paper investigates the impact of delays and trade-offs between a campaign's coverage and its timeliness.

SIAs are generally run in countries with endemic measles transmission after one birth cohort of susceptibles has accumulated [9]. This is often assessed as a balance between births, RI, and previous immunization campaigns [10,11]. Additionally, the impact of disease-induced immunity can be incorporated via epidemiological modeling [12]. Broadly speaking, these campaigns are run at a cadence of 2 to 5 years, depending on RI rates [13]. Campaigns are usually targeted to children in age cohorts likely to be susceptible because they have not been previously vaccinated via RI or SIAs or been infected with measles.

It is possible to find and study examples of delayed SIA campaigns for specific countries (e.g., [14,15]), but with no comprehensive database it is instructive to consider the relative timing of campaigns and periods of high measles transmission when outbreaks are most likely to occur. Measles seasonality is well studied [6,16–20] and historical case data reveal a propensity for outbreaks in the spring and winter months. Figure 1 shows these peak seasons for measles transmission estimated from the World Health Organization's (WHO) monthly measles data from 2000 to 2020 for 174 countries (see Section 2.1 for more details). However, historical SIA data from the WHO's SIA calendar for the same time period reveal a more even distribution across the seasons of national campaign timings. The two distributions are significantly different from what one would expect based on epidemiological timing (KS test, $p = 1.1 \times 10^{-6}$). Furthermore, the resulting distribution of offsets from campaign timing to the estimated peak seasonality shows that there are many campaigns run during the peak season as well as a few months after.

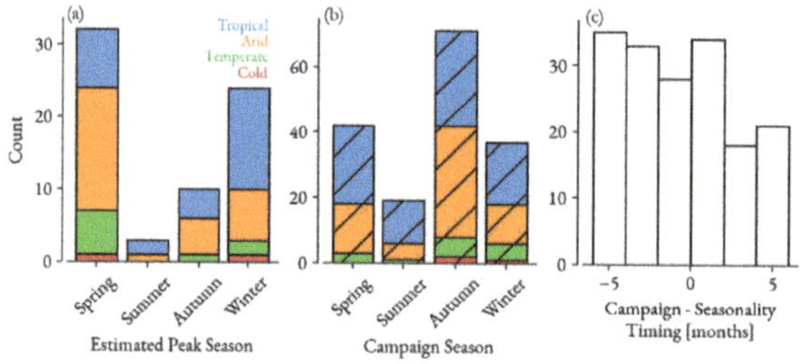


**Figure 1.** (**a**) Estimated measles peak seasons at the national level and further aggregated by Köppen–Geiger climate classification [21]. (**b**) The aggregated timing of SIA campaigns from 2000 to 2020. (**c**) The resulting offset distribution between campaign timing and the estimated seasonality.

Epidemiology is only one important component of deciding when to schedule campaigns along with a number of other considerations including resource availability, weather, and community factors [9]. The timeline for planning these campaigns is complex and involved; the WHO field guide details over 85 pages, with the steps involved including macroplanning, budgeting, microplanning, training, social mobilization, and monitoring [9]. Potential delays in any of these steps could propagate to a delay in the overall execution of the campaign. Although the highest quality campaign is always desired, there is a trade-off between a well-timed but potentially lower quality campaign and a higher quality campaign that is mistimed. This analysis provides quantitative assessments looking at near-term measles incidence as well as longer term patterns.

## 2. Materials and Methods

### 2.1. Seasonality Estimation

The monthly seasonality of measles transmission is roughly estimated for countries represented in the WHO's monthly measles cases data by looking at the phase offset for the yearly periodic signal in the case data's Fourier transform from 2000 to 2010; it is selected for countries who have had at least 100 cases over the time series. The monthly estimates are aggregated to seasons as reproduced in Figure 1. The results are consistent whether seasonality is estimated from the Fourier transform or the maximum monthly cases aggregated over the 20-year time series. The seasonality and campaign timing are compared by offsetting the campaign by 4 months and then performing a KS test.

### 2.2. Transmission Model and Building the SIA Calendar

Measles transmission dynamics were simulated using the Generic branch of EMOD ([22], v2.21). Simulations of a well-mixed population with varying RI were given the the model initialization and inputs described at the end of this section. This software has been calibrated and applied for country-specific models including measles [23], polio [24], malaria [25], and rubella [26]. For this analysis, a generalized model not calibrated to a single country but varied across parameters relevant for a broad range of locations was chosen. The model produces dynamic outbreak behavior where the periodicity and severity of outbreaks can maintain long-term stability or fluctuate over time. These dramatic changes in the transmission patterns are consistent with observations of measles and our mathematical understanding [18,27]. However, this causes a challenge for incorporating SIAs since the simulation parameters do not consistently determine the outbreak periodicity and behavior.

To build the SIA calendar, each simulation is initially run for 15 years. In post-processing, the first outbreak to occur after a 5 year period is identified as when the number of current infections exceeds the 95th percentile of active infections that occur over the entire simulation run. This metric is used throughout to identify the start of outbreaks in the simulation. A following round of simulations are launched that follow the initial transmission trajectory but with a rapidly implemented (1-day duration) SIA [9] scheduled 4 months before the start of the outbreak. This process can then be repeated to generate a calendar of effective SIAs.

SIA doses are age-targeted to children between 9 months and 5 years. Doses are first allocated to children who have received a dose via RI, reflecting an underlying assumption that children already reached by RI are also most accessible to outreach activities. This is an assumption that produces conservative bounds on the impact of SIA delays. Surveys suggest that the performance of SIAs in reaching children who are not immunized through the RI system varies between settings [28].

For the analysis, two values of RI coverage (30% and 70%) are considered to highlight the differences between low- and higher-coverage settings [29]. SIA coverage values are run at 50%, 70%, and 95%. The highest SIA coverage reflects the current recommendation of 95% coverage both on aggregate and in each district [9], which is more stringent than measles elimination strategies that aim for 95% coverage in combination between RI and SIAs [30,31].

The setting is initialized with 1 million individuals with an age distribution equilibrated for a given crude birth rate and the age-based mortality of Nigeria. A reproductive number, $R_0$, of 14 is assumed, consistent with a exponential infectivity distribution with daily rate equal to 14/8 and a Gaussian infectious period with mean of 8 days and standard deviation of 2 days. The latent period is assumed to be normally distributed with mean of 10 days and standard deviation of 2 days. Maternal protection was incorporated with initial susceptibility following the sigmoid $1/(1+\exp((50-\text{age in days})/50))$.

The model includes a constant rate of imported infections, and daily values of 0.03 and 0.1 are considered for a sensitivity analysis. The results are shown for a value of 0.1, but qualitative results do not change with the lower importation rate. Crude birth rates were chosen randomly from a range of 25 to 40 per 1 thousand people in the population. Transmission seasonality was incorporated as a sinusoidal forcing factor on infectivity, with amplitude varying between 20% and 100%. Note that for the upper bound of 100%, infectivity approaches zero for a small time during the year. Analyses performed with an amplitude ranges of 0% to 50% had the same qualitative results. There were 256 simulations run over this space for each scenario analyzed.

SIA dose allocation was carried out such that children reached by RI would receive an SIA dose before a child who did not receive an RI dose. There is no MCV2 dose incorporated into the simulation. At MCV1 rates of 30% and 70%, and given an MCV1 seroconversion probability of 85% at 8 months [32], susceptibility is dominated by zero-dose children, not

MCV1 recipients who failed to seroconvert. MCV2 is thus not expected to qualitatively change the results presented here.

## 3. Results

Measles transmission dynamics were simulated in a well-mixed population with routine immunization, vital dynamics, and an optimized calendar of SIAs. The trade-off between SIA coverage and timeliness in Figure 2 is assessed by two different metrics. The top two panels show the outbreak size as measured by the total number of people infected over the next year after the SIA was scheduled to occur. The bottom two panels show the outbreak intensity as measured by the maximum peak daily incidence over that year. These metrics are calculated for each simulation as the SIA is delayed by 1, 2, 4, and 6 months. The results for 50%, 70%, and 95% coverage SIAs are visualized with added noise in the x-dimension (time) for the visualization. The mean trend over the entire set of simulations is depicted by the solid line; shaded regions correspond to the 95% confidence intervals. For the 30% RI coverage scenario, the 50% SIA delayed by 1 month has a smaller and less intense outbreak than the 95% SIA delayed by 6 months. This trade-off only reverses after 5 months of delay for the 50% SIA. For the 70% RI coverage scenario, the 50% and 70% SIAs do not change appreciably with the delay due to our modeling assumption that SIA doses are administered first to children who have received a dose via RI (see Section 2.2).

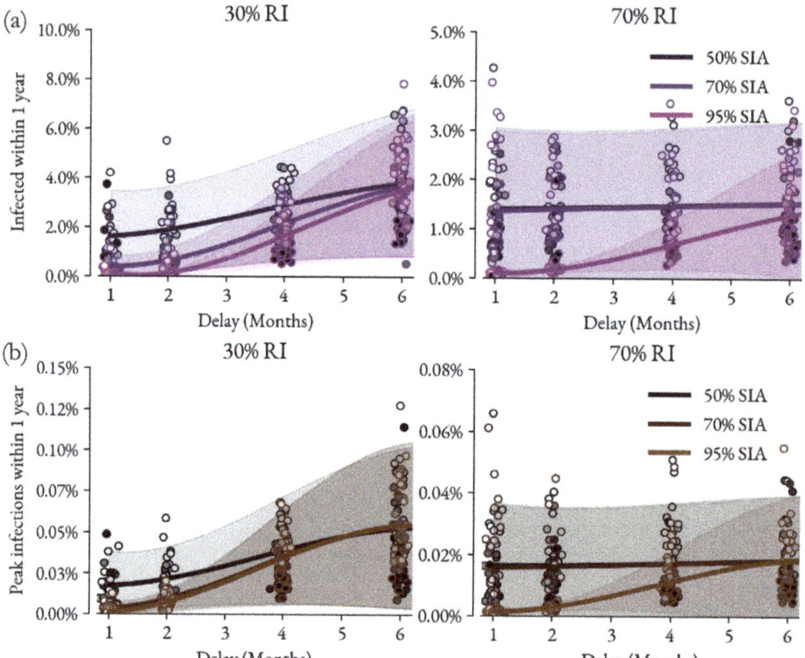


**Figure 2.** Resulting outbreak size (number of infections for a year following when the SIA was planned) and intensity (peak number of infections for that same time period) are measured in both total infections (**a**) and peak number of infections (**b**). Each circle represents a simulation (N = 256) with the circle's shading indicating the birth rate (scaling from 25 to 40 per 1 k people per year). Curves are Gaussian process regression fits to the simulation results and shaded regions are 95% CIs from the fit; 70% and 95% lines are indistinguishable for a 70% RI coverage scenario.

The importance of the dose association assumption is explored in Figure 3. The absolute difference in outbreak size (calculated as percentage of the population) is shown between the 95% SIA delayed by 6 months and the 50% SIA as it is delayed by 1, 2, 4, and 6 months. However, the mean trend is compared across the simulation suite for two bounding assumptions: (1) SIA doses first go to children who have received a dose via RI and (2) all children are equally likely to receive an SIA dose. This calculation shows how the lower-coverage, timely SIA will outperform the higher-coverage, delayed SIA in higher RI coverage settings if the campaign is able to effectively reach zero-dose children, specifically children who have not received a measles vaccine.

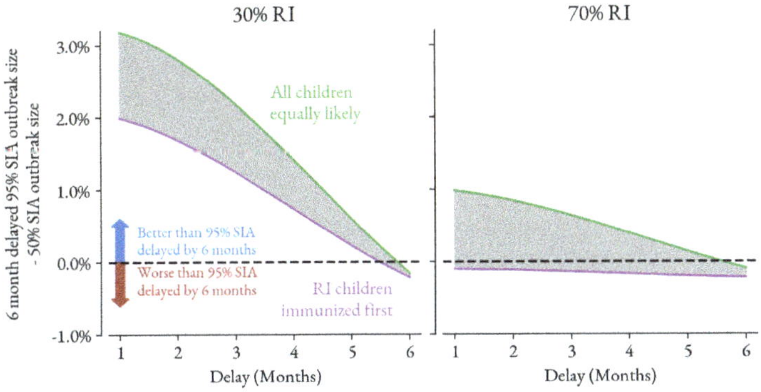


**Figure 3.** Different dose associations for previous immunization will impact how much, if at all, the well-timed but lower-coverage SIA will perform compared to the delayed, higher-coverage SIA. In these figures, the difference in outbreak size between the 95% coverage SIA delayed by 6 months and the 50% SIA delayed between 1 and 6 months is plotted for two bounding assumptions. The purple line shows the results for SIA doses going first to children who received a dose via RI. The green line shows results for all children being equally likely to receive a dose during the SIA.

The last metric considered is how the cost-effectiveness of the high-coverage SIA is affected by delay. Figure 4 shows the infections averted per 100 campaign doses as the 95% SIA is delayed by 1, 2, 4, and 6 months. The cost-effectiveness of the 95% SIA is reduced by almost a factor of 3 as it is delayed by 1 to 6 months. This is due to the fact that the campaign doses arrive too late to avoid the outbreak and are administered to children who have been infected and therefore acquired natural immunity.

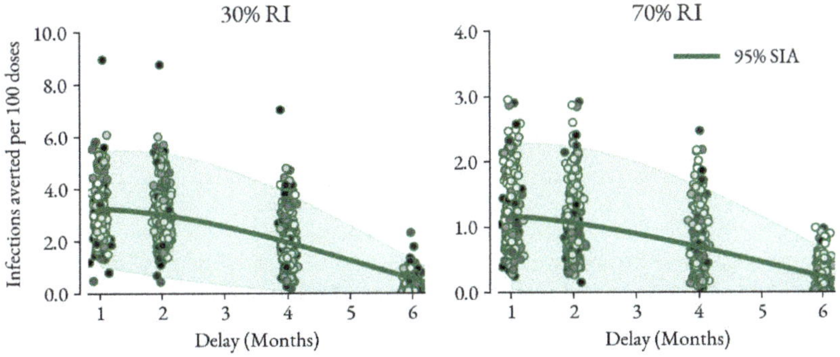


**Figure 4.** Dosage impact of the 95% coverage SIA as measured by infections averted per 100 campaign doses as it is delayed from 1 to 6 months. The infections were counted over the year following the planned SIA compared to if no SIA was executed. The impact per dose of the SIA is reduced by a factor of almost 3 when moving from a 1- to 6-month delay.

Along with the immediate effect of the SIA in reducing the next year's infections, longer-term effects are considered by showing the number of years until the next outbreak in Figure 5. Each individual sub-panel shows results for RI and SIA coverage level combinations. Each simulation is plotted as an individual circle whose color indicates the number of years until the next outbreak. These SIAs are not delayed. As seen in Figure 2, an SIA coverage of less than 70% has limited effect for the higher RI coverage scenario (70%). This produces the counter-intuitive result that simulations with 30% RI and 70% SIA coverage have more time between outbreaks than simulations with 70% RI and (essentially useless due the dose association assumption) 50% or 70% SIAs. However, looking across the different coverage scenarios, higher-coverage and timely SIAs will not only reduce burden for the coming year (Figure 2) but also increase the number of years until the next outbreak. A dependence on birth rate can also be observed. Both of these results are consistent with previous studies (e.g., [13]).

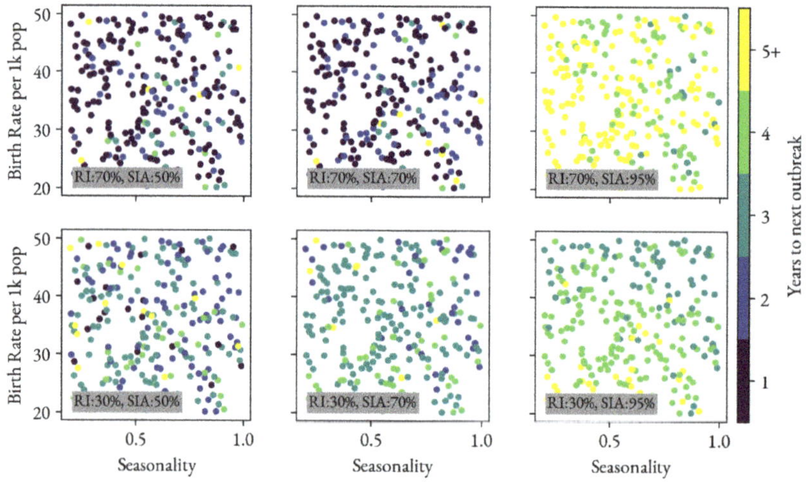


**Figure 5.** Period in years between the SIA and the next outbreak depicted across the range of simulations considered in this analysis.

## 4. Discussion

SIAs are a proven and trusted tool for measles outbreak prevention where sub-optimal RI leaves immunity gaps. However, a tool can only be as good as its application. In the case of endemic measles transmission, it must be applied in a timely manner. This analysis demonstrates how SIAs performed on time outperform delayed SIAs even if the timely SIA has significantly lower coverage. The cost-effectiveness of the high-coverage SIA is also greatly reduced by delay. These results suggest that coverage is not necessarily the only metric that should be considered to evaluate SIA performance and impact. Furthermore, coverage should be considered within the larger context of transmission patterns to duly evaluate how effective the SIA is at reducing susceptibility. This becomes increasingly important given the recent backslide in observed RI systems and surveillance [33]. However, it is important to keep in mind that a substantial reduction in measles mortality over the past decade is well documented, although rarely incorporating epi-linked case and RI histories (e.g., [34]). Vaccination, through RI systems and SIAs, plays an important role, but other interventions (targeting, e.g., improved women's health, management of acute malnutrition, and early breastfeeding) can also have a significant impact on reducing measles mortality and morbidity [34].

There are several limitations to this analysis. First, the role of MCV2 is not considered for clarity of the discussion and interpretation. Second, clustering or transmission correlation between susceptible groups that might arise from low-coverage settings (e.g., geographic, communal) is not included. This could be investigated via a setting-specific model calibrated to observed transmission patterns. The choice to use a more generic model to investigate general trends and patterns sacrificed the ability to capture this issue. Heterogeneity in coverage, whether it is derived from remoteness [35], conflict [36], or intersectional factors [37], would also impact the corresponding impact of the SIA. Finally, the simulation setup was designed such that there was complete certainty about the imminence of a measles outbreak, and thereby maximizes the observed effects of delay. In practice, campaigns must be planned over long horizons; measles outbreaks often fall into periodic patterns [38,39] and the 1-birth-cohort-unvaccinated rule of thumb provides a good proxy for susceptibility sufficient to support an outbreak, since measles outbreaks are not perfectly predictable. However, timeliness remains a necessary component for an effective SIA.

Reaching zero-dose and under-immunized children is an important goal and necessary component of measles outbreak prevention and control. Not only is this an equitable aim, it is central to reducing measles morbidity and mortality world-wide. As part of the IA2030 strategy, the prioritization of zero-dose children for SIA campaigns remains critical [40]. However, in the case of measles SIAs in outbreak-prone settings, this analysis strongly suggests that coverage and timeliness are intricately intertwined. Higher-coverage SIAs will naturally outperform lower-coverage ones in a strict comparison. However, if epidemiological analyses indicate that outbreaks may be imminent and the necessary planning steps to achieve higher coverage would incur significant delays, it may be better to prioritize timeliness for coverage.

**Author Contributions:** Conceptualization, K.A.R. and K.A.M.; methodology, K.A.R. and K.F.; software, K.F.; validation, K.A.R.; formal analysis, K.A.R.; investigation, K.A.R.; data curation, K.A.R.; writing—original draft preparation, K.A.R.; writing—review and editing, K.A.R., K.F. and K.A.M.; visualization, K.A.R.; project administration, K.A.M. All authors have read and agreed to the published version of the manuscript.

**Funding:** This work is based on research conducted by the Institute for Disease Modeling, a research group within, and solely funded by, the Bill and Melinda Gates Foundation.

**Institutional Review Board Statement:** Not applicable.

**Informed Consent Statement:** Not applicable.

**Data Availability Statement:** Scripts and simulation outputs will be available on zenodo: https://doi.org/10.5281/zenodo.7764622. Source code for EMOD is available on GitHub: https://github.com/InstituteforDiseaseModeling/EMOD-Generic (accessed on 1 July 2024).

**Acknowledgments:** We thank the IVIR-AC members Natasha Crowcroft, Kendall Krause, Niket Thakkar, Natalia Corona, and Maike Sonnewald for their feedback. We also thank the reviewers and editors for their critiques.

**Conflicts of Interest:** The funders had no role in the analysis, or interpretation of the data; the preparation, review, or approval of the report; or the decision to submit the manuscript for publication. All authors are employees of the Bill and Melinda Gates Foundation; however, this study does not necessarily represent the views of the Bill and Melinda Gates Foundation.

## Abbreviations

The following abbreviations are used in this manuscript:

| | |
|---|---|
| EMOD | Epidemiological MODeling software |
| MCV | Measles-Containing Vaccine |
| RI | Routine Immunization |
| SIA | Supplementary Immunization Activity |
| WHO | World Health Organization |

## References


1. Minta, A.A.; Ferrari, M.; Antoni, S.; Portnoy, A.; Sbarra, A.; Lambert, B.; Hatcher, C.; Hsu, C.H.; Ho, L.L.; Steulet, C.; et al. Progress Toward Measles Elimination—Worldwide, 2000–2022. *MMW. Morb. Mortal. Wkly. Rep.* **2023**, *72*, 1262–1268. [CrossRef] [PubMed]
2. World Health Organization. Measles vaccines: WHO position paper, April 2017—Recommendations. *Vaccine* **2019**, *37*, 219–222. [CrossRef] [PubMed]
3. Moss, W.J.; Strebel, P.M. Chapter 38 measles vaccines. In *Plotkin's Vaccines*, 8th ed.; Elsevier: Philadelphia, PA, USA, 2023; pp. 629–663.
4. Grassly, N.C.; Fraser, C. Seasonal infectious disease epidemiology. *Proc. R. Soc. B Biol. Sci.* **2006**, *273*, 2541–2550. [CrossRef]
5. Grais, R.F.; Conlan, A.J.K.; Ferrari, M.J.; Djibo, A.; Le Menach, A.; Bjørnstad, O.N.; Grenfell, B.T. Time is of the essence: Exploring a measles outbreak response vaccination in Niamey, Niger. *J. R. Soc. Interface/R. Soc.* **2008**, *5*, 67–74. [CrossRef] [PubMed]
6. Thakkar, N.; Gilani, S.S.A.; Hasan, Q.; McCarthy, K.A. Decreasing measles burden by optimizing campaign timing. *Proc. Natl. Acad. Sci. USA* **2019**, *116*, 11069–11073. [CrossRef] [PubMed]
7. Thakkar, N.; Abubakar, A.H.A.; Shube, M.; Jama, M.A.; Derow, M.; Lambach, P.; Ashmony, H.; Farid, M.; Sim, S.Y.; O'Connor, P.; et al. Estimating the Impact of Vaccination Campaigns on Measles Transmission in Somalia. *Vaccines* **2024**, *12*, 314. [CrossRef] [PubMed]
8. Minetti, A.; Kagoli, M.; Katsulukuta, A.; Huerga, H.; Featherstone, A.; Chiotcha, H.; Noel, D.; Bopp, C.; Sury, L.; Fricke, R.; et al. Lessons and challenges for measles control from unexpected large outbreak, Malawi. *Emerg. Infect. Dis.* **2013**, *19*, 202. [CrossRef] [PubMed]
9. WHO. *Planning and Implementing High-Quality Supplementary Immunization Activities for Injectable Vaccines Using an Example of Measles and Rubella Vaccines: Field Guide*; Technical report; World Health Organization: Geneva, Switzerland, 2016.
10. Measles Programmatic Risk Assessment Tool. 2017. Available online: https://www.who.int/teams/immunization-vaccines-and-biologicals/immunization-analysis-and-insights/surveillance/measles-programmatic-risk-assessment-tool (accessed on 1 July 2024).
11. Lam, E.; Schluter, W.W.; Masresha, B.G.; Teleb, N.; Bravo-Alcántara, P.; Shefer, A.; Jankovic, D.; McFarland, J.; Elfakki, E.; Takashima, Y.; et al. Development of a District-Level Programmatic Assessment Tool for Risk of Measles Virus Transmission. *Risk Anal.* **2017**, *37*, 1052–1062. [CrossRef] [PubMed]
12. Cutts, F.; Dansereau, E.; Ferrari, M.; Hanson, M.; McCarthy, K.; Metcalf, C.; Takahashi, S.; Tatem, A.; Thakkar, N.; Truelove, S.; et al. Using models to shape measles control and elimination strategies in low- and middle-income countries: A review of recent applications. *Vaccine* **2020**, *38*, 979–992. [CrossRef]
13. Verguet, S.; Johri, M.; Morris, S.K.; Gauvreau, C.L.; Jha, P.; Jit, M. Controlling measles using supplemental immunization activities: A mathematical model to inform optimal policy. *Vaccine* **2015**, *33*, 1291–1296. [CrossRef]
14. Kisangau, N.; Sergon, K.; Ibrahim, Y.; Yonga, F.; Langat, D.; Nzunza, R.; Borus, P.; Galgalo, T.; Lowther, S.A. Progress towards elimination of measles in Kenya, 2003-2016. *Pan Afr. Med. J.* **2018**, *31*, 65. [CrossRef]
15. Cutts, F.T.; Lessler, J.; Metcalf, C.J. Measles elimination: Progress, challenges and implications for rubella control. *Expert Rev. Vaccines* **2013**, *12*, 917–932. [CrossRef]
16. Fine, P.; Clarkson, J. Measles in England and Wales—I: An Analysis of Factors Underlying Seasonal Patterns. *Int. J. Epidemiol.* **1982**, *11*, 5–14. [CrossRef]
17. Duncan, C.J.; Duncan, S.R.; Scott, S. The Dynamics of Measles Epidemics. *Theor. Popul. Biol.* **1997**, *52*, 155–163. [CrossRef]
18. Ferrari, M.J.; Grais, R.F.; Bharti, N.; Conlan, A.J.K.; Bjørnstad, O.N.; Wolfson, L.J.; Guerin, P.J.; Djibo, A.; Grenfell, B.T. The dynamics of measles in sub-Saharan Africa. *Nature* **2008**, *451*, 679–684. [CrossRef]
19. Bharti, N.; Tatem, A.J.; Ferrari, M.J.; Grais, R.F.; Djibo, A.; Grenfell, B.T. Explaining Seasonal Fluctuations of Measles in Niger Using Nighttime Lights Imagery. *Science* **2011**, *334*, 1424–1427. [CrossRef]
20. Thakkar, N.; Jindal, S.; Rosenfeld, K. Seasonality and susceptibility from measles time series. *arXiv* **2024**, arXiv:2405.09664.
21. Beck, H.E.; McVicar, T.R.; Vergopolan, N.; Berg, A.; Lutsko, N.J.; Dufour, A.; Zeng, Z.; Jiang, X.; van Dijk, A.I.J.M.; Miralles, D.G. High-resolution (1 km) Köppen-Geiger maps for 1901–2099 based on constrained CMIP6 projections. *Sci. Data* **2023**, *10*, 724. [CrossRef] [PubMed]
22. Bershteyn, A.; Gerardin, J.; Bridenbecker, D.; Lorton, C.W.; Bloedow, J.; Baker, R.S.; Chabot-Couture, G.; Chen, Y.; Fischle, T.; Frey, K.; et al. Implementation and applications of EMOD, an individual-based multi-disease modeling platform. *Pathog. Dis.* **2018**, *76*, fty059. [CrossRef] [PubMed]
23. Zimmermann, M.; Frey, K.; Hagedorn, B.; Oteri, A.J.; Yahya, A.; Hamisu, M.; Mogekwu, F.; Shuaib, F.; McCarthy, K.A.; Chabot-Couture, G. Optimization of frequency and targeting of measles supplemental immunization activities in Nigeria: A cost-effectiveness analysis. *Vaccine* **2019**, *37*, 6039–6047. [CrossRef]
24. McCarthy, K.A.; Chabot-Couture, G.; Shuaib, F. A spatial model of Wild Poliovirus Type 1 in Kano State, Nigeria: Calibration and assessment of elimination probability. *BMC Infect. Dis.* **2016**, *16*, 521. [CrossRef] [PubMed]
25. Gerardin, J.; Bever, C.A.; Bridenbecker, D.; Hamainza, B.; Silumbe, K.; Miller, J.M.; Eisele, T.P.; Eckhoff, P.A.; Wenger, E.A. Effectiveness of reactive case detection for malaria elimination in three archetypical transmission settings: A modelling study. *Malar. J.* **2017**, *16*, 248. [CrossRef] [PubMed]
26. Cheng, A.; Frey, K.; Mwamba, G.N.; McCarthy, K.A.; Hoff, N.A.; Rimoin, A.W. Examination of scenarios introducing rubella vaccine in the Democratic Republic of the Congo. *Vaccine X* **2021**, *9*, 100127. [CrossRef] [PubMed]

27. Earn, D.J.D.; Rohani, P.; Bolker, B.M.; Grenfell, B.T. A Simple Model for Complex Dynamical Transitions in Epidemics. *Science* **2000**, *287*, 667–670. [CrossRef] [PubMed]
28. Portnoy, A.; Jit, M.; Helleringer, S.; Verguet, S. Impact of measles supplementary immunization activities on reaching children missed by routine programs. *Vaccine* **2018**, *36*, 170–178. [CrossRef] [PubMed]
29. Sbarra, A.N.; Rolfe, S.; Nguyen, J.Q.; Earl, L.; Galles, N.C.; Marks, A.; Abbas, K.M.; Abbasi-Kangevari, M.; Abbastabar, H.; Abd-Allah, F.; et al. Mapping routine measles vaccination in low- and middle-income countries. *Nature* **2021**, *589*, 415–419. [CrossRef]
30. *Measles Elimination by 2020: A Strategy for the African Region*; Technical Report AFR/RC61/R1; World Health Organization Regional Office for Africa: Brazzaville, Congo, 2011; p. 2.
31. World Health Organization Regional Office for South-East Asia. *Measles and Rubella Elimination by 2023*; Technical Report SEA/RC72/R3; World Health Organization Regional Office for South-East Asia: New Delhi, India, 2019.
32. Nic Lochlainn, L.M.; de Gier, B.; van der Maas, N.; Strebel, P.M.; Goodman, T.; van Binnendijk, R.S.; de Melker, H.E.; Hahné, S.J.M. Immunogenicity, effectiveness, and safety of measles vaccination in infants younger than 9 months: A systematic review and meta-analysis. *Lancet Infect. Dis.* **2019**, *19*, 1235–1245. [CrossRef] [PubMed]
33. Durrheim, D.N.; Andrus, J.K.; Tabassum, S.; Bashour, H.; Githanga, D.; Pfaff, G. A dangerous measles future looms beyond the COVID-19 pandemic. *Nat. Med.* **2021**, *27*, 360–361. [CrossRef] [PubMed]
34. Naghavi, M.; Ong, K.L.; Aali, A.; Ababneh, H.S.; Abate, Y.H.; Abbafati, C.; Abbasgholizadeh, R.; Abbasian, M.; Abbasi-Kangevari, M.; Abbastabar, H.; et al. Global burden of 288 causes of death and life expectancy decomposition in 204 countries and territories and 811 subnational locations, 1990–2021: A systematic analysis for the Global Burden of Disease Study 2021. *Lancet* **2024**, *403*, 2100–2132. [CrossRef]
35. Metcalf, C.J.E.; Tatem, A.; Bjornstad, O.N.; Lessler, J.; O'Reilly, K.; Takahashi, S.; Cutts, F.; Grenfell, B. Transport networks and inequities in vaccination: Remoteness shapes measles vaccine coverage and prospects for elimination across Africa. *Epidemiol. Infect.* **2015**, *143*, 1457–1466. [CrossRef]
36. Grundy, J.; Biggs, B.A. The Impact of Conflict on Immunisation Coverage in 16 Countries. *Int. J. Health Policy Manag.* **2018**, *8*, 211–221. [CrossRef] [PubMed]
37. Shearer, J.C.; Nava, O.; Prosser, W.; Nawaz, S.; Mulongo, S.; Mambu, T.; Mafuta, E.; Munguambe, K.; Sigauque, B.; Cherima, Y.J.; et al. Uncovering the Drivers of Childhood Immunization Inequality with Caregivers, Community Members and Health System Stakeholders: Results from a Human-Centered Design Study in DRC, Mozambique and Nigeria. *Vaccines* **2023**, *11*, 689. [CrossRef] [PubMed]
38. Brownlee, J. Periodicities of Epidemics of Measles in the Large Towns of Great Britain and Ireland. *Proc. R. Soc. Med.* **1919**, *12*, 77–120. [CrossRef] [PubMed]
39. Bartlett, M.S. Measles Periodicity and Community Size. *J. R. Stat. Soc. Ser. A* **1957**, *120*, 48–70. [CrossRef]
40. *Immunization Agenda 2030: A Global Strategy to Leave No One Behind*; Technical report; World Health Organization: Geneva, Switzerland, 2020.

*vaccines*

MDPI

*Review*

# Vaccination Week in the Americas: An Ongoing Initiative to Strengthen and Sustain Measles and Rubella Elimination in the Region

**Alba Maria Ropero, Hannah Kurtis, Lauren Vulanovic, Pamela Bravo-Alcántara, Maite Vera Antelo and Margherita Ghiselli ***

Pan American Health Organization, Washington, DC 20037, USA; roperoal@paho.org (A.M.R.); kurtisha@paho.org (H.K.); brownlau@paho.org (L.V.); bravopam@paho.org (P.B.-A.); veraanmai@paho.org (M.V.A.)
* Correspondence: ghisellmar@paho.org

**Abstract:** Vaccination Week in the Americas (VWA) is a yearly regional initiative that promotes the benefits of vaccination to all persons in the region. In its 22-year history, more than 1.15 billion people have been reached under the framework of VWA across more than 40 countries and territories. This review examines multiple PAHO and WHO data points, documents and reports related to measles/rubella vaccination coverage and VWA since its inception. Its goal is to document the impact that the VWA has had in maintaining and accelerating measles and rubella disease elimination, in the context of PAHO's Disease Elimination Initiative. The results suggest that VWA's contributions to measles and rubella elimination have been substantial. Every year, VWA promotes (a) renewed political commitment to the immunization program from the highest political authorities of Member States; (b) vaccination operations to close immunity gaps, recover under-vaccinated persons, and reach chronically underserved populations; and (c) the dissemination of messages on the benefits of vaccination through regional and national communications campaigns. VWA will continue to be an important contributor to disease elimination efforts in the Americas, even as new targets are set in response to the evolving epidemiological landscape.

**Keywords:** measles; rubella; elimination; immunity gap; Vaccination Week in the Americas

## 1. Introduction

Vaccination Week in the Americas (VWA) is the Americas' yearly initiative for the promotion of the regional immunization program and the closure of the most urgent immunity gaps. Launched in 2003, it serves as a coordinated and flexible platform for countries to offer vaccines and promote the benefits of immunization to health workers and the public. Over the years, countries have taken advantage of this event to complement the operations of the routine immunization program or launch mass vaccination campaigns and mop-up operations. This review documents the extensive contributions of the VWA to achieve and sustain the elimination of measles, rubella and congenital rubella syndrome (CRS) in the Americas.

This review considered the results of the VWA as reported in each year's final report for the event, as well as the yearly data presented in the reports to the Regional Measles-Rubella Elimination Monitoring and Re-verification Commission, the PAHO electronic joint reporting form (eJRF) and the WHO/UNICEF Estimates of National Immunization Coverage (WUENIC). This review aims to describe the contributions of the VWA in maintaining and accelerating measles and rubella disease elimination, in the context of PAHO's Elimination Initiative [1]. We conclude by presenting some limitations of the platform, as well as lessons learned to further the goal of measles/rubella disease elimination in the Americas.

## 2. History of the Vaccination Week in the Americas

Vaccination Week in the Americas (VWA) is an annual initiative that has been celebrated in the Americas for the last 22 years. As reported previously [2–4], an outbreak of measles linked to endemic transmission emerged along the border between Venezuela and Colombia in 2002. In response to this crisis, the ministers of health of the Andean Region and then-Director of the Pan American Health Organization (PAHO) Dr. George A. O. Alleyne signed the Sucre Agreement, which specified several actions to prevent future outbreaks, including the establishment of a coordinated, multi-country vaccination week among Andean countries.

The first VWA was celebrated in June 2003, with the participation of 19 countries and territories across the Americas, resulting in the vaccination of more than 16 million people [4]. In September 2003, during PAHO's 44th Directing Council, health ministers endorsed Resolution CD44.R1 "Sustaining Immunization Programs-Elimination of Rubella and Congenital Rubella Syndrome (CRS)", which included language supporting "the implementation of an annual hemispheric Vaccination Week [. . .] targeting high-risk population groups and underserved areas." [5]. This resolution was significant since it provided the political mandate for countries' participation in VWA in the years to come.

Also, the VWA served as an inspiration for the creation of World Immunization Week (WIW) by the World Health Organization (WHO). Following the example of the Americas, other WHO regions created their own regional vaccination weeks (EURO in 2005; EMRO in 2010; AFRO in 2011; WPRO in 2011; and SEARO in 2012). During the 56th World Health Assembly in May 2012, Resolution WHA 65.18. called on "Member States to designate the last week of April, when appropriate, as World Immunization Week", with the aim to prioritize and fully fund immunization programs, ensure access to vaccines for individuals throughout the life course, encourage vaccine-related innovation, and inspire vaccine advocacy efforts [6].

In its 22-year history, more than 1.15 billion people have been vaccinated under the framework of VWA. Of note, this figure includes the administration of at least 78.8 million doses of measles and rubella-containing vaccine (MMR or MR), of which more than 40.5 million were adult doses.

## 3. Contributions to the Measles/Rubella Global Elimination Initiative

### *3.1. A Platform to Accelerate PAHO's Elimination Initiative*

Since its inception, the VWA has included several elements that actively promote, accelerate and maintain the target of vaccine-preventable disease (VPD) control and measles/rubella elimination in the Americas. These include the following:

1. The annual opportunity to revitalize political and financial commitment towards sustaining VPD control and measles/rubella elimination across the region.
    (a) Targeted vaccination operations designed to close the most urgent immunity gaps and reduce the pool of susceptible persons.
    (b) Flexibility to adapt the VWA platform to the national context and address the most urgent immunity gaps, in accordance with the country's epidemiological situation and public health priorities. This is often done through outreach activities, mass vaccination campaigns and mop-up operations.
    (c) Offer of equitable access to vaccination services for remote and chronically underserved populations.
2. Cooperation between countries to promote shared health goals such as measles/rubella elimination, including joint cross-border vaccination operations between Member States.
3. Widespread dissemination of messages and communication materials at both the country and regional level, which promote the benefits of vaccines to health workers and the public.

Furthermore, in 2019, the PAHO Member States approved the Resolution PAHO Disease Elimination Initiative during the 57th Directing Council. This policy provides a common and sustainable framework with prioritized lines of action to orient and guide countries of the region as they work toward the elimination of a group of 30 priority communicable diseases—including measles and rubella—and related conditions. The framework is strategic, inclusive, standardized, and multisectoral, and can be adopted, adapted, and implemented in a staged manner by the countries of the region according to their national and local contexts and priorities [1,7]. Given its flexibility and wide, sustained implementation across the region, the VWA was quickly included among the strategies that countries implement to advance this Initiative.

As with the global switch from trivalent to bivalent oral polio vaccine (OPV) in 2016 and the introduction of the COVID-19 vaccine in 2021, Member States can now use the VWA to accelerate the implementation of this Initiative in their own territories. Its regular implementation allows all countries to prepare their advocacy and vaccination activities in a timely fashion, as well as to tailor interventions and coordinate cross-border operations where vaccination coverage rates are weakest.

### 3.2. Political Priority on the National Agenda of Member States

One of the main strategic objectives of the VWA is to maintain the topic of immunization at the forefront of the political agenda of Member States, partners and donors.

At the regional level, the yearly launching ceremony of the VWA is hosted by the PAHO Director and represents an opportunity to engage directly the Ministries of Health, civil societies and partners of the region and advocate in favor of a strong, well-financed regional immunization program. Each year, Ministers of Health of select countries and representatives of strategic partnerships are invited to share messages in support of immunization programs, so the Director's message is amplified across the region. Also, the ceremony serves as a call to action to governments to increase vaccination coverage rates by investing in all aspects of the national immunization program, including human resource capacity and integration of vaccination services into the primary healthcare system.

These same objectives are replicated in each country through the national-level VWA launching ceremonies. Here, governments, civil societies and their partners publicly renew their commitment to the national immunization program. In the months leading up to VWA, the leadership of the immunization program and the staff of the PAHO Country Offices engage national authorities at the highest levels to ensure their vocal support and advocacy in favor of vaccination operations and programs. The successful participation of heads of state, their spouses and ministers of health has been a key outcome of these events. On occasion, political commitment to national immunization programs has been showcased through the creation of ministerial declarations, which are signed during a VWA launching ceremony to bring maximum visibility to the event. A recent example occurred during VWA 2023, when the countries of the Caribbean agreed to strengthen national immunization programs through the Declaration of Nassau [8]. These statements often attract opportunities for cooperation and collaboration between governments, partners and the private sector, which may translate into financial or in-kind support towards national vaccination activities.

Finally, the PAHO Director holds a press conference the week prior to the VWA to discuss vaccines and the benefits of vaccination with the wider public, as well as to address the most urgent questions related to the regional immunization program.

### 3.3. Vaccination Operations

The VWA is designed to be flexible in how it is implemented country-to-country and year-to-year. Countries set their own goals within the regional strategic framework, so the initiative becomes an annual opportunity to advance public health priorities and close the most urgent gaps within the performance of the national EPI. Below we describe some of the strategies that have been implemented under the auspices of the VWA to bring vaccination services closer to the public and close the most urgent immunity gaps.

#### 3.3.1. Outreach Efforts

Vaccination outreach efforts are one of the hallmark activities carried out by countries during the celebration of the VWA. In the context of VPD control and measles/rubella elimination, this has taken the form of special efforts to ensure that isolated or vulnerable populations are offered vaccination services at convenient times and places. For example, countries such as Argentina, Brazil, Bolivia, Colombia, Ecuador, Nicaragua, Paraguay, Peru and Venezuela have used VWA to vaccinate indigenous groups against measles and rubella, with outreach teams often traveling by boat, plane and foot to reach the most remote villages.

Another essential contribution of VWA to VPD control and measles/rubella elimination is cross-border vaccination activities. For example, Honduras, Guatemala, Nicaragua and Panama carried out synchronized measles follow-up vaccination campaigns as part of their VWA celebrations in 2008. These campaigns were combined with a series of consecutive VWA launching ceremonies organized in border areas between the United States and Mexico and across Central America around the theme of a "Caravan for Health" and the shared slogan "Get on Board, Get Vaccinated". Common themes mentioned during these ceremonies included the need for international cooperation and solidarity to prevent VPD spread. Finally, in 2024, cross-border vaccination activities were organized between Mexico, Belize and Guatemala; between Brazil and Colombia; and between Brazil and Paraguay.

Also, countries have used the VWA to reach individuals whose profession puts them at higher risk for measles/rubella exposure, compared to the general population. Many countries—including Bolivia, Grenada, Jamaica, Panama, St. Kitts and Nevis and Trinidad and Tobago—used the VWA to intensify their vaccination activities against measles and rubella among health workers. Countries with a high influx of tourists (ex., Caribbean territories, the Dominican Republic, Mexico) targeted professionals who are in close contact with travelers, including taxi drivers and baggage handlers. For example, Anguilla vaccinated immigration, police and customs officers, while the Dominican Republic vaccinated individuals working in the tourism industry. Peru vaccinated airport workers and hotel staff.

Countries have used the VWA platform to make the vaccination setting more friendly for the public. The province of Cordoba in Argentina hosts the annual *La Noche de las Vacunas* ("Vaccination Night"), where local hospitals open their doors around 8:00 pm for an all-night party where thousands of people of all ages can play games, listen to live music, watch performances, have dinner and get vaccinated [9]. Countries like Belize, Bolivia, Costa Rica, Dominican Republic, Jamaica and Trinidad and Tobago completed MR vaccination operations in schools and daycare centers, while countries like Argentina, Brazil and Trinidad and Tobago set up mobile routine vaccination services at town squares, concert venues, shopping malls, metro stations, senior centers, banks and other public spaces. Intensified efforts to peri urban areas are hallmarks of the VWA, in its effort to reach chronically underserved populations.

Finally, migrant populations have benefited from VWA events. For example, the Ministry of Health of the Dominican Republic has worked with non-governmental organizations and community groups to reach migrant populations who have limited or no access to routine health services within the country, but whose vulnerable situations places them at high risk for contracting VPDs if they remain susceptible. Also, Trinidad and Tobago used the VWA to expand vaccination service hours and make routine immunization more accessible to all persons, including migrant populations. The countries of St. Kitts and Nevis and Turks and Caicos implemented outreach operations in migrant communities to encourage vaccination for all persons.

#### 3.3.2. Mass Vaccination Campaigns and Mop-Up Operations against Measles/Rubella

Current PAHO recommendations state that the measles-containing vaccine should be administered at 12 and at 18 months of age [10]. With regional vaccination coverage rates fluctuating between 85% and 91% from 2017 to 2022 [11]—well below the 95% target set for the region—an accumulation of non-immune children has resulted over time [11]. This includes both children who were never vaccinated and those who were vaccinated but failed to respond to the vaccine. With each successive birth cohort, the number of children susceptible to measles increases. This build-up is the most serious obstacle to measles elimination. High vaccination coverage through routine health services is essential, yet alone it is clearly not sufficient to reach and maintain measles elimination.

Mass vaccination campaigns are a rapid and resource-intensive strategy to close the immunity gaps left by the routine immunization program, quickly reduce the number of susceptible persons and maintain the elimination targets that the Americas already achieved. As part of the VWA's 22-year history, 25 high-quality "follow-up" campaigns were implemented at least 14 countries implemented high-quality "follow-up" mass campaigns against measles/rubella among children younger than five years, with the purpose of providing a second vaccination opportunity to the entire cohort. Through these campaigns, close to 49 million children were vaccinated with measles-containing vaccines. The most frequent targeted group was children 1–4 years old (52%), while 28% of the campaigns targeted older children (up to 14 years). Administrative coverage rates ranged from 73% to 114%, with a median of 96% (Table 1).

**Table 1.** Follow-up mass vaccination campaigns carried out during Vaccination Week of the Americas, 2003–2023.

| | First Campaign | | | | Second Campaign | | | | Third Campaign | | | | Fourth Campaign | | | |
|---|---|---|---|---|---|---|---|---|---|---|---|---|---|---|---|---|
| Countries | Year | Age Group | Coverage (%) | Vaccinated | Year | Age Group | Coverage (%) | Vaccinated | Year | Age Group | Coverage (%) | Vaccinated | Year | Age Group | Coverage (%) | Vaccinated |
| Bolivia | 2003 | 1–4 yo | 95 | 894,634 | | | | | | | | | | | | |
| Paraguay | 2003 | 1–4 yo | 93 | 551,993 | 2014 | 1–5 yo | 73 | 738,619 | | | | | | | | |
| Honduras | 2004 | 1–4 yo | 94 | 714,207 | 2008 | 1–4 yo | 97 | 687,966 | 2012 | 2–4 yo | 84 | 710,166 | | | | |
| Nicaragua | 2008 | 1–4 yo | 95 | 375,781 | 2012 | 1–4 yo | 107 | 559,985 | 2016 | 1–4 yo | 101 | 541,836 | 2022 | 1–6 yo | 114 | 823,127 |
| Venezuela | 2006 | 1–4 yo | 99 | 2,673,972 | 2014 | 1–5 yo | 99 | 2,466,543 | | | | | | | | |
| Guatemala | 2008 | 1–6 yo | 95 | 1,992,185 | | | | | | | | | | | | |
| Panama | 2008 | 1–4 yo | 94 | 230,116 | 2018 | 1–4 yo | 98 | 288,274 | | | | | | | | |
| Dominican Republic | 2010 | 1–8 yo | 96 | 1,532,705 | 2015 | 1–4 yo | 95 | 742,792 | 2022 | 1–5 yo | 95 | 934,329 | | | | |
| Costa Rica | 2011 | 2–9 yo | 93 | 585,121 | | | | | | | | | | | | |
| Ecuador | 2012 | 6 m–14 yo | 101 | 4,700,526 | | | | | | | | | | | | |
| Haiti | 2012 | 9 m–9 yo | 99 | 2,963,911 | 2016 | 1–4 yo | 99 | 1,279,526 | | | | | | | | |
| Colombia | 2021 | 1–10 yo | 95 | 7,752,514 | | | | | | | | | | | | |
| Mexico | 2021 | 1–9 yo | 96 | 11,202,785 | | | | | | | | | | | | |
| Ecuador | 2023 | 1–12 yo | 98 | 3,119,470 | | | | | | | | | | | | |
| TOTAL | | | | 39,289,920 | | | | 6,763,705 | | | | 2,186,331 | | | | 823,127 |

Source: electronic Joint Reporting Form (eJRF), World Health Organization.

During this same period, six countries used the VWA platform to implement "speed-up" campaigns, a one-time mass intervention targeting adolescents and adults aged 25–39 years to eliminate rubella and CRS, as well as advance towards measles elimination. In these campaigns, close to 45 million individuals were vaccinated with the MR vaccine. The coverage rate achieved ranged from 98% to 99%, with a median of 99% (Table 2). Also, multiple countries and territories in the Caribbean carried out an intensification of vaccination activities to target different age groups and ensure that all receive one or two doses of the MMR vaccine. This outreach strategy contributes to achieving high and homogeneous population immunity rates.

With the support of PAHO, countries of Latin America implemented synchronized speed-up campaigns in a short timespan: 89% of these campaigns were conducted between 2004–2008, while 38% were launched or implemented during VWA.

Table 2. Speed-up mass vaccination campaigns carried out during Vaccination Week of the Americas.

| Countries | Year | Age Group | Coverage (%) | Vaccinated |
|---|---|---|---|---|
| Ecuador | 2004 | 16–39 yo | 98 | 4,982,760 |
| El Salvador | 2004 | 15–39 yo | 98 | 2,796,391 |
| Paraguay | 2005 | 5–39 yo | 99 | 3,753,392 |
| Bolivia | 2006 | 15–39 yo | 98 | 4,015,554 |
| Guatemala | 2007 | 9–39 yo | 99 | 7,172,847 |
| Mexico | 2008 | 19–29 yo | 99 | 22,231,820 |
| Total individuals vaccinated | | | | 44,952,764 |

Source: electronic Joint Reporting Form (eJRF), World Health Organization.

#### 3.3.3. Response Operations against the 2017 and 2018 Outbreaks in Venezuela and Brazil

In July 2017, Venezuela reported a measles outbreak in the southern state of Bolivar. Since the country was not able to close the outbreak within 12 months from the notification of the first confirmed case, it was reclassified as having reestablished endemic measles virus transmission. As a result, the whole region lost the measles-free status it had achieved in 2016. By February 2018, the virus spread to Roraima state in Brazil, which borders Bolivar. By 2019, Venezuela had reported 7054 confirmed cases: 727 in 2017; 5799 in 2018; and 1722 in 2019.

During the VWA in April 2018, Venezuela implemented an outbreak response intervention by intensifying MR vaccination activities among children between ages 6 months to 15 years, with a focus in the nine states with the highest proportion of confirmed cases and highest cumulative incidence rates. Additionally, this campaign was an opportunity to offer the tetanus and adult diphtheria (Td) vaccine to persons ages 7 to 15 years to close the ongoing diphtheria outbreak. The mass vaccination campaign was eventually expanded to all 24 states of Venezuela. Between April 2018 and May 2019, 8.9 million children received the MR vaccine, for a national coverage rate of 104%.

By April 2018, only 3 of the 27 states of Brazil had been affected by the measles outbreak. Therefore, the country selected to implement its follow-up MR vaccination campaign in August 2018, outside the framework of the VWA, to allow for additional time to implement micro-planning exercises as well as complete large procurement and distribution operations for vaccines and supplies. In the three affected states, the VWA focused its MR vaccination activities among migrant populations found in shelters or at border posts.

#### 3.3.4. Communications and Community Engagement

Each year, PAHO develops a regional VWA communication campaign. Materials include a slogan that reflects current events and priorities; digital and print materials (including posters, banners, stickers, gifs, videos, and images), public service announcement (PSA) infographics, and a social media package with content tailored for a variety of platforms. Countries can adapt these materials to meet the goals and targets of their own VWA campaign and ensure that all images and messages reflect the ethnic and linguistic composition of their populations. Over the years, many countries adapted these materials and slogans to promote the mass vaccination campaign they implement against measles and rubella.

While the option for adaptation remains available to countries, there have been several years where the regional communication campaign materials included a specific call to action centered around measles and rubella elimination activities. This concentration of efforts around a specific topic has occurred mostly in years when the Americas have hosted international sporting events or have contributed a significant number of players to the game. For example, in 2014 and 2018—both FIFA World Cup years—the VWA regional communication campaign themes used soccer slogans and graphics to focus on strengthening surveillance operations and vaccination activities to prevent measles and rubella outbreaks. For the 2007 Cricket World Cup—hosted in the West Indies—Caribbean countries used the VWA to bolster their epidemiological surveillance operations to identify any suspected cases of measles or rubella among participants or spectators. At the same time, communication campaigns in the hosting countries emphasized the importance of vaccination to prevent the spread of measles and rubella.

Community engagement is another critical element of VWA communications campaigns. Over the years, countries developed multiple approaches to engage with different audiences at the local level in order to promote vaccination against measles/rubella. For example, collaboration with church leaders has allowed the VWA to promote key vaccination messages among their congregations. In other cases, high-level health professionals or political leaders have been invited to speak about vaccination opportunities during religious services. Often, churches serve as the location for health fairs and MR vaccination during the VWA week.

A pivotal moment was the introduction of COVID-19 vaccines in the region of the Americas in January 2021. At this time of uncertainly and high pressure for rapid vaccine introduction, the novelty of the vaccine itself raised considerable doubts about the vaccines' safety and effectiveness. In multiple countries, these doubts threatened to spread to antigens of the routine immunization program, such as measles-containing vaccines. PAHO used the VWA as an opportunity to engage with the public, health workers and local opinion leaders, answer questions and concerns, address rumors and debunk myths. The communication materials of the VWA were designed to provide consistent and up-to-date answers to the most frequent questions around the region.

## 4. Lessons Learned

### 4.1. Political Priority

The main lesson learned from the VWA is the importance of a periodic, well-coordinated and flexible opportunity for governments and heads of state to address the importance of vaccines and vaccination operations, regardless of other political priorities or events. Indeed, the VWA often served as an opportunity to showcase how vaccines can alleviate the outcomes of a public health emergency. This yearly appointment allows all Member States to remind their populations of the risk of vaccine-preventable diseases and of the importance of routine vaccines for the health and well-being of all communities.

Another lesson learned is the convenience of the VWA as a well-established platform to facilitate and accelerate the implementation of region-wide public health interventions. As with the trivalent–bivalent OPV switch in 2016 and the introduction of the COVID-19 vaccines in 2021, the VWA can ease these moments of transition by presenting them within a familiar and reliable framework to both the health workforce and the public.

### 4.2. Vaccination Operations

The VWA provides a platform to implement synchronized and massive vaccination campaigns, thus increasing population immunity levels quickly. Each year, the VWA underscores the need to "reach the unreached" by focusing efforts to bring vaccines to vulnerable and chronically underserved populations. This effort is a cornerstone of the elimination strategy of measles and rubella.

Flexibility is another attribute of the VWA platform. Countries set their own vaccination goals, so the initiative becomes an annual opportunity to advance national public health priorities. At the same time, by maintaining measles and rubella elimination as a regional target, PAHO provides ongoing guidance and support to countries and partners to achieve this common goal while allowing space for Member States to implement the vaccination tactics that work best for their context.

### *4.3. Communications and Community Engagement*

In the area of communications, there are two main lessons learned. The first is the importance of allowing countries to adapt the VWA communications materials (both print and digital media). Regional VWA materials already reflect the ethnic diversity of the Americas, so countries have multiple options to select the images that best reflect their populations. Also, all information materials developed by the regional level (for example, talking points on measles/rubella surveillance and vaccination activities, MR coverage rates, number of suspected and confirmed cases) are designed so that countries can easily replace region-level data with their own national and local information and can further tailor the materials to speak to their own priorities.

The second lesson learned is to use the VWA platform to increase the public's risk perception of measles and rubella disease while decreasing the risk perception associated with the safety and effectiveness of MR vaccination. This can be done by emphasizing the risk of severe illness, hospitalization, encephalitis, pneumonia, birth defects, miscarriage and death—all of which can be prevented through vaccination. Also, communication materials have been used to highlight the safety and effectiveness of the measles-containing vaccines, which have been consistently proven over decades of use in the general population. The VWA provides multiple opportunities for public health experts to promote these points, as well as to meaningfully engage with health workers and the public on MR vaccination, address doubts and provide reliable and updated information.

### *4.4. Limitations*

Upon review of the VWA documentation, we notice two main limitations to its contributions of the measles and rubella disease elimination initiative. First, since the VWA is always celebrated the last week of April, its operations cannot be timed to address public health emergencies. An example is the measles outbreak that was declared between Venezuela and Brazil in July 2017. Both affected and neighboring countries had to implement rapid response operations outside the context of the VWA to prevent further transmission. Also, the fact that the VWA serves as both an outreach activity to vaccinate zero-dose children and as a mop-up operation for under-vaccinated persons means that the target population for a specific antigen is often larger than the one specified for routine immunization activities. In the case of MR vaccination, the mass vaccination follow-up campaigns organized for the VWA often reached all children younger than five years, while the national immunization program recommends vaccinating children at 12 and at 18 months of age. Therefore, we cannot ascertain that VWA vaccination operations closed the immunity gaps left by the routine immunization programs of Venezuela and Brazil. Nonetheless, we presented strong evidence that VWA operations in both affected and neighboring countries contributed to shrinking the pool of persons susceptible to measles and rubella in the Americas—thus possibly preventing additional outbreaks.

A second limitation is the arrival of the COVID-19 pandemic to the Americas in 2020. While most VWA events at the national and regional level continued uninterrupted, Colombia had to extend its mass campaign vaccination operations throughout 2020 to achieve its MR coverage targets. Also, Honduras, Bolivia and Paraguay postponed their MR follow-up vaccination campaigns originally scheduled for 2021. Furthermore, since the 2020 VWA was limited in scope and the 2021 VWA was dedicated mostly to COVID-19 vaccine introduction, the countries of the Americas have had limited opportunity to date to employ this platform as an extension of the PAHO Elimination Initiative. Future iterations of the VWA will likely be more explicit in promoting the platform for this purpose.

## 5. Conclusions

For the last 22 years, the countries and territories of the Americas have used the VWA to renew their political and financial commitment to the regional immunization program, advance in the elimination of vaccine-preventable diseases—including measles and rubella—and remind the public of the benefits of vaccines for the health and well-being of all communities. Its consistent implementation during the last week of April allowed countries to join this yearly appointment through coordinated operations and messages and offers the public a familiar interface with the national vaccination program. In its next iterations, the VWA will continue to support the PAHO Elimination Initiative while it contributes to closing the most urgent immunity gaps.

**Author Contributions:** Creation of Vaccination Week in the Americas (A.M.R.); Acquisition of data related to the history of Vaccination Week in the Americas (A.M.R. and H.K.); Acquisition, analysis and interpretation of data related to communications operations and community engagement activities (H.K., L.V. and M.V.A.); Acquisition, analysis and interpretation of data related to mass vaccination campaigns and mop-up operations (P.B.-A.); Development of the structure of the article; Acquisition, analysis and interpretation of data related to political advocacy; Compilation and analysis of limitations and lessons learned (M.G.). All authors have approved the submitted version; and all agree to be personally accountable for his/her own contributions and for ensuring that questions related to the accuracy or integrity of any part of the work, even ones in which the author was not personally involved, are appropriately investigated, resolved, and documented in the literature. All authors have read and agreed to the published version of the manuscript.

**Funding:** This publication was supported by the Grant or Cooperative Agreement Number NU66GH002171, funded by the Centers for Disease Control and Prevention. Its contents are solely the responsibility of the authors and do not necessarily represent the official views of the Centers for Disease Control and Prevention or the Department of Health and Human Services.

**Acknowledgments:** We express our sincere gratitude for the tireless effort and dedication to the immunization staff. Their commitment to public health remained strong even in the most challenging moments of the pandemic. Their collaboration and commitment have been fundamental to confront this global crisis. The solidarity and cooperation they demonstrated reflects the strength of our region and are inspiring examples of Pan-Americanism.

**Conflicts of Interest:** The authors declare no conflicts of interest.

## References

1. Pan American Health Organization. CD57/7—PAHO Disease Elimination Initiative: A Policy for an Integrated Sustainable Approach to Communicable Diseases in the Americas. Available online: https://iris.paho.org/handle/10665.2/51612 (accessed on 5 July 2024).
2. Pan American Health Organization. Vaccination Week in the Americas. *EPI Newsl.* **2003**, *25*, 3–4.
3. Ropero Alvarez, A.M.; Kurtis, H.J.; Vulanovic, L.; Hasan, H.; Ruiz, C.; Thrush, E. The evolution of Vaccination Week in the Americas. *Rev. Panam. Salud. Publica* **2017**, *41*, e150. [CrossRef] [PubMed]
4. Pan American Health Organization. *Vaccination: An Act of Love. 10 Years of Vaccination Week in the Americas = Vacunación: Un Gesto de Amor. 10 Años de la Semana de Vacunación en Las Américas*; PAHO: Washington, DC, USA, 2012. Available online: https://iris.paho.org/handle/10665.2/34317 (accessed on 15 May 2024).
5. Pan American Health Organization. *Resolution CD44.R1. Sustaining Immunization Programs-Elimination of Rubella and Congenital Rubella Syndrome (CRS)*; 44th Directing Council: Washington, DC, USA, 2003. Available online: https://www1.paho.org/english/gov/cd/cd44-r1-e.pdf (accessed on 12 May 2024).
6. World Health Organization. *Resolution WHA 65.18 World Immunization Week*; 65th World Health Assembly; World Health Organization: Geneva, Switzerland, 2012. Available online: https://apps.who.int/gb/ebwha/pdf_files/WHA65-REC1/A65_REC1-en.pdf#page=25 (accessed on 12 May 2024).
7. Pan American Health Organization. *Elimination Initiative*; PAHO: Washington, DC, USA, 2019. Available online: https://www.paho.org/en/elimination-initiative (accessed on 11 July 2024).
8. Countries of the Caribbean Agree to Strengthen National Immunization Programs through Declaration of Nassau. Available online: https://www.paho.org/en/news/27-4-2023-countries-caribbean-agree-strengthen-national-immunization-programs-through (accessed on 31 May 2024).
9. "Vaccine Night", a Health Festival. Available online: https://www.paho.org/es/historias/noche-vacunas-fiesta-salud (accessed on 31 May 2024).

10. Pan American Health Organization. *Measles Elimination: Field Guide*, 2nd ed.; PAHO: Washington, DC, USA, 2005. Available online: https://www3.paho.org/hq/dmdocuments/2010/FieldGuide_Measles_2ndEd_e.pdf (accessed on 2 May 2024).
11. Pan American Health Organization. Immunization throughout the Life Course in the Americas. Available online: https://paho-cim.shinyapps.io/immunization-dashboard/# (accessed on 31 May 2024).

MDPI AG
Grosspeteranlage 5
4052 Basel
Switzerland
Tel.: +41 61 683 77 34

*Vaccines* Editorial Office
E-mail: vaccines@mdpi.com
www.mdpi.com/journal/vaccines

www.ingramcontent.com/pod-product-compliance
Lightning Source LLC
Chambersburg PA
CBHW061458220926
51850CB00004B/122
*9783725842131*